MARINO'S

The ICU

Book

FOURTH EDITION

Paul L. Marino, MD, PhD, FCCM

Clinical Associate Professor
Weill Cornell Medical College
New York, New York

Illustrations by Patricia Gast

MARINO'S

The ICU Book

FOURTH EDITION

Wolters Kluwer | Lippincott Williams & Wilkins
Health
Philadelphia • Baltimore • New York • London
Buenos Aires • Hong Kong • Sydney • Tokyo

Acquisitions Editor: Keith Donnellan
Product Development Editor: Nicole Dernoski
Production Project Manager: Bridgett Dougherty
Manufacturing Manager: Beth Welsh
Marketing Manager: Dan Dressler
Creative Director: Doug Smock
Production Services: Aptara, Inc.

© 2014 by Wolters Kluwer Health/Lippincott Williams & Wilkins
Two Commerce Square
2001 Market St.
Philadelphia, PA 19103
LWW.com

3rd Edition © 2007 by Lippincott Williams & Wilkins - a Wolters Kluwer Business
2nd Edition © 1998 by LIPPINCOTT WILLIAMS & WILKINS

Printed in the USA

Library of Congress Cataloging-in-Publication data available on request from the publisher.

ISBN-13: 978-1-4511-2118-6

Care has been taken to confirm the accuracy of the information presented and to describe generally accepted practices. However, the authors, editors, and publisher are not responsible for errors or omissions or for any consequences from application of the information in this book and make no warranty, expressed or implied, with respect to the currency, completeness, or accuracy of the contents of the publication. Application of this information in a particular situation remains the professional responsibility of the practitioner.

The authors, editors, and publisher have exerted every effort to ensure that drug selection and dosage set forth in this text are in accordance with current recommendations and practice at the time of publication. However, in view of ongoing research, changes in government regulations, and the constant flow of information relating to drug therapy and drug reactions, the reader is urged to check the package insert for each drug for any change in indications and dosage and for added warnings and precautions. This is particularly important when the recommended agent is a new or infrequently employed drug.

Some drugs and medical devices presented in this publication have Food and Drug Administration (FDA) clearance for limited use in restricted research settings. It is the responsibility of the health care provider to ascertain the FDA status of each drug or device planned for use in their clinical practice.

To purchase additional copies of this book, call our customer service department at (800) 638-3030 or fax orders to (301) 223-2320. International customers should call (301) 223-2300.

Visit Lippincott Williams & Wilkins on the Internet: at LWW.com. Lippincott Williams & Wilkins customer service representatives are available from 8:30 am to 6 pm, EST.

10 9 8 7 6 5 4 3

To Daniel Joseph Marino,
my 26-year-old son,
who has become
the best friend
I hoped he would be.

I would especially commend the physician who,
in acute diseases,
by which the bulk of mankind are cut off,
conducts the treatment better than others.

HIPPOCRATES

Preface to Fourth Edition

The fourth edition of *The ICU Book* marks its 23rd year as a fundamental sourcebook for the care of critically ill patients. This edition continues the original intent to provide a "generic textbook" that presents fundamental concepts and patient care practices that can be used in any adult intensive care unit, regardless of the specialty focus of the unit. Highly specialized topics, such as obstetrical emergencies, burn care, and traumatic injuries, are left to more qualified specialty textbooks.

This edition has been reorganized and completely rewritten, with updated references and clinical practice guidelines included at the end of each chapter. The text is supplemented by 246 original illustrations and 199 original tables, and five new chapters have been added: Vascular Catheters (Chapter 1), Occupational Exposures (Chapter 4), Alternate Modes of Ventilation (Chapter 27), Pancreatitis and Liver Failure (Chapter 39), and Nonpharmaceutical Toxidromes (Chapter 55). Each chapter ends with a brief section entitled "A Final Word," which highlights an insight or emphasizes the salient information presented in the chapter.

The ICU Book is unique in that it represents the voice of a single author, which provides a uniformity in style and conceptual framework. While some bias is inevitable in such an endeavor, the opinions expressed in this book are rooted in experimental observations rather than anecdotal experiences, and the hope is that any remaining bias is tolerable.

Acknowledgements

Acknowledgements are few but well deserved. First to Patricia Gast, who is responsible for all the illustrations and page layouts in this book. Her talent, patience, and counsel have been an invaluable aid to this author and this work. Also to Brian Brown and Nicole Dernoski, my longtime editors, for their trust and enduring support.

Contents

SECTION V
Cardiac Emergencies

SECTION VI
Blood Components

SECTION VII
Acute Respiratory Failure

SECTION VIII
Mechanical Ventilation

SECTION IX
Acid-Base Disorders

SECTION X
Renal and Electrolyte Disorders

VASCULAR ACCESS

He who works with his hands is a laborer.
He who works with his head and his hands is a craftsman.

Louis Nizer
Between You and Me
1948

Chapter 1

VASCULAR CATHETERS

It is not a bad definition of man to describe him as a tool-making animal.

Charles Babbage (1791 – 1871)

One of the most dramatic events in medical self-experimentation took place in a small German hospital during the summer of 1929 when a 25 year old surgical resident named Werner Forssman inserted a plastic urethral catheter into the basilic vein in his right arm and then advanced the catheter into the right atrium of his heart (1). This was the first documented instance of central venous cannulation using a flexible plastic catheter. Although a success, the procedure had only one adverse consequence; i.e., Dr. Forssman was immediately dismissed from his residency because he had acted without the consent of his superiors, and his actions were perceived as reckless and even suicidal. Upon dismissal, he was told that "such methods are good for a circus but not for a respected hospital"(1). Forssman went on to become a country doctor, but his achievement in vascular cannulation was finally recognized in 1956 when he was awarded the Nobel Prize in Medicine for performing the first right-heart catheterization in a human subject.

Werner Forssman's self-catheterization was a departure from the standard use of needles and rigid metal cannulas for vascular access, and it marked the beginning of the modern era of vascular cannulation, which is characterized by the use of flexible plastic catheters like the ones described in this chapter.

CATHETER BASICS

Catheter Material

Vascular catheters are made of synthetic polymers that are chemically inert, biocompatible, and resistant to chemical and thermal degradation. The most widely used polymers are polyurethane and silicone.

Polyurethane

Polyurethane is a versatile polymer that can act as a solid (e.g., the solid tires on lawn mowers are made of polyurethane) and can be modified to exhibit elasticity (e.g., Spandex fibers used in stretchable clothing are made of modified polyurethane). The polyurethane in vascular catheters provides enough tensile strength to allow catheters to pass through the skin and subcutaneous tissues without kinking. Because this rigidity can also promote vascular injury, polyurethane catheters are used for short-term vascular cannulation. Most of the vascular catheters you will use in the ICU are made of polyurethane, including peripheral vascular catheters (arterial and venous), central venous catheters, and pulmonary artery catheters.

Silicone

Silicone is a polymer that contains the chemical element silicon together with hydrogen, oxygen, and carbon. Silicone is more pliable than polyurethane (e.g., the nipple on baby bottles is made of silicone), and this reduces the risk of catheter-induced vascular injury. Silicone catheters are used for long-term vascular access (weeks to months), such as that required for prolonged administration of chemotherapy, antibiotics, and parenteral nutrition solutions in outpatients. The only silicone-based catheters inserted in the ICU setting are peripherally-inserted central venous catheters (PICCs). Because of their pliability, silicone catheters cannot be inserted percutaneously without the aid of a guidewire or introducer sheath.

Catheter Size

The size of vascular catheters is determined by the *outside diameter* of the catheter. There are two measures of catheter size: the gauge size and the "French" size.

Gauge Size

The gauge system was introduced (in England) as a sizing system for iron wires, and was later adopted for hollow needles and catheters. Gauge size varies inversely with outside diameter (i.e., the higher the gauge size, the smaller the outside diameter); however, there is no fixed relationship between gauge size and outside diameter. The International Organization for Standardization (ISO) has proposed the relationships shown in Table 1.1 for gauge sizes and corresponding outside diameters in peripheral catheters (2). Note that each gauge size is associated with a range of outside diameters (actual OD), and further that there is no fixed relationship between the actual (measured) and nominal outside diameters. Thus, the only way to determine the actual outside diameter of a catheter is to consult the manufacturer. Gauge sizes are typically used for peripheral catheters, and for the infusion channels of multilumen catheters.

French Size

The French system of sizing vascular catheters (named after the country of origin) is superior to the gauge system because of its simplicity and uniformity. The French scale begins at zero, and each increment of one French unit represents an increase of 1/3 (0.33) millimeter in outer diameter (3): i.e., French size × 0.33 = outside diameter (mm). Thus, a catheter that is 5 French units in size will have an outer diameter of 5 × 0.33 = 1.65 mm. (A table of French sizes and corresponding outside diameters is included in Appendix 2 in the rear of the book.) French sizes can increase indefinitely, but most vascular catheters are between 4 French and 10 French in size. French sizes are typically used for multilumen catheters and for large-bore single lumen catheters (like introducer sheaths, described later in the chapter).

Table 1.1	Gauge Sizes & Outside Diameters for Peripheral Catheters[†]	
Gauge	Range of Actual OD (mm)	Nominal OD (mm)
24	0.65 – 0.749	0.7
22	0.75 – 0.949	0.8, 0.9
20	0.95 – 1.149	1.0, 1.1
18	1.15 – 1.349	1.2, 1.3
16	1.55 – 1.849	1.6, 1.7, 1.8
14	1.85 – 2.249	1.9, 2.0, 2.1, 2.2

[†]From the International Organization for Standardization; ISO 10555-5; 1996 (available at www.iso.org). OD = outside diameter.

Catheter Flow

Steady flow (Q) through a hollow, rigid tube is proportional to the pressure gradient along the length of the tube ($P_{in} - P_{out}$, or ΔP), and the constant of proportionality is the resistance to flow (R):

$$Q = \Delta P \times 1/R \qquad (1.1)$$

The properties of flow through rigid tubes was first described by a German physiologist (Gotthif Hagen) and a French physician (Jean Louis Marie Poiseuille) working independently in the mid-19th century. They both observed that flow (Q) through rigid tubes is a function of the inner radius of the tube (r), the length of the tube (L) and the viscosity of the fluid (μ). Their observations are expressed in the equation shown below, which is known as the *Hagen-Poiseuille equation* (4).

$$Q = \Delta P \times (\pi r^4 / 8\mu L) \qquad (1.2)$$

This equation states that the steady flow rate (Q) in a rigid tube is directly related to the fourth power of the inner radius of the tube (r^4), and is inversely related to the length of the tube (L) and the viscosity of the fluid (μ). The term enclosed in parentheses ($\pi r^4/8\mu L$) is equivalent to the reciprocal of resistance (1/R, as in equation 1.1), so the resistance to flow can be expressed as $R = 8\mu L/\pi r^4$.

Since the Hagen-Poiseuille equation applies to flow through rigid tubes, it can be used to describe flow through vascular catheters, and how the dimensions of a catheter can influence the flow rate (see next).

Inner Radius and Flow

According to the Hagen-Poiseuille equation, the inner radius of a catheter has a profound influence on flow through the catheter (because flow is directly related to the fourth power of the inner radius). This is illustrated in Figure 1.1, which shows the gravity-driven flow of blood through catheters of similar length but varying outer diameters (5). (In studies such as this, changes in inner and outer diameter are considered to be equivalent.) Note that the relative change in flow rate is three times greater than the relative change in catheter diameter (Δ flow$/\Delta$ diameter$=3$). Although the magnitude of change in flow in this case is less than predicted by the Hagen-Poiseuille equation (a common observation, with possible explanations that are beyond the scope of this text), the slope of the graph in Figure 1.1 clearly shows that changes in catheter diameter have a marked influence on flow rate.

Catheter Length and Flow

The Hagen-Poiseuille equation indicates that flow through a catheter will decrease as the length of the catheter increases, and this is shown in

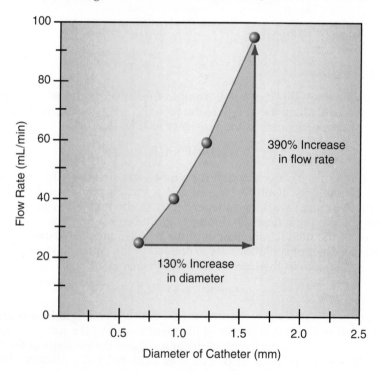

FIGURE 1.1 Relationship between flow rate and outside diameter of a vascular catheter. From Reference 5.

Figure 1.2. (6) Note that flow in the longest (30 cm) catheter is less than half the flow rate in the shortest (5 cm) catheter; in this case, a 600% increase in catheter length is associated with a 60% reduction in catheter flow (Δflow/Δlength = 0.1). Thus, the influence of catheter length on flow rate is proportionately less than the influence of catheter diameter on flow rate, as predicted by the Hagen-Poiseuille equation.

The comparative influence of catheter diameter and catheter length, as indicated by the Hagen-Poiseuille equation and the data in Figures 1.1 and 1.2, indicates that *when rapid volume infusion is necessary, a large-bore catheter is the desired choice, and the shortest available large-bore catheter is the optimal choice.* (See Chapter 11 for more on this subject.) The flow rates associated with a variety of vascular catheters are presented in the remaining sections of this chapter.

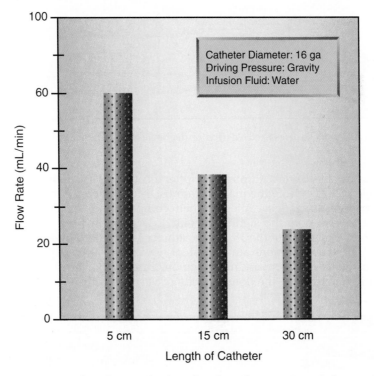

FIGURE 1.2 The influence of catheter length on flow rate. From Reference 6.

COMMON CATHETER DESIGNS

There are three basic types of vascular catheters: peripheral vascular catheters (arterial and venous), central venous catheters, and peripherally inserted central catheters.

Peripheral Vascular Catheters

The catheters used to cannulate peripheral blood vessels in adults are typically 16–20 gauge catheters that are 1–2 inches in length. Peripheral catheters are inserted using a catheter-over-needle device like the one shown in Figure 1.3. The catheter fits snugly over the needle and has a tapered end to prevent fraying of the catheter tip during insertion. The needle has a clear hub to visualize the "flashback" of blood that occurs when the tip of the needle enters the lumen of a blood vessel. Once flashback is evident, the catheter is advanced over the needle and into the lumen of the blood vessel.

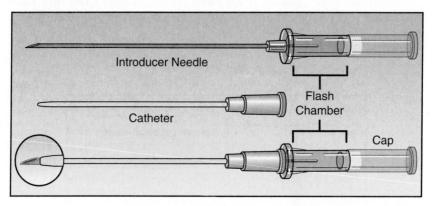

FIGURE 1.3 A catheter-over-needle device for the cannulation of peripheral blood vessels.

The characteristics of flow through peripheral catheters are demonstrated in Table 1.2 (7,8). Note the marked (almost 4-fold) increase in flow in the larger-bore 16 gauge catheter when compared to the 20 gauge catheter and also note the significant (43%) decrease in flow rate that occurs when the length of the 18 gauge catheter is increased by less than one inch. These observations are consistent with the relationships in the Hagen-Poiseuille equation, and they demonstrate the power of catheter diameter in determining the flow capacity of vascular catheters.

Table 1.2	Flow Characteristics in Peripheral Vascular Catheters		
Gauge Size	Length	Flow Rate mL/min	L/hr
16	30 mm (1.2 in)	220	13.2
18	30 mm (1.2 in)	105	6.0
	50 mm (2 in)	60	3.6
20	30 mm (1.2 in)	60	3.6

From References 6 and 7. All flow rates are for gravity-driven flow of water.

Central Venous Catheters

Cannulation of larger, more centrally placed veins (i.e., subclavian, internal jugular, and femoral veins) is often necessary for reliable vascular access in critically ill patients. The catheters used for this purpose, commonly known as *central venous catheters*, are typically 15 to 30 cm (6 to 12 inches) in length, and have single or multiple (2–4) infusion channels. Multilumen catheters are favored in the ICU because the typical ICU patient recquires a multitude of parenteral therapies (e.g., fluids, drugs, and nutrient mixtures), and multilumen catheters make it possible to deliver these therapies using a single venipuncture. The use of multiple infusion channels does not increase the incidence of catheter-related infections (9), but the larger diameter of multilumen catheters creates an increased risk of catheter-induced thrombosis (10).

Triple-lumen catheters like the one shown in Figure 1.4 are the consensus favorite for central venous access. These catheters are available in diameterss of 4 French to 9 French, and the 7 French size (outside diameter = 2.3 mm) is a popular choice in adults. Size 7 French triple lumen catheters typically have one 16 gauge channel and two smaller 18 gauge channels. To prevent mixing of infusate solutions, the three outflow ports are separated as depicted in Figure 1.4.

The features of triple lumen catheters (7 French size) from one manufacturer are shown in Table 1.3. Note the much slower flow rates in the 16 gauge and 18 gauge channels when compared to the 16 and 18 gauge peripheral catheters in Table 1.2. This, of course, is due to the much longer length of central venous catheters, as predicted by the Hagen-Poiseuille

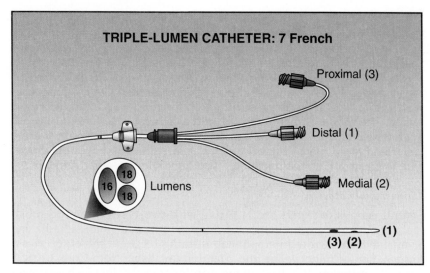

FIGURE 1.4 A triple-lumen central venous catheter showing the gauge size of each lumen and the outflow ports at the distal end of the catheter.

equation. There are 3 available lengths for the triple lumen catheter: the shortest (16 cm) catheters are intended for right-sided catheter insertions, while the longer (20 cm and 30 cm) catheters are used in left-sided cannulations (because of the longer path to the superior vena cava). The 20 cm catheter is long enough for most left-sided cannulations so (to limit catheter length tand thereby preserve flow), it seems wise to avoid central venous catheters that are longer than 20 cm, if possible.

Table 1.3	Selected Features of Triple-Lumen Central Venous Catheters			
Size	**Length**	**Lumens**	**Lumen Size**	**Flow Rate (L/hr)†**
7 Fr	16 cm (6 in)	Distal	16 ga	3.4
		Medial	18 ga	1.8
		Proximal	18 ga	1.9
7 Fr	20 cm (8 in)	Distal	16 ga	3.1
		Medial	18 ga	1.5
		Proximal	18 ga	1.6
7 Fr	30 cm (12 in)	Distal	16 ga	2.3
		Medial	18 ga	1.0
		Proximal	18 ga	1.1

†All flow rates are for gravity-driven flow of isotonic saline from a height of 40 inches above the catheters. Fr = French size; ga = gauge size.
From Arrow International (www.arrowintl.com); accessed 8/1/2011.

Insertion Technique

Central venous catheters are inserted by threading the catheter over a guidewire (a technique introduced in the early 1950s and called the Seldinger technique after its founder). This technique is illustrated in Figure 1.5. A small bore needle (usually 20 gauge) is used to probe for the target vessel. When the tip of the needle enters the vessel, a long, thin wire with a flexible tip is passed through the needle and into the vessel lumen. The needle is then removed, and a catheter is advanced over the guidewire and into the blood vessel. When cannulating deep vessels, a larger and more rigid "dilator catheter" is first threaded over the guidewire to create a tract that facilitates insertion of the vascular catheter.

Antimicrobial Catheters

Central venous catheters are available with two types of antimicrobial coating: one uses a combination of chlorhexidine and silver sulfadiazine (available from Arrow International, Reading PA), and the other uses a combination of minocycline and rifampin (available from Cook Critical Care, Bloomington, IN). Each of these antimicrobial catheters has proven effective in reducing the incidence of catheter-related septicemia (11,12).

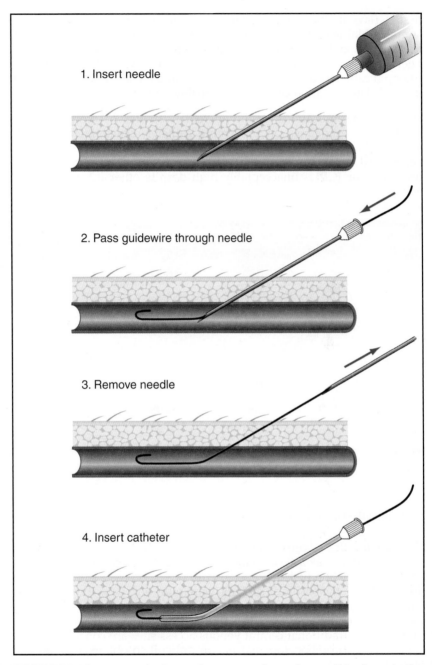

FIGURE 1.5 The steps involved in guidewire-assisted cannulation of blood vessels (the Seldinger technique).

A single multicenter study comparing both types of antimicrobial coating showed superior results with the minocycline-rifampin catheters (13). A design flaw in the chlorhexidine-silver sulfadiazine catheter (i.e., no antimicrobial activity on the luminal surface of the catheter) has since been corrected, but a repeat comparison study has not been performed. Therefore, the evidence at the present time favors the minocycline rifampin catheters as the most effective antimicrobial catheters in clinical use (12). This situation could (and probably will) change in the future.

What are the indications for antimicrobial catheters? According to the most recent guidelines on preventing catheter-related infections (14), antimicrobial catheters should be used if the expected duration of central venous catheterization is > 5 days and if the rate of catheter-related infections in your ICU is unacceptably high despite other infection control efforts.

Table 1.4	Selected Features of Peripherally Inserted Central Catheters			
Size	**Length**	**Lumens**	**Lumen Size**	**Flow Rate (L/hr)†**
5 Fr	50 cm (195 in)	Single	16 ga	1.75
5 Fr	70 cm (27.5 in)	Single	16 ga	1.30
5 Fr	50 cm (19.5 in)	Distal	18 ga	0.58
		Proximal	20 ga	0.16
5 Fr	70 cm (27.5 in)	Distal	18 ga	0.44
		Proximal	20 ga	0.12

†All flow rates are for gravity-driven flow of isotonic saline from a height of 40 inches above the catheters. Fr = French size; ga = gauge size.
From Arrow International (www.arrowintl.com); accessed 8/1/2011.

Peripherally Inserted Central Catheters

Concern for the adverse consequences of central venous cannulation (e.g., pneumothorax arterial puncture, poor patient acceptance) prompted the introduction of *peripherally inserted central catheters* (PICCs), which are inserted in the basilic or cephalic vein in the arm (just above the antecubital fossa) and advanced into the superior vena cava (15). (Insertion of PICCs is described in the next chapter). In the ICU, PICCs are used primarily when traditional central venous access sites are considered risky (e.g., severe thrombocytopenia) or are difficult to obtain (e.g., morbid obesity).

The characteristics of PICC devices from one manufacturer are shown in Table 1.4. These catheters are smaller in diameter than central venous catheters because they are introduced into smaller veins. However, the major distinction between PICCs and central venous catheters is their length; i.e., the length of the catheters in Table 1.4 (50 cm and 70 cm) is at least double the length of the triple lumen catheters in Table 1.3. The tradeoff for this added length is a reduction in flow capacity, which is evident when comparing the flow rates in Table 1.4 and Table 1.3. Flow is particularly sluggish in the double lumen PICCs because of the smaller diameter of the infusion channels. The flow limitation of PICCs (especially the double lumen catheters) makes them ill-suited for aggressive volume therapy.

SPECIALTY CATHETERS

The catheters described in this section are designed to perform specific tasks, and are otherwise not used for patient care. These specialty devices include hemodialysis catheters, introducer sheaths, and pulmonary artery catheters.

Hemodialysis Catheters

One of the recognized benefits of intensive care units is the ability to provide emergent hemodialysis for patients with acute renal failure, and this is made possible by a specially designed catheter like the one shown in Figure 1.6. The features of this catheter are shown in Table 1.5.

Table 1.5	Selected Features of Hemodialysis Catheters			
Size	**Length**	**Lumens**	**Lumen Size**	**Flow Rate (L/hr)[†]**
12 Fr	12 cm (6 in)	Proximal	12 ga	23.7
		Distal	12 ga	17.4
12 Fr	20 cm (8 in)	Proximal	12 ga	19.8
		Distal	12 ga	15.5

[†]All flow rates are for gravity-driven flow of isotonic saline from a height of 40 inches above the catheters. Fr = French size; ga = gauge size.
From Arrow International (www.arrowintl.com); accessed 8/1/2011.

Hemodialysis catheters are the wide-body catheters of critical care, with diameters up to 16 French (5.3 mm), and they are equipped with dual 12 gauge infusion channels that can accommodate the high flow rates (200–300 mL/min) needed for effective hemodialysis. One channel carries blood from the patient to the dialysis membranes, and the other channel returns the blood to the patient.

Hemodialysis catheters are usually placed in the internal jugular vein and are left in place until alternate access is available for dialysis. Cannulation of the subclavian vein is forbidden because of the propensity for subclavian vein stenosis (16), which hinders venous outflow from the ipsilateral arm and thereby prevents the use of that arm for chronic hemodialysis access with an arteriovenous shunt.

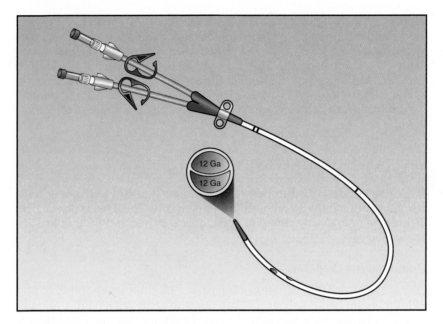

FIGURE 1.6 Large-bore double lumen catheter for short-term hemodialysis.

Introducer Sheaths

Introducer sheaths are large-bore (8–9 French) catheters that serve as conduits for the insertion and removal of temporary vascular devices. In the ICU, they are used primarily to facilitate the placement of pulmonary artery (PA) catheters (see Figure 8.1 for an illustration of an introducer sheath and its companion PA catheter). The introducer sheath is first placed in a large, central vein, and the PA catheter is then threaded through the sheath and advanced into the pulmonary artery. The placement of PA catheters often requires repeated trials of advancing and retracting the catheter to achieve the proper position in the pulmonary artery, and the introducer sheath facilitates these movements. When the PA catheter is no longer needed, the introducer sheath allows the catheter to be removed and replaced with a central venous catheter, if needed, without a new venipuncture.

Rapid Infusion

Introducer sheaths can also serve as stand-alone infusion devices by virtue of a side infusion port on the hub of the catheter. The large diameter of introducer sheaths has made them popular as rapid infusion devices for the management of acute blood loss. When introducer sheaths are used with pressurized infusion systems, flow rates of 850 mL/min have been reported (17). The use of introducer sheaths for rapid volume infusion is revisited in Chapter 11.

Pulmonary Artery Catheters

Pulmonary artery balloon-flotation catheters are highly specialized devices capable of providing as many as 16 measures of cardiovascular function and systemic oxygenation. These catheters have their own chapter (Chapter 8), so proceed there for more information.

A FINAL WORD

The performance of vascular catheters as infusion devices is rooted in the Hagen–Poiseuille equation, which describes the influence of catheter dimensions on flow rate. The following statements from this equation are part of the "essential knowledge base" for vascular catheters.

1. Flow rate is directly related to the inner radius of a catheter (i.e., both vary in the same direction), and is inversely related to the length of the catheter (i.e., vary in opposite directions).
2. The inner radius (lumen size) of a catheter has a much greater influence on flow rate than the length of the catheter.
3. For rapid infusion, a large bore catheter is essential, and a short, large bore catheter is optimal.

As for the performance of individual catheters, each ICU has its own stock of vascular catheters, and you should become familiar with the sizes and flow capabilities of the catheters that are available.

REFERENCES

1. Mueller RL, Sanborn TA. The history of interventional cardiology: Cardiac catheterization, angioplasty, and related interventions. Am Heart J 1995; 129:146–172.

Catheter Basics

2. International Standard ISO 10555–5. Sterile, single-use intravascular catheters. Part 5: Over-needle peripheral catheters. 1996:1–3.
3. Iserson KV. J.-F.-B. Charriere: The man behind the "French" gauge. J Emerg Med 1987; 5:545–548.
4. Chien S, Usami S, Skalak R. Blood flow in small tubes. In Renkin EM, Michel CC (eds). Handbook of Physiology. Section 2: The cardiovascular system. Volume IV. The microcirculation. Bethesda: American Physiological Society, 1984:217–249.
5. de la Roche MRP, Gauthier L. Rapid transfusion of packed red blood cells: effects of dilution, pressure, and catheter size. Ann Emerg Med 1993; 22:1551–1555.

6. Mateer JR, Thompson BM, Aprahamian C, et. al. Rapid fluid infusion with central venous catheters. Ann Emerg Med 1983; 12:149–152.

Common Catheter Designs

7. Emergency Medicine Updates (http://emupdates.com); accessed 8/1/2011.

8. Dula DJ, Muller A, Donovan JW. Flow rate variance of commonly used IV infusion techniques. J Trauma 1981; 21:480–481.

9. McGee DC, Gould MK. Preventing complications of central venous catheterization. New Engl J Med 2003; 348:1123–1133.

10. Evans RS, Sharp JH, Linford LH, et. al., Risk of symptomatic DVT associated with peripherally inserted central catheters. Chest 2010; 138:803–810.

11. Casey AL, Mermel LA, Nightingale P, Elliott TSJ. Antimicrobial central venous catheters in adults: a systematic review and meta-analysis. Lancet Infect Dis 2008; 8:763–776.

12. Ramos ER, Reitzel R, Jiang Y, et al. Clinical effectiveness and risk of emerging resistance associated with prolonged use of antibiotic-impregnated catheters. Crit Care Med 2011; 39:245–251.

13. Darouche RO, Raad II, Heard SO, et al. A comparison of antimicrobial-impregnated central venous catheters. New Engl J Med 1999; 340:1–8.

14. O'Grady NP, Alexander M, Burns LA, et al, and the Healthcare Infection Control Practices Advisory Committee (HICPAC). Guidelines for the prevention of intravascular catheter-related infection. Clin Infect Dis 2011; 52:e1–e32.
(Available at www.cdc.gov/hipac/pdf/guidelines/bsi-guidelines-2011.pdf; accessed 4/15/2011)

15. Ng P, Ault M, Ellrodt AG, Maldonado L. Peripherally inserted central catheters in general medicine. Mayo Clin Proc 1997; 72:225–233.

Specialty Catheters

16. Hernandez D, Diaz F, Rufino M, et al. Subclavian vascular access stenosis in dialysis patients: Natural history and risk factors. J Am Soc Nephrol 1998; 9:1507–1510.

17. Barcelona SL, Vilich F, Cote CJ. A comparison of flow rates and warming capabilities of the Level 1 and Rapid Infusion System with various-size intravenous catheters. Anesth Analg 2003; 97:358–363.

Chapter 2

CENTRAL VENOUS ACCESS

Good doctors leave good tracks.

J. Willis Hurst, MD

Vascular access in critically ill patients often involves the insertion of long, flexible catheters (like those described in the last chapter) into large veins entering the thorax or abdomen; this type of *central venous access* is the focus of the current chapter. The purpose of this chapter is not to teach you the technique of central venous cannulation (which must be mastered at the bedside), but to describe the process involved in establishing central venous access and the adverse consequences that can arise.

PRINCIPLES & PREPARATIONS

Small vs. Large Veins

Catheters placed in small, peripheral veins have a limited life expectancy because they promote localized inflammation and thrombosis. The inflammation is prompted by mechanical injury to the blood vessel and by chemical injury to the vessel from caustic drug infusions. The thrombosis is incited by the inflammation, and is propagated by the sluggish flow in small, cannulated veins. (The viscosity of blood varies inversely with the rate of blood flow, and thus the low flow in small, cannulated veins is associated with an increase in blood viscosity, and this increases the propensity for thrombus formation.)

Large veins offer the advantages of a larger diameter and higher flow rates. The larger diameter allows the insertion of larger bore, multilumen catheters, which increases the efficiency of vascular access (i.e., more infusions per venipuncture). The higher flow rates reduce the damaging effects of infused fluids and thereby reduce the propensity for local thrombosis. The diameters and flow rates of some representative large and small veins are shown in Table 2.1. Note that the increase in flow rate is far greater than the increase in vessel diameter; e.g., the diameter of the subclavian vein is about three times greater than the diameter of the metacarpal veins, but the flow rates in the subclavian vein are as much as 100 times higher than flow rates in the metacarpal veins. This relationship between flow rate and vessel diameter is an expression of the Hagen-Poiseuille equation described in Chapter 1 (see Equation 1.2).

Table 2.1	Comparative Size and Flow Rates for Large and Small Veins		
	Vein	**Diameter**	**Flow Rate[†]**
Upper Body:			
	Superior Vena Cava	18 – 22 mm	1800 – 2000 mL/min
	Internal Jugular Vein	10 – 22 mm	500 – 1400 mL/min
	Subclavian Vein	7 – 12 mm	350 – 800 mL/min
	Metacarpal Veins	2 – 5 mm	8 – 10 mL/min
Lower Body:			
	Inferior Vena Cava	27 – 36 mm	1200 – 2000 mL/min
	Femoral Vein	8 – 16 mm	700 – 1100 mL/min

[†]Flow rates are for healthy adults.

Indications

The major indications for central venous access are summarized as follows (1):

1. When peripheral venous access is difficult to obtain (e.g., in obese patients or intravenous drug abusers) or difficult to maintain (e.g., in agitated patients).
2. For the delivery of vasoconstrictor drugs (e.g., dopamine, norepinephrine), hypertonic solutions (e.g., parenteral nutrition formulas), or multiple parenteral medications (taking advantage of the multilumen catheters described in Chapter 1).
3. For prolonged parenteral drug therapy (i.e., more than a few days).
4. For specialized tasks such as hemodialysis, transvenous cardiac pacing, or hemodynamic monitoring (e.g., with pulmonary artery catheters).

Contraindications

There are no absolute contraindications to central venous cannulation (1), including the presence or severity of a coagulation disorder (2,3). However, there are risks associated with cannulation at a specific site, and these are described later in the chapter.

Infection Control Measures

Infection control is an essential part of vascular cannulation, and the preventive measures recommended for central venous cannulation are shown in Table 2.2 (4,5). When used together (as a "bundle"), these five measures have been effective in reducing the incidence of catheter-related bloodstream infections (6,7). The following is a brief description of these preventive measures.

Table 2.2	The Central Line Bundle
Components	**Recommendations**
Hand Hygiene	Use an alcohol-based handrub or a soap and water handwash before and after inserting or manipulatng catheters.
Barrier Precautions	Use maximal barrier precautions, including cap, mask, sterile gloves, sterile gown, and sterile full body drape, for catheter insertion or guidewire exchange.
Skin Antisepsis	Apply a chlorhexadine-based solution to the catheter insertion site and allow 2 minutes to air-dry.
Cannulation Site	When possible, avoid femoral vein cannulation, and cannulate the subclavian vein rather than the internal jugular vein.
Catheter Removal	Remove catheter promptly when it is no longer needed.

From the Institute for Healthcare Improvement (5). Adherence to all recommendations in this bundle has been shown to reduce the incidence of catheter-related bloodstream infections (6,7).

Skin Antisepsis

Proper hand hygiene is considered one of the most important, and most neglected, methods of infection control. Alcohol-based hand rubs are preferred if available (4,8); otherwise, handwashing with soap (plain or antimicrobial soap) and water is acceptable (4). Hand hygiene should be performed before and after palpating catheter insertion sites, and before and after glove use (4).

The skin around the catheter insertion site should be decontaminated just prior to cannulation, and the preferred antiseptic agent is chlorhexidine (4–7). This preference is based on clinical studies showing that chlorhexidine is superior to other antiseptic agents for limiting the risk of catheter-associated infections (9). The enhanced efficacy of chlorhexidine is attributed to its prolonged (residual) antimicrobial activity on the skin, which lasts for at least 6 hours after a single application (10). Anti-microbial activity is maximized if chlorhexidine is allowed to air-dry on the skin for at least two minutes (4).

Barriers

All vascular cannulation procedures, except those involving small peripheral veins, should be performed using full sterile barrier precautions, which includes caps, masks, sterile gloves, sterile gowns, and a sterile drape from head to foot (4). The only barrier precaution advised for peripheral vein cannulation is the use of gloves, and nonsterile gloves are acceptable as long as the gloved hands do not touch the catheter (4).

Site Selection

According to the current guidelines for preventing catheter-related infections (4), femoral vein cannulation should be avoided, and cannulating the subclavian vein is preferred to cannulating the internal jugular vein. These recommendations are based on the perceived risk of catheter-related infections at each site (i.e., the highest risk from the femoral vein and the lowest risk from the subclavian vein). However, there are other considerations that can influence the preferred site of catheter insertion; e.g., the subclavian vein is the least desirable site for insertion of hemodialysis catheters (for reasons explained later). Hence the qualifying term "when possible" is added to the recommendation for catheter insertion site in the central line bundle. The special considerations for each central venous access site are presented later in the chapter.

AIDS TO CANNULATION

Ultrasound Guidance

Since its introduction in the early 1990s, the use of real-time ultrasound imaging to locate and cannulate blood vessels has added considerably to the success rate and safety of vascular cannulation (11,12). The following is a brief description of ultrasound-guided vascular cannulation.

Ultrasound Basics

Ultrasound imaging is made possible by specialized transducers (gray scale adapters) that convert the amplitude of reflected ultrasound waves (echoes) into colors representing shades of gray in the black-white continuum. Higher amplitude echoes produce brighter or whiter images, while lower amplitude echoes produce darker or blacker images. This methodology is knows as B-mode (brightness-mode) ultrasound, and it produces two-dimensional, gray-scale images. The frequency of the ultrasound waves is directly related to the resolution of the ultrasound image, and is inversely related to the depth of tissue penetration; i.e., higher frequency waves produce higher resolution images, but the area visualized is smaller.

Ultrasound waves pass readily through fluids, so fluid-filled structures like blood vessels have a dark gray or black interior on the ultrasound image.

Vascular Ultrasound

Vascular ultrasound uses probes that emit high-frequency waves to produce high-resolution images, but visualization is limited to only a few centimeters from the skin. Ultrasound images are used in real time to

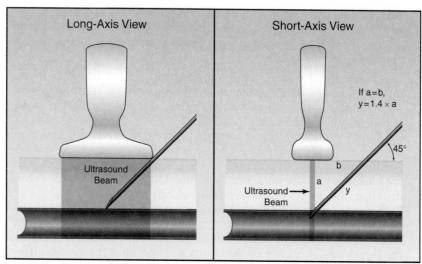

FIGURE 2.1 Orientation of the ultrasound beam in the long-axis and short-axis view. See text for further explanation.

locate the target vessel and assist in guiding the probe needle into the target vessel. This process in influenced by the orientation of the ultrasound beam, as depicted in Figure 2.1.

LONG-AXIS VIEW: The panel on the left in Figure 2.1 shows the ultrasound beam aligned with the long axis of the blood vessel. In this orientation, the probe needle and the blood vessel are in the plane of the ultrasound beam, and both will appear in a longitudinal (long-axis) view on the ultrasound image. This is demonstrated in Figure 2.2, which shows a long-axis view of the internal jugular vein with a visible probe needle advancing towards the vein (12). The ability to visualize the path of the probe needle in this view makes it easy to guide the needle into the lumen of the target vessel.

SHORT-AXIS VIEW: The panel on the right in Figure 2.1 shows the ultrasound beam running perpendicular to the long axis of the blood vessel. This orientation creates a cross-sectional (short-axis) view of the blood vessel, like the images in Figures 2.3. Note that the probe needle does not cross the ultrasound beam until it reaches the target vessel, so it is not possible to visualize the path of the probe needle in this view. Note also that when the needle does reach the ultrasound beam, it will be visible only as a small, high-intensity dot (that may not be readily apparent) on the ultrasound image.

Despite the limitation in visualizing the probe needle, the short-axis view is often favored (particularly by novices) because blood vessels are easier to locate when the ultrasound beam is perpendicular to the long axis of the vessel. The following measures can help to guide the probe needle when the short-axis view is used for ultrasound imaging.

1. Advance the needle using short, stabbing movements to displace tissue along the path of the needle. This displacement is often evident on the ultrasound image, and can provide indirect evidence of the path taken by the needle.

2. Determine the distance that the probe needle must travel to reach the target vessel. This can be done by visualizing a right-angle triangle similar to the one shown in Figure 2.1 (right panel). One side of this triangle is the vertical distance from the ultrasound probe to the target vessel (a), the other side of the triangle is the distance from the ultrasound probe to the insertion point of the probe needle (b), and the hypotenuse of the triangle (y) is the distance to the blood vessel when the needle is inserted at an angle of 45°. This distance (the length of the hypotenuse) can be calculated using the Pythagorean equation ($y^2 = a^2 + b^2$); if the two sides of the triangle are equal in length (a = b), the equation can be reduced to: $y = 1.4 \times a$. Using this relationship, the distance the needle must travel to reach the target vessel (y) can be determined using only the vertical distance to the target vessel (a), which is easily measured on the ultrasound image.

Example: If the vertical distance from the ultrasound probe to the target vessel is 5 cm (a = 5 cm), the insertion point for the probe needle should be 5 cm from the ultrasound probe (b = 5 cm). If the needle is then inserted at a 45° angle, the distance to the blood vessel should be $1.4 \times 5 = 7$ cm.

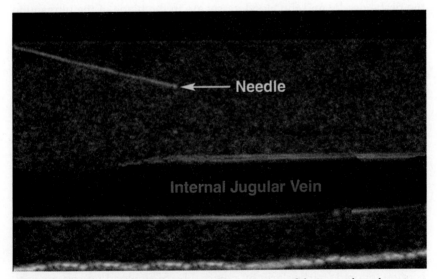

FIGURE 2.2 Ultrasound image showing a long-axis view of the internal jugular vein, with a visible probe needle advancing towards the vein. From Reference 12. (Image digitally enhanced.)

Body Tilt

Tilting the body so the head is below the horizontal plane (the Trendelenburg position) will distend the large veins entering the thorax from above to facilitate cannulation of the subclavian vein and internal jugular vein. In healthy subjects, head-down body tilt to 15° below horizontal is associated with a diameter increment of 20–25% in the internal jugular vein (14), and 8–10% in the subclavian vein (15). Further increases in the degree of body tilt beyond 15° produces little or no incremental effect (14). Thus, the full benefit of the head-down position is achieved with small degrees of body tilt, which is advantageous because it limits the undesirable effects of the head-down position (e.g., increased intracranial pressure and increased risk of aspiration). The head-down body tilt is not necessary in patients with venous congestion (e.g., from left or right heart failure), and is not advised in patients with increased intracranial pressure.

CENTRAL VENOUS ACCESS ROUTES

The following is a brief description of central venous cannulation at four different access sites: i.e., the internal jugular vein, the subclavian vein, the femoral vein, and the veins emerging from the antecubital fossa. The focus here is the location and penetration of the target vessel; once this is accomplished, cannulation proceeds using the Seldinger technique, which is described in Chapter 1 (see Figure 1.5).

Internal Jugular Vein

Anatomy

The internal jugular vein is located under the sternocleidomastoid muscle on either side of the neck, and it runs obliquely down the neck along a line drawn from the pinna of the ear to the sternoclavicular joint. In the lower neck region, the vein is often located just anterior and lateral to the carotid artery, but anatomic relationships can vary (16). At the base of the neck, the internal jugular vein joins the subclavian vein to form the innominate vein, and the convergence of the right and left innominate veins forms the superior vena cava. The supine diameter of the internal jugular vein varies widely (from 10 mm to 22 mm) in healthy subjects (14).

The right side of the neck is preferred for cannulation of the internal jugular vein because the vessels run a straight course to the right atrium. The right side is particularly well suited for the placement of temporary pacer wires, hemodialysis catheters, and pulmonary artery catheters.

Positioning

A head-down body tilt of 15° will distend the internal jugular vein and facilitate cannulation, as described earlier. The head should be turned slightly in the opposite direction to straighten the course of the vein, but turning the head beyond 30° from midline is counterproductive because it stretches the vein and reduces the diameter (16).

Ultrasound Guidance

The internal jugular vein is well suited for ultrasound imaging because it is close to the skin surface and there are no intervening structures to interfere with transmission of the ultrasound waves. A short-axis view of the internal jugular vein and carotid artery on the right side of the neck is shown in Figure 2.3. (This image was obtained by placing the ultrasound probe across the triangle created by the two heads of the sternocleidomastoid muscle, which is shown in Figure 2.4.) The image on the left shows the large jugular vein situated anterior and lateral to the smaller carotid artery. The image on the right shows the vein collapsing when a compressive force is applied to the overlying skin; this is a popular maneuver for determining if a blood vessel is an artery or vein.

When ultrasound guidance is used for internal jugular vein cannulation, there is an increased success rate, fewer cannulation attempts, a shorter time to cannulation, and a reduced risk of carotid artery puncture (16–18). As a result of these benefits, ultrasound guidance has been recommended as a standard practice for cannulation of the internal jugular vein (16).

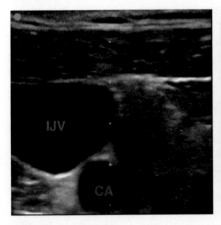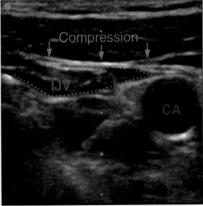

FIGURE 2.3 Ultrasound images (short-axis view) of the author's internal jugular vein (IJV) and carotid artery (CA) on the right side of the neck. The image on the right shows collapse of the vein when downward pressure is applied to the overlying skin. The green dots mark the lateral side of each image. (Images courtesy of Cynthia Sullivan, R.N. and Shawn Newvine, R.N.).

Landmark Method

When ultrasound imaging is not available, cannulation of the internal jugular vein is guided by surface landmarks. There are two approaches to the internal jugular vein using surface landmarks, as described next.

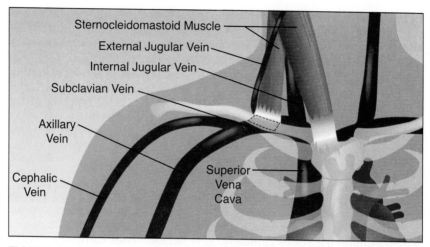

FIGURE 2.4 Anatomic relationships of the internal jugular vein and subclavian vein.

ANTERIOR APPROACH: For the anterior approach, the operator first identifies the triangular area at the base of the neck created by the separation of the two heads of the sternocleidomastoid muscle (see Figure 2.4). The internal jugular vein and carotid artery run through this triangle. The operator first locates the carotid artery pulse in this triangle; once the artery is located by palpation, it is gently retracted toward the midline and away from the internal jugular vein. The probe needle is then inserted at the apex of the triangle (with bevel facing up) and the needle is advanced toward the ipsilateral nipple at a 45° angle from the skin. If the vein is not entered by a depth of 5 cm, the needle should be drawn back and advanced again in a more lateral direction.

POSTERIOR APPROACH: For the posterior approach, the insertion point for the probe needle is 1 cm above the point where the external jugular vein crosses over the lateral edge of the sternocleidomastoid muscle (see Figure 2.4). The probe needle is inserted at this point (with the bevel at 3 o'clock) and then advanced along the underbelly of the muscle in a direction pointing to the suprasternal notch. The internal jugular vein should be encountered 5 to 6 cm from the insertion point.

Complications

Accidental puncture of the carotid artery is the most feared complication of jugular vein cannulation, and has a reported prevalence of 0.5–11% when anatomic landmarks are used (17,19,20), and 1% when ultrasound imaging is employed (17). If the artery is punctured by the small-bore probe needle, it is usually safe to remove the needle and compress the site for at least 5 minutes (double the compression time for patients with a coagulopathy). Insertion of a catheter into the carotid artery is more of a problem because removing the catheter can be fatal (20,21). If confronted with a catheterized carotid artery, leave the catheter in place and consult a vascular surgeon *pronto* (21).

OTHERS: Accidental puncture of the pleural space (resulting in hemothorax and/or pneumothorax) is not expected at the internal jugular vein site because it is located in the neck. However, this complication is reported in 1.3% of internal jugular vein cannulations using the landmark approach (19). The principal complication of indwelling jugular vein catheters is septicemia, which has a reported incidence that varies from zero to 2.3 cases per 1000 catheter days (22,23). Catheters in the internal jugular vein are considered a greater infectious risk than catheters in the subclavian vein (4,5), but this is not supported by some clinical surveys (22).

Comment

The internal jugular vein should be the favored site for central venous access when ultrasound imaging is available (16), and the right internal jugular vein is the preferred site for insertion of transvenous pacemaker wires, pulmonary artery catheters, and hemodialysis catheters. Awake patients often complain of discomfort and limited neck mobility from indwelling jugular vein catheters, so other sites should be considered for central venous access in conscious patients. (Peripherally inserted central catheters, which are described later, may be a better choice for central venous access in conscious patients.)

The Subclavian Vein

Anatomy

The subclavian vein is a continuation of the axillary vein as it passes over the first rib (see Figure 2.4). It runs most of its course along the underside of the clavicle (sandwiched between the clavicle and first rib), and at some points is only 5 mm above the apical pleura of the lungs. The underside of the vein sits on the anterior scalene muscle along with the phrenic nerve, which comes in contact with the vein along its posteroinferior side. Situated just deep to the vein, on the underside of the anterior scalene muscle, is the subclavian artery and brachial plexus. At the thoracic inlet, the subclavian vein meets the internal jugular vein to form the innominate vein. The subclavian vein is 3–4 cm in length, and the diameter is 7–12 mm in the supine position (24). The diameter of the subclavian vein does not vary with respiration (unlike the internal jugular vein), which is attributed to strong fascial attachments that fix the vein to surrounding structures and hold it open (24). This is also the basis for the claim that volume depletion does not collapse the subclavian vein (25), which is an unproven claim.

Positioning

The head-down body tilt distends the subclavian vein (24) and can facilitate cannulation. However, other maneuvers used to facilitate cannulation, such as arching the shoulders or placing a rolled towel under the shoulder, actually cause a paradoxical decrease in the cross-sectional area of the vein (24,26).

Ultrasound Guidance

Ultrasound imaging can improve the success rate and reduce the adverse consequences of subclavian vein cannulation (25). However, the subclavian vein is not easily visualized because the overlying clavicle blocks transmission of ultrasound waves. Because of this technical difficulty, ultrasound guidance is not currently popular for subclavian vein cannulation.

Landmark Method

The subclavian vein can be located by identifying the portion of the sternocleidomastoid muscle that inserts on the clavicle (see Figure 2.4). The subclavian vein lies just underneath the clavicle at this point, and the vein can be entered from above or below the clavicle. This portion of the clavicle can be marked with a small rectangle, as shown in Figure 2.4, to guide insertion of the probe needle.

INFRACLAVICULAR APPROACH: The subclavian vein is typically entered from below the clavicle. The probe needle is inserted at the lateral border of the rectangle marked on the clavicle, and the needle is advanced (with the bevel at 12 o'clock) along the underside of the clavicle in a direction that would bisect the rectangle into two triangles. The needle should enter the subclavian vein within a few centimeters from the surface. It is important to keep the needle on the underside of the clavicle to avoid puncturing of the subclavian artery, which lies deep to the subclavian vein. When the needle enters the subclavian vein, the bevel of the needle should be rotated to 3 o'clock so the guidewire will advance in the direction of the superior vena cava.

SUPRACLAVICULAR APPROACH: Identify the angle formed by the lateral margin of the sternocleidomastoid muscle and the clavicle. The probe needle is inserted so that it bisects this angle. Keep the bevel of the needle at 12 o'clock and advance the needle along the underside of the clavicle in the direction of the opposite nipple. The vein should be entered at a distance of 1 to 2 cm from the skin surface (the subclavian vein is more superficial in the supraclavicular approach). When the vein is entered, turn the bevel of the needle to 9 o'clock so the guidewire will advance in the direction of the superior vena cava.

Complications

The immediate complications of subclavian vein cannulation include puncture of the subclavian artery ($\leq 5\%$), pneumothorax ($\leq 5\%$), brachial plexus injury ($\leq 3\%$), and phrenic nerve injury ($\leq 1.5\%$) (19,25). All are less frequent when ultrasound guidance is used (25).

Complications associated with indwelling catheters include septicemia and subclavian vein stenosis. The incidence of septicemia in one survey was less than one case per 1000 catheter days (22). Stenosis of the subclavian vein appears days or months after catheter removal, and has a reported incidence of 15–50% (27). The risk of stenosis is the principal reason to avoid cannulation of the subclavian vein in patients who might require a hemodialysis access site (e.g., arteriovenous fistula) in the ipsilateral arm (27).

Comment

The major advantage of the subclavian vein site is patient comfort after catheters are placed. The claim that infections are less frequent with subclavian vein catheters (4,5) is not supported by some clinical studies (22).

Femoral Vein

Anatomy

The femoral vein is a continuation of the long saphenous vein in the groin, and is the main conduit for venous drainage of the legs. It is located in the femoral triangle along with the femoral artery and nerve, as shown in Figure 2.5. The superior border of the femoral triangle is formed by the inguinal ligament, which runs from the anterior superior iliac spine to the pubic symphysis, just beneath the inguinal crease on the skin. At the level of the inguinal ligament (crease), the femoral vein lies just medial to the femoral artery, and is only a few centimeters from the skin. The vein is easier to locate and cannulate when the leg is placed in abduction.

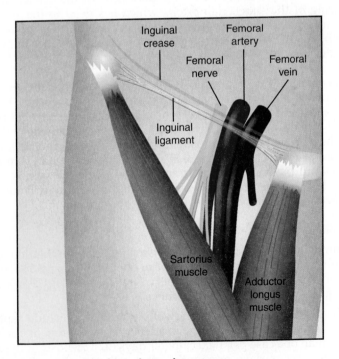

FIGURE 2.5 Anatomy of the femoral triangle.

Ultrasound Imaging

Ultrasound visualization of the femoral artery and vein is possible by placing the ultrasound probe over the femoral artery pulse, which is typically located just below and medial to the midpoint of the inguinal crease. A cross-sectional (short-axis) view of the femoral artery and femoral vein in this location is shown in Figure 2.6. In the image on the left, the femoral artery and vein are identified by their lateral and medial positions, respectively. In the image on the right, the color Doppler mode of ultrasound is used to distinguish between the femoral artery (red color) and femoral vein (blue color). (The red and blue colors do not identify arterial vs. venous flow, but indicate the direction of flow in relation to the ultrasound probe. The red color indicates movement towards the probe, and the blue color indicates movement away from the probe, as indicated by the color legend to the left of the color Doppler image.)

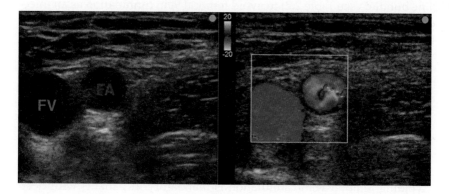

FIGURE 2.6 Ultrasound images (short-axis view) of the femoral vein (FV) and femoral artery (FA) in the left groin. The image on the right identifies the femoral vein (blue color) and femoral artery (red color) using the color Doppler mode of ultrasound. The color legend indicates the directional color assignment for the color Doppler image. The green dots mark the lateral side of each image.

Landmark Method

To cannulate the femoral vein when ultrasound imaging is not available, begin by locating the femoral artery pulse (as described in the prior section) and insert the probe needle (with the bevel at 12 o'clock) 1 to 2 cm medial to the pulse; the vein should be entered at a depth of 2 to 4 cm from the skin. If the femoral artery pulse is not palpable, draw an imaginary line from the anterior superior iliac crest to the pubic tubercle, and divide the line into three equal segments. The femoral artery should be just underneath the junction between the middle and medial segments, and the femoral vein should be 1 to 2 cm medial to this point. This method of locating the femoral vein results in successful cannulation in over 90% of cases (28).

Complications

The major concerns with femoral vein cannulation include puncture of the femoral artery, femoral vein thrombosis, and septicemia. Thrombus formation from indwelling catheters is more common than suspected, but is clinically silent in most cases. In one study of indwelling femoral vein catheters, thrombosis was detected by ultrasound in 10% of patients, but clinically evident thrombosis occurred in less than 1% of patients (23).

The incidence of septicemia from femoral vein catheters is 2 to 3 infections per 1000 catheter days, which is no different than the incidence of septicemia from indwelling catheters in the subclavian vein or internal jugular vein (22,23). This is contrary to the claim that femoral vein catheters have the highest risk of infection amongst central venous catheters (4), and it does not support the recommendation in the "central line bundle" (see Table 2.2) to avoid femoral vein cannulation as an infection control measure.

Comment

The femoral vein is generally regarded as the least desirable site for central venous access, but the observations just presented indicate that the negative publicity directed at femoral vein catheters do not seem justified. The femoral vein is a favored site for temporary hemodialysis catheters (23), and for central venous access during cardiopulmonary resuscitation (because it does not disrupt resuscitation efforts in the chest) (29). However, the use of leg veins for vascular access is not advised during cardiac arrest because drug delivery may be delayed (30). Avoiding femoral vein cannulation is mandatory in patients with deep vein thrombosis of the legs, and in patients with penetrating abdominal trauma (because of the risk of vena cava disruption) (1).

Peripherally Inserted Central Catheters

Catheters can be advanced into the superior vena cava from peripheral veins located just above the antecubital fossa in the arm. These *peripherally inserted central catheters* (PICCs) are described in Chapter 1 (see Table 1.4). There are two veins that emerge from the antecubital fossa, as shown in Figure 2.7. The basilic vein runs up the medial aspect of the arm, and the cephalic vein runs up the lateral aspect of the arm. The basilic vein is preferred for PICC placement because it has a larger diameter than the cephalic vein, and it runs a straighter course up the arm.

PICC Placement

PICC insertion is performed with ultrasound guidance. Once the basilic vein is located and cannulated, the catheters are advanced a predetermined distance to place the catheter tip in the lower third of the superior vena cava, just above the right atrium. The distance the catheter must be advanced is estimated by measuring the distance from the antecubital fossa to the shoulder, then from the shoulder to the right sternoclavicular

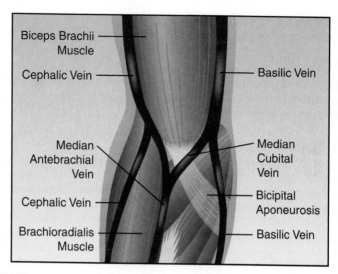

FIGURE 2.7 Anatomy of the major veins in the region of the antecubital fossa in the right arm.

joint, then down to the right 3rd intercostal space. In an average sized adult, the distance from the right antecubital fossa to the right atrium is 52–54 cm, and the distance from the left antecubital fossa to the right atrium is 56–58 cm. When the catheter has been advanced the desired distance, a portable chest x-ray is obtained to locate the catheter tip. Malposition of the catheter tip is reported in 6–7% of PICC insertions (31).

Complications

The most common complication of PICC insertion is catheter-induced thrombosis, which most often involves the axillary and subclavian veins (32). Occlusive thrombosis with swelling of the upper arm has been reported in 2–11% of patients with indwelling PICC devices (32,33); the highest incidence occurs in patients who have a history of venous thrombosis (32) and in cancer patients (33). Septicemia from PICCs occurs at a rate of one infection per 1000 catheter days (31), which is similar to the rate of infection from central venous catheters.

Comment

PICCs are very appealing for central venous access for the following reasons. First, they eliminate many of the risks associated with cannulation of the subclavian vein and internal jugular vein (e.g., puncture of a major artery, pneumothorax). Second, PICC insertion is relatively easy (thanks to ultrasound) and causes less discomfort than cannulation at other central venous access sites. Third, PICCs can be left in place for prolonged periods of time (several weeks) with only a minimal risk of infection. These features make PICC insertion a desirable choice for central venous access in the ICU.

IMMEDIATE CONCERNS

Venous Air Embolism

Air entry into the venous circulation is an uncommon but potentially lethal complication of central venous cannulation. The following is a brief description of this feared complication.

Pathophysiology

Pressure gradients that favor the movement of air into the venous circulation are created by the negative intrathoracic pressure generated during spontaneous breathing, and by gravitational gradients between the site of air entry and the right atrium (i.e., when the site of air entry is vertically higher than the right atrium). A pressure gradient of only 5 mm Hg across a 14 gauge catheter (internal diameter = 1.8 mm) can entrain air at a rate of 100 mL per second, and this is enough to produce a fatal venous air embolism (35). Both the volume of air and the rate of entry determine the consequences of venous air embolism.

The consequences can be fatal when air entry reaches 200–300 mL (3–5 mL/kg) over a few seconds (35). The adverse consequences of venous air embolism include acute right heart failure (from an air lock in the right ventricle) that can progress to cardiogenic shock, leaky-capillary pulmonary edema, and acute embolic stroke from air bubbles that pass through a patent foramen ovale (35).

Prevention

Prevention is the most effective approach to venous air embolism. Positive-pressure mechanical ventilation reduces the risk of air entry through central venous catheters by creating a positive pressure gradient from the central veins to the atmosphere. Other preventive measures include the Trendelenburg position (head-down body tilt) for insertion and removal of internal jugular vein and subclavian vein catheters, and a supine or semirecumbent position for insertion and removal of femoral vein catheters. These measures will reduce, but not eliminate, the risk of venous air embolism. In one study employing appropriate body positions for 11,500 central venous cannulation procedures (34), 15 cases of venous air embolism were observed (incidence = 0.13%).

Clinical Presentation

Venous air embolism can be clinically silent (34). In symptomatic cases, the earliest manifestation is sudden onset of dyspnea, which may be accompanied by a distressing cough. In severe cases, there is rapid progression to hypotension, oliguria, and depressed consciousness (from cardiogenic shock). In the most advanced cases, the mixing of air and blood in the right ventricle can produce a drum-like, mill wheel murmur just prior to cardiovascular collapse (35).

Venous air embolism is usually a clinical diagnosis, but there are some diagnostic aids. Transesophageal echocardiography is the most sensitive method of detecting air in the right heart chambers, and precordial Doppler ultrasound is the most sensitive noninvasive method of detecting air in the heart (35). (Doppler ultrasound converts flow velocities into sounds, and air in the cardiac chambers produces a characteristic high-pitched sound.) The drawback of these diagnostic modalities is limited availability in emergency situations.

Management

The management of venous air embolism includes measures to prevent air entrainment, and general cardiorespiratory support. The first step is to make sure that there is no disruption in the catheter or intravenous tubing that could introduce air into the circulation. If air entrainment is suspected through an indwelling catheter, you can attach a syringe to the hub of the catheter and attempt to aspirate air from the bloodstream. Placing the patient in the left lateral decubitus position is a traditional recommendation aimed at relieving an air lock blocking outflow from the right ventricle, but the value of this maneuver has been questioned (35). Chest compressions can help to force air out of the pulmonary outflow tract and into the pulmonary circulation, but the clinical benefits of this maneuver are unproven (35). Pure oxygen breathing is used to reduce the volume of air in the bloodstream by promoting the movement of nitrogen out of the air bubbles in the blood. However, the efficacy of this maneuver is also unproven.

Pneumothorax

Pneumothorax is an infrequent event during central venous cannulation, and most cases are associated with subclavian vein cannulation. When pneumothorax is suspected, the chest x-ray should be obtained in the upright position and after a forced exhalation (if possible). The forced exhalation will decrease lung volume but will not decrease the volume of air in a pneumothorax; the result is an increase in the relative size of the pneumothorax on the chest x-ray, which can facilitate detection. Unfortunately, few patients in an ICU may be capable of performing a forced exhalation.

The Supine Pneumothorax

Critically ill patients are often unable to sit upright, so chest x-rays are frequently taken in the supine position. This creates a problem for the detection of a pneumothorax. The problem is the distribution of pleural air in the supine position (36); i.e., pleural air does not collect at the apex of the lungs in the supine position, but instead collects anteriorly (because the anterior thorax is the nondependent region in the supine position). Pleural air in this location will be in front of the lungs on the supine chest x-ray, and it can go undetected because of the lung markings behind the pneumothorax. Clinical studies have shown that portable chest x-rays fail to detect 25 to 50% of pneumothoraces when patients are in the supine position (37–39). B-mode ultrasound is superior to portable chest x-rays for detecting supine pneumothoraces (38,39). (An example of a supine pneumothorax that is not apparent on a portable chest x-ray is shown in Chapter 27.)

Delayed Pneumothorax

Pneumothoraces from central venous cannulation may not be radi-ographically evident for 24 to 48 hours (40), and these will be missed on chest x-rays obtained immediately after catheter insertion. However, serial chest x-rays over the first 48 hours post-insertion are not necessary if patients remain asymptomatic.

Catheter Tip Location

Post-insertion chest x-rays are also used to identify the location of the catheter tip, which should be positioned in the distal one-third of the supe-rior vena cava, 1–2 cm above the junction of the right atrium. The appro-priate position for a central venous catheter is shown in Figure 2.8. The cannulation site in this case is the right internal jugular vein, and the catheter follows a straight course down the mediastinum, within the long axis of the superior vena cava shadow. The tip of the catheter is just above the carina, which is the bifurcation of the trachea to form the right

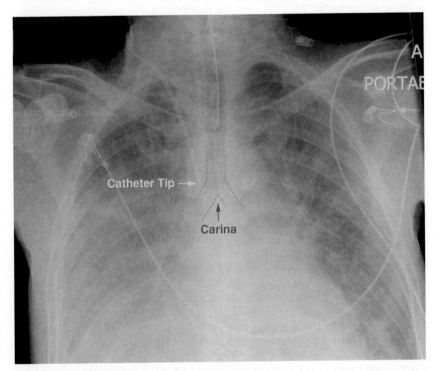

FIGURE 2.8 Portable chest x-ray showing the proper placement of an internal jugular vein catheter with the tip of the catheter located at the level of the carina, where the tra-chea bifurcates to form the right and left mainstem bronchi. The dotted lines are used to highlight the region of the tracheal bifurcation. (Catheter image digitally enhanced.)

and left mainstem bronchi. The carina is located just above the junction between the superior vena cava and the right atrium, so a catheter tip that is at the level of the carina, or slightly above it, is appropriately positioned in the distal superior vena cava. The carina is thus a useful landmark for evaluating catheter tip location (41).

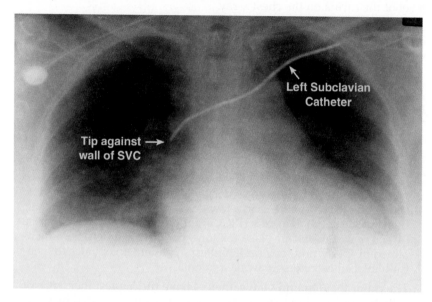

Left Subclavian
Catheter

Tip against →
wall of SVC

FIGURE 2.9 Malposition of a left subclavian vein catheter with the tip abutting the lateral wall of the superior vena cava (SVC). (Catheter image digitally enhanced.)

Misplaced catheters are found in 5% to 25% of cannulations involving central venous catheters and PICC devices (19,31,39). The following are some aberrant catheter tip positions that can prove harmful.

Tip Abuts the Wall of the Vena Cava

Catheters inserted from the left side must make an acute turn downward when they enter the superior vena cava from the left innominate vein. Catheters that do not make this turn can end up in a position like the one shown in Figure 2.9. The tip of the catheter is at the lateral edge of the superior vena cava shadow, suggesting that the catheter tip is in contact with the lateral wall of the superior vena cava. In this position, any forward movement of the catheter (e.g., from shrugging the left shoulder) could puncture the vessel wall and produce a hemothorax (see Figure 3.1). Catheters in this position should be withdrawn into the innominate vein.

Catheter Tip in Right Atrium

As mentioned earlier, the tip of a central venous catheter will be in the right atrium if it is located below the level of the carina on a chest x-ray. This is a common occurrence; e.g., in one study, one of every four central venous catheters was positioned with the tip in the right atrium (39). This malposition creates a risk of right atrial perforation and cardiac tamponade, which is fatal in over 50% of cases (42). Fortunately, this complication occurs only rarely (42), and the risk of cardiac perforation can be eliminated entirely by repositioning catheters when the tip is below the level of the carina on the chest x-ray.

A FINAL WORD

The following points related to central venous cannulation deserve emphasis.

1. Success in central venous cannulation is most likely when real-time ultrasound imaging is used to locate and cannulate the target vessels. Ultrasound-guided vascular cannulation is the most useful innovation in critical care practice in the past 10 or 15 years, and the benefits from mastering this technique can be considerable.

2. For patients who are hemodynamically stable and are expected to stay in the ICU for more than a few days, consider using peripherally inserted central catheters (PICCs) for daily infusion needs. These catheters can be left in place for long periods of time when maintained properly, and they rank highest in patient acceptance for centrally placed catheters in awake patients.

3. The claim that femoral vein catheters have the highest incidence of catheter-related bloodstream infections (2) is not supported by some clinical studies (22,23), and thus the recommendation to avoid femoral vein cannulation as an infection control measure (see Table 2.2) should be questioned. The femoral vein is an acceptable site for temporary hemodialysis catheters, and it is also an acceptable site for central venous cannulation when catheter insertion at other sites is problematic.

Finally, the You Tube website has several instructional videos showing the insertion of central venous catheters in the internal jugular vein, subclavian vein and femoral vein using both ultrasound guidance and surface landmarks. To access these videos, enter "central venous catheterization" in the search box.

REFERENCES

Ultrasound Texts

Levitov A, Mayo P, Slonim A, eds. Critical Care Ultrasonography. New York: McGraw-Hill, 2009.

Noble VE, Nelson BP. Manual of Emergency and Critical Care Ultrasound. 2nd ed., New York: Cambridge University Press, 2011.

Principles and Preparations

1. Taylor RW, Palagiri AV. Central venous catheterization. Crit Care Med 2007; 35:1390–1396.

2. Doerfler M, Kaufman B, Goldenberg A. Central venous catheter placement in patients with disorders of hemostasis. Chest 1996; 110:185–188.

3. Fisher NC, Mutimer DJ. Central venous cannulation in patients with liver disease and coagulopathy – a prospective audit. Intensive Care Med 1999; 25:481–485.

4. O'Grady NP, Alexander M, Burns LA, et. al. and the Healthcare Infection Control Practices Advisory Committee (HICPAC). Guidelines for the Prevention of Intravascular Catheter-related Infections. Clin Infect Dis 2011; 52:e1–e32. (Available at ww.cdc.gov/hicpac/pdf/guidelines/bsi-guidelines-2011.pdf)

5. Institute for Healthcare Improvement. Implement the central line bundle. www.ihi.org/knowledge/Pages/Changes/ImplementtheCentralLineBundle.aspx (Accessed November 5, 2011)

6. Pronovost P, Needham D, Berenholtz S, et al. An intervention to decrease catheter-related bloodstream infections in the ICU. N Engl J Med 2006; 355:2725–2732.

7. Furuya EY, Dick A, Perencevich EN, et al. Central line bundle implementation in U.S. intensive care units and impact on bloodstream infection. PLoS-ONE 2011; 6(1):e15452. (Open access journal available at www.plosone.org; accessed November 5, 2011.)

8. Tschudin-Sutter S, Pargger H, and Widmer AF. Hand hygiene in the intensive care unit. Crit Care Med 2010; 38(Suppl):S299–S305.

9. Chaiyakunapruk N, Veenstra DL, Lipsky BA, et al. Chlorhexidine compared with povidone-iodine solution for vascular catheter-site care: a meta-analysis. Annals Intern Med 2002; 136:792–801.

10. Larson EL. APIC Guideline for hand washings and hand antisepsis in healthcare settings. Am J Infect Control 1995; 23:251–269.

Aids to Cannulation

11. Noble VE, Nelson BP. Vascular access. In: Manual of Emergency and Critical Care Ultrasound. 2nd ed., New York: Cambridge University Press, 2011:273–296.

12. Abboud PAC, Kendall JL. Ultrasound guidance for vascular access. Emerg Med Clin North Am 2004; 22:749–773.

13. Costantino TG, Parikh AK, Satz WA, Fojtik JP. Ultrasonography-guided peripheral intravenous access versus traditional approaches in patients with difficult intravenous access. Ann Emerg Med 2005; 46:456–461.

14. Clenaghan S, McLaughlin RE, Martyn C, et al. Relationship between Trendelenburg tilt and internal jugular vein diameter. Emerg Med J 2005; 22:867–868.

15. Fortune JB, Feustel P. Effect of patient position on size and location of the subclavian vein for percutaneous puncture. Arch Surg 2003; 138:996–1000.

Central Venous Access Routes

16. Feller-Kopman D. Ultrasound-guided internal jugular access. Chest 2007; 132:302–309.

17. Hayashi H, Amano M. Does ultrasound imaging before puncture facilitate internal jugular vein cannulation? Prospective, randomized comparison with landmark-guided puncture in ventilated patients. J Cardiothorac Vasc Anesth 2002; 16:572–575.

18. Leung J, Duffy M, Finckh A. Real-time ultrasonographically-guided internal jugular vein catheterization in the emergency department increases success rate and reduces complications: A randomized, prospective study. Ann Emerg Med 2006; 48:540–547.

19. Ruesch S, Walder B, Tramer M. Complications of central venous catheters: internal jugular versus subclavian access – A systematic review. Crit Care Med 2002; 30:454–460.

20. Reuber M, Dunkley LA, Turton EP, et al. Stroke after internal jugular venous cannulation. Acta Neurol Scand 2002; 105:235–239.

21. Shah PM, Babu SC, Goyal A, et al. Arterial misplacement of large-caliber cannulas during jugular vein catheterization: Case for surgical management. J Am Coll Surg 2004; 198:939–944.

22. Deshpande K, Hatem C, Ulrich H, et al. The incidence of infectious complications of central venous catheters at the subclavian, internal jugular, and femoral sites in an intensive care unit population. Crit Care Med 2005; 33:13–20.

23. Parienti J-J, Thirion M, Megarbane B, et al. Femoral vs jugular venous catheterization and risk of nosocomial events in adults requiring acute renal replacement therapy. JAMA 2008; 299:2413–2422.

24. Fortune JB, Feustel. Effect of patient position on size and location of the subclavian vein for percutaneous puncture. Arch Surg 2003; 138:996–1000.

25. Fragou M, Gravvanis A, Dimitriou V, et al. Real-time ultrasound-guided subclavian vein cannulation versus the landmark method in critical care patients: A prospective randomized study. Crit Care Med 2011; 39:1607–1612.

26. Rodriguez CJ, Bolanowski A, Patel K, et al. Classic positioning decreases cross-sectional area of the subclavian vein. Am J Surg 2006; 192:135–137.

27. Hernandez D, Diaz F, Rufino M, et al. Subclavian vascular access stenosis in dialysis patients: Natural history and risk factors. J Am Soc Nephrol 1998; 9:1507–1510.

28. Getzen LC, Pollack EW. Short-term femoral vein catheterization. Am J Surg 1979; 138:875–877.

29. Hilty WM, Hudson PA, Levitt MA, Hall JB. Real-time ultrasound-guided femoral vein catheterization during cardiopulmonary resuscitation. Ann Emerg Med 1997; 29:311–316.

30. Cummins RO (ed). ACLS Provider Manual. Dallas, TX; American Heart Association, 2001: pp. 38–39.

31. Ng P, Ault M, Ellrodt AG, Maldonado L. Peripherally inserted central catheters in general medicine. Mayo Clin Proc 1997; 72:225–233.

32. Evans RS, Sharp JH, Linford LH, et al. Risk of symptomatic DVT associated with peripherally inserted central catheters. Chest 2010; 138:803–810.

33. Hughes ME. PICC-related thrombosis: pathophysiology, incidence, morbidity, and the effect of ultrasound guided placement technique on occurrence in cancer patients. JAVA 2011; 16:8–18.

Immediate Concerns

34. Vesely TM. Air embolism during insertion of central venous catheters. J Vasc Interv Radiol 2001; 12:1291–1295.

35. Mirski MA, Lele AV, Fitzsimmons L, Toung TJK. Diagnosis and treatment of vascular air embolism. Anesthesiology 2007; 106:164–177.

36. Tocino IM, Miller MH, Fairfax WR. Distribution of pneumothorax in the supine and semirecumbent critically ill adult. Am J Radiol 1985;144:901–905.

37. Blaivas M, Lyon M, Duggal S. A prospective comparison of supine chest radiography and bedside ultrasound for the diagnosis of traumatic pneumothorax. Acad Emerg Med 2005; 12:844–849.

38. Ball CG, Kirkpatrick AW, Laupland KB, et al. Factors related to the failure of radiographic recognition of occult posttraumatic pneumothoraces. Am J Surg 2005; 189:541–546.

39. Vezzani A, Brusasco C, Palermo S, et al. Ultrasound localization of central vein catheter and detection of postprocedural pneumothorax: an alternative to chest radiography. Crit Care Med 2010; 38:533–538.

40. Collin GR, Clarke LE. Delayed pneumothorax: a complication of central venous catheterization. Surg Rounds 1994;17:589–594.

41. Stonelake PA, Bodenham AR. The carina as a radiological landmark for central venous catheter tip position. Br J Anesthesia 2006; 96:335–340.

42. Booth SA, Norton B, Mulvey DA. Central venous catheterization and fatal cardiac tamponade. Br J Anesth 2001; 87:298–302.

Chapter 3

THE INDWELLING VASCULAR CATHETER

My dear Watson, you see but you do not observe.

Sir Arthur Conan Doyle,
Scandal in Bohemia,
1891

Every patient in the ICU is equipped with at least one indwelling vascular catheter, and attention to the maintenance and adverse consequences of these devices is part of everyday patient care. This chapter describes the routine care and troublesome complications of indwelling vascular catheters. Many of the recommendations in this chapter are taken from the clinical practice guidelines listed at the end of the chapter (1–3).

ROUTINE CATHETER CARE

The recommendations for routine catheter care are summarized in Table 3.1.

Catheter Site Dressing

Catheter insertion sites should be covered with a sterile dressing for the life of the catheter. The sterile dressing can be a covering of sterile gauze pads, or an adhesive, transparent plastic membrane (called occlusive dressings). The transparent membrane in occlusive dressings is semipermeable, and allows the loss of water vapor, but not liquid secretions, from the underlying skin. This prevents excessive drying of the underlying skin to promote wound healing. Occlusive dressings are favored because the transparent membrane allows daily inspection of the catheter insertion site. Sterile gauze dressings are preferred when the catheter insertion site is difficult to keep dry (1).

Table 3.1	Recommendations for Routine Catheter Care
	Recommendations
Sterile Dressings	Adhesive transparent dressings are favored because they allow inspection of the catheter insertion site.
	Sterile gauze dressings are used for skin areas that are difficult to keep dry.
	Adhesive transparent dressings and sterile gauze dressings provide equivalent protection against catheter colonization.
Antimicrobial Gels	Do not apply antimicrobial gels to catheter insertion sites, except for hemodialysis catheters.
Replacing Catheters	Regular replacement of central venous catheters is not recommended.
Flushing Catheters	Avoid using heparin in catheter flush solutions.

From the clinical practice guidelines in Reference 1.

Sterile gauze dressings and occlusive dressings are roughly equivalent in their ability to limit catheter colonization and infection (1,4–6). However, occlusive dressings can promote colonization and infection when moisture accumulates under the sealed dressing (4,6), so occlusive dressings should be changed when fluid accumulates under the transparent membrane.

Antimicrobial Gels

The application of antimicrobial gels to the insertion site of central venous catheters does not reduce the incidence of catheter-related infections (1), with the possible exception of hemodialysis catheters (7). As a result, topical antimicrobial gels are recommended only for hemodialysis catheters (1), and are applied after each dialysis.

Replacing Catheters

Peripheral Vein Catheters

The major concern with peripheral vein catheters is phlebitis (from the catheter or infusate), which typically begins to appear after 3–4 days (1,8). Catheter replacement is thus recommended every 3–4 days (1), but peripheral catheters are usually left in place as long as there is no evidence of localized phlebitis (i.e., pain, erythema and swelling around the insertion site).

Central Venous Catheters

Replacing central venous catheters at regular intervals, using either guidewire exchange or a new venipuncture site, does not reduce the incidence of catheter-related infections (9), and can actually promote complications (both mechanical and infectious) (10). One study showed a 7% complication rate associated with replacement of central venous catheters (11). The combination of no benefit and added risk is the reason that routine replacement of indwelling central venous catheters is not recommended (1). This recommendation also applies to peripherally inserted central catheters (PICCs), hemodialysis catheters, and pulmonary artery catheters (1). Catheter replacement is also not necessary when there is erythema around the catheter insertion site, since erythema alone is not evidence of infection (12).

Flushing Catheters

Vascular catheters are flushed at regular intervals to prevent thrombotic obstruction, although this may not be necessary for peripheral catheters that are used intermittently (13). The standard flush solution is heparinized saline (with heparin concentrations ranging from 10 to 1,000 units/mL) (14). Catheters that are used only intermittently are filled with heparinized saline and capped when not in use; this is known as a *heparin lock*. Arterial catheters are flushed continuously at a rate of 3 mL/hour using a pressurized bag to drive the flush solution through the catheter (15).

Alternatives to Heparin

The use of heparin in catheter flush solutions has two disadvantages: i.e., cost (considering all the catheter flushes performed in the hospital each day) and the risk of heparin-induced thrombocytopenia (see Chapter 19). These disadvantages can be eliminated by using heparin-free flush solutions. Saline alone is as effective as heparinized saline for flushing venous catheters (14), but this is not the case for arterial catheters (15), where 1.4% sodium citrate is a suitable alternative to heparinized saline for maintaining catheter patency (16).

NONINFECTIOUS COMPLICATIONS

The noninfectious complications of indwelling central venous catheters include catheter occlusion, thrombotic occlusion of the cannulated central vein, and perforation of the superior vena cava or right atrium.

Catheter Occlusion

Occlusion of central venous catheters can be the result of sharp angles or kinks in the catheter (usually created during insertion), thrombosis (from backwash of blood into the catheter), insoluble precipitates in the infusates (from medications or inorganic salts), and lipid residues (from propofol or total parenteral nutrition). Thrombosis is the most common cause of catheter obstruction, and is reported in up to 25% of central venous catheters (17). Occlusion from insoluble precipitates can be the result of water-insoluble drugs (e.g., diazepam, digoxin, phenytoin, trimethoprim-sulfa) or anion–cation complexes (e.g., calcium phosphate) that precipitate in an acid or alkaline solution (18).

Restoring Patency

Every effort should be made to restore patency and avoid replacing the catheter. Advancing a guidewire to dislodge an obstructing mass is not advised because of the risk of embolization. Chemical dissolution of the obstructing mass (described next) is the preferred intervention.

THROMBOTIC OCCLUSION: Since thrombosis is the most common cause of catheter obstruction, the initial attempt to restore patency should involve the local instillation of a thrombolytic agent. Alteplase (recombinant tissue plasminogen activator) is currently the favored thrombolytic agent for restoring catheter patency, and the regimen shown in Table 3.2 can restore patency in 80–90% of occluded catheters (19,20). There are no reports of abnormal bleeding associated with this regimen (19).

Table 3.2	Protocol for Restoring Patency in Occluded Vascular Catheters
Drug	Alteplase (recombinant tissue plasminogen activator)
Preparation	Cathflo Activase (Genentech Inc.) available as a powder in 2 mg vials of alteplase Add 2 mL sterile water to each vial for a drug concentration of 1 mg/mL.
Regimen	1. Instill 2 mL (2 mg) of drug solution into the occluded catheter and cap the hub of the catheter. 2. Wait 30 minutes and attempt to withdraw blood from the catheter. 3. If the occlusion persists, wait another 90 minutes (total dwell time=120 min) and attempt to withdraw blood from the catheter. 4. If the occlusion persists, prepare a second dose of alteplase (2 mg) and repeat steps 1–3. 5. If patency is restored, withdraw 5 mL of blood through the catheter to remove the drug solution and any residual clot. 6. If alteplase instillation does not restore patency, consider instilling 0.1N HCL for drug or calcium phosphate precipitates, or 70% ethanol if lipid residues are suspected.

From References 19, 20

NON-THROMBOTIC OCCLUSION: Dilute acid will promote the dissolution of occlusive precipitates (e.g., calcium phosphate precipitates), and catheter occlusion that is refractory to thrombolysis is occasionally relieved after instillation of 0.1N hydrochloric acid (21). If lipid residues are suspected as a cause of catheter occlusion (e.g., from propofol infusions or lipid emulsions used for parenteral nutrition), instillation of 70% ethanol can restore catheter patency (18).

Venous Thrombosis

Thrombus formation is common around the intravascular segment of indwelling catheters, but the thrombosis is clinically silent in most cases. When patients with indwelling central venous catheters are routinely tested with ultrasonography or contrast venography, thrombosis involving the catheter tip is found in as many as 40% of the catheters (22). However, catheter-associated thrombosis is clinically silent in more than 95% of cases (22–24). Symptomatic thrombosis is reported most often with femoral vein catheters (3.4%) and peripherally inserted central catheters (3%) (23,24).

Catheter-associated thrombosis is much more common in cancer patients, where as many as two-thirds of patients have evidence of catheter-associated thrombosis when routinely tested (25), and as many as one-third of patients have symptomatic thrombosis (25). The greater risk of thrombosis in cancer patients is explained by three factors: i.e., the prolonged duration of catheterization, infusion of chemotherapeutic agents, and the hypercoagulable state that accompanies many cancers.

Upper Extremity Thrombosis

About 10% of cases of deep vein thrombosis (DVT) involve the upper extremities, and an estimated 80% of upper extremity DVTs are attributed to central venous catheters (26). Thrombotic occlusion of the axillary and subclavian veins produces swelling of the upper arm, which can be accompanied by paresthesias and arm weakness (26). These thrombi can also propagate into the superior vena cava, but thrombotic occlusion of the superior vena cava and the subsequent *superior vena cava syndrome* (with facial swelling, headache, etc.) occurs rarely in catheter-related DVT of the upper extremities (27). Finally, fewer than 10% of upper extremity DVTs are accompanied by symptomatic pulmonary emboli (26).

DIAGNOSIS: Compression ultrasonography is the diagnostic test of choice for upper extremity DVT (see Figure 2.3 for an example of this method). A positive test (i.e., clot-filled veins do not collapse with compression) has a sensitivity of 97% and a specificity of 96% for upper extremity DVT (26). D-dimer levels are not reliable for screening suspected cases of upper extremity DVT because critically ill patients often have elevated D-dimer levels.

MANAGEMENT: Surprisingly, removal of the offending catheter is not mandatory in upper extremity DVT, and is recommended only when arm swelling is severe or painful, or when anticoagulant therapy is contraindicated (26). Anticoagulant therapy has not been adequately studied in upper extremity DVT, and the anticoagulant regimens used for lower extremity DVT have been adopted for the upper extremity (26). These regimens are described in Chapter 6.

Lower Extremity Thrombosis

As mentioned earlier, symptomatic DVT of the lower extremity develops in about 3% of femoral vein cannulations (24). The diagnosis and management of lower extremity DVT is described in Chapter 6.

Vascular Perforation

Catheter-induced perforation of the superior vena cava or right atrium is uncommon but has potentially life-threatening complications of central venous cannulation, as described at the end of Chapter 2. These perforations are avoidable with vigilance and prompt correction of misplaced catheters.

Superior Vena Cava Perforation

Perforation of the superior vena cava is most often caused by left-sided central venous catheters that enter the superior vena cava but do not make the acute turn downward toward the right atrium. The tip of the catheter then abuts the lateral wall of the superior vena cava, as shown in Figure 2.9 in the last chapter. Most perforations occur within 7 days of catheter placement (28). The clinical symptoms (substernal chest pain, cough, and dyspnea) are nonspecific, and suspicion of perforation is often prompted by the sudden appearance of mediastinal widening or a pleural effusion on a chest x-ray, like the one in Figure 3.1. The unexpected appearance of a pleural effusion in a patient with a left-sided central venous catheter should always raise suspicion of superior vena cava perforation.

DIAGNOSIS: The pleural effusions associated with catheter-induced perforation of the superior vena cava are the result of intravenous fluids flowing into the pleural space. Thoracentesis will thus support the diagnosis of vena cava perforation if the pleural fluid is similar in composition to the intravenous infusion fluid. Pleural fluid glucose levels can be useful if a parenteral nutrition formula was infusing through the catheter. The perforation can be confirmed by injecting radiocontrast dye through a catheter in the superior vena cava and noting the presence of dye in the mediastinum.

MANAGEMENT: When vena cava perforation is first suspected, the infusion should be stopped immediately. If the diagnosis is confirmed, the catheter should be removed immediately (this does not provoke mediastinal bleeding) (28). Antibiotic therapy is not necessary unless there is evidence of infection in the pleural fluid (28).

Cardiac Tamponade

The most life-threatening complication of central venous catheterization is cardiac tamponade from catheter-induced perforation of the right atrium. Although considered rare, the actual incidence of this complication is not known (29). The first sign of tamponade is usually the abrupt onset

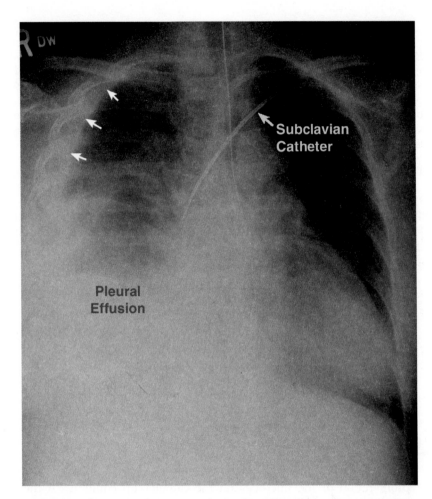

FIGURE 3.1 Chest x-ray of a patient with a perforated superior vena cava caused by a left-sided subclavian catheter (which is positioned like the catheter in Figure 2.9). Image courtesy of John E. Heffner, MD (from Reference 27).

of dyspnea, which can progress to cardiovascular collapse within an hour. The diagnosis requires ultrasound evidence of a pericardial effusion with diastolic collapse of the right heart, and immediate pericardiocentesis is necessary to relieve the tamponade. Emergency thoracotomy may also be necessary if there is a large tear in the wall of the heart.

Catheter-associated pericardial tamponade is often overlooked, and the mortality rate varies from 40% to 100% in published reports (29). The most effective approach to this condition is prevention, which requires proper positioning of central venous catheters so the tip is at, or slightly above, the tracheal carina. The proper position of a central venous catheter is shown in Figure 2.8 in the last chapter.

CATHETER-RELATED BLOODSTREAM INFECTIONS

Pathogenic organisms can colonize the intravascular portion of central venous catheters, and dissemination of these organisms in the bloodstream (i.e., *catheter-related bloodstream infections*) can be fatal in up to 25% of cases (30). Fortunately, the incidence of these infections has declined by almost 60% over the past decade (31), presumably as a result of preventive measures like those in Table 2.3 in the last chapter. The following is a description of the etiology and management of these infections.

Pathogenesis

Sources of Infection

The sources of catheter-related bloodstream infections are indicated in Figure 3.2. Each is described below using the corresponding numbers in the illustration.

1. Microbes can gain access to the bloodstream via contaminated infusates (e.g., blood products), but this occurs rarely.

2. Contamination of the internal lumen of vascular catheters can occur through break points in the infusion system, such as catheter hubs. This may be a prominent route of infection for catheters inserted through subcutaneous tunnels.

3. Microbes on the skin can migrate along the subcutaneous tract of an indwelling catheter and eventually reach (and colonize) the intravascular portion of the catheter. This is considered the principal route of infection for percutaneous (non-tunneled) catheters, which includes most of the catheters inserted in the ICU .

4. Microorganisms in circulating blood can attach to the intravascular portion of an indwelling catheter. This is considered a secondary seeding of the catheter from a source of septicemia elsewhere, but proliferation of the microbes on the catheter tip could reach the point where the catheter becomes a source of septicemia.

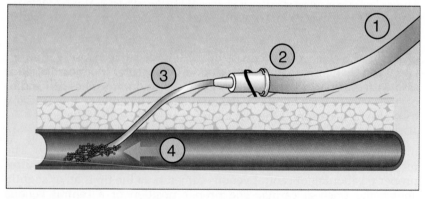

FIGURE 3.2 Sources of microbial colonization at the distal end of vascular catheters. See text for explanation.

(For a contrary view of the importance of skin microbes in catheter-related infections, see the very last section of the chapter: *A Final Word*.)

Biofilms

Microbes are not freely moving organisms, and have a tendency to congregate on inert surfaces. When a microbe comes in contact with a surface, it releases adhesive molecules (called *adhesins*, of course) that firmly attach it to the surface. The microbe then begins to proliferate, and the newly formed cells release polysaccharides that coalesce to form a matrix known as *slime* (because of its physical properties), which then encases the proliferating microbes. The encasement formed by the polysaccharide matrix is called a *biofilm*. Biofilms are protective barriers that shield microbes from the surrounding environment, and this protected environment allows microbes to thrive and proliferate (32).

Biofilms are ubiquitous in nature, and predominate on surfaces that are exposed to moisture (the slippery film that covers rocks in a stream is a familiar example of a biofilm). They also form on indwelling medical devices such as vascular catheters (33). In fact, the organism that is most frequently involved in catheter-related infections, *Staphylococcus epidermidis*, shows a propensity for adherence to polymer surfaces and slime production (34). A biofilm of *S. epidermidis* is shown in Figure 3.3.

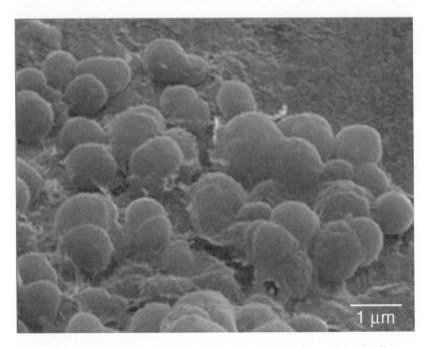

FIGURE 3.3 Electron micrograph of *Staphylococcus epidermidis* encased in a biofilm. Image courtesy of Jeanne VanBriesen, Ph.D., Carnegie Mellon University. Image colorized digitally.

BIOFILM RESISTANCE: Biofilms on medical devices are problematic because they show a resistance to host defenses and antibiotic therapy. Phagocytic cells are unable to ingest organisms that are embedded in a biofilm, and *antibiotic concentrations that eradicate free-living bacteria must be 100 to 1,000 times higher to eradicate bacteria in biofilms* (35). Chemical substances that disrupt biofilms, such as tetrasodium EDTA, may have a prominent role in the eradication of biofilms on medical devices (36).

Incidence

Each day that a catheter remains in place carries a risk of infection, so the frequency of catheter-related infections is expressed in terms of the total number of catheter-days. The incidence of catheter-associated infections in Table 3.3 is expressed as the number of infections per 1,000 catheter-days. The information in this table, which is organized by type of specialty ICU, is from the National Healthcare Safety Network Report of 2010, which includes data from about 2,500 hospitals in the United States (37). The most striking feature of this data is the *remarkably low incidence of catheter-associated infections* in all the ICUs, regardless of specialty Furthermore, this data overestimates the actual incidence of infection, as described next.

Table 3.3	Incidence of Catheter-Associated Bloodstream Infections (CABI) in the United States in 2010	
Type of ICU	**Infections per 1,000 catheter-days**	
	Pooled Mean	**Range (10–90%)**
Burn Units	3.5	0 – 8.0
Trauma Units	1.9	0 – 4.0
Medical ICUs	1.8	0 – 3.5
Surgical ICUs	1.4	0 – 3.2
Med/Surg ICUs	1.4	0 – 3.1
Coronary Care Units	1.3	0 – 2.7
Neurosurgical ICUs	1.3	0 – 2.7
Cardiothoracic ICUs	0.9	0 – 2.0

From the National Healthcare Safety Network Report (37). Includes only ICUs in major teaching hospitals.

Associated vs. Related Infections

The following two definitions are used to identify infections attributed to central venous catheters:

Catheter-*Associated* Bloodstream Infections (CABI) are bloodstream infections that have no apparent source other than a vascular catheter in patients who either have an indwelling catheter or have had one within 48 hours of the positive blood culture. This is the definition used in epidemiological surveys (like the one in Table 3.3), and it requires no evidence of microbial growth on the suspected catheter.

Catheter-*Related* Bloodstream Infections (CRBI) are bloodstream infections where the organism identified in peripheral blood is also present in significant quantities on the tip of the catheter or in a blood sample drawn through the catheter (the criteria for a significant quantity is presented later). This is the definition used in clinical practice, and it requires evidence of catheter involvement with the same organism present in peripheral blood.

The diagnostic criteria for CABI (which are used in clinical surveys) are far less rigorous than the diagnostic criteria for CRBI (which are used in clinical practice), so the incidence of CABI (like the one in Table 3.3) can overestimate the incidence of CRBI (the actual incidence in clinical practice). In one comparison study, the incidence of CABI exceeded that of CRBI by one infection per 1,000 catheter-days (38). If this difference is applied to the data in Table 3.3 (i.e., subtract one from the incidences in the table), the mean incidence of catheter-related infections falls to less than one per 1,000 catheter days in most of the ICUs.

Clinical Features

Catheter-related infections do not appear in the first 48 hours after catheter insertion (which presumably is the time required for colonization of the catheter tip). When they do appear, the clinical manifestations are typically non-specific signs of systemic inflammation (e.g., fever, leukocytosis). Inflammation at the catheter insertion site has no predictive value the presence of septicemia (12), and purulent drainage from the catheter insertion site is uncommon, and can be a manifestation of an exit-site infection without bloodstream invasion (2). The diagnosis of CRBI is thus not possible on clinical grounds, and one of the culture methods described next is required to conform or exclude the diagnosis.

Diagnosis

There are three culture-based approaches to the diagnosis of CRBI, and these are included in Table 3.4. The culture method you select in each case will be determined by the decision to retain or replace the suspect catheter.

Catheter Management

The evaluation of suspected CRBI requires one of three possible decisions for the suspect catheter:

1. Remove the catheter and insert a new catheter at a new venipuncture site.
2. Replace the catheter over a guidewire using the same venipuncture site.
3. Leave the catheter in place.

The first option (remove the catheter and insert a new one at a new site) is recommended for patients with neutropenia, a prosthetic valve, indwelling pacemaker wires, evidence of severe sepsis or septic shock, or purulent drainage from the catheter insertion site (2). Otherwise, catheters can be left in place or replaced over a guidewire. Option #3 (leave the catheter alone) is desirable because most evaluations for CRBI do not confirm the diagnosis (so replacing the catheter is not necessary), and because guidewire exchanges can have adverse effects (10,11).

Table 3.4	Culture Methods & Diagnostic Criteria for Catheter-Related Bloodstream Infections (CRBI)
Culture Method	**Diagnostic Criteria for CRBI**
Semiquantitative Culture of Catheter Tip	Same organism on catheter tip and in peripheral blood, and growth from the catheter tip >15 colony-forming units (cfu) in 24 hours.
Differential Quantitative Blood Cultures	Same organism in peripheral blood & catheter blood, and colony count from catheter blood ≥3 times greater than colony count from peripheral blood.
Differential Time to Positive Culture	Same organism in peripheral blood & catheter blood, and onset of growth in catheter blood at least two hours before onset of growth in peripheral blood.

From the clinical practice guidelines in Reference 2.

Semiquantitative Culture of Catheter Tip

The standard approach to suspected CRBI is to remove the catheter and culture the tip, as outlined below.

1. Before the catheter is removed, swab the skin around the catheter insertion site with an antiseptic solution.

2. Remove the catheter using sterile technique and sever the distal 5 cm (2 inches) of the catheter. Place the severed segment in a sterile culturette tube for transport to the microbiology laboratory, and request a semiquantitative or roll-plate culture (the tip of the catheter will be rolled across a culture plate, and the number of colonies that appear in 24 hours will be recorded). If an antimicrobial-impregnated catheter is removed, inform the lab of such so they can add the appropriate inhibitors to the culture plate.

3. Draw 10 mL of blood from a peripheral vein for a blood culture.

4. The diagnosis of CRBI is confirmed if the same organism is isolated from the catheter tip and the blood culture, and growth from the catheter tip exceeds 15 colony forming units (cfu) in 24 hours.

Because the outer surface of the catheter is cultured, this method will not detect colonization on the inner (luminal) surface of the catheter (which is the surface involved if microbes are introduced via the hub of the catheter). Nevertheless, semiquantitative catheter tip cultures are considered the "gold standard" method for the diagnosis of CRBI.

Differential Quantitative Blood Cultures

This method is designed for catheters that are left in place, and is based on the expectation that when the catheter is the source of a bloodstream infection, blood withdrawn through the catheter will have a higher microbial density than blood obtained from a peripheral vein. This requires a quantitative assessment of microbial density in the blood, where the results are expressed as number of colony forming units per mL (like urine cultures). This method is outlined below.

1. Obtain specialized Isolator culture tubes (Isolator Culture System, Dupont, Wilmington, DE) from the microbiology laboratory. These tubes contain a substance that lyses cells to release intracellular organisms.

2. Decontaminate the hub of the catheter with an antiseptic solution (use the distal lumen in multilumen catheters) and draw 10 mL of blood through the catheter and directly into the Isolator culture tube.

3. Draw 10 mL of blood from a peripheral vein using the Isolator culture tube.

4. Send both specimens to the microbiology lab for quantitative cultures. The blood will be processed by lysing the cells to release microorganisms, separating the cell fragments by centrifugation, and adding broth to the supernatant. This mixture is placed on a culture plate and allowed to incubate for 72 hours. Growth is recorded as the number of colony forming units per milliliter (cfu/mL).

5. The diagnosis of CRBI is confirmed if the same organism is isolated from the catheter blood sample and the peripheral blood sample, and the colony count in the catheter blood sample is at least 3 times greater than the colony count in peripheral blood.

An example of the comparative growth density in a case of CRBI is shown in Figure 3.4.

Because blood is withdrawn through the lumen of the catheter, this method may not detect microbes on the outer surface of the catheter. However, the diagnostic accuracy of this method is 94% when compared with catheter tip cultures (the gold standard) (39).

Differential Time to Positive Culture

This method is also designed for catheters that remain in place, and is based on the expectation that when a catheter is the source of a bloodstream infection, the blood withdrawn through the catheter will show microbial growth earlier than blood obtained from a peripheral vein. This

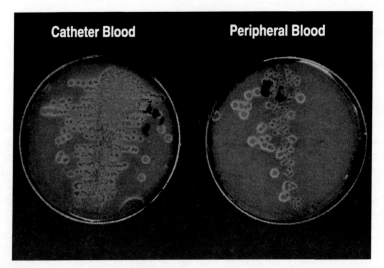

FIGURE 3.4 Culture plates showing colonies of bacterial growth from blood drawn from a central venous catheter (*Catheter Blood*) and a peripheral vein (*Peripheral Blood*). The denser growth from catheter blood is evidence of catheter-related septicemia. (From Curtas S, Tramposch K. Culture methods to evaluate central venous catheter sepsis. Nutr Clin Pract 1991;6:43). Image colorized digitally.

method uses routine (qualitative) blood cultures; and requires 10 mL of blood drawn through the catheter, and 10 mL of blood from a peripheral vein. The diagnosis of CRBI is confirmed if the same organism is isolated from the catheter blood and peripheral blood, and growth is first detected at least 2 hours earlier in the catheter blood. This approach is technically easier and less costly than comparing quantitative blood cultures, but the diagnostic accuracy is lower (39).

The Microbial Spectrum

The organisms involved in CRBI are (in order of prevalence) coagulase-negative staphylococci, Gram-negative aerobic bacilli (*Pseudomonas aeruginosa, Klebsiella pneumoniae, E. coli,* etc), enterococci, *Staphylococcus aureus* and *Candida species* (40). Coagulase-negative staphylococci (mostly *Staphylococcus epidermidis*) are responsible for about one-third of infections, while Gram-negative bacilli and other organisms that inhabit the bowel (enterococci and *Candida* species) are involved in about half the infections. This microbial spectrum is important to consider when selecting empiric antimicrobial therapy.

Management

Empiric Antibiotic Therapy

Empiric antibiotic therapy is recommended for all ICU patients with suspected CRBI, and should be started immediately after cultures are obtained. The recommendations for empiric antibiotic coverage from published guidelines (2) are shown in Table 3.5.

Table 3.5	Empiric Antibiotics for Common Isolates in Catheter-Related Bloodstream Infections	
Organism	**Antibiotic**	**Comment**
Staphylococci	Vancomycin	If MRSA isolates with MIC>2 mg/mL are prevalent, use daptomycin.
Enterococci	Vancomycin	If vancomycin resistance is a concern, use daptomycin.
Gram-Negative Bacilli	Carbepenem[a] or Cefepime or Pipericillin-Tazobactam	Add aminoglycoside for neutropenia or concern for multidrug-resistant organisms.
Candida species	Echinocandin[b]	Indications: Femoral catheter, TPN hematologic malignancy, prolonged antibiotic Rx, recent transplant, or Candida sp. elsewhere.
Cardiothoracic ICUs	0.9	0 – 2.0

From the clinical practice guidelines in Reference 2. See Chapter 52 for antibiotic dosing.
[a]Carbapenems include imipenem,meropenem, and doripenem.
[b]Echinocandins include caspofungin, micafungin, and anidulafungin.

Vancomycin is the backbone of the empiric antibiotic regimen because it is the most active agent against staphylococci (including coagulase-negative and methicillin-resistant strains), and enterococci, which together are responsible for about 50% of catheter-related infections (40). Daptomycin can substitute for vancomycin if there is a risk of infection with vancomycin-resistant enterococci. Empiric coverage for enteric Gram-negative bacilli is advised because these organisms are the second most common isolates in ICU patients with CRBI (40). The antibiotics best-suited for empiric Gram-negative coverage include the carbepenems (e.g., meropenem), the fourth-generation cephalosporins (e.g., cefepime), and the β-lactam/β-lactamase inhibitor combinations (e.g., pipericillin/tazobactam). Additional Gram-negative coverage (with an aminoglycoside) is recommended for patients with neutropenia, and when multidrug- resistant Gram-negative bacilli are possible offenders.

Empiric coverage for candidemia is recommended when the conditions listed in Table 3.5 are present. The echinocandins (e.g., caspofungin) are favored over the azoles (e.g., fluconazole) for empiric coverage because some Candida species (i.e., Candida krusei and Candida glabrata) are resistant to azoles. The dosing of antifungal agents is described in Chapter 52.

Culture-Confirmed Infections

If the culture results confirm the diagnosis of CRBI, further antibiotic therapy is dictated by the identified organisms and antibiotic susceptibilities. The pathogen-specific antibiotic recommendations from the most recent guidelines on CRBI (2) are shown in Table 3.6.

Table 3.6	Pathogen-Specific Antibiotic Recommendations	
Pathogens	**Preferred Antibiotics**	**Alternative Antibiotics**
I. Staphylococci		
Methicillin-sensitive	Nafcillin or Oxacillin	Cefazolin or Vancomycin
Methicillin-resistant	Vancomycin	Daptomycin or Linezolid
II. Enterococci		
Ampicillin-sensitive	Ampicillin	Vancomycin
Ampicillin-resistant, Vancomycin-sensitive	Vancomycin	Daptomycin or Linezolid
Ampicillin-resistant, Vancomycin-resistant	Daptoomycin, or Linezolid	Quinupristin/Dalfopristin
III. Gram-negative bacilli		
Acinetobacter sp.	Carbepenem[a]	Ampicillin-Sulbactam
E. coli & *Klebsiella* sp.	Carbepenem[a]	Aztreonam
Enterobacter sp.	Carbepenem[a]	Cefepime
Pseudomonas aeruginosa	Carbepenem[a], or Cefepime, or Pipericillin-Tazobactam	Carbepenem[a], or Cefepime, or Pipericillin-Tazobactam
IV. *Candida* sp.μμ		
Candida albicans	Fluconazole	Echinocandin[b]
Candida krusei and *Candida glabrata*	Echinocandin[b]	Amphotericin B

From the clinical practice guidelines in Reference 2. See Chapter 52 for antibiotic dosing.
[a]Carbapenems include imipenem, meropenem, and doripenem.
[b]Echinocandins include caspofungin, micafungin, and anidulafungin.

CATHETER MANAGEMENT: When the diagnosis of CRBI is confirmed, catheters that were left in place or changed over a guidewire should be removed and reinserted at a new venipuncture site, unless the offending organism is a coagulase-negative staphylococcus (e.g., *S. epidermidis*) or an enterococcus, and the patient shows a favorable response to empiric antimicrobial therapy (2).

Decontamination of catheters that are left in place can be difficult with systemic antibiotic therapy (probably because of biofilm resistance), and recurrent infections are common (41). Instillation of concentrated antibiotic solutions into indwelling catheters (*antibiotic lock therapy*) enhances the ability to disrupt biofilms and eradicate persistent organisms (see next).

Antibiotic Lock Therapy

Antibiotic lock therapy is recommended for all catheters that are left in place during systemic antibiotic therapy (2). The antibiotic lock solution contains the same antibiotic used systemically, in a concentration of 2–5 mg/mL in heparinized saline. This solution is injected into each lumen of the indwelling catheter and allowed to dwell for 24 hours, and the solution is then replaced every 24 hours for the duration of systemic antibiotic therapy. If the catheter is never idle and antibiotic lock therapy is not possible, then the systemic antibiotic(s) should be delivered through the suspect lumen. (For a list of pathogen-specific antibiotic lock solutions, see the clinical practice guidelines in Reference 2.)

Duration of Treatment

The duration of antibiotic therapy is determined by the offending pathogen, the status of the catheter (i.e., replaced or retained), and the clinical response. For patients who show a favorable response in the first 72 hours of systemic antibiotic therapy, the recommended duration of treatment is as follows (2):

1. If coagulase-negative staphylococci are involved, antibiotic therapy is continued for 5–7 days if the catheter is removed, and for 10–14 days if the catheter is left in place.
2. If *S. aureus* is the culprit, antibiotic therapy can be limited to 14 days if the catheter is removed *and* the following conditions are satisfied: the patient is not diabetic or immunosuppressed, there are no intravascular prosthetic devices in place, and there is no evidence of endocarditis on transesophageal ultrasound (2). (Some recommend that all cases of *S. aureus* bacteremia include an evaluation for endocarditis with transesophageal ultrasound, which should be performed 5–7 days after the onset of bacteremia.) If any of these conditions are present, 4–6 weeks of antibiotic therapy is recommended (2).
3. For infections caused by enterococci or Gram-negative bacilli, 7–14 days of antibiotic therapy is recommended, regardless of whether the catheter is replaced or retained (2).
4. For uncomplicated *Candida* infections, antifungal therapy should be continued for 14 days after the first negative blood culture (2).

Persistent Sepsis

Continued signs of sepsis or persistent septicemia after 72 hours of antimicrobial therapy should prompt an evaluation for the following conditions.

Suppurative Thrombophlebitis

As mentioned earlier, thrombus formation on indwelling catheters is common, and these thrombi can trap microbes from a colonized catheter. Proliferation of these microbes can then transform the thrombus into an intravascular abscess. This condition is known as *suppurative thrombophlebitis*, and the most common offending organism is *Staphylococcus aureus* (2). Clinical manifestations are often absent, but can include purulent drainage from the catheter insertion site, limb swelling from thrombotic venous occlusion, multiple cavitary lesions in the lungs from septic emboli, and embolic lesions of the hand if arterial catheters are involved.

The diagnosis of septic thrombophlebitis requires evidence of thrombosis in the cannulated blood vessel (e.g., by ultrasound) and persistent septicemia with no other apparent source. Treatment includes catheter removal and systemic antibiotic therapy for 4–6 weeks (2). Surgical excision of the infected thrombus is usually not necessary, and is reserved for cases of refractory septicemia. There is no consensus on the use of heparin anticoagulation in suppurative thrombophlebitis; according to the most recent guidelines on catheter-related infections (2), heparin therapy is a consideration (not a requirement) for this condition.

Endocarditis

Nosocomial endocarditis is uncommon; the reported incidence in university teaching hospitals is 2–3 cases annually (42,43). Vascular catheters are implicated in 30 to 50% of cases, and staphylococci (mostly *S. aureus*) are the offending organisms in up to 75% of cases (42,43). Methicillin-resistant strains of *S. aureus* (MRSA) predominate in some reports (44).

Typical manifestations of endocarditis (e.g., new or changing cardiac murmur) can be absent in as many as two-thirds of patients with nosocomial endocarditis involving *Staphylococcus aureus* (44). As a result, endocarditis should be considered in all cases of *S. aureus* bacteremia, including patients who appear to respond to antimicrobial therapy (2). The diagnostic procedure of choice for endocarditis is transesophageal (not transthoracic) ultrasound. Diagnostic findings include valvular vegetations, new-onset mitral regurgitation, and perivalvular abscess.

Antimicrobial therapy for 4–6 weeks is standard recommendation for endocarditis. Unfortunately, despite our best efforts for antibiotic therapy, about 30% of patients do not survive the illness (42–44).

A FINAL WORD

A Contrary View

One of the central themes in catheter-related bloodstream infections (CRBI) is the notion that most of these infections arise from microbes on the skin that travel along the catheter and colonize the intravascular portion of the catheter. This is the basis for the antiseptic practices (e.g., skin decontamination, sterile dressings) that are mandated for the care of catheterized patients. The belief that CRBIs originate from the skin is based on the observation that staphylococci are prevalent in CRBIs, combined with the assumption that staphylococci exist only on the skin. This assumption is problematic because staphylococci also inhabit mucosal surfaces (45) and they are prominent inhabitants of the bowel during prolonged antibiotic therapy (46) and in critically ill patients (47). In fact, *Staphylococcus epidermidis* (the most frequent isolate in CRBIs) is *one of the most common organisms found in the upper GI tract of patients with multiorgan failure* (47). Thus, the prevalence of staphylococci in CRBIs is not evidence of a skin locus of origin. The following observations suggest that CRBIs do not originate from the skin:

1. Gram-negative bacilli and enterococci are found in over 50% of colonized central venous catheters (48), and these organisms are inhabitants of the bowel, not the skin.

2. There is a poor correlation between cultures of the skin around the catheter insertion site and cultures of the catheter tip in cases of CRBI (49).

3. Decontamination of the skin around the catheter insertion site does not reduce the incidence of CRBIs (1).

4. Finally, if skin microbes are a major source of CRBIs, then why is there no risk of CRBIs from peripheral catheters (where the distance from the skin to the catheter tip is much shorter than with central venous catheters)?

It is quite possible that transient septicemia from sites other than the skin could lead to colonization of indwelling catheters (the colonized catheters could then disseminate organisms into the bloodstream and act as a primary source of septicemia). An intravascular route of colonization would explain why CRBIs are associated with central venous catheters (where a relatively long segment of catheter is in the bloodstream) and not peripheral catheters.

The prevalence of enteric organisms (Gram-negative bacilli) on colonized catheters suggests that the bowel is an important source of microbes that colonize vascular catheters (50). The gastrointestinal tract is home to an enormous population of microbes, and these organisms are known to enter the systemic circulation by *translocation* across the bowel mucosa. (The role of the bowel as an occult source of septicemia is described in more detail in Chapter 5 and Chapter 40.)

Why is this so important? Because if the skin is not the principal site of origin for catheter colonization, then we are spending a lot of time and money decontaminating the wrong surface.

REFERENCES

Clinical Practice Guidelines

1. O'Grady NP, Alexander M, Burns LA, et. al. and the Healthcare Infection Control Practices Advisory Committee (HICPAC). Guidelines for the Prevention of Intravascular Catheter-related Infections. Clin Infect Dis 2011; 52:e1–e32. (Available at www.cdc.gov/hicpac/pdf/guidelines/bsi-guidelines-2011.pdf)

2. Mermel LA, Allon M, Bouza E, et al. Clinical practice guidelines for the diagnosis and management of intravascular catheter-related infection: 2009 update by the Infectious Diseases Society of America. Clin Infect Dis 2009; 49:1–45.

3. Debourdeau P, Chahmi DK, Le Gal G, et al. 2008 guidelines for the prevention and treatment of thrombosis associated with central venous catheters in patients with cancer: report from the working group. Ann Oncol 2009; 20:1459–1471.

Routine Catheter Care

4. Hoffman KK, Weber DJ, Samsa GP, et al. Transparent polyurethane film as intravenous catheter dressing. A meta-analysis of infection risks. JAMA 1992; 267:2072–2076.

5. Gillies D, O'Riordan E, Carr D, et al. Central venous catheter dressings: a systematic review. J Adv Nurs 2003; 44:623–632.

6. Maki DG, Stolz SS, Wheeler S, Mermi LA. A prospective, randomized trial of gauze and two polyurethane dressings for site care of pulmonary artery catheters: implications for catheter management. Crit Care Med 1994; 22:1729–1737.

7. Lok CE, Stanle KE, Hux JE, et ak. Hemodialysis infection prevention with polysporin ointment. J Am Soc Nephrol 2003; 14:169–179.

8. Lai KK. Safety of prolonging peripheral cannula and IV tubing use from 72 hours to 96 hours. Am J Infect Control 1998; 26:66–70.

9. Cook D, Randolph A, Kernerman P, et al. Central venous replacement strategies: a systematic review of the literature. Crit Care Med 1997; 25:1417–1424.

10. Cobb DK, High KP, Sawyer RP, et al. A controlled trial of scheduled replacement of central venous and pulmonary artery catheters. N Engl J Med 1992; 327:1062–1068.

11. McGee DC, Gould MK. Preventing complications of central venous catheterization. New Engl J Med 2003; 348:1123–1133.

12. Safdar N, Maki D. Inflammation at the insertion site is not predictive of catheter-related bloodstream infection with short-term, noncuffed central venous catheters. Crit Care Med 2002; 30:2632–2635.

13. Walsh DA, Mellor JA. Why flush peripheral intravenous cannulae used for intermittent intravenous injection? Br J Clin Pract 1991; 45:31–32.

14. Peterson FY, Kirchhoff KT. Analysis of research about heparinized versus nonheparinized intravascular lines. Heart Lung 1991; 20:631–642.

15. American Association of Critical Care Nurses. Evaluation of the effects of heparinized and nonheparinized flush solutions on the patency of arterial pressure monitoring lines: the AACN Thunder Project. Am J Crit Care 1993; 2:3–15.

16. Branson PK, McCoy RA, Phillips BA, Clifton GD. Efficacy of 1.4% sodium citrate in maintaining arterial catheter patency in patients in a medical ICU. Chest 1993; 103:882–885.

Obstructions & Perforations

17. Jacobs BR. Central venous catheter occlusion and thrombosis. Crit Care Clin 2003; 19:489–514.

18. Trissel LA. Drug stability and compatibility issues in drug delivery. Cancer Bull 1990; 42:393–398.

19. Deitcher SR, Fesen MR, Kiproff PM, et. al. Safety and efficacy of alteplase for restoring function in occluded central venous catheters: results of the cardio-vascularthrombolytic to open occluded lines trial. J Clin Oncol 2002; 20:317–324.

20. Cathflo Activase (Alteplase) Drug Monograph. San Francisco, CA: Genentech, Inc, 2005.

21. Shulman RJ, Reed T, Pitre D, Laine L. Use of hydrochloric acid to clear obstructed central venous catheters. J Parent Ent Nutr 1988; 12:509–510.

22. Timsit J-F, Farkas J-C, Boyer J-M, et al. Central vein catheter-related thrombosis in intensive care patients. Chest 1998; 114:207–213.

23. Evans RS, Sharp JH, Linford LH, et al. Risk of symptomatic DVT associated with peripherally inserted central catheters. Chest 2010; 138:803–810.

24. Joynt GM, Kew J, Gomersall CD, et al. Deep venous thrombosis caused by femoral venous catheters in critically ill adult patients. Chest 2000; 117:178–183.

25. Verso M, Agnelli G. Venous thromboembolism associated with long-term use of central venous catheters in cancer patients. J Clin Oncol 2003; 21:3665–3675.

26. Kucher N. Deep-vein thrombosis of the upper extremities. N Engl J Med 2011; 364:861–869.

27. Otten TR, Stein PD, Patel KC, et al. Thromboembolic disease involving the superior vena cava and brachiocephalic veins. Chest 2003; 123:809–812.

28. Heffner JE. A 49-year-old man with tachypnea and a rapidly enlarging pleural effusion. J Crit Illness 1994; 9:101–109.

29. Booth SA, Norton B, Mulvey DA. Central venous catheterization and fatal cardiac tamponade. Br J Anesth 2001; 87:298–302.

Catheter-Related Infections

30. CDC. Guidelines for the prevention of intravascular catheter-related infections. MMWR 2002; 51: No. RR-10.

31. Srinivasan A, Wise M, Bell M, et al. Vital signs: central line-associated blood-stream infections — United States, 2001, 2008, and 2009. MMWR 2011; 60:243–248.

32. O'Toole G, Kaplan HB, Kolter R. Biofilm formation as microbial development. Annual Rev Microbiol 2000; 54:49–79.

33. Passerini L, Lam K, Costerton JW, King EG. Biofilms on indwelling vascular catheters. Crit Care Med 1992; 20:665–673.

34. von Eiff C, Peters G, Heilman C. Pathogenesis of infections due to coagulase-negative staphylococci. Lancet Infect Dis 2002; 2:677–685.

35. Gilbert P, Maira-Litran T, McBain AJ, et al. The physiology and collective recalcitrance of microbial biofilm communities. Adv Microbial Physiol 2002; 46:203–256.

36. Percival SL, Kite P, Easterwood K, et al. Tetrasodium EDTA as a novel central venous catheter lock solution against biofilm. Infect Control Hosp Epidemiol 2005; 26:515-519.

37. Dudeck MA, Horan TC, Peterson KD, et al. National Healthcare Safety Network (NHSN) Report, data summary for 2010, device-associated module. Am J Infect Control 2011; 39:798–816.

38. Sihler KC, Chenoweth C, Zalewski C, et al. Catheter-related vs catheter-associated blood stream infections in the intensive care unit: incidence, microbiology, and implications. Surg Infect 2010; 11:529–534.

39. Bouza E, Alvaredo N, Alcela L, et al. A randomized and prospective study of 3 procedures for the diagnosis of catheter-related bloodstream infection without catheter withdrawal. Clin Infect Dis 2007; 44:820–826.

40. Richards M, Edwards J, Culver D, Gaynes R. Nosocomial infections in medical intensive care units in the United States. Crit Care Med 1999; 27:887–892.

41. Raad I, Davis S, Khan A, et al. Impact of central venous catheter removal on the recurrence of catheter-related coagulase-negative staphylococcal bacteremia. Infect Control Hosp Epidemiol 1992; 154:808–816.

42. Martin-Davila P, Fortun J, Navas E, et al. Nosocomial endocarditis in a tertiary hospital. Chest 2005; 128:772–779.

43. Gouello JP, Asfar P, Brenet O, et al. Nosocomial endocarditis in the intensive care unit: an analysis of 22 cases. Crit Care Med 2000; 28:377–382.

44. Fowler VG, Miro JM, Hoen B, et al. *Staphylococcus aureus* endocarditis: a consequence of medical progress. JAMA 2005; 293:3012–3021.

45. von Eiff C, Becker K, Machka K, et; al. Nasal carriage as a source of *Staphylococcus aureus* bacteremia. N Engl J Med 2001; 344:11-16.

46. Altemeier WA, Hummel RP, Hill EO. Staphylococcal enterocolitis following antibiotic therapy. Ann Surg 1963; 157:847–858.

47. Marshall JC, Christou NV, Horn R, Meakins JL. The microbiology of multiple organ failure. Arch Surg 1988; 123:309–315.

48. Mrozek N, Lautrette A, Aumeran C, et al. Bloodstream infection after positive catheter cultures: what are the risks in the intensive care unit when catheters are routinely cultured on removal. Crit Care Med 2011; 39:1301–1305.

49. Atela I, Coll P, Rello J, et al. Serial surveillance cultures of skin and catheter hub specimens from critically ill patients with central venous catheters: Molecular epidemiology of infection and implications for clinical management and research. J Clin Microbiol 1997; 35:1784–1790.

50. Sing R, Marino PL. Bacterial trasnslocation: an occult cause of catheter-related sepsis. Infect Med 1993; 10:54–57.

PREVENTIVE PRACTICES IN THE ICU

The only thing necessary for the triumph of evil is for good men to do nothing.

Edmund Burke
1770

Chapter 4

OCCUPATIONAL EXPOSURES

The risk of nosocomial (hospital-acquired) infections is not limited to the patient population; i.e., hospital workers are also at risk of acquiring infections from occupational exposure to bloodborne and airborne pathogens. The bloodborne pathogens include the human immunodeficiency virus (HIV), and the hepatitis B and C viruses, while the airborne pathogens include *Mycobacterium tuberculosis,* and the respiratory viruses (e.g., the influenza virus). This chapter describes the modes and risks of disease transmission, and the recommended protective measures, for these potentially harmful occupational exposures. Most of the recommendations in this chapter are from the clinical practice guidelines listed at the end of the chapter (1–5).

BLOODBORNE PATHOGENS

The transmission of bloodborne pathogens occurs primarily by accidental puncture wounds from contaminated needles, and less frequently by exposure of mucous membranes and nonintact skin to splashes of infected blood. The risk of transmission for each of the bloodborne pathogens is summarized in Table 4.1.

Table 4.1	Average Risk of Transmission for Bloodborne Pathogens		
Type of Exposure	**Source**	**Risk per Exposure**	**Exposures per Infection**
Needlestick Injury	HBV (+) Blood	22 – 31%	3 – 4.5
Needlestick Injury	HCV (+) Blood	1.8%	56
Needlestick Injury	HIV (+) Blood	0.3%	333
Mucous Membrane	HIV (+) Blood	0.09%	1,111

From the clinical practice guidelines in References 2 and 3.
HBV = hepatitis B virus; *HCV* = hepatitis C virus; *HIV* = human immunodeficiency virus.

Needlestick Injuries

Each year, about 10% of hospital workers experience an accidental puncture wound from a hollow-bore needle or suture needle; i.e., a *needlestick injury* (5,6). High-risk activities include the manipulation of suture needles, and the recapping and disposal of used hollow-bore needles. The incidence of needlestick injuries is highest in staff surgeons and surgical trainees; e.g., in one survey of 17 surgical training programs, 99% of the residents claimed at least one needlestick injury by the last year of training, and 53% of the injuries involved high-risk patients (7). Over half of the needlestick injuries in this survey were not reported, which is consistent with other studies showing that needlestick injuries are often dismissed as insignificant events (8).

Safety Devices

The emergence of HIV in the 1980s created concern for needlestick injuries and, in the year 2000, the United States Congress passed the Needlestick Safety and Prevention Act that mandates the use of "safety-engineered" needles in all American healthcare facilities. An example of a safety-engineered needle is shown in Figure 4.1. The needle is equipped with a rigid, plastic housing that is attached by a hinge joint to the hub of the needle. The protective housing is normally positioned away from the needle so it does not interfere with normal use. After the needle is used, it is locked into the protective housing as shown in the illustration. The needle and attached syringe are then placed in a puncture-proof "sharps container" for eventual disposal. (Sharps containers are found in every room in the ICU.) This procedure avoids any contact between the hands and the needle, thereby eliminating the risk of needlestick injury.

One-Handed Recapping Technique

Once the needle is locked in its protective housing, it is not possible to remove it for further use. In situations where a needle may need to be reused (e.g., for repeated lidocaine injections during a prolonged procedure), the needle can be rendered harmless when idle by recapping it with the one-handed "scoop technique" shown in Figure 4.2. With the syringe still attached, the needle is advanced into the needle cap and then rotated vertically until it is perpendicular to the horizontal surface. The needle is then pushed into the cap until it locks in place. The hands never touch the needle while it is recapped , thereby eliminating the risk of a needlestick injury.

Human Immunodeficiency Virus (HIV)

Occupational transmission of HIV is a universally feared but infrequent occurrence. From 1981 through December 2002, there were 57 documented cases of HIV transmission to healthcare workers (9). Of these 57 cases, 19 cases (33.3%) involved laboratory personnel and 2 cases (3.5%) involved housekeeping and maintenance workers, leaving only 36 cases involving hospital personnel that work at the bedside. These 36 cases

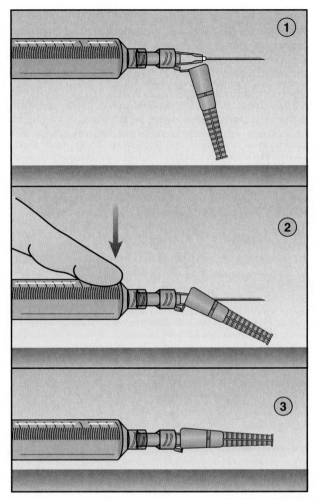

FIGURE 4.1 A safety-engineered needle that allows the needle to be locked into a rigid plastic housing after it is used. The hands never touch the needle, thereby eliminating the risk of a needlestick injury.

represent an average of only 1.6 cases annually over the 22-year survey period. If all these cases occurred in the 6,000 ICUs in this country, the average yearly risk of HIV transmission in an ICU setting would be about one case per 3,750 ICUs. Not much of a risk.

Needlestick Exposures

A needlestick puncture from a hollow needle will transfer an average of one microliter (10^{-6} L) of blood (10). During the viremic stages of HIV infection, there are as many as 5 infectious particles per microliter of blood (11). Therefore, puncture of the skin with a hollow needle that contains HIV-infected blood is expected to transfer at least a few infectious particles. Fortunately, this is not enough to transmit the disease in most cases. As shown in Table 4.1, *the average risk for HIV transmission from a single needlestick injury with HIV-infected blood is 0.3%* (2,3), which translates to one infection for every 333 needlestick injuries involving HIV-infected blood. The likelihood of HIV transmission is greater in the following circumstances: when the source patient has advanced HIV disease, when the skin puncture is deep, when there is visible blood on the needle, and in cases where the needle entered an artery or vein in the source patient (12).

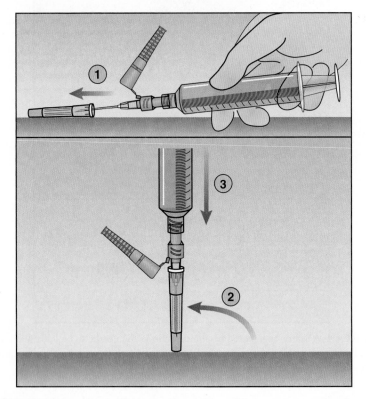

FIGURE 4.2 The one-handed "scoop technique" for safely recapping needles that may need to be reused.

Mucous Membrane Exposures

Exposure of mucous membranes to HIV-infected blood (e.g., a blood splash to the face) is much less likely to result in HIV transmission than a needlestick injury. As shown in Table 4.1, *the average risk for HIV transmission from a single mucous membrane exposure to HIV-infected blood is 0.09%* (2,3), which translates to one infection for every 1,111 mucous membrane exposures to HIV-infected blood (i.e., a one-in-a-thousand chance of disease transmission).

Postexposure Management

The postexposure management of needlestick injuries or mucous membrane exposures is determined by the HIV status of the source patient. If the HIV status is unknown, this can be quickly resolved in the hospital setting by performing a rapid HIV-antibody test on a blood sample from the source patient. This is an enzyme-linked immunoabsorbent assay (ELISA) that yields results in only 10 to 15 minutes. A negative test does not eliminate the possibility of HIV infection (because it takes 4–6 weeks for antibodies to appear in plasma after the onset of infection), but it does obviate the need for postexposure drug prophylaxis. A positive ELISA test in the source patient is an indication to begin postexposure drug prophylaxis, but the result must be confirmed by another test; i.e., a Western Blot or immunofluorescent antibody assay. The recommendations for postexposure prophylaxis are shown in Table 4.2 (3). When indicated, prophylactic drugs should be started within 36 hours of the exposure (12).

Table 4.2	Postexposure Prophylaxis for HIV Infection		
	HIV Status of Source Patient		
Exposure Type	**HIV(+): Class 1[†]**	**HIV(+): Class 2[†]**	**HIV(−)**
Needlestick Injuries			
Less Severe[1]	2 drugs	≥ 3 drugs	No drugs
More Severe[1]	3 drugs	≥ 3 drugs	No drugs
Mucous Membrane Exposures			
Small Volume[2]	2 drugs (?)[§]	2 drugs	No drugs
Large Volume[2]	2 drugs	≥ 3 drugs	No drugs

From the clinical practice guidelines in Reference 3. See text for the recommended drug combinations.
[†]HIV(+): Class 1 – asymptomatic HIV infection or viral load <1,500 copies/mL
[†]HIV(+): Class 2 – symptomatic HIV infection or viral load >1,500 copies/mL, or acute seroconversion
[§]Drugs are optional.
[1]Less Severe: solid needle or superficial injury. More Severe: deep puncture, visible blood on the needle, or a needle that entered an artery or vein of the source patient.
[2]Small Volume: a few drops. Large Volume: a major blood splash.

Postexposure Drug Regimens

The standard two-drug regimen is a combination of two nucleoside reverse transcriptase inhibitors: zidovudine (300 mg BID) and lamivudine (150 mg BID). These two drugs are available in a combination tablet (Combivir, containing 300 mg zidovudine and 150 mg lamivudine per tablet), which is taken twice daily. If additional drugs are indicated, the preferred regimen is a combination of two protease inhibitors: lopinavir/ritinovir (400 mg/100 mg), available as a single tablet (Kaletra) taken three times daily (3). In high-risk exposures, 28 days of drug therapy is recommended. However, as many as 50% of hospital workers who receive antiretroviral drugs following HIV exposure are unable to complete the four-week treatment period because of adverse drug effects (3).

ADVERSE DRUG EFFECTS: Side effects are common with antiretroviral drug therapy, and the frequency of side effects is higher when the drugs are taken for postexposure prophylaxis. The most frequent side effects include nausea, malaise, fatigue, and diarrhea (3). More serious drug toxicities include pancreatitis and lactic acidosis from nucleoside reverse transcriptase inhibitors, and severe hypertriglyceridemia from protease inhibitors (3).

DRUG INTERACTIONS: Protease inhibitors have a number of serious drug interactions. Drugs that are contraindicated during therapy with protease inhibitors include midazolam and triazolam (enhanced sedation), cisapride (risk of cardiac arrhythmias), statins (potential for severe myopathy and rhabdomyolysis), and rifampin (can reduce plasma levels of protease inhibitors by as much as 90%) (3).

(For more information on the use of antiretroviral drugs for postexposure prophylaxis, see References 3 and 12.)

CAVEAT: Although drug prophylaxis has become the standard of care for occupational exposure to HIV, it is important to emphasize that over 99% of healthcare workers who are exposed to HIV-infected blood do not develop HIV infection, even in the absence of postexposure drug prophylaxis (12). This is an important consideration in light of the adverse reactions associated with antiretroviral drugs.

Postexposure Surveillance

Antibody responses to HIV infection can take at least 4 to 6 weeks to develop. Following documented exposure to HIV infection, serial assays for HIV antibodies are recommended at 6 weeks, 3 months, and 6 months after the exposure (3). More prolonged testing is not warranted unless the exposed person develops symptoms compatible with HIV infection.

Postexposure Hotline

The National Clinicians' Postexposure Prophylaxis Hotline (PEP line) is a valuable resource for the latest information on postexposure prophylaxis for HIV infection. The toll-free number is 888-448-4911.

Hepatitis B Virus

The hepatitis B virus (HBV) is the most transmissible of the bloodborne pathogens. During an acute infection, one microliter (10^{-6} L) of blood can have as many as one million infectious particles (compared to 5 or fewer infectious particles per microliter for HIV-infected blood). As shown in Table 4.1, *the average risk for disease transmission from a single needlestick exposure to HBV-infected blood is 22–31%* (2), which translates to one infection for every 3 to 5 exposures to HBV-infected blood. (This transmission rate is for blood that contains both the hepatitis B surface antigen and the e antigen of hepatitis B; the presence of both antigens in blood indicates an infection that is highly contagious.)

Another feature of HBV that favors transmission is the ability of the virus to remain viable in dried blood at room temperatures for up to one week (13). This increases the risk of viral transmission from cuts or bruises (i.e., nonintact skin) that come in contact with dried blood on environmental surfaces.

Hepatitis B Vaccination

An effective vaccine is available for hepatitis B, and immunization is advised for all hospital workers who have contact with blood, body fluids, or sharp instruments (which is virtually everyone who works in an ICU). Most hospitals provide the vaccine free-of-charge to high-risk employees. The only contraindication to vaccination is a prior history of anaphylaxis from baker's yeast (2). The vaccine is a recombinant form of the hepatitis B surface antigen (HBsAg) that is administered in three doses according to the following schedule (2,14):

1. The first two doses are given 4 weeks apart, and the 3rd dose is administered 5 months after the 2nd dose. All doses are administered by deep IM injection.

2. If the vaccination series is interrupted (which is common because of the prolonged time between doses), it is not necessary to repeat the entire sequence. If the second dose is missed, it is given as soon as possible, and the 3rd dose is administered at least 2 months later. If the 3rd dose is missed, it is administered as soon as possible to complete the vaccination.

Completion of the triple-dose vaccination schedule produces lifetime immunity against HBV infection in over 90% of healthy adults ≤ 40 years of age (14). Efficacy declines with age, reaching 75% by 60 years of age (14). Vaccination is also less effective in immunocompromised patients, particularly those with HIV infection. Immunity is the result of an antibody to the hepatitis B surface antigen (anti-HBs). Blood levels of anti-HBs must reach ≥ 10 mIU/mL to achieve full immunity, and this usually requires 4–6 weeks after the vaccination is completed. When the first vaccination series does not achieve full immunity, a second series is effective in 30% to 50% of cases (2). If immunity is not achieved by the second vaccination series, the subject is considered a nonresponder and receives no further immunizations. Responders do not require a booster dose of the vaccine, even though antibody levels wane with time (2).

Since most healthy adults achieve immunity after completion of the first vaccination series, postvaccination anti-HBs levels are not measured routinely. The principal indications for postvaccination anti-HBs levels are occupational exposure to HBV-infected blood, and high-risk occupations (e.g., hemodialysis technicians).

Postexposure Management

The management strategies following possible exposure to HBV are outlined in Table 4.3. Management decisions are dictated by the immune status of the exposed individual, and the HBV status of the source patient (as determined by the presence or absence of hepatitis B surface antigen in the blood).

Table 4.3	Postexposure Prophylaxis for Hepatitis B Virus (HBV)	
Vaccination Status	**HBV Status of Source Patient**	
Exposure Type	**HBsAG(+)**	**HBsAg(−)**
Not vaccinated	HBIG (0.06 mL/kg IM) and start HBV vaccination	Start HBV vaccination
Vaccinated and Immune[†]	No treatment	No treatment
Vaccinated and Not Immune[†]	HBIG (0.06 mL/kg IM) and repeat HBV vaccination* or HBIG ×2[§]	Repeat HBV vaccination*

From the clinical practice guidelines in Reference 2.

HBsAg = hepatitis B surface antigen; *HBIG* = hepatitis B immune globulin.

[†]Immunity requires the presence in blood of the antibody to hepatitis B surface antigen (antiHBs) at a concentration ≥10 mIU/mL.

*If immunity is not achieved after 2 courses of HBV vaccination, no further immunization is warranted.

[§]*HBIG* ×2 = Hepatitis B immune globulin in two intramuscular doses of 0.06 mIU/mL each. This regimen is reserved for subjects who don't achieve immunity after 2 courses of HBV vaccination.

Following exposure to HBV-infected blood (i.e., the blood of the source patient is positive for hepatitis B surface antigen), exposed individuals who have not achieved immunity to HBV (either because they did not receive the vaccination series or because the post-vaccination anti-HBs levels are < 10 mIU/mL) should receive hepatitis B immune globulin (HBIG) by deep intramuscular injection at a dose of 0.06 mL/kg, along with the first dose of HBV vaccine. The HBV vaccination series is recommended for all nonimmune individuals who are exposed to HBV-positive blood, except for individuals who are nonresponders after two completed immunizations. This latter group of subjects (i.e., nonresponders) should receive two injections of HBIG (0.06mL/kg for each injection).

Hepatitis C Virus

Transmission of the hepatitis C virus (HCV) is considered a rare event in the hospital setting, with the possible exception of the hemodialysis suite. As shown in Table 4.1, *the average risk for disease transmission from a single needlestick exposure to HCV-infected blood is 1.8%* (2), which translates to one infection per 56 exposures. Transmission from mucous membrane exposure is rare, and there are no documented cases of HCV transmission through nonintact skin.

The antibody produced in response to HCV infection (anti-HCV) is not protective (2), which means there is no vaccine for HCV and no effective antibody prophylaxis following exposure to HCV-infected blood. When a hospital worker sustains a needlestick injury, the HCV status of the source patient can be determined by the presence or absence of anti-HCV in blood. If the source patient has evidence of HCV infection (i.e., has a positive assay for anti-HCV), serial determinations of anti-HCV antibody in the exposed subject is recommended for 6 months following the exposure (2). A positive assay for anti-HCV in the exposed individual is evidence of HCV transmission.

AIRBORNE PATHOGENS

Pathogens that are transmitted through the air are generated by coughing or sneezing (one cough or sneeze can produce 3,000 airborne particles), and by procedures such as airway suctioning, endotracheal intubation, and cardiopulmonary resuscitation. The transmission of these pathogens is classified according to the size of the dispersed particles and the mode of transmission. Figure 4.3 shows a summary of the types of transmission, the pathogens involved, and the infection control measures recommended to prevent transmission.

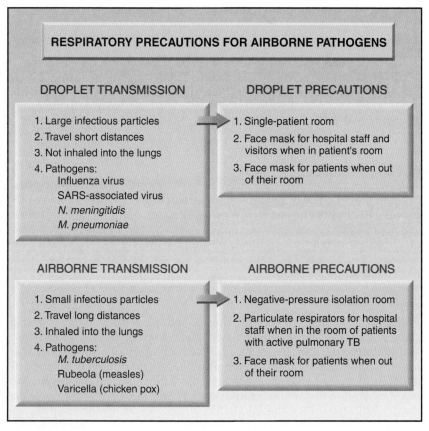

FIGURE 4.3 Respiratory precautions for pathogens that are dispersed in the air.

Droplet Transmission

Droplets are relatively large particles (> 5 microns in diameter) that do not travel far from the source (typically < 3 feet). These particles are transmitted by impact on the nasal mucosa and oral mucosa, and are not inhaled into the lungs. The principal pathogens that are transmitted via the droplet route are respiratory viruses, including the influenza virus and the corona virus responsible for Severe Acute Respiratory Syndrome (SARS), along with *Mycoplasma pneumoniae, Nisseria meningiditis,* and *Bordetella pertussis* (the causative agent for diphtheria).

Droplet Precautions

The recommendations for preventing droplet transmission include: a private room for the patient if possible, masks for hospital workers and visitors while in the patient's room, and a mask for the patient whenever outside the room (1). Either surgical masks or procedure masks (i.e., the ones with elastic loops for the ears) are sufficient for this purpose. If a private room is not available, the patient's bed should be separated from other beds by a curtain and a distance of at least 3 feet (1).

Airborne Transmission

Airborne transmission is the term used to describe the transmission of small infectious particles (< 5 microns in diameter) that are suspended in the air and can reach distances that extend well beyond the patient's room. These particles are also small enough to be inhaled into the lungs. The principal pathogen transmitted via the airborne route in adults is *Mycobacterium tuberculosis.*

Airborne Precautions

The features that distinguish airborne precautions from droplet precautions include the use of negative-pressure isolation rooms to prevent the movement of airborne pathogens out of the room, and the use of *particulate respirators* to prevent inhalation of airborne pathogens (1). For cases of active pulmonary tuberculosis, these precautions are continued until there are 3 consecutive sputum samples that are devoid of acid-fast bacilli on microscopic exam (1).

Masks vs. Respirators

Protective face masks (surgical masks and procedure masks) are designed to prevent large infectious droplets from impacting on the nasal and oral mucosa, and do not block inhalation of small airborne particles into the lungs. Respirators, on the other hand, are designed to block inhalation of pathogenic material into the lungs; particulate respirators block inhalation of small (< 5µ in diameter) infectious particles, while gas mask respirators block the inhalation of toxic gases. In the hospital setting, particulate respirators are recommended primarily for protection against *Mycobacterium tuberculosis* (1). The Centers for Disease Control

(CDC) currently recommends the "N95" respirator for this use (15); the "N" indicates that the mask will block non-oil based or aqueous aerosols (the type that transmits the tubercle bacillus), and the "95" indicates the mask will block 95% of airborne infectious particles. Respirators must create a tight seal around the nose and mouth to be effective, and they are usually fit-tested before use.

Atypical Pulmonary TB

It is important to distinguish infections caused by *Mycobacterium tuberculosis* from those caused by atypical mycobacteria (e.g., *Mycobacterium avium* complex) because there is no evidence for person-to-person transmission of atypical mycobacteria. This obviates the need for respiratory precautions (i.e., droplet precautions and airborne precautions) when caring for patients with atypical pulmonary tuberculosis (1).

A FINAL WORD

There are two take-home messages in this chapter.

1. Vaccination against hepatitis B virus (HBV) virtually eliminates the risk of HBV transmission in the typical hospital worker (i.e., not elderly and not immunocompromised), so avoiding HBV immunization is both foolish and dangerous.

2. HIV is rarely transmitted in the hospital setting, and over 99% of healthcare workers who are exposed to HIV-infected blood are not expected to acquire the illness, even in the absence of postexposure prophylaxis with antiretroviral drugs (12). This should help to relieve the trepidation that often accompanies a needlestick injury with a blood-stained needle from an HIV-infected patient.

REFERENCES

Clinical Practice Guidelines

1. Siegel JD, Rhinehart E, Jackson M, Chiarello L, and the Healthcare Infection Control Practices Advisory Committee. 2007 Guideline for Isolation Precautions: Preventing Transmission of Infectious Agents in Healthcare Settings. Available at http://www.cdc.gov/ncidod/dhqp/pdf/isolation2007.pdf. Accessed 1/31/12.

2. Centers for Disease Control and Prevention. Updated U.S. Public Health Service Guidelines for the management of occupational exposures to HBV, HCV, and HIV and recommendations for postexposure prophylaxis. MMWR 2001; 50 (No. RR-11):1–52.

3. Centers for Disease Control and Prevention. Updated U.S. Public Health Service guidelines for the management of occupational exposures to HIV and recommendations for postexposure prophylaxis. MMWR 2005; 54 (No. RR-9):1–17.

4. Centers for Disease Control and Prevention. Immunization of health-care workers: Recommendations of the Advisory Committee on Immunization Practices (ACIP) and the Hospital Infection Control Practices Advisory Committee (HICPAC). MMWR 1997, 46(RR-18): 1–42.

5. National Institute for Occupational Safety and Health. Preventing needle-stick injuries in health care settings. DHHS (NIOSH) Publication Number 2000-108; November, 1999. http://www.cdc.gov/niosh/docs/2000-108.pdf. Accessed 1/31/12.

Bloodborne Pathogens

6. Panlilo AL, Orelien JG, Srivastava PU, et. al.; NaSH Surveillance Group; EPINet Data Sharing Network. Estimate of the annual number of percuta-neous injuries among hospital-based healthcare workers in the United States, 1997-1998. Infect Control Hosp Epidemiol 2004; 25:556–562.

7. Makary MA, Al-Attar A, Holzmueller CG, et al. Needlestick injuries among surgeons in training. N Engl J Med 2007; 356:2693–2699.

8. Henderson DK. Management of needlestick injuries. A house officer who has a needlestick. JAMA 2012; 307:75–84.

9. National Insitutes for Occupational Safety and Health. Worker Health Chartbook, 2004. NIOSH Publication No. 2004-146. Accessed from the CDC website on 2/2/12.

10. Berry AJ, Greene ES. The risk of needlestick injuries and needlestick-trans-mitted diseases in the practice of anesthesiology. Anesthesiology 1992; 77:1007–10021.

11. Moran GJ. Emergency department management of blood and body fluid exposures. Ann Emerg Med 2000; 35:47–62.

12. Landovitz RJ, Currier JS. Postexposure prophylaxis for HIV infection. N Engl J Med 2009; 361:1768–1775.

13. Bond WW, Favero MS, Petersen NJ, et al. Survival of hepatitis B virus after drying and storage for one week. Lancet 1981; 1:550–551.

14. Mast EE, Weinbaum CM, Fiore AE, et. al., for the Advisory Committee on Immunization Practices (ACIP). A comprehensive immunization strategy to eliminate transmission of Hepatitis B infection in the United States. MMWR 2006; 55(RR16):1–25.

15. Fennelly KP. Personal respiratory protection against mycobacterium tuber-culosis. Clin Chest Med 1997; 18:1–17.

Chapter 5

ALIMENTARY PROPHYLAXIS

We are told the most fantastic biological tales. For example,
that it is dangerous to have acid in your stomach.

JBS Haldane (1939)

Standard antiseptic practices are designed to prevent microbial invasion from the skin, but (as mentioned at the end of Chapter 3) the skin is not the only body surface that can be breached by microbes. The alimentary tract, which extends from the mouth to the rectum, is outside the body (like the hole in a donut), and the mucosal lining of the alimentary tract is the largest body surface area in contact with the outside world (about 300 m², or about the size of a tennis court). This mucosa serves as a barrier to microbial invasion, just like the skin. However, unlike the skin, which is multilayered and covered with a keratinized surface, the mucosa of the alimentary tract is a single layer of columnar epithelial cells that is only 0.1 mm thick. Considering this paper-thin "inner skin," and the unfathomable number of infectious organisms in the alimentary tract (i.e., up to one *trillion* microbes in each gram of stool), it seems that the real threat of microbial invasion comes from the alimentary tract, not the skin.

This chapter will introduce you to the importance of the alimentary tract as a source of infection in critically ill patients, and what can be done to reduce the risk of infection from the mouth all the way down to the rectum. Included is a section on stress-related mucosal injury in the stomach, and the measures used to prevent troublesome bleeding from this condition.

MICROBIAL INVASION FROM THE BOWEL

Microbial organisms are aquatic creatures that require moisture to thrive, and the moisture-rich environment in the alimentary tract is ideal for microbial proliferation. The alimentary tract in adults is home to 400-500 species of bacteria and fungi (1,2), with a total mass of about 2 kg (4.4 pounds) (3). The distribution of this mass of microbes is not uniform, as depicted in Figure 5.1 (1). The rectum is the most populated region of the alimentary tract (with up to one trillion microbes per gram of stool), and the stomach is the least populated region (with less than 1,000 organisms per mL of gastric contents). The reason for this uneven distribution will be explained shortly.

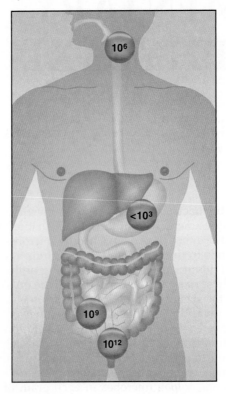

FIGURE 5.1 The population density of microorganisms in different regions of the alimentary tract. Numbers indicate colony forming units per gram or mL of luminal contents. (From Reference 1)

Protective Mechanisms

There are three levels of infection control in the alimentary tract.

1. The first level takes place in the stomach, where the antimicrobial actions of gastric acid eradicates microorganisms swallowed in food and saliva and maintains a relatively sterile environment in the upper GI tract.

2. The second level of protection occurs at the bowel wall, where the mucosal lining of the bowel acts as a physical barrier that blocks the movement of enteric pathogens and proinflammatory substances (e.g., endotoxin) into the systemic circulation.

3. The third level of protection takes place on the extraluminal side of the bowel wall, where the reticuloendothelial system traps and destroys microbes that breach the mucosal barrier. About two-thirds of the reticuloendothelial system in the body is located in the abdomen (4), which suggests that microbial invasion across the bowel wall may be a frequent occurrence.

Failure of any of these protective mechanisms can lead to the systemic spread of enteric pathogens, as depicted in Figure 5.2. The movement of enteric microbes across the bowel wall is known as *translocation* (5), and it plays an important role in the pathogenesis of ICU-acquired bloodstream infections (described later) and progressive multiorgan failure (described next).

Multiorgan Failure

Multiorgan failure is a life-threatening (and often lethal) condition characterized by persistent systemic inflammation and progressive dysfunction in two or more major organs (6). Septicemia may or may not be present. The unrelenting systemic inflammation in this condition is the source of the multiorgan injury, and the driving force for this inflammation is the translocation of enteric pathogens and proinflammatory substances (e.g., endotoxin) across a disrupted mucosal barrier in the GI tract (6,7).

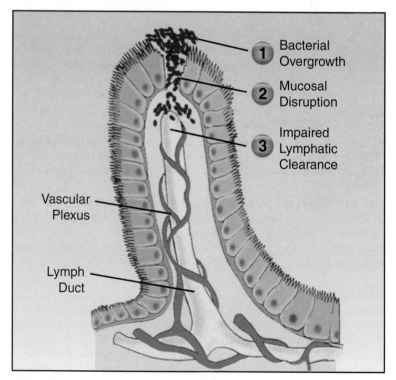

FIGURE 5.2 Illustration of an intestinal villus depicting three conditions that promote the systemic spread of enteric pathogens.

THE GI TRACT AS SITE OF ORIGIN: According to the "gut hypothesis" of multiorgan failure, the problem begins with a period of splanchnic hypoperfusion (e.g., from hypovolemia or hypotension) that leads to ischemic injury of the GI mucosa. The damaged mucosa then permits enteric pathogens and/or proinflammatory triggers to gain access to the systemic circulation. This initiates a systemic inflammatory response (e.g., fever, leukocytosis), which is accompanied by hemodynamic changes (i.e., sympathetic nervous system activation with splanchnic vasoconstriction) that promotes further splanchnic hypoperfusion and mucosal injury. The result is a self-sustaining process that drives systemic inflammation to the point of widespread inflammatory injury and progressive multiorgan failure. According to this scenario (and to borrow a popular phrase), *the GI tract is the 'motor' of multiorgan failure* (7).

Gastric Acid

Gastric acid is often misperceived as a digestive aid. An acid environment in the stomach facilitates the absorption of iron and calcium, and triggers the production of pepsin; however, patients with achlorhydria (inability to acidify gastric secretions) are not troubled by malabsorption (8). The principal function of gastric acid is not to facilitate digestion, but to serve as an antimicrobial defense mechanism, as described next.

Historical Note

The benefits of antisepsis were first recognized in the mid-nineteenth century by a British surgeon named Joseph Lister, who treated penetrating skin wounds with a chemical agent that was used to treat sewage, and observed a marked decline in suppurative wound infections. Lister's observations were published in 1867 in a treatise entitled *On the Antiseptic Principle in the Practice of Surgery* (9). In the following excerpt from this treatise, Lister describes the chemical agent that he used:

> The material which I have employed is carbolic acid, a volatile compound which appears to exercise a peculiarly destructive influence upon low forms of life, and hence is the most powerful antiseptic with which we are at present acquainted.

As indicated, the very first antiseptic agent used in clinical medicine was an acid. Thus, Joseph Lister not only discovered the benefits of antisepsis in preventing infections, he also discovered the benefits of acids in eradicating infectious microbes. (In recognition of Lister's discoveries, his name is now immortalized by a mouthwash, Listerine!)

Antiseptic Effects of Gastric Acid

The influence of gastric pH on the growth of a pathogenic organism is shown in Figure 5.3 (10). The pathogen in this case is *Salmonella typhimurium*, a common cause of infectious enteritis in humans. The graph in Figure 5.3 shows the survival of *S. typhimurium* in gastric juice at three different pH levels. The organism thrives at a pH of 4. However, survival begins to decline at a pH of 3, and the organism is almost completely eradicated at a pH of 2. These survival curves indicate that gastric secretions are bactericidal when the pH falls below 4. The normal pH of gastric secretions is well within this range.

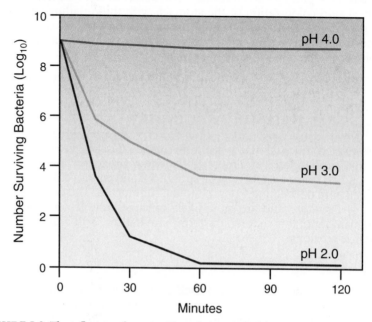

FIGURE 5.3 The influence of gastric pH on the survival of *Salmonella typhimurium*, a common cause of infectious enteritis. (From Reference 10)

Considering the bactericidal effects of gastric acidity, it is likely that *gastric acid serves as an antimicrobial guardian that protects the GI tract from unwanted pathogens*. The benefits of gastric acid as an infection control device are summarized below.

1. Gastric acid eradicates pathogens that are ingested in contaminated food products. This is demonstrated in studies showing that reduced gastric acidity is associated with an increased incidence of infectious gastroenteritis from *Salmonella* and *Campylobacter* species (8,10–13). Food processing techniques do not always remove infectious organisms, and gastric acid serves as a built-in backup mechanism for disinfecting the food we eat.

2. Gastric acid can block the transmission of illnesses via the fecal-oral route. This is demonstrated by the association of gastric-acid suppressing drugs with *Clostridium difficile* enterocolitis (14). This is an important and often-overlooked complication of drugs that suppress gastric acidity, and will be described in more detail later in the chapter.

3. Gastric acid eradicates microorganisms that are swallowed in saliva, which explains the marked drop in microbial density between the mouth and stomach in Figure 5.1. Loss of gastric acidity leads to colonization of the stomach with microbes that are swallowed in sali-

va. This may have little consequence in healthy subjects, who have harmless saprophytes in their saliva. However, critically ill patients often have pathogenic Gram-negative bacilli in their saliva (described later), and colonization of the stomach with these pathogens can promote Gram-negative septicemia (from translocation across the gastric mucosa) (15), as well as lung infections (from aspiration of infected gastric secretions into the airways) (16).

The antiseptic benefits of gastric acid will resurface in the next section.

STRESS-RELATED MUCOSAL INJURY

Stress-related mucosal injury is a term used to describe erosions in the gastric mucosa that occur in almost all patients with acute, life-threatening illness (18,19). These erosions can be superficial and confined to the mucosa, or they can bore deeper and extend into the submucosa. The deeper lesions are called *stress ulcers*, and are more likely to cause troublesome bleeding. For the remainder of this chapter, the term "stress ulcer" will indicate both types of gastric erosions.

Pathogenesis

The gastric mucosa must protect itself against injury from the acid environment in the stomach, and gastric mucosal blood flow is considered to play an important part in this protection (by supplying nutrients to maintain the functional integrity of the mucosa). The importance of mucosal blood flow is demonstrated by the fact that 70 to 90% of the blood supply to the stomach is delivered to the gastric mucosa (20). Splanchnic vasoconstriction and hypoperfusion is common in critically ill patients, and the resultant decrease in gastric mucosal blood flow is considered the principal cause of gastric erosions (18–20). Once the gastric mucosa is disrupted, the acidity in the gastric lumen can aggravate the surface lesions.

Table 5.1	Risk Factors for Stress Ulcer Bleeding
Highest-Risk Conditions	**Other High-Risk Conditions**
1. Mechanical Ventilation (> 48 h)	1. Circulatory Shock

2. Coagulopathy
  a. platelets < 50,000 or
  b. INR > 1.5 or
  c. PTT > 2x control
	2. Severe Sepsis
	3. Multisystem Trauma
	4. Traumatic Brain & Spinal Cord Injury

3. Burns involving > 30% of the body surface	5. Renal Failure 6. Steroid Therapy

Clinical Consequences

Erosions are visible on luminal surface of the stomach in 75% to 100% of patients within 24 hours of admission to the ICU (19). These lesions often ooze blood from eroding into superficial capillaries, but clinically significant bleeding (i.e., results in a significant drop in blood pressure or a drop in hemoglobin >2 g/dL) is observed in less than 5% of ICU patients (18,19,21).

Risk Factors

The conditions that predispose to stress ulcer bleeding are listed in Table 5.1 (18,21). The independent risk factors (i.e., require no other risk factors to promote bleeding) include mechanical ventilation for longer than 48 hours, and a significant coagulopathy (i.e., platelets < 50,000, INR > 1.5, or activated PTT > twice control) (21). However, all of the conditions in Table 5.1 are indications for prophylaxis to prevent stress ulcer bleeding.

Preventive Measures

The goal of prophylaxis for stress ulcers is not to prevent their appearance (since they appear almost immediately after ICU admission), but to prevent clinically significant bleeding from these lesions. Surveys indicate that about 90% of ICU patients receive some form of prophylaxis for stress ulcer bleeding (22), but this is excessive. Prophylaxis is primarily indicated for the conditions listed in Table 5.1, and is especially important for patients who are ventilator-dependent for longer than 48 hours, or have a significant coagulopathy.

Table 5.2	Drugs Used for Prophylaxis of Stress Ulcer Bleeding		
Drug	**Type**	**Usual Route**	**Usual Dose[1]**
Famotidine	H$_2$ Blocker	IV	20 mg every 12 hr.[2]
Ranitidine[1]	H$_2$ Blocker	IV	50 mg every 8 hr.[2]
Lansoprazole	PPI	NG	30 mg once daily
Omeprazole	PPI	NG	20 mg once daily
Pantoprazole	PPI	IV	40 mg once daily
Sucralfate	Protectant	NG	1 gram every 6 hr.

The dose of gastric acid-suppressing drugs may need to be adjusted to maintain pH ≥4 in gastric aspirates.

[2]Dose reduction is necessary in renal failure.

Abbreviations: PPI = proton pump inhibitor; NG = nasogastric instillation.

Methods of Prophylaxis

The principal method of prophylaxis for stress ulcer bleeding is to block the production of gastric acid using histamine type-2 receptor antagonists or proton pump inhibitors, and maintain a pH $\geq$ 4 in gastric aspirates. The other method of prophylaxis involves the use of a cytoprotective agent (sucralfate) that protects damaged areas of the gastric mucosa without altering gastric acidity. The individual drugs that are used for prophylaxis of stress ulcer bleeding are shown in Table 5.2.

[1]Histamine H2 - Receptor Antagonists

Inhibition of gastric acid secretion with histamine H_2-receptor antagonists (H_2 blockers) is the most popular method of stress ulcer prophylaxis (22). The drugs most frequently used for this purpose are ranitidine and famotidine; both drugs are typically given as an intravenous bolus in the doses shown in Table 5.2. Ranitidine is the most studied gastric acid–suppressing drug for stress ulcer prophylaxis. A single 50 mg dose of ranitidine given as an IV bolus will reduce gastric acidity (pH > 4) for 6–8 hrs. (24), so the typical ranitidine dosing regimen is 50 mg IV every 8 hours. Famotidine has a longer duration of action; i.e., a single 20 mg dose of famotidine given as an IV bolus will reduce gastric acidity (pH > 4) for 10–15 hours (23), so the typical famotidine dosing regimen is 20 mg IV every 12 hours.

DOSE ADJUSTMENTS: Intravenous doses of famotidine and ranitidine are largely excreted unchanged in the urine, and accumulation of these drugs in renal failure can produce a neurotoxic condition characterized by confusion, agitation and even seizures (23,24). Reduced dosing is therefore advised in patients with renal insufficiency.

BENEFITS AND RISKS: H_2 blockers are effective in reducing the incidence of clinically important bleeding from stress ulcers, but the benefit occurs primarily in patients with one or more of the risk factors in Table 5.1 (25). Prolonged use of H_2 blockers is accompanied by a decrease in their ability to maintain a pH $\geq$ 4 in gastric aspirates, but this does not influence their ability to prevent stress ulcer-related bleeding (17).

The principal risks associated with H_2 blockers are related to reduced gastric acidity. As mentioned earlier, these risks include an increased incidence of infectious gastroenteritis, including *Clostridium difficile* enterocolitis (14), and an increased incidence of pneumonia from aspiration of infectious gastric secretions into the airways (16,17). These risks, however, may be greater with the class of drugs described next.

Proton Pump Inhibitors (PPIs)

Proton pump inhibitors (PPIs) are potent acid-suppressing drugs that reduce gastric acidity by binding to the membrane pump responsible for hydrogen ion secretion by gastric parietal cells (26). These drugs are actually prodrugs, and must be converted to the active form within gastric parietal cells. Once activated, these drugs bind irreversibly to the membrane pump and produce complete inhibition of gastric acid secretion. The PPIs that are used for stress ulcer prophylaxis are included in Table 5.2.

PHARMACOLOGICAL ADVANTAGES: PPIs have several advantages over H_2 blockers. First, they produce a greater reduction in gastric acidity and have a longer duration of action, often requiring only a single daily dose. Secondly, the responsiveness to PPIs does not diminish with continued usage (26). Finally, PPIs are metabolized in the liver, and do not require a dose adjustment in renal failure. As a result of these advantages, PPIs are gradually replacing H_2 blockers for stress ulcer prophylaxis in hospitalized patients (22).

COMPARATIVE BENEFITS AND RISKS: Despite their enhanced potency, PPIs have not shown any advantage over H_2 blockers for prophylaxis of stress ulcer bleeding (27). Furthermore, the enhanced gastric acid suppression with PPIs may create a greater risk of infection than with H_2 blockers. This is supported by studies showing a higher incidence of hospital-acquired pneumonia with PPIs compared to H_2 blockers (28), and a higher incidence of *Clostridium difficile* enterocolitis in outpatients treated with PPIs instead of H_2 blockers (14). The overall risk-benefit accounting for PPIs is in favor of avoiding these drugs for the prophylaxis of stress ulcer bleeding.

PPIS AND CLOPIDOGREL: The popular antiplatelet agent, clopidogrel, is a prodrug that is converted to its active form by the same (cytochrome P-450) pathway in the liver that metabolizes PPIs. Therefore, PPIs can impede clopidogrel activation in the liver (by competitive inhibition) and reduce its antiplatelet activity (29). This effect is evident with in vitro tests of platelet aggregation, but the clinical significance of this interaction is unclear. Nevertheless, the Food and Drug Administration advises avoiding PPIs, if possible, in patients taking clopidogrel.

Sucralfate

Sucralfate is an aluminum salt of sucrose sulfate that adheres primarily to damaged areas of the gastric mucosa (via electrostatic bonds with exposed proteins) and forms a viscous covering that shields the denuded surface from luminal acids and pepsin proteolysis. It is classified as a *protectant* or cytoprotective agent, and has no effect on gastric acid secretion (30). Sucralfate promotes the healing of gastric and duodenal ulcers, and reduces the incidence of clinically important bleeding from stress ulcers (25).

Sucralfate is available as a tablet (1 gram per tablet) or a suspension (1g/10 mL), and is most effective when given as a suspension (tablets can be crushed and dissolved in water, if necessary). The dosing of sucralfate for stress ulcer prophylaxis is shown in Table 5.2. A single dose of sucralfate (1 mg) will remain adherent to the damaged mucosa for about 6 hours, so dosing at 6-hour intervals is advised.

DRUG INTERACTIONS: Sucralfate binds the following drugs in the lumen of the bowel (30): ciprofloxacin, digoxin, ketoconazole, norfloxacin, phenytoin, ranitidine, thyroxin, tetracycline, theophylline, and warfarin. (The interactions with ciprofloxacin and norfloxacin are considered the most significant.) When these drugs are given orally or via feeding tube, sucralfate dosing should be separated by at least 2 hours to avoid any drug interactions.

ALUMINUM CONTENT: The sucralfate molecule contains 8 aluminum hydroxide moieties that are released when sucralfate reacts with gastric acid. The aluminum can bind phosphate in the bowel, but hypophosphatemia is rare (31). Nevertheless, sucralfate is not advised for patients with persistent or severe hypophosphatemia. Sucralfate does not elevate plasma aluminum levels, even with prolonged use (32).

Sulcrafate vs. Gastric Acid Suppression

Sucralfate is appealing because it does not alter gastric acidity, and should not create the increased risk of infection that accompanies acid-suppressing drugs. Several clinical trials have compared sucralfate with an acid-suppressing drug (ranitidine) for stress ulcer prophylaxis, and Figure 5.4 shows the combined results from 10 clinical trials involving ventilator-dependent patients (17). Clinically significant bleeding (defined earlier) occurred less frequently with ranitidine, while pneumonia occurred less frequently with sucralfate. When the incidence of bleeding and pneumonia are combined (as shown in the center box), there are fewer adverse events with sucralfate. Although not shown, the mortality rate was the same with both drugs.

There are two possible interpretations of the results in Figure 5.4, based on the desired outcome. If the desired result is fewer episodes of bleeding, then ranitidine is superior to sucralfate. However if the desired result is fewer adverse events (bleeding and pneumonia), then sucralfate is superior to ranitidine. It seems that the goal of any preventive strategy is fewer adverse events, in which case the results in Figure 5.4 would favor sucralfate over ranitidine (i.e., gastric acid suppression) for prophylaxis of stress ulcer bleeding.

PHYSICIAN PREFERENCE: The most recent survey of critical care physicians showed that 64% used H_2 blockers, 23% used proton pump inhibitors, and only 12% used sucralfate for stress ulcer prophylaxis (22). However, only 30% of the physicians based their preferences on the efficacy and side effects of the drugs (!).

Gastric Acid Suppression and C. difficile

One of the most compelling reasons for avoiding gastric acid–suppressing drugs is the increased risk of Clostridium difficile enterocolitis associated with these drugs. This has been reported in both outpatients (14,33) and inpatients (34,35), and is a greater risk with proton pump inhibitors than with H_2 blockers (14,34). In fact, the increase in C. difficile enterocolitis that has been observed in recent years coincides with the increased use of proton pump inhibitors in both outpatients and inpatients. It is very possible that the increasing incidence of C. difficile enterocolitis in hospitalized patients is not the result of increased antibiotic usage (since antibiotics

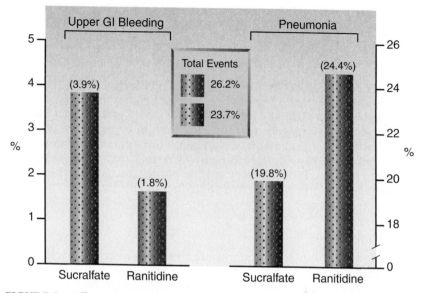

FIGURE 5.4 Effects of stress ulcer prophylaxis with ranitidine and sucralfate on the incidence of clinically significant upper GI bleeding and pneumonia in ventilator-dependent patients. The height of the columns in each graph are significantly different at the p < 0.01 level. (From Reference 17)

have always been overused), but instead is a consequence of the escalating use of gastric acid suppression for stress ulcer prophylaxis.

Enteral Feeding

Enteral tube feedings exert a trophic effect on the GI mucosa that helps to maintain the structural and functional integrity of the mucosal surface (see Chapter 48). Enteral feeding solutions also raise the pH in the lumen of the stomach. Both of these effects should protect against stress ulcer bleeding. The benefit of enteral tube feedings is revealed in the combined results of three clinical studies, which showed that the ability of H$_2$ blockers to reduce stress ulcer bleeding was lost when patients received a full regimen of enteral tube feedings (36). These results suggest that patients who receive enteral tube feedings do not require any further prophylactic measures for stress ulcer bleeding. Unfortunately, more studies are required before the experts will commit to tube feedings as a suitable method of stress ulcer prophylaxis.

Occult Blood Testing

Monitoring occult blood in gastric aspirates has no predictive value for identifying patients who will develop clinically significant bleeding from stress ulcers because gastric aspirates almost always contain occult blood in the presence of stress ulcers (37). For cases where testing for occult blood in gastric aspirates is performed, guaiac and Hemoccult tests are not reliable because of false-positive and false-negative results when the test fluid has a pH < 4 (38). The Gastroccult test (Smith, Kline Laboratories) is not influenced by pH (38), and is a more reliable test for occult blood in gastric aspirates.

DECONTAMINATION OF THE ALIMENTARY TRACT

The microbes that normally inhabit the oral cavity and GI tract seem to live in peaceful coexistence with us. However, in the presence of severe or chronic illness, the alimentary tract becomes populated by more pathogenic organisms capable of causing invasive infections. This section describes two methods for combating this pathogenic colonization. Both methods haven proven effective in reducing the incidence hospital-acquired infections.

Oral Decontamination

The aspiration of mouth secretions into the upper airways is believed to be the inciting event in most cases of hospital-acquired pneumonia. An average of 1 billion (10^9) microorganisms are present in each milliliter of saliva (39), so aspiration of one microliter (10^{-3} mL) of saliva will introduce about one million (10^6) microbes into the airways. Fortunately, the microbes that normally inhabit the mouth are harmless saprophytes (e.g., lactobacillus and α-hemolytic streptococci) that show little tendency to produce invasive infection. Critically ill patients are not as fortunate, as described next.

Colonization of the Oral Cavity

The oral cavity in hospitalized patients is often colonized with pathogenic organisms, most notably aerobic Gram-negative bacilli like *Pseudomonas aeruginosa* (40,41). The change in microflora is not environmentally driven, but is directly related to the severity of illness in each patient. This is demonstrated in Figure 5.5 (41). Note that healthy subjects were not colonized with aerobic Gram-negative bacilli, regardless of the environment. This highlights the importance of host-specific factors in the colonization of body surfaces.

BACTERIAL ADHERENCE: The specific organisms that colonize body surfaces are determined by specialized receptor proteins on epithelial cells that bind to adhesion proteins (called adhesins) on the surface of bacteria. These receptors are specific for certain groups or species of microorganisms, and this determines the microbes that can attach to the body surface. In healthy subjects, the epithelial cells in the mouth have receptors that bind harmless saprophytes (e.g., lactobacillus), while in seriously ill patients, the same epithelial cells have receptors that bind pathogenic organisms (e.g., *Pseudomonas aeruginosa*). The presence of a serious illness somehow induces the epithelial cells to express a different receptor for bacterial adherence; identifying the mechanism for this change is the first step towards the goal of manipulating epithelial cell receptors to prevent pathogenic colonization and infection in seriously ill patients.

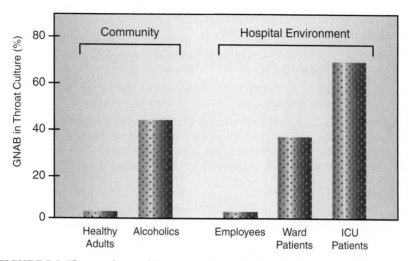

FIGURE 5.5 The prevalence of Gram-negative aerobic bacilli (GNAB) in cultures of the oral cavity in the specified groups of subjects. (From Reference 41)

Colonization of the oral mucosa with aerobic Gram-negative bacilli can be viewed as a prelude to pneumonia because Gram-negative bacilli are the most common cause of nosocomial pneumonia (see Chapter 29). This is the basis for efforts to decontaminate the oral cavity, as described next

Chlorhexidine

Chlorhexidine is an antiseptic agent that is popular for skin antisepsis because of its prolonged residual activity (6 hours), as described in Chapter 2. It has also been adopted for antisepsis in the mouth, primarily in ventilator-dependent patients, but has had limited success. Only 4 of 7 clinical trials have shown that routine oral care with chlorhexidine is effective in reducing the risk of ventilator-associated pneumonia (42). Postoperative cardiac surgery patients seem to benefit the most from oral decontamination with chlorhexidine (42), and the CDC guidelines for preventing healthcare-associated pneumonia includes a recommendation for oral rinses with chlorhexidine gluconate (0.12%) in the perioperative period for cardiac surgery (43). These guidelines also state that oral rinses with chlorhexidine can not be recommended in other patient populations.

The limited benefit of oral decontamination with chlorhexidine could be related to the limited antibacterial spectrum of chlorhexidine; i.e., it is effective primarily against Gram-positive organisms (44), while Gram-negative organisms are the predominant microbes in the oropharynx of critically ill patients (41), as shown in Figure 5.5.

Nonabsorbable Antibiotics

The direct application of nonabsorbable antibiotics to the oral mucosa is a more effective method of oral decontamination than chlorhexidine. The following is a popular antibiotic regimen for oral decontamination in ventilator-dependent patients (45):

Preparation: A mixture of 2% gentamicin, 2% colistin, and 2% vancomycin in Orabase gel. (Prepared by the pharmacy).

Regimen: Apply the paste to the buccal mucosa with a gloved finger every 6 hours until the patient is extubated.

This regimen is designed to eradicate staphylococci, Gram-negative aerobic bacilli, and *Candida* species from the oropharynx. There is little activity against normal mouth flora. Because of the selective nature of the antimicrobial activity, this regimen is known as *selective oral decontamination* (SOD).

EFFICACY: Clinical studies using SOD in ventilator-dependent patients have yielded results like those in Figure 5.6, where SOD was associated with a 57% (relative) decline in the incidence of tracheal colonization, and a 67% (relative) decrease in the incidence of (ventilator-associated) pneumonia (45). These results have been corroborated in other studies (46).

Another benefit from SOD is a reduction in ICU-acquired bacteremias involving Gram-negative bacilli (47,48). This is shown in Fig. 5.7 (47). Both graphs in this figure show that SOD was associated with a 33% (relative) decrease in the incidence of Gram-negative bacteremias.

The influence of oral decontamination on Gram-negative bacteremia is an unanticipated observation, and indicates that *the mouth is a source of*

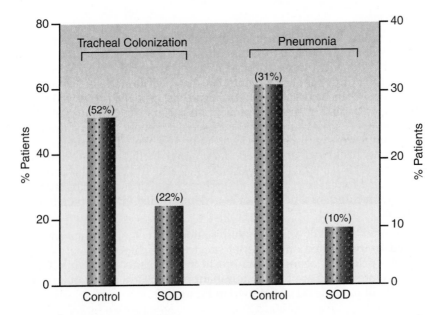

FIGURE 5.6 The effects of selective oral decontamination (SOD) on the incidence of tracheal colonization and pneumonia in ventilator-dependent patients. The height of the columns in each graph are significantly different at the p = 0.01 level. (From Reference 45)

bacteremia in ICU patients. Since brushing your teeth can result in bacteremia, it is possible that movements of endotracheal tubes and nasogastric tubes (e.g., with head movements) can damage the oropharyngeal mucosa and promote bacterial translocation in the mouth.

RESISTANCE: Despite dramatic effects like those in Figure 5.6, oral decontamination with nonabsorbable antibiotics is largely ignored in the United States (not so in Europe) because of concerns about the possible emergence of antibiotic-resistant organisms. However, there is no evidence of antibiotic resistance in any of the reports of antibiotic-based oral decontamination.

Selective Digestive Decontamination

Selective digestive decontamination (SDD) is essentially an extension of SOD to include the entire alimentary canal. One popular SDD regimen is shown below (49).

Oral cavity: A paste containing 2% polymyxin, 2% tobramycin, and 2% amphotericin is applied to the inside of the mouth with a gloved finger every 6 hours.

GI tract: A 10-mL solution containing 100 mg polymyxin E, 80 mg tobramycin, and 500 mg amphotericin is given via a nasogastric tube every 6 hours.

Systemic: Intravenous cefuroxime, 1.5 grams every 8 hours, for the first four days.

Note that the same drug combination used for SOD is also used to decontaminate the oral cavity and the GI tract. This nonabsorbable antibiotic regimen is designed to eradicate staphylococci, Gram-negative aerobic bacilli, and fungal species, while sparing the normal inhabitants of the bowel (mostly anaerobes) to prevent colonization with opportunistic pathogens like *Clostridium difficile.* The intravenous antibiotic provides systemic protection while the bowel regimen begins to take effect (decontamination of the bowel takes about one week). The SDD regimen is intended for all patients who will stay in the ICU longer than 72 hours, and is administered from admission until the patient is well enough to be discharged from the ICU.

Clinical Efficacy

Several studies have shown a significant reduction in ICU-acquired infections associated with SDD (47-49). The results of one of these studies is shown in Figure 5.7 (47). This was a large, randomized trial that evaluated the influence of SOD and SDD on ICU-acquired bacteremias involving Gram-negative bacilli. Both bar graphs show that SDD patients had 69% drop in the incidence of Gram-negative bacteremias when compared with control patients. Although not shown in the figure, the SDD effect was accompanied by a decrease in mortality. Improved survival in patients receiving SDD has also been observed in other studies (50).

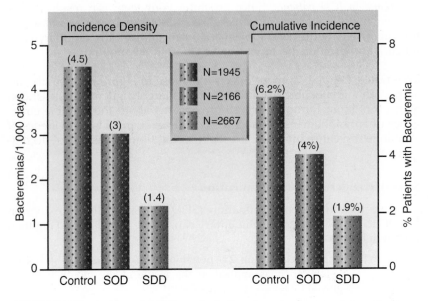

FIGURE 5.7 The incidence of ICU-acquired, Gram-negative bacteremia in patients randomized to receive selective oral decontamination (SOD), selective digestive decontamination (SDD), or standard care (control). The graph on the left shows the number of bacteremias per 1,000 days (incidence density), and the graph on the right shows the percentage of patients with bacteremia (cumulative incidence). N is the number of patients in each study group. (From Reference 47)

Antibiotic Resistance

The principal fear with SDD is possible emergence of antibiotic-resistant organisms. However, this fear is not supported by clinical observations. (50,51).

Resistance to SDD

Numerous clinical studies over the past 25 years have shown that SDD is an effective method for preventing ICU-acquired infections, yet SDD is rarely used in the United States. Some of the resistance to SDD is based on an unfounded fear of antibiotic resistance, as just described. Another concern is a lack of consistent survival benefit with SDD. Early studies of SDD typically showed no survival benefit, but more recent and larger clinical trials have shown a significant improvement in survival associated with SDD (48,50). Thus, there is little justification for the continued disregard of SDD.

A FINAL WORD

One of the recurring themes in this book is the importance of the alimentary tract as a source of infection in critically ill patients. The summary statements and recommendations listed below are designed to assist you in limiting the risk of infection from this important site.

1. Prophylaxis for stress ulcer bleeding is overused in the ICU (22), and should be limited to the conditions in Table 5.1.

2. Gastric acid suppression is overused as a method of stress ulcer prophylaxis, and this has probably contributed to the surge in *C. difficile* infections in recent years (34,35).

3. Proton pump inhibitors should be avoided for stress ulcer prophylaxis because they are not more effective than H_2 blockers (27), and they are more likely to promote unwanted infections (14,28).

4. Recent evidence suggests that total enteral nutrition is an effective method of stress ulcer prophylaxis (36).

5. Oral decontamination is advised for all ventilator-dependent patients, and the use of non-absorbable antibiotics provides better antimicrobial coverage than chlorhexidine (44), and has more proven efficacy for preventing ventilator-associated pneumonia (45,46).

6. Selective digestive decontamination (SDD) is a proven method for reducing the incidence of ICU-acquired infections (47-50), and there is no evidence that it promotes the emergence of antibiotic-resistant organisms (50,51). As a result, SDD deserves much more consideration for the prevention of ICU-acquired infections.

REFERENCES

Books

Marston A, Bulkley GB, Fiddian-Green RG, Haglund UH, eds. Splanchnic Ischemia and Multiple Organ Failure. St. Louis: C.V. Mosby, 1989.

Microbial Invasion From the Bowel

1. Simon GL, Gorbach SL. Intestinal microflora. Med Clin North Am 1982; 66:557–574.

2. Borriello SP. Microbial flora of the gastrointestinal tract. In: Microbial metabolism in the digestive tract. Boca Raton, FL: CRC Press, 1989; 2–19.

3. Bengmark S. Gut microbial ecology in critical illness: is there a role for prebiotics, probiotics, and synbiotics? Curr Opin Crit Care 2002; 8:145–151.

4. Langkamp-Henken B, Glezer JA, Kudsk KA. Immunologic structure and function of the gastrointestinal tract. Nutr Clin Pract 1992; 7:100–108.

5. Alexander JW, Boyce ST, Babcock GF, et al. The process of microbial translocation. Ann Surg 1990; 212:496–510.

6. Deitch EA. Multiple organ failure. Pathophysiology and potential future therapy. Ann Surg 1992; 216:117–134.

7. Meakins JL, Marshal JC. The gastrointestinal tract: the 'motor' of MOF. Arch Surg 1986; 121:197–201.

8. Howden CW, Hunt RH. Relationship between gastric secretion and infection. Gut 1987; 28:96–107.

9. Lister J. On the antiseptic principle in the practice of surgery. Br Med J 1867; ii:246-250. Reprinted in Clin Orthop Relat Res 2010; 468:2012–2016.

10. Gianella RA, Broitman SA, Zamcheck N. Gastric acid barrier to ingested microorganisms in man: studies in vivo and in vitro. Gut 1972; 13:251–256.

11. Wingate DL. Acid reduction and recurrent enteritis. Lancet 1990; 335:222.

12. Neal KR, Scott HM, Slack RCB, Logan RFA. Omeprazole as a risk factor for campylobacter gastroenteritis: case-control study. Br Med J 1996; 312:414–415.

13. Cook GC. Infective gastroenteritis and its relationship to reduced acidity. Scand J Gastroenterol 1985; 20(Suppl 111):17–21.

14. Dial S, Delaney JAC, Barkun AN, Suissa S. Use of gastric acid-suppressing agents and the risk of community-acquired Clostridium difficile-associated disease. JAMA 2005; 294:2989–2994.

15. MacFie J, Reddy BS, Gatt M, et al. Bacterial translocation studied in 927 patients over 13 years. Br J Surg 2006; 93:87–93.

16. Gulmez SE, Holm A, Frederiksen H, et al. Use of proton pump inhibitors and the risk of community-acquired pneumonia. Arch Intern Med 2007; 167:950–955.

17. Huang J, Cao Y, Liao C, et al. Effect of histamine-2-receptor antagonists versus sucralfate on stress ulcer prophylaxis in mechanically ventilated patients: A meta-analysis of 10 randomized controlled trials. Crit Care 2010; 14:R194–R204.

Stress-Related Mucosal Injury

18. Steinberg KP. Stress-related mucosal disease in the critically ill patient: Risk factors and strategies to prevent stress-related bleeding in the intensive care unit. Crit Care Med 2002; 30(Suppl):S362–S364.

19. Fennerty MB. Pathophysiology of the upper gastrointestinal tract in the critically ill patient: rationale for the therapeutic benefits of acid suppression. Crit Care Med 2002; 30(Suppl):S351–S355.

20. O'Brien PE. Gastric acidity: the gastric microvasculature and mucosal disease. In Marston A, Bulkley GB, Fiddian-Green RG, Hagland UH, eds. Splanchnic Ischemia and Multiple Organ Failure. St. Louis: C.V. Mosby, 1989:145–158.

21. Cook DJ, Fuller MB, Guyatt GH. Risk factors for gastrointestinal bleeding in critically ill patients. N Engl J Med 1994; 330:377–381.

22. Daley RJ, Rebuck JA, Welage LS, et al. Prevention of stress ulceration: current trends in critical care. Crit Care Med 2004; 32:2008–2013.

23. Ranitidine. AHFS Drug Information, 2011. Bethesda, MD: American Society of Health System Pharmacists, 2011:2983–2990.

24. Famotidine. AHFS Drug Information, 2011. Bethesda, MD: American Society of Health System Pharmacists, 2011:2977–2983.

25. Cook DJ, Reeve BK, Guyatt GH. Stress ulcer prophylaxis in critically ill patients. JAMA 1996; 275:308–314.

26. Pisegna JR. Pharmacology of acid suppression in the hospital setting: focus on proton pump inhibition. Crit Care Med 2002; 30(Suppl): S356–S361.

27. Lin P-C, Chang C-H, Hsu P-I, et al. The efficacy and safety of proton pump inhibitors vs histamine-2 receptor antagonists for stress ulcer bleeding prophylaxis among critical care patients: A meta-analysis. Crit Care Med 2010; 38:1197–1205.

28. Herzig SJ, Howell MD, Ngo LH, Marcantonio ER. Acid-suppressive medication use and the risk for hospital-acquired pneumonia. JAMA 2009; 301:2120–2128.

29. Egred M. Clopidogrel and proton-pump inhibitor interaction. Br J Cardiol 2011; 18:84–87.

30. Sucralfate. AHFS Drug Information, 2011. Bethesda, MD: American Society of Health System Pharmacists, 2011:2996–2998.

31. Miller SJ, Simpson J. Medication–nutrient interactions: hypophosphatemia associated with sucralfate in the intensive care unit. Nutr Clin Pract 1991; 6:199–201.

32. Tryba M, Kurz-Muller K, Donner B. Plasma aluminum concentrations in long-term mechanically ventilated patients receiving stress ulcer prophylaxis with sucralfate. Crit Care Med 1994; 22:1769–1773.

33. Lowe DO, Mamdani MM, Kopp A, et. al. Proton pump inhibitors and hospitalization for *Clostridium difficile*-associated disease: a population-based study. Clin Infect Dis 2006; 43:1272–1276.

34. Dial S, Alrasadi K, Manoukian C, et. al. Risk of *Clostridium-difficile* diarrhea among hospitalized patients prescribed proton pump inhibitors: cohort and case-control studies. Canad Med Assoc J 2004; 171:33–38.

35. Aseri M, Schroeder T, Kramer J, Kackula R. Gastric acid suppression by proton pump inhibitors as a risk factor for *Clostridium difficile*-associated diarrhea in hospitalized patients. Am J Gastroenterol 2008; 103:2308–2313.

36. Marik PE, Vasu T, Hirani A, Pachinburavan M. Stress ulcer prophylaxis in the new millenium: a systematic review and meta-analysis. Crit Care Med 2010; 38:2222–2228.

37. Maier RV, Mitchell D, Gentiello L. Optimal therapy for stress gastritis. Ann Surg 1994; 220:353–363.

38. Rosenthal P, Thompson J, Singh M. Detection of occult blood in gastric juice. J Clin Gastroenterol 1984; 6:119.

Decontamination of the Alimentary Tract

39. Higuchi JH, Johanson WG. Colonization and bronchopulmonary infection. Clin Chest Med 1982; 3:133–142.

40. Estes RJ, Meduri GU. The pathogenesis of ventilator-associated pneumonia: I. Mechanisms of bacterial transcolonization and airway inoculation. Intensive Care Med 1995; 21:365–383.

41. Johanson WG, Pierce AK, Sanford JP. Changing pharyngeal bacterial flora of hospitalized patients. Emergence of gram-negative bacilli. N Engl J Med 1969; 281:1137–1140.

42. Chlebicki MP, Safdar N. Topical chlorhexidine for prevention of ventilator-associated pneumonia: a meta-analysis. Crit Care Med 2007; 35:595–602.

43. Tablan OC, Anderson LJ, Besser r, et. al. Guidelines for preventing health-care-associated pneumonia, 2003: recommendations of CDC and the Health-care Infection Control Practices Advisory Committee. MMWR 2004; 53(N0. RR-3):1–40.

44. Emilson CG. Susceptibility of various microorganisms to chlorhexidine. Scand J Dent Res 1977; 85:255–265.

45. Bergmans C, Bonten M, Gaillard C, et al. Prevention of ventilator-associated pneumonia by oral decontamination. Am J Respir Crit Care Med 2001; 164:382–388.

46. van Nieuwenhoven CA, Buskens E, Bergmans DC, et al. Oral decontamination is cost-saving in the prevention of ventilator associated pneumonia in intensive care units. Crit Care Med 2004; 32:126–130.

47. Oostdijk EA, de Smet AM, Kesecioglu J, et. al. The role of intestinal colonization with Gram-negative bacteria as a source for intensive care unit-acquired bacteremia. Crit Care Med 2011; 39:961–966.

48. de Smet AMGA, Kluytmans JAJW, Cooper BS, et al. Decontamination of the digestive tract and oropharynx in ICU patients. N Engl J Med 2009; 360:20–31.

49. Stoutenbeek CP, van Saene HKF, Miranda DR, Zandstra DF. The effect of selective decontamination of the digestive tract on colonization and infection rate in multiple trauma patients. Intensive Care Med 1984; 10:185–192.

50. de Jonge E, Schultz MJ, Spanjaard L, et al. Effects of selective decontamination of digestive tract on mortality and acquisition of resistant bacteria in intensive care: a randomized controlled trial. Lancet 2003; 362:1011–1016.

51. Ochoa-Ardila ME, Garcia-Canas A, Gomez-Mediavilla K, et al. Long-term use of selective decontamination of the digestive tract does not increase antibiotic resistance: a 5-year prospective cohort study. Intensive Care Med 2011; 37:1458–1465.

Chapter 6

VENOUS THROMBO- EMBOLISM

Two words best characterize the mortality and morbidity due to venous thromboembolism in the United States: substantial and unacceptable.

Kenneth M. Moser, MD

The threat of pulmonary embolism is a daily concern in ICU patients, who typically have one or more risk factors for venous thrombosis (the precursor of pulmonary embolism). Thrombus formation occurs most frequently in proximal leg veins, and becomes apparent only when a portion of the thrombus breaks loose and travels to the lungs to become a pulmonary embolus. This progression from silent leg thrombosis to symptomatic pulmonary embolism is a significant, and preventable, problem in hospitalized patients. In fact, pulmonary embolism is considered the most common preventable cause of death in hospitalized patients, and the prevention of venous thrombosis is considered the single most important measure for ensuring patient safety during hospitalization (see Federal Reports in bibliography).

This chapter presents the current practices for the prevention, diagnosis, and treatment of venous thrombosis and pulmonary embolism (i.e., venous thromboembolism) in the ICU patient population. Several clinical practice guidelines and reviews of this subject are included in the bibliography at the end of the chapter (1–8).

RISK FACTORS

Several conditions promote venous thromboembolism (VTE) in hospitalized patients, and these are listed in Table 6.1 (1). One or more of these conditions is present in almost all ICU patients, and thus VTE is considered a universal risk in critically ill patients (1,5). The incidence of VTE in

97

different groups of patients, which is shown in Figure 6.1 (1), can be used to estimate of the likelihood of VTE in individual ICU patients. The presence of additional risk factors (e.g., prior VTE) will add further to the risk of VTE in any of the clinical groups shown in Figure 6.1.

Table 6.1	Risk Factors for Venous Thromboembolism in Hospitalized Patients
Surgery	Major surgery, especially cancer-related surgery, hip and knee surgery
Trauma	Multisystem trauma, especially spinal cord injury and fractures of the spine
Malignancy	Any malignancy, active or occult Chemotherapy and radiotherapy
Acute Medical Illness	Stroke, right-sided heart failure, sepsis, inflammatory bowel disease, nephrotic syndrome, myeloproliferative disorders
Drugs	Erythropoiesis-stimulating drugs, estrogen-containing compounds
Patient-Specific Factors	Prior thromboembolism, obesity, increasing age, pregnancy
ICU-Related Factors	Prolonged mechanical ventilation, neuromuscular paralysis, severe sepsis, vasopressors, platelet transfusions, immobility

From References 1 and 5.

Major Surgery

Major surgery (i.e., surgery performed under general or spinal anesthesia that lasts longer than 30 minutes) is the most recognized cause of VTE in hospitalized patients, and autopsy studies have shown that VTE is responsible for about 10% of postoperative deaths (9). The propensity for VTE after major surgery is primarily due to thromboplastin release during the surgical procedure, which produces a generalized hypercoagulable state. The risk of VTE is particularly high following cancer-related surgery (1,5).

Orthopedic Surgery

The highest incidence of postoperative VTE occurs after major orthopedic procedures involving the hip and knee (1,5). Vascular injury in the lower extremities contributes to the enhanced risk of VTE following hip and knee surgery.

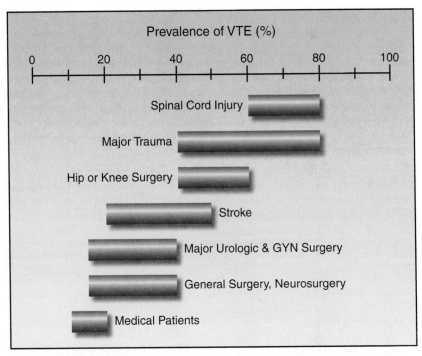

FIGURE 6.1 The prevalence of venous thromboembolism in different groups of hospitalized patients. From Reference 4.

Major Trauma

The risk of VTE is highest following major or multisystem trauma. Victims of major trauma have a greater than 50% chance of developing VTE, and pulmonary embolism is the third leading cause of death in those who survive the first day (1). The trauma conditions with the highest risk of VTE are brain and spinal cord injuries, spinal fractures, and fractures of the hip and pelvis (1,5). Several factors contribute to the propensity for VTE after major trauma, including thromboplastin release from injured tissues, vascular injury, and prolonged immobility.

Acute Medical Illness

Hospitalization for acute medical illness is associated with an eightfold increase in the risk of VTE (10). Although VTE is less common in medical patients than in postoperative patients or trauma victims (see Figure 6.1), the majority (70% to 80%) of deaths from VTE occur in medical patients (1). Medical conditions with a particularly high risk of VTE include cancer, acute stroke with lower extremity weakness, and right-sided heart failure. In a Medical ICU, additional risk factors for VTE can include mechanical ventilation, severe sepsis, and prolonged immobility.

THROMBOPROPHYLAXIS

Autopsy studies in critically ill patients reveal pulmonary emboli in as many as 27% of patients (5), and in the majority of these cases there is no clinical suspicion of venous thrombosis or pulmonary embolism prior to death (5). Because of the insidious nature of VTE, prevention is the best means of limiting the adverse consequences of this condition. In fact, preventive strategies for VTE should have the greatest impact on patient safety in the ICU setting because of the ubiquitous presence of risk factors for VTE in critically ill patients.

This section describes the methods that are used to prevent thrombus formation in critically ill patients. The preventive measures that are recommended in a variety of conditions are included in Table 6.2, and the prophylactic anticoagulant dosing regimens are shown in Table 6.3.

Table 6.2	Thromboprophylaxis for Selected Conditions in the ICU
Conditions	**High-Risk Regimens[1]**
Acute Medical Illness	LDUH or LMWH
Major Abdominal Surgery	(LDUH or LMWH) + (GCS or IPC)
Thoracic Surgery	(LDUH or LMWH) + (GCS or IPC)
Cardiac Surgery with Complications	(LDUH or LMWH) + IPC
Craniotomy	IPC
Hip or Knee Surgery	LMWH
Major Trauma	LDUH or LMWH or IPC
Head or Spinal Cord Injury	(LDUH or LMWH) + IPC
Any of the above + active bleeding or high risk of bleeding	IPC

From Reference 1. Abbreviations: LDUH = low-dose unfractionated heparin; LMWH = low-molecular weight heparin; GCS = graded compression stockings; IPC = intermittent pneumatic compression.

[1]Critically ill patients are considered to be in the high-risk category for each of the conditions listed.

Unfractionated Heparin

Heparin is a mucopolysaccharide molecule that varies in size, anticoagulant activity, and pharmacokinetic properties. The standard or *unfractionated* heparin preparation is a heterogeneous mix of molecules that can vary in size by a factor of 10, and only one-third of the molecules have anticoagulant activity.

Properties

Heparin is an indirect-acting drug that must bind to a cofactor (antithrombin III or AT) to produce its anticoagulant effect. The heparin-AT complex is capable of inactivating several coagulation factors, but the strongest interactions involve the inhibition of factor IIa (thrombin) and factor Xa (3). The anti-IIa (antithrombin) activity is 10 times more sensitive than the anti-Xa activity (3).

Heparin also binds to plasma proteins, endothelial cells, and macrophages. Heparin binding to plasma proteins determines bioavailability, and variations in plasma protein levels are responsible for the variable anticoagulation effects of heparin. The binding of heparin to endothelial cells and macrophages promotes clearance from the bloodstream.

PLATELET BINDING: Heparin binds to a specific protein on platelets to form an antigenic complex that induces the formation of IgG antibodies. These antibodies can cross-react with the platelet binding site and activate platelets, thereby promoting thrombosis and a consumptive thrombocytopenia. This is the mechanism for *heparin-induced thrombocytopenia*, which is described in detail in Chapter 19.

Low-Dose Unfractionated Heparin

The highly sensitive antithrombin activity of the heparin-AT complex allows low doses of heparin to inhibit thrombogenesis without producing systemic anticoagulation. The standard regimen of low-dose unfractionated heparin (LDUH) is 5,000 units given by subcutaneous injection twice daily (every 12 hours) or three times daily (every 8 hours). Clinical studies of LDUH in ICU patients (11) and postoperative patients (12) have shown a 50% to 60% reduction in the incidence of leg vein thrombosis in patients who received LDUH (although most cases were asymptomatic). The risk of major bleeding is less than 1% with both dosing regimens (13), so there is no need to monitor laboratory tests of anticoagulation during LDUH prophylaxis.

OBESITY: Fixed doses of heparin may be less effective in obese patients because of the increased volume of drug distribution in obesity. For this reason, the recommended dosing for LDUH in obesity (defined as a body mass index or BMI $\geq$ 30 kg/m^2) is 5,000 units every 8 hours for a BMI of 30 to 49.9 kg/m^2, and 7,500 units every 8 hours for a BMI $\geq$ 50 kg/m^2 (14), as shown in Table 6.3. (Appendix 2 includes equations and tables for determining BMI.)

INDICATIONS: As shown in Table 6.2, LDUH can be used for thromboprophylaxis in most conditions except hip and knee surgery (1). There is no evidence that the two dosing regimens for LDUH (every 8 hrs. and every 12 hrs.) differ in preventing VTE (4,13), so the twice-daily LDUH regimen is the more prudent choice.

Table 6.3	Anticoagulant Regimens for Thromboprophylaxis

Unfractionated Heparin

	Usual Dose:	5,000 Units SC every 12 hrs. or 5,000 Units SC every 8 hrs.
	Obesity:	5,000 Units SC every 8 hrs. (BMI<50) 7,500 Units SC every 8 hrs. (BMI ≥50)

Enoxaparin (LMWH)

	Usual Dose:	40 mg SC once daily or 30 mg SC twice daily
	Obesity:	0.5 mg/kg SC once daily (BMI > 40)
	Renal Failure:	30 mg once daily (for CrCL < 30 ml/min)

Dalteparin (LMWH)

	Usual Dose:	2,500 Units SC once daily or 5,000 Units SC once daily
	Renal Failure:	No recommended dose adjustment

From References 4, 14, 17–19.

Low-Molecular-Weight Heparin

Low-molecular-weight heparin (LMWH) is produced by enzymatic cleavage of heparin molecules, which produces smaller molecules of more uniform size. The average molecular weight of LMWH is about one-third that of unfractionated heparin. LMWH must still bind to antithrombin III to produce its anticoagulant effects, but the anti-IIa (antithrombin) activity of the LMWH-AT complex is much reduced relative to the anti-Xa activity; i.e., the anti-Xa activity of LMWH is 2–4 times greater than the antithrombin activity (3).

Comparative Features

LMWH does not bind as readily to plasma proteins, endothelial cells, macrophages, or platelets as unfractionated heparin, and this gives LMWH the following advantages (3):

1. As a result of reduced binding to plasma proteins, LMWH is a more potent anticoagulant than unfractionated heparin, and has a more predictable dose-response relationship. This latter feature obviates the need for routine laboratory tests of anticoagulant effect during therapy with LMWH (3).

2. Reduced binding to endothelial cells and macrophages gives LMWH a longer duration of action than unfractionated heparin. As a result, LMWH requires less frequent dosing than unfractionated heparin.

3. Reduced binding to platelets by LMWH results in a lower risk of heparin-induced thrombocytopenia (15,16). This is a major advan-

tage, and one of the principal reasons that LMWH is favored over unfractionated heparin.

The major drawback with LMWH is its clearance by the kidneys, which creates the need for dosage adjustments in patients with renal failure. However, the tendency to accumulate in renal failure varies with individual LMWH preparations (see later).

LMWH vs. Low-Dose Unfractionated Heparin

Clinical studies comparing thromboprophylaxis with LMWH and low-dose unfractionated heparin (LDUH) have shown the following:

1. LMWH is equivalent to LDUH for most conditions encountered in the ICU, including acute medical illnesses, major, non-orthopedic surgery, and cancer-related surgery (16). This is reflected in Table 6.2, which shows LMWH as an alternative to LDUH for most of the conditions listed.

2. LMWH is superior to LDUH for major orthopedic procedures involving the hip and knee (1,5). As a result, LMWH is preferred method of thromboprophylaxis for hip and knee surgery. The first dose of LMWH should not be given sooner than 12 hours after the procedure to limit the risk of bleeding (1).

3. The incidence of heparin-induced thrombocytopenia with LMWH (0.2%) is less than 10% of the incidence with LDUH (2.6%) (15). This is an important distinction, and is the reason for the proposal that LMWH should be favored over LDUH for all cases where anticoagulant prophylaxis is required (5).

Dosing Regimens

There are several LMWH preparations available for clinical use, and each one has a unique dosage and pharmacokinetic profile. The LMWHs used most often in the United States are enoxaparin (Lovenox) and dalteparin (Fragmin), and Table 6.3 shows the prophylactic dosing regimens for each of these agents.

ENOXAPARIN: Enoxaparin was the first LMWH approved for use in the United States (in 1993), and the clinical experience with this LMWH is the most extensive. The standard enoxaparin dose for thromboprophylaxis is 40 mg given by subcutaneous injection once daily (4,17). In conditions with a very high risk of VTE (e.g., major trauma, hip and knee surgery), the dose is 30 mg by subcutaneous injection twice daily (17). The prophylactic dose of enoxaparin in renal failure (i.e., creatinine clearance < 30 mL/min) is 30 mg once daily by subcutaneous injection (17). In patients with morbid obesity (i.e., BMI > 40 kg/m^2), an enoxaparin dose of 0.5 mg/kg once daily by subcutaneous injection has been shown to provide safe and effective thromboprophylaxis (18).

DALTEPARIN: The dosing recommendations for dalteparin are shown in Table 6.3. Dalteparin has two advantages over enoxaparin. First, dalteparin is given only once daily, even in high-risk doses (19). More importantly, there is evidence that dalteparin prophylaxis can be continued without dose reduction in patients with renal failure (20). The appropriate dose of dalteparin in morbid obesity is not known.

Neuraxial Analgesia

Anticoagulant prophylaxis can promote hematoma formation during the insertion and removal of intrathecal and epidural catheters. This is a feared complication because spinal and epidural hematomas can compress the spinal cord and produce paralysis. To limit the risk of this complication, the insertion and removal of intrathecal and epidural catheters should be performed at a time when anticoagulant effects are minimal; e.g., if a twice daily dosing regimen is used, these procedure should be delayed at least 12 hours after the prior anticoagulant dose, and for a once-daily dosing regimen, the delay should be at least 24 hours after the prior anticoagulant dose (4). In addition, at least 2 hours should elapse after these procedures before an anticoagulant dose is administered (4).

Mechanical Thromboprophylaxis

External compression of the lower extremities can be used to promote venous outflow from the legs and reduce the risk of VTE from immobility. This method of mechanical thromboprophylaxis is typically used as a replacement for anticoagulant drugs in patients who are bleeding or have a high risk of bleeding, but it can also be used as an adjunct to prophylaxis with anticoagulant drugs (see Table 6.2). There are two methods of external leg compression: graded compression stockings and intermittent pneumatic compression.

Graded Compression Stockings

Graded compression stockings (also known as thromboembolism-deterrent or TED stockings) are designed to create 18 mm Hg external pressure at the ankles and 8 mm Hg external pressure in the thigh (21). The resulting 10 mm Hg pressure gradient acts as a driving force for venous outflow from the legs. These stockings have been shown to reduce the incidence of VTE by 50% when used alone after major surgery (22). However, they are the least effective method of thromboprophylaxis, and are never used as sole means of prevention in critically ill patients.

Intermittent Pneumatic Compression

Intermittent pneumatic compression (IPC) is achieved with inflatable bladders that are wrapped around the lower extremities and connected to a pneumatic pump. Bladder inflation promotes venous outflow from the legs by creating 35 mm Hg external compression at the ankle and 20 mm Hg external compression at the thigh (21), and repeated inflation and deflation creates a pumping action that further augments venous outflow from the legs.

The IPC method is more effective than graded compression stockings (1,5), and can be used alone for thromboprophylaxis in the early period following craniotomy (1). IPC is the favored method of mechanical prophylaxis used in the ICU, but there are some shortcomings; i.e., the inflatable bladders restrict mobility and can macerate the skin, and the repeated inflation and deflation of the bladders is often annoying for awake patients. Therefore, IPC should be discontinued as soon as it is no longer necessary.

DIAGNOSTIC EVALUATION

As mentioned earlier, thrombosis in the deep veins of the legs is often clinically silent, and VTE is suspected only when a symptomatic pulmonary embolus appears. The diagnostic approach to pulmonary embolism is accurately described by the following quote from a recent review of the topic (6):

> The one certainty surrounding the issue of thromboembolism diagnosis in critically ill patients is that considerable uncertainty remains.

In patients who are evaluated for possible pulmonary embolism, the diagnosis is confirmed in as few as 10% of cases (23), and when physicians have a highest degree of certainty that a patient has a pulmonary embolism, they are correct in only 17–25% of the patients (23). What this means is that when you suspect a pulmonary embolus, it usually isn't there. It also means that the diagnostic evaluation of pulmonary embolism serves prïimarily to exclude the diagnosis rather than confirm it.

The Clinical Evaluation

The clinical presentation of acute pulmonary embolism (PE) includes nonspecific manifestations such as dyspnea, tachypnea, tachycardia, and hypoxemia. The predictive value of clinical and laboratory findings in suspected cases of PE is shown in Table 6.4 (24). Note that none of the findings provides more than a 50% chance of identifying pulmonary embolism (i.e., the positive predictive value), and further that the absence of these findings does not exclude PE (i.e., the negative predictive value should be ≥ 98% to exclude the presence of a condition). Of particular interest is the negative predictive value of 70% for hypoxemia, which means that 30% of patients with a pulmonary embolus have a normal arterial PO_2. Although not included in Table 6.4, the alveolar–arterial PO_2 (A–a PO_2) gradient can also be normal in patients with pulmonary emboli (25).

D-Dimer Assay

Active thrombosis is accompanied by some degree of clot lysis, and this produces cross-linked fibrin monomers, also called fibrin D-dimers or D-dimers. Plasma D-dimer levels are elevated in patients with VTE, and the D-dimer assay has become a popular screening test for suspected VTE in non-ICU patients. However, D-dimer levels have little predictive value in ICU patients. The problem is the multitude of other conditions that can elevate plasma D-dimer levels, including sepsis, malignancy, pregnancy, heart failure, renal failure, and even advanced age (26). As a result, a majority (up to 80%) of ICU patients have elevated plasma D-dimer levels in the absence of VTE (27). This is reflected in the poor positive predictive value of the D-dimer assay in Table 6.4. Because of the high prevalence of elevated D-dimer levels in critically ill patients, the D-dimer assay is not considered a useful test for VTE in the ICU setting.

Table 6.4	Predictive Value of Clinical and Laboratory Findings in Suspected Pulmonary Embolism	
Findings	**Positive Predictive Value**[†]	**Negative Predictive Value**[§]
Dyspnea	37%	75%
Tachycardia	47%	86%
Tachypnea	48%	75%
Pleuritic Chest Pain	39%	71%
Hemoptysis	32%	67%
Pulmonary Infiltrate	33%	71%
Pleural Effusion	40%	69%
Hypoxemia	34%	70%
Elevated D-Dimer[1]	27%	92%

[†]Positive predictive value is the percentage of patients with the finding who have a pulmonary embolus.
[§]Negative predictive value is the percentage of patients without the finding who do not have a pulmonary embolus.
[1]From Reference 26. Other data from Reference 24.

Summary

The information just presented shows that *there are no clinical or laboratory findings that will confirm or exclude the presence of a pulmonary embolus.* As a result, the diagnostic approach to PE requires specialized tests, which are included in the flow diagram shown in Figure 6.2.

Venous Ultrasound

Pulmonary emboli originate primarily from thrombi in proximal leg veins (28), so the evaluation of suspected PE can begin with a search for thrombosis in the proximal leg veins using ultrasound imaging at the bedside. The basics of vascular ultrasound are described in Chapter 2.

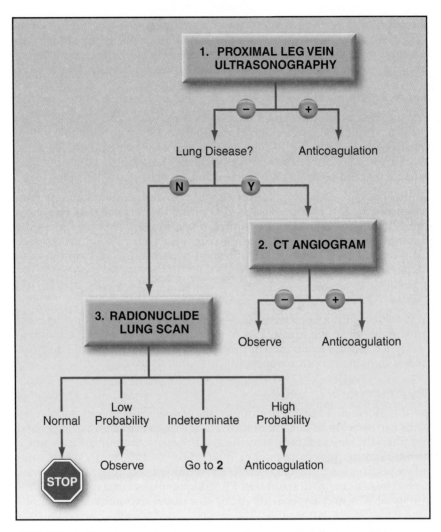

FIGURE 6.2 Flow diagram for the evaluation of suspected pulmonary embolism.

Methodology

There are two ultrasound methods for identifying venous thrombosis. The principal method is *compression ultrasound*, where a compressive force is applied to the skin overlying the target vein. This will normally compress the underlying vein and obliterate its lumen (see Figure 2.3). However, when a vein is filled with blood clots (which are often not visualized by ultrasound), external compression does not compress the vein. Therefore, an incompressible vein is used as evidence of a clot-filled vein (29).

The *color Doppler mode* of ultrasound can be used as an adjunct to compression ultrasonography. This method converts flow velocities into color images, and the flow in arteries and veins can be identified by the direction of flow in relation to the ultrasound probe (see Figure 2.6 in Chapter 2). The presence of thrombosis will be identified by sluggish or absent flow in the visualized (and incompressible) vein. The combination of compression and Doppler ultrasound is known as *duplex ultrasound*.

Test Performance

For the detection of proximal deep vein thrombosis (proximal DVT) in the legs, duplex ultrasound has a sensitivity ≥ 95%, a specificity ≥ 97%, a positive predictive value as high as 97%, and a negative predictive value as high as 98% (29). These numbers indicate that duplex ultrasound is a reliable method of confirming and excluding proximal DVT in the legs.

Unlike the high sensitivity for proximal DVT, duplex ultrasound is non-diagnostic in 32% to 55% of cases of DVT below the knee (30). However, calf DVT is not considered a source of pulmonary emboli unless the thrombi propagate into the larger proximal leg veins. Therefore, a search for proximal DVT is the principal task of venous ultrasound in the evaluation of suspected PE.

Yield

In patients with documented PE, venous ultrasound shows evidence of proximal DVT in the legs in 45% of patients (31). This yield is enough to justify ultrasound evaluation of proximal leg veins as the initial diagnostic test in patients with suspected PE.

Upper Extremity DVT

As described in Chapter 3, thrombosis of the axillary and subclavian veins can develop as a result of indwelling subclavian vein catheters and peripherally inserted central catheters (PICCs). Although PE is not a common consequence of upper extremity DVT (< 10% of cases) (32), careful inspection for catheter-associated swelling of the upper arms is warranted in patients with suspected PE. Venous ultrasonography has s sensitivity of 97% and a specificity of 96% for upper extremity DVT (32).

The Diagnostic Evaluation

If venous ultrasound shows evidence of proximal leg vein DVT, no further evaluation for PE is necessary (since the treatment of DVT and PE is essentially the same). However, *a negative evaluation for DVT does not exclude the diagnosis of acute PE*. When the search for leg vein thrombosis is unrevealing, the next step in the evaluation is determined by the presence or absence of lung disease (see Figure 6.2).

CT Angiography

In patients with lung disease (i.e., most patients in the ICU), the next step in the evaluation of suspected PE is to visualize the pulmonary arteries with computed tomographic (CT) angiography. This is a specialized method of CT that uses a spiral or helical scanner that rotates around the patient to produce a "volumetric" two-dimensional view of the lungs

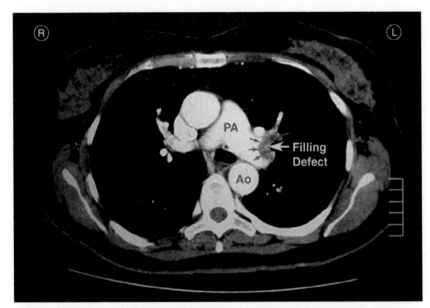

FIGURE 6.3 CT angiogram showing a pulmonary embolus (filling defect) in the left main pulmonary artery (PA). AO = aorta. Image digitally retouched.

(33). When spiral CT is combined with the peripheral injection of a contrast agent, the central pulmonary arteries can be visualized. Pulmonary emboli appear as filling defects, as shown in Figure 6.3.

Test Performance

In studies using newer, multidetector CT scans, CT angiography (CTA) has a sensitivity of 83%, a specificity of 96%, a positive predictive value of 86%, and a negative predictive value of 95% for the diagnosis of PE (34). Sensitivity is highest (> 90%) for detecting clots in the main pulmonary arteries, while, emboli in smaller, subsegmental vessels can be missed. However, the importance of detecting smaller, subsegmental emboli is questionable because withholding anticoagulant therapy based on a negative CT scan does not seem to adversely affect clinical outcomes (35).

One of the shortcomings of CTA is the risk of nephrotoxicity from the radiocontrast dye. This is particularly relevant in ICU patients, who often have one or more risk factors for dye-induced nephropathy (e.g., renal insufficiency, diabetes, volume depletion, etc.). In one study that included non-ICU patients, 18% of the patients with suspected pulmonary embolism were not eligible for CTA because of elevated serum creatinine levels (34). If CTA is necessary in a patient with mild renal compromise (a creatinine clearance > 60 mL/min) volume expansion and N-acetylcysteine can help to limit the risk of dye-induced nephrotoxicity (if you can convince the radiologist to perform the procedure). See Chapter 34 for more information on dye-induced renal injury.

Radionuclide Lung Scan

Ventilation-perfusion lung scans are widely used in the evaluation of suspected PE, but they secure the diagnosis in only about 25% to 30% of cases (36). The problem is the presence of lung disease (particularly infiltrative disease), which produces an abnormal scan in about 90% of cases (36). Lung scans are most helpful in patients with no underlying lung disease (which, unfortunately, excludes most ICU patients). If the decision is made to proceed with a lung scan, the results can be used as follows (36):

1. A normal lung scan excludes the presence of a pulmonary embolus, whereas a high-probability lung scan carries a 90% probability that a pulmonary embolus is present.

2. A low-probability lung scan does not reliably exclude the presence of a PE. However, when combined with a negative ultrasound evaluation of the legs, a low-probability scan is sufficient reason to stop the diagnostic workup and observe the patient.

3. An intermediate-probability or indeterminate lung scan has no value in predicting the presence or absence of a pulmonary embolus. In this situation, the options include spiral CT angiography (see Figure 6.2) or conventional pulmonary angiography (see next).

Conventional Pulmonary Angiography

Conventional pulmonary angiography is considered the most accurate method for detecting pulmonary emboli, and is reserved for cases where the other diagnostic tests are unable to confirm or exclude a pulmonary embolism that is highly suspected *and* associated with significant morbidity. Conventional angiography is rarely performed, in part because the other diagnostic tests are considered sufficient in most cases, and in part because the procedure is time-consuming and can be risky (i.e., in patients with right heart failure or renal insufficiency).

MANAGEMENT

The initial treatment of VTE that is not life-threatening is anticoagulation with one of the heparin preparations. The pharmacology and comparative features of unfractionated heparin and low-molecular-weight heparin (LMWH) have been described earlier in the chapter.

Unfractionated Heparin

For full anticoagulation, unfractionated heparin is administered as an intravenous bolus followed by a continuous infusion. Dosing based on body weight, like the regimen in Table 6.5, achieves more rapid anticoagulation than fixed-dosing regimens (37). The anticoagulant effect is monitored with the activated partial thromboplastin time (PTT); the target PTT is 46–70 seconds, or a PTT ratio (test/control) between 1.5 and 2.5 (3).

Table 6.5	Weight-Based Heparin Dosing Regimen

1. Give initial bolus dose of 80 IU/kg and follow with continuous infusion of 18 IU/kg/hr. (Use actual body weight.)

2. Check PTT 6 hrs. after start of infusion, and adjust heparin dose as indicated below.

PTT (sec)	PTT Ratio	Bolus Dose	Continuous Infusion
<35	<1.2	80 IU/kg	Increase by 4 IU/kg/hr
35–45	1.3–1.5	40 IU/kg	Increase by 2 IU/kg/hr
46–70	1.5–2.3	—	—
71–90	2.3–3.0	—	Decrease by 2 IU/kg/hr
>90	>3	—	Stop infusion for 1 hr. then decrease by 3 IU/kg/hr

3. Check PTT 6 hrs. after each dose adjustment. When in the desired range (46–70 sec), monitor daily.

From Reference 37.

Obesity

The weight-based dosing regimen in Table 6.5 was derived in patients weighing less than 130 kg (286 lbs.). For body weights in excess of 130 kg, this regimen can result in excessive anticoagulation (38). To avoid this problem, the adjusted body weight shown here is recommended for patients with morbid obesity (i.e., a body mass index or BMI $\geq$ 40 kg/m^2) (14).

$$\text{Adjusted weight (kg)} = \text{IBW} + 0.4 \times (\text{actual weight} - \text{IBW})$$

$$\text{Men: IBW (kg)} = 50 + 2.3 \times (\text{height} > 60 \text{ in})$$

$$\text{Women: IBW (kg)} = 45 + 2.3 \times (\text{height} > 60 \text{ in})$$

The adjusted body weight is almost halfway between the ideal body weight (IBW) and the actual body weight.

Heparin-Induced Thrombocytopenia

An antibody-mediated thrombocytopenia can appear 5–10 days after initiation of heparin therapy (or sooner with prior heparin exposure), and the resultant platelet clumping can lead to symptomatic venous and arterial thrombosis. This condition is described in detail in Chapter 19.

Reversing Heparin Anticoagulation

The anticoagulation effects of heparin can be rapidly reversed with protamine sulfate, a protein (from fish sperm) that binds to heparin and forms an inactive compound. An intravenous protamine dose of 1 mg will neutralize about 100 units of heparin within 5 minutes (3). The following are some recommendations for heparin reversal with protamine:

1. For IV-bolus heparin: if only a few minutes have elapsed, give 1 mg of protamine IV per 100 units of heparin administered; if 30 minutes have elapsed, give 0.5 mg of protamine IV per 100 units of heparin; if ≥2 hours have elapsed, give 0.25–0.375 mg of protamine IV per 100 units heparin administered (39).

2. For continuous-infusion heparin: use the heparin dose infused over the prior 2 hours and give 1 mg of protamine IV per 100 units heparin infused (3).

Protamine should be administered slowly (over 10 minutes) to minimize the risk of bradycardia and hypotension. Efficacy can be determined with an activated PTT drawn 5–15 minutes after drug administration (39). Hypersensitivity-like reactions (including anaphylaxis) can occur, and are more common in patients with allergic reactions to fish products or prior exposure to protamine-insulin preparations.

Low-Molecular-Weight Heparin

LMWH is an effective alternative to unfractionated heparin for treating DVT and PE (7). The therapeutic dose of the LMWH studied most extensively is shown below:

Enoxaparin: 1 mg/kg by subcutaneous injection every 12 hours. Reduce dose by 50% in patients with a creatinine clearance <30 mL/min; e.g., 1 mg/kg once daily (3).

As mentioned earlier, the predictable anticoagulant effects of LMWH obviates the need for routine monitoring of anticoagulant activity. In cases where anticoagulant monitoring may be necessary (e.g., in patients with renal failure or morbid obesity), the laboratory test of choice is the heparin-Xa (anti-Xa) level in plasma, which should be measured four hours after LMWH administration. The desired anti-Xa level is 0.6 to 1.0 units/mL for twice-daily enoxaparin dosing, and >1 unit/mL for once-daily enoxaparin dosing (3).

Although LMWH has several advantages over unfractionated heparin, continuous-infusion unfractionated heparin is preferred for treating VTE in the ICU because it is rapidly acting, can be reversed promptly with protamine, and does not require dose adjustment in patients with renal insufficiency. LMWH is more appropriate for non-ICU patients and outpatients.

Reversing LMWH Anticoagulation

There is no proven method of reversing anticoagulation with LMWH because protamine has variable efficacy in reversing the anti-Xa effects of LMWH. The following approach is recommended (3,39):

1. If less than 8 hours have elapsed since the last dose of LMWH, give IV protamine in a dose of 1 mg per 100 anti-Xa units of LMWH up to a maximum dose of 50 mg. (For enoxaparin, 1 mg is equivalent to

100 anti-Xa units.) If bleeding continues, a second protamine dose of 0.5 mg per 100 anti-Xa units of LMWH can be given.

2. If more than 8 hours have elapsed since the last dose of LMWH, give IV protamine in a dose of 0.5 mg per 100 anti-Xa units of LMWH (39).

Warfarin

Oral anticoagulation with warfarin should be started as soon as possible after the start of heparin anticoagulation. The initial dose is 5–10 mg daily for the first 2 days, with subsequent dosing tailored to the international normalized ratio (INR). The target INR is 2–3. When the INR reaches the therapeutic range, anticoagulation with unfractionated heparin or LMWH can be discontinued. Warfarin anticoagulation is primarily an outpatient management issue, and will not be described here. The management of warfarin-associated hemorrhage is described in Chapter 19. (For more information on warfarin anticoagulation, see Reference 40.)

Table 6.6	Thrombolytic Therapy in Acute Pulmonary Embolism

Indications:
    1. Pulmonary embolism with obstructive shock
    2. Pulmonary embolism with right ventricular dysfunction (?)
    3. No contraindication to thrombolytic therapy

Therapeutic Regimen:
    1. Continuous infusion heparin is used in conjunction with lytic therapy. Infusion can be continued during lytic drug delivery.
    2. Standard thrombolytic regimen:
        Alteplase: 100 mg infused over 2 hrs..
    3. Regimens aimed at accelerated clot lysis:
        Alteplase: 0.6 mg/kg infused over 15 min.
        Reteplase: 10 U by IV bolus and repeat in 30 min.
    4. Systemic drug administration is preferred to pulmonary artery instillation

Complications:
    1. Major hemorrhage: 9–12%
    2. Intracranial hemorrhage: 1–2%

From References 7, 8, 42, and 43.

Thrombolytic Therapy

Anticoagulation therapy for acute PE is aimed at preventing clot extension and recurrent embolism, but has little effect on disrupting the in situ embolus. In patients with life-threatening PE, clot dissolution with thrombolytic agents is a more appealing approach than anticoagulation, but has had limited success. Thrombolytic therapy can reduce right heart strain (8), but there is little or no improvement in survival (41). At the present time, thrombolytic therapy for patients with life-threatening PE is prompted more by desperation than by anticipation of a successful outcome.

The general features of thrombolytic therapy in acute PE are summarized in Table 6.6. The consensus indication for thrombolytic therapy is hemodynamic deterioration (obstructive shock), but thrombolytic therapy is also popular for patients with PE and right ventricular dysfunction (7,8). The standard thrombolytic regimen is a 2-hour infusion of alteplase (recombinant tissue plasminogen activator) (2,7). However, there are other drug regimens that may be better suited for rapid clot lysis, and these are included in Table 6.6 (42,43). Continuous-infusion heparin is used in conjunction with thrombolytic therapy, and the infusion can be continued during the thrombolytic treatment period (although it is frequently stopped and restarted after the lytic agents are given). Heparin therapy is particularly advantageous after thrombolysis because clot dissolution releases thrombin, and this can lead to thrombotic reocclusion of the involved vessel (44).

About 10–12% of patients experience a major bleeding episode after thrombolytic therapy, and 1–2% develop intracranial hemorrhage (7,8). However, the risk of major hemorrhage is usually not a concern when confronted with a PE that is an immediate threat to life.

Embolectomy

If you're lucky enough to work in a medical center with an experienced team that is readily available around-the-clock, embolectomy (either surgical or catheter-based) is an option for life-threatening PE, particularly when there is a contraindication to thrombolytic therapy (2). Survival rates of 83% have been reported with emergency embole ctomy (45).

Vena Cava Interruption

Mesh-like filters can be placed in the inferior vena cava to trap thrombi that break loose from leg veins and prevent them from travelling to the lungs (46). The clinical situations where these devices are used is described next.

Clinical Uses

Vena cava interruption is used in all the conditions listed below (44), which include recommended indications (A-1,A-2), reasonable indications (A-2, A-3), and debated indications (B).

  A. Patient has proximal DVT in the legs plus one of the following:

  1. An absolute contraindication to anticoagulation.

2. Pulmonary embolization during full anticoagulation.

3. A large, free-floating thrombus (i.e., the leading edge of the thrombus is not adherent to the vessel wall).

4. Limited cardiopulmonary reserve (i.e., unlikely to tolerate a pulmonary embolus).

B. Patient does not have a proximal DVT in the legs, but has a high risk of VTE and a high risk of hemorrhage from anticoagulant prophylaxis (e.g., traumatic brain or spinal cord injury).

Most of the debate about vena cava interruption concerns its use as a preventive measure in high-risk patients (condition B). The issues in this debate are beyond the reach of this text, and are described in references 46 and 47.

Design Features

Inferior vena cava (IVC) filters come in a variety of structural designs, and can be permanent, temporary, or optional (i.e., permanent or temporary). The grandfather of modern IVC filters is the Greenfield Filter shown in Figure 6.4, which was introduced in 1973 and continues to be used today (Boston Scientific, Natick, MA). Note the elongated, conical shape (like a badminton birdie), which allows the basket to fill to 75% of its capacity without compromising the cross-sectional area of the vena cava. This limits the risk of vena cava obstruction and leg edema, which was common with earlier "umbrella-shaped" IVC filters. The Greenfield Filter is a per-

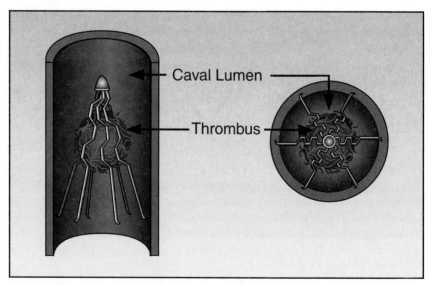

FIGURE 6.4 The Greenfield Filter. The struts have hooked ends to anchor the filter to the wall of the vena cava, and the elongated, conical shape allows the filter to trap blood clots without obstructing blood flow.

manent device, with hooked ends on the struts that anchor the filter to the wall of the vena cava. Removable IVC filters were introduced in 2003 (46).

IVC filters are inserted percutaneously, usually through the internal jugular vein or femoral vein, and are placed below the renal veins, if possible. Removable filters can be retrieved when the condition responsible for the insertion (e.g., bleeding from anticoagulation) is no longer present.

The Clinical Experience

Although not devoid of risk, IVC filters are remarkably safe and effective. The incidence of symptomatic PE after filter placement is about 5% (48), and troublesome complications (e.g., migration of the filter) are reported in less than 1% of cases (48). One of the intriguing features of IVC filters (which receives little attention) is the fact that they never seem to get infected, even when exposed to bacteremia.

A FINAL WORD

The experience with venous thromboembolism, which is far from satisfying, can be summarized as follows:

1. When you think it's there, it usually isn't (i.e., when a pulmonary embolism is suspected, the diagnosis is confirmed in as few as 10% of cases).

2. When you don't think it's there, it can be (i.e., in most cases of pulmonary embolism, the venous thrombosis is clinically silent prior to the embolic event).

3. When you finally find it, it may be too late (i.e., in massive pulmonary embolism, there is no treatment that consistently improves survival).

4. Because of the conditions stated above, the best approach to venous thromboembolism is to prevent it.

REFERENCES

Federal Reports

Shojania KG, Duncan BW, McDonald KM, et al, eds. Making healthcare safer: a critical analysis of patient safety practices. Evidence report/technology assessment No. 43. AHRQ Publication No. 01-E058. Rockville, MD: Agency for Healthcare Research and Quality, July, 2001.

Clinical Practice Guidelines

1. Guyatt GH, Aki EA, Crowther M, et al. Executive summary: Antithrombotic Therapy and Prevention of Thrombosis, 9th ed: American College of Chest Physicians Evidence-Based Clinical Practice Guidelines. Chest 2012; 141(Suppl):7S–47S.

2. Kearon C, Akl EA, Comerota AJ, et al. Antithrombotic therapy for VTE disease. Antithrombotic Therapy and Prevention of Thrombosis, 9th ed: American College of Chest Physicians Evidence-Based Clinical Practice Guidelines. Chest 2012; 141(Suppl):e419S–e494S.

3. Garcia DA, Baglin TP, Weitz JI, Samama MM. Parenteral anticoagulants. Antithrombotic Therapy and Prevention of Thrombosis, 9th ed: American College of Chest Physicians Evidence-Based Clinical Practice Guidelines. Chest 2012; 141(Suppl):e24S–e43S.

4. Geerts WH, Bergqvist D, Pineo GF, et. al. Prevention of venous thromboembolism. American College of Chest Physicians Evidence-Based Clinical Practice Guidelines (8th edition). Chest 2008; 133(Suppl):381S–453S.

Reviews

5. McLeod AG, Geerts W. Venous thromboembolism prophylaxis in critically ill patients. Crit Care Clin 2011; 27:765–780.

6. Magana M, Bercovitch R, Fedullo P. Diagnostic approach to deep venous thrombosis and pulmonary embolism in the critical care setting. Crit Care Clin 2011; 27:841–867.

7. Tapson VF. Treatment of pulmonary embolism: anticoagulation, thrombolytic therapy, and complications of therapy. Crit Care Clin 2011; 27:825–839.

8. Wood KE. Major pulmonary embolism. Crit Care Clin 2011; 27:885–906.

9. Linblad B, Eriksson A, Bergqvist D. Autopsy-verified pulmonary embolism in a surgical department: analysis of the period from 1951 to 1988. Br J Surg 1991; 78:849–852.

10. Heit JA, Silverstein MD, Mohr DM, et al. Risk factors for deep vein thrombosis and pulmonary embolism: a population-based case-control study. Arch Intern Med 2000; 160:809–815.

11. Cade JF. High risk of the critically ill for venous thromboembolism. Crit Care Med 1982; 10:448–450.

12. Collins R, Scrimgeour A, Yusuf S. Reduction in fatal pulmonary embolism and venous thrombosis by perioperative administration of subcutaneous heparin: overview of results of randomized trials in general, orthopedic, and urologic surgery. N Engl J Med 1988; 318:1162–1173.

13. King CS, Holley AB, Jackson JL, et al. Twice vs. three times daily heparin dosing for thromboembolism prophylaxis in the general medical population. A meta-analysis. Chest 2007; 131:507–516.

14. Medico CJ, Walsh P. Pharmacotherapy in the critically ill obese patient. Crit Care Clin 2010; 26:679–688.

15. Martel N, Lee J, Wells PS. The risk of heparin-induced thrombocytopenia with unfractionated and low-molecular-weight heparin thromboprophylaxis: a meta-analysis. Blood 2005; 106:2710–2715.

16. The PROTECT Investigators. Dalteparin versus unfractionated heparin in critically ill patients. N Engl J Med 2011; 364:1304–1314.

17. Enoxaparin. AHFS Drug Information, 2012. Bethesda, MD: American Society of Health System Pharmacists, 2012:1491–1501.

18. Rondina MT, Wheeler M, Rodgers GM, et al. Weight-based dosing of enoxaparin for VTE prophylaxis in morbidly obese, medical patients. Thromb Res 2010; 125:220–223.

19. Dalteparin. AHFS Drug Information, 2012. Bethesda, MD: American Society of Health System Pharmacists, 2012:1482–1491.

20. Douketis J, Cook D, Meade M, et al. Prophylaxis against deep vein thrombosis in critically ill patients with severe renal insufficiency with the low-molecular-weight heparin dalteparin: an assessment of safety and pharmacokinetics. Arch Intern Med 2008; 168:1805–1812.

21. Goldhaber SZ, Marpurgo M, for the WHO/ISFC Task Force on Pulmonary Embolism. Diagnosis, treatment and prevention of pulmonary embolism. JAMA 1992; 268:1727–1733.

22. Sachdeva A, Dalton M, Amarigiri SV, Lees T. Graduated compression stockings for prevention of deep vein thrombosis. Cochrane Database Syst Rev 2010; 7: CD001484

23. Kabrhel C, Camargo CA, Goldhaber SZ. Clinical gestalt and the diagnosis of pulmonary embolism. Chest 2005; 127:1627–1630.

24. Hoellerich VL, Wigton RS. Diagnosing pulmonary embolism using clinical findings. Arch Intern Med 1986; 146:1699–1704.

25. Stein PD, Goldhaber SZ, Henry JW. Alveolar-arterial oxygen gradient in the assessment of acute pulmonary embolism. Chest 1995; 107:139–143.

26. Kelly J, Rudd A, Lewis RR, Hunt BJ. Plasma D-dimers in the diagnosis of venous thromboembolism. Arch Intern Med 2002; 162:747–756.

27. Kollef MH, Zahid M, Eisenberg PR. Predictive value of a rapid semiquantitative D-dimer assay in critically ill patients with suspected thromboembolism. Crit Care Med 2000; 28:414–420.

28. Hyers TM. Venous thromboembolism. Am J resp Crit Care Med 1999; 159:1–14.

29. Tracey JA, Edlow JA. Ultrasound diagnosis of deep venous thrombosis. Emerg Med Clin N Am 2004; 22:775–796.

30. Gaitini D. Current approaches and controversial issues in the diagnosis of deep vein thrombosis via duplex doppler ultrasound. J Clin Ultrasound 2006; 34:289–297.

31. Girard P, Sanchez O, Leroyer C, et al. Deep venous thrombosis in patients with acute pulmonary embolism. Prevalence, risk factors, and clinical significance. Chest 2005; 128:1593–1600.

32. Kucher N. Deep-vein thrombosis of the upper extremities. N Engl J Med 2011; 364:861–869.

33. Remy-Jardin M, Remy J, Wattinine L, Giraud F. Central pulmonary thromboembolism: diagnosis with spiral volumetric CT with the single-breath-hold technique – comparison with pulmonary angiography. Radiology 1992; 185:381–387.

34. Stein PD, Fowler SE, Goodman LR, et al. Multidetector computed tomography for acute pulmonary embolism. N Engl J Med 2006; 354:2317–2327.

35. Quiroz R, Kucher N, Zou KH, et al. Clinical validity of a negative computed tomography scan in patients with suspected pulmonary embolism. JAMA 2005; 293:2012–2017.

36. The PIOPED Investigators. Value of the ventilation/perfusion scan in acute pulmonary embolism. Results of the prospective investigation of pulmonary embolism diagnosis (PIOPED). JAMA 1990; 263:2753–2759.

37. Raschke RA, Reilly BM, Guidry JR, et al. The weight-based heparin dosing nomogram compared with a "standard care" nomogram. Ann Intern Med 1993; 119:874–881.

38. Holliday DM, Watling SM, Yanos J. Heparin dosing in the morbidly obese patient. Ann Pharmacother 1994; 28:1110–1111.

39. Protamine Sulfate. AHFS Drug Information, 2012. Bethesda, MD: American Society of Health System Pharmacists, 2012:1618–1620.

40. Ageno W, Gallus AS, Wittkowsky A, et al. Oral anticoagulant therapy. Antithrombotic Therapy and Prevention of Thrombosis, 9th ed: American College of Chest Physicians Evidence-Based Clinical Practice Guidelines. Chest 2012; 141(Suppl):e44S–e88S.

41. Todd JL, Tapson VF. Thrombolytic therapy for acute pulmonary embolism: A critical appraisal. Chest 2005; 135:1321–1329.

42. Goldhaber SZ, Agnelli G, Levine MN. Reduced-dose bolus alteplase vs. conventional alteplase infusion for pulmonary embolism thrombolysis: an international multicenter randomized trial: the Bolus Alteplase Pulmonary Embolism Group. Chest 1994; 106:718–724.

43. Tebbe U, Graf A, Kamke W, et al. Hemodynamic effects of double bolus reteplase versus alteplase infusion in massive pulmonary embolism. Am Heart J 1999; 138:39–44.

44. Topol EJ. Acute myocardial infarction: thrombolysis. Heart 2000; 83:122–126.

45. Sareyyupoglu B, Greason KL, Suri RM et al. A more aggressive approach to emergency embolectomy for acute pulmonary embolism. Mayo Clin Proc 2010; 85:785–790.

46. Fairfax LM, Sing RF. Vena Cava Interruption. Crit Care Clin 2011; 27:781–804.

47. Young T, Tang H, Hughes R. Vena cava filters for the prevention of pulmonary embolism. Cochrane Database Syst Rev. 2010; 2:CD006212.

48. Athanasoulis CA, Kaufman JA, Halpern EF, et al. Inferior vena cava filters: review of 26-year single-center clinical experience. Radiology 2000; 216:54–66.

HEMODYNAMIC MONITORING

Not everything that counts can be counted.
And not everything that can be counted counts.

Albert Einstein

Chapter 7

ARTERIAL PRESSURE MONITORING

It should be clearly recognized that arterial pressure cannot be measured with precision by means of sphygmomanometers.

Committee for Arterial Pressure Recording,
American Heart Association, 1951

About 60 years have elapsed since the warning in the introductory quote, yet the same imprecise method continues to be the accepted standard for the measurement of arterial blood pressure (1). (This is not good news for the 75 million people in the United States with hypertension, who have a diagnosis that is based on a flawed measurement.) The accuracy of the standard (noninvasive) blood pressure measurement is even more of a problem in patients who are hemodynamically unstable (for reasons described later), and blood pressure monitoring in these patients often requires direct intra-arterial pressure recordings. This chapter describes the indirect and direct methods of blood pressure monitoring, and the problems associated with each method.

INDIRECT METHODS

Although the blood pressure measurement is one of the most frequently performed measurements in clinical practice, observational studies have shown that almost no one measures the blood pressure properly (i.e., according to the guidelines of the American Heart Association). In surveys that included primary care physicians, nurses, medical specialists, and surgeons (3), none of the examinees measured the blood pressure correctly (2,3). In one of these studies (3), only 3% of the general practitioners and 2% of the nurses obtained blood pressure measurements that were reliable (3).

The American Heart Association publishes guidelines for the indirect blood pressure measurement, and these are included in the bibliography at the end of this chapter (1). The principal recommendations from these guidelines are included in this section.

Sphygmomanometry

The indirect blood pressure is measured with a device called a *sphygmo-manometer* (sphygmos is the Greek term for pulse, and manometer is a pressure measuring device) which consists of an inflatable bladder covered by a cloth sleeve, and a gauge or column of mercury to measure pressure. The cloth sleeve is wrapped around the upper arm or thigh in an area that overlies a major artery (usually the brachial artery), and the bladder in the sleeve is inflated to compress the underlying artery.

The effects of arterial compression are illustrated in Figure 7.1. As the cuff pressure increases and the underlying artery is compressed, the pulsations in the artery gradually increase and then decrease until the artery is occluded. These "counterpulsations" produce oscillations in cuff pressure (as shown in the figure), and measuring these pressure oscillations is the basis for the *oscillometric method* of blood pressure recording. Counterpulsations can also be converted into sound waves, which is the basis for the *auscultation method* of measuring blood pressure.

Dimensions of the Bladder

Counterpulsations are more reproducible, and blood pressure measurements are more reliable, when an artery is compressed uniformly. The

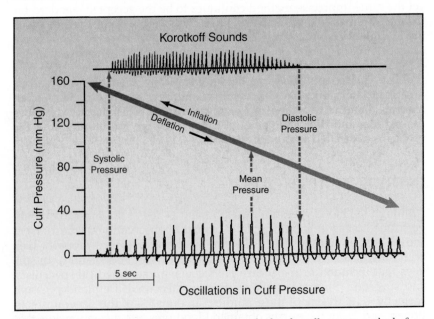

FIGURE 7.1 Comparison of the auscultation method and oscillometric method of blood pressure measurement. See text for explanation.

tendency for cuff inflation to produce uniform compression of an under-lying artery is determined by the dimensions of the inflatable bladder in the cuff and the circumference of the upper arm or thigh. The optimal relationships between the dimensions of the cuff bladder and the circum-ference of the upper arm are shown in Figure 7.2. To produce uniform arterial occlusion, the length of the bladder should be at least 80% of the circumference of the upper arm (measured midway between the shoul-der and elbow), and the width of the bladder should be at least 40% of the upper arm circumference (1). *If the cuff bladder is too small for the size of the upper arm, the pressure measurements will be falsely elevated* (1). Errors in measurement are much less pronounced when the cuff bladder is inap-propriately large relative to arm circumference.

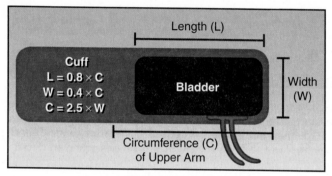

FIGURE 7.2 Optimal relationships between the width (W) and length (L) of the cuff bladder and the circumference (C) of the upper arm.

Miscuffing

A mismatch between cuff size and limb size (called miscuffing) *is the most common source of error in indirect blood pressure measurements* (1–4). To indi-cate the magnitude of this problem, one study showed that 97% of pri-mary care physicians routinely used blood pressure cuffs of inappropri-ate size (2). Most cases (80–90%) of miscuffing involve cuffs that are too small for the size of the upper arm (1,2). As an aid in selecting the appro-priate cuff size, Table 7.1 shows the recommended cuff sizes for upper arm circumferences ranging from 22 cm (about 9 inches) to 52 cm (about 21 inches). An easier way to determine the appropriate cuff size is de-scribed next.

Simple Method to Assess Cuff Size

Align the cuff so that the long axis runs along the long axis of the arm. Then turn the cuff over so the bladder on the underside is facing you, and wrap the cuff around the upper arm. The bladder (width) should encir-cle close to half (40%) of the upper arm (circumference). If the bladder encircles less than half of the upper arm, the cuff is too small, and the blood pressure measurement will be spuriously elevated. No change in cuff size is needed if the cuff bladder is too big (i.e., if it encircles more than half of the upper arm) because the errors in measurement in this situation are small or nonexistent (1).

Table 7.1	Appropriate Size of Blood Pressure Cuff in Relation to Upper Arm Circumference	
Upper Arm Circumference	**Blood Pressure Cuff**	
	Size	**Dimensions**
22 to 26 cm	Small Adult	12 × 24 cm
27 to 34 cm	Adult	16 × 30 cm
35 to 44 cm	Large Adult	16 × 36 cm
45 to 52 cm	Adult Thigh	16 × 42 cm

From Reference 1.

Auscultation Method

The auscultatory method used today is the same one introduced in 1904 by a Russian surgeon named Nicolai Korotkoff (5). This method is being replaced by the oscillometric method for noninvasive blood pressure measurements in the ICU, so it will not be described in detail here. The following are some salient points about the auscultatory method from the American Heart Association guidelines (1).

1. If the patient is in the sitting position, the arm and the back should be supported. Otherwise, the diastolic pressure reading can be falsely elevated.

2. Use the bell-shaped head of the stethoscope to listen for the sounds generated during cuff deflation (called Korotkoff sounds). These sounds have a very low frequency (25 to 50 Hz) (6), and the bell-shaped head of a stethoscope is a low-frequency transducer.

3. Don't place the head of the stethoscope under the blood pressure cuff, as this creates sounds during cuff deflation that will interfere with detection of the Korotkoff sounds.

4. The rate of cuff deflation should not exceed 2 mm Hg/sec. More rapid deflation rates can lead to underestimation of the systolic pressure and overestimation of diastolic pressure.

5. The disappearance of the Korotkoff sounds (Phase V) is used as the diastolic pressure. However, in high-output conditions (e.g., anemia, pregnancy), the sounds can continue long after cuff deflation. When this occurs, the diastolic pressure is indeterminate. In pregnancy, some recommend that the point where the Korotkoff sounds become muffled (Phase IV) be used as the diastolic pressure.

Oscillometric Method

First introduced in the mid-1970s, automated oscillometric devices have become the standard method of blood pressure monitoring in all areas of the hospital (including ICUs). As mentioned earlier, the oscillometric method is designed to measure pulsatile pressure changes that appear during arterial compression and decompression. As in the auscultation method, a cuff is wrapped around the upper arm and inflated to occlude the underlying brachial artery. As the cuff deflates and the artery re-opens, the pulsatile pressure changes illustrated in Figure 7.1 are transmitted from the artery to the blood pressure cuff. The pulsatile cuff pressures are then processed electronically to determine the mean, systolic, and diastolic pressures (7). The conversion of pulsatile pressures into the standard measures of blood pressure (i.e., systolic, diastolic, and mean pressures) is accomplished by proprietary algorithms that are developed by the companies that manufacture oscillometric recording devices. These algorithms can vary with each manufacturer, and their proprietary nature makes them unavailable for critical evaluation. This lack of standardization is a major problem with the oscillometric technique (7,8).

The most accurate measurement provided by the oscillometric method is the *mean arterial pressure*, which corresponds to the point where the pulsatile pressures reach maximum amplitude (see Figure 7.1). Mean pressures determined with the *maximum-amplitude algorithm* are often within 5 mm Hg of the intraarterial pressures (7). However, in patients with noncompliant arteries (e.g., elderly patients and those with peripheral vascular disease), mean pressures measured by oscillometry can be 40% lower than intraarterial pressures (1,7).

There is less agreement about the relationship of the systolic and diastolic pressures to the oscillations in cuff pressure. As a result, the systolic and diastolic pressures are less reliable than the mean pressure. The diastolic pressure is the most problematic because the arterial pulsations do not disappear at the diastolic pressure (unlike the disappearance of the Korotkoff sounds at the diastolic pressure), so it is difficult to determine exactly when the diastolic pressure occurs in relation to the oscillating cuff pressures.

Accuracy

The limited accuracy of indirect blood pressure measurements is magnified in critically ill patients, and this is demonstrated in Figure 7.3. The data in this figure is from two studies comparing direct intraarterial pressures with pressures obtained with the auscultation method (in patients with circulatory shock) and with the oscillometric method (in unselected ICU patients) (4,9). All auscultatory pressures differed from the intraarterial pressures by more than 10 mm Hg (which is the threshold for an unacceptable difference), and the discrepancy was more than 20 mm Hg in almost three-quarters of the measurements (auscultatory pressures were always lower than intraarterial pressures). The discrepancy for oscillometric pressures was unacceptable in 61% of measurements.

The particularly poor performance of the auscultatory method in patients with circulatory shock is the result of reduced systemic flow (from hypotension and vasopressors), which curtails the arterial counterpulsations and reduces the intensity of the Korotkoff sounds. Since reliable blood pressure measurements are essential in the management of circulatory shock (e.g., to guide fluid resuscitation), direct measurements of intraarterial pressure is the consensus recommendation.

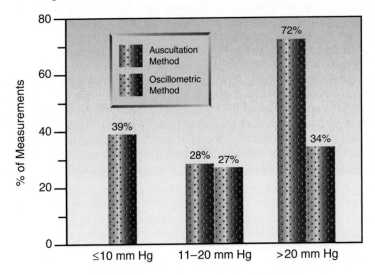

Discrepancy Between Indirect and Direct Measurements

FIGURE 7.3 Discrepancy between indirect and direct blood pressure measurements in critically ill patients. From References 4 and 9.

DIRECT MEASUREMENTS

Intraarterial pressure is typically measured from the radial, brachial, axillary, or femoral arteries. The arterial cannulation technique is not described here, but many of the practices related to arterial cannulation are similar to those described in Chapter 2 for central venous cannulation.

Systolic Amplification

The contour of the arterial pressure waveform changes as it moves away from the proximal aorta. This is shown in Figure 7.4. Note that as the pressure wave moves toward the periphery, the systolic pressure gradually increases and the systolic portion of the waveform narrows. The systolic pressure can increase as much as 20 mm Hg from the proximal aorta to the radial or femoral arteries (10). This increase in peak systolic pressure is offset by the narrowing of the systolic pressure wave, so the mean arterial pressure (described later) remains unchanged.

Reflected Waves

The increase in systolic pressure in peripheral arteries is the result of pressure waves that are reflected back from vascular bifurcations and narrowed blood vessels (11). Reflected waves move faster when the arteries are stiff, and they reach the arterial pressure waveform before it has time to decrement; the convergence of antegrade and retrograde pressure waves serves to heighten the peak of the antegrade pressure waveform. (You can see this effect when ocean waves meet from opposing directions, and this effect has been implicated in the formation of "monster waves".) *Amplification of the systolic pressure by reflected waves is the mechanism for systolic hypertension in the elderly* (11). Because systolic amplification is the result of retrograde pressure waves, it does not promote systemic blood flow.

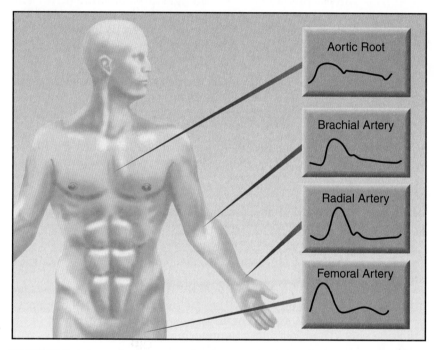

FIGURE 7.4 Arterial pressure waveforms at specific points along the arterial circulation.

Mean Arterial Pressure

The mean arterial pressure (MAP) is the time-averaged pressure in the major arteries, and is *the principal driving force for systemic blood flow* (10,12). The MAP is measured electronically as the area under the arterial pressure wave, divided by the duration of the cardiac cycle. When invasive monitoring is not available, MAP is often derived from the systolic and diastolic blood pressures (SBP and DBP) as follows (10): MAP = $\frac{1}{3}$ SBP + $\frac{2}{3}$ DBP. However, this relationship is based on the assumption that diastole accounts for two-thirds of the cardiac cycle, which occurs only when the heart rate is 60 beats/minute; a rarity in critically ill patients. Therefore, calculation of MAP is not advised in the ICU setting.

Determinants of Mean Pressure

Steady flow (Q) through a closed hydraulic circuit is directly related to the pressure gradient across the circuit ($P_{in} - P_{out}$), and inversely related to the resistance to flow (R) through the circuit. This relationship is described by the simplified equation shown below (which is the hydraulic equivalent of Ohm's Law).

$$Q = (P_{in} - P_{out}) / R \qquad (7.2)$$

If the hydraulic circuit is the circulatory system, volumetric flow becomes cardiac output (CO), the inflow pressure is the mean arterial pressure (MAP), the outflow pressure is the mean right atrial pressure (RAP), and the resistance to flow is the systemic vascular resistance (SVR). The equivalent relationships in the circulatory system are as follows:

$$CO = (MAP - RAP) / SVR \qquad (7.3)$$

Rearranging the terms then identifies the determinants of mean arterial pressure

$$MAP = (CO \times SVR) + RAP \qquad (7.4)$$

Right atrial pressure is negligible in most patients, and thus the RAP is often eliminated from the equation (when there is no right heart failure).

Circulatory Shock

The determinants of MAP in equation 7.4 are the basis for the three general types of circulatory shock; i.e.,

a. Low RAP = hypovolemic shock.

b. Low CO = cardiogenic shock

c. Low SVR = vasogenic shock (e.g., septic shock)

As such, the determinants of MAP are the central focus of the diagnostic approach to hypotension and circulatory shock. The management of circulatory shock requires close monitoring of MAP, preferably with intraarterial pressure recordings. A MAP ≥ 65 mm Hg is one of the endpoints of management (10,12).

Recording Artifacts

Fluid-filled recording systems can produce artifacts that further distort the arterial pressure waveform. Failure to recognize these artifacts can lead to errors in blood pressure management.

Resonant Systems

Vascular pressures are transmitted through fluid-filled plastic tubes that connect the arterial catheter to the pressure transducer. This fluid-filled system can oscillate spontaneously, and the oscillations can distort the arterial pressure waveform (13,14).

The performance of a resonant system is defined by two factors: the resonant frequency and the damping factor. The resonant frequency is the frequency of oscillations that occur when the system is disturbed. When the frequency of an incoming signal approaches the resonant frequency of the system, the resident oscillations add to the incoming signal and amplify it. This type of system is called an *underdamped* system. The damping factor is a measure of the tendency for the system to attenuate the incoming signal. A resonant system with a high damping factor is called an *overdamped* system.

Waveform Distortion

Three waveforms from different recording systems are shown in Figure 7.5. The waveform in panel *A*, with the rounded peak and the dicrotic notch, is the normal waveform expected from a recording system with no distortion. The waveform in panel *B*, with the sharp systolic peak, is from an underdamped recording system. Underdamped systems are popular for pressure recording because of their rapid response characteristics, but these systems can amplify the systolic pressure by as much as 25 mm Hg (15). The final waveform in panel *C* has an attenuated peak and a narrow

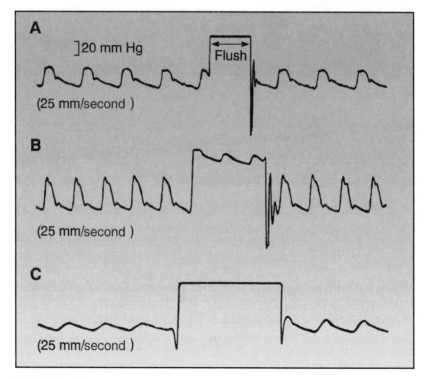

FIGURE 7.5 The rapid flush test. Panel *A*: Normal response; Panel *B*: Underdamped response; Panel *C*: Overdamped response. See text for explanation.

pulse pressure. This waveform is from an overdamped system. Overdamping reduces the gain of the system and attenuates the pressure waveform. Overdamping can be the result of partial obstruction of the catheter with a thrombus, or air bubbles in the recording circuit.

Fast Flush Test

A pressurized flush of the catheter-tubing system can also help to identify a recording circuit that is distorting the pressure waveform (14,15). Most commercially available transducer systems are equipped with a one-way valve that can be used to deliver a flush from a pressurized source. Figure 7.5 shows the results of a flush test in three different situations; the response when the flush is released will help characterize the system In panel *A*, the flush release is followed by a high-frequency burst. This is the normal behavior of a fluid-filled system. In panel *B*, the flush release produces a more sluggish frequency response. This is characteristic of an underdamped system, which will produce some degree of systolic amplification (as suggested by the narrowed peak on the pressure waveforms). The flush release in panel *C* does not produce oscillations. This is a sign of an overdamped system, which will attenuate the arterial pressure waveform and produce a spuriously low systolic pressure.

A FINAL WORD

> *Most ignorance is vincible ignorance; we don't know because*
> *we don't want to know.*
>
> Aldous Huxley

The most disturbing feature of indirect blood pressure (BP) measurements is not their limited accuracy, but the universal lack of competence in the methodology. In two studies presented earlier in the chapter (2,3), *no one* measured the blood pressure correctly! This is perplexing, unacceptable, and dangerous.

Because BP measurements are performed so frequently, the impact of false readings can be enormous. For example, about 85% of adults in the United States (about 180 million) have a BP measurement at least once yearly—if 3% of the measurements are falsely elevated (a common error), then as many as 5.4 million new cases of hypertension will be created each year. This would explain why there are currently 74.6 *million* adults in the United States with hypertension (17) (more than the entire population of France!).

The American Heart Association publishes guidelines for indirect blood pressure measurements (1), and you are urged to read these guidelines. And then read them again.

REFERENCES

Clinical Practice Guidelines

1. Pickering TG, Hall JE, Appel LJ, et al. Recommendations for blood pressure measurement in humans and experimental animals: Part 1: Blood pressure measurement in humans: a statement for professionals from the Sub-committee of Professional and Public Education of the American Heart Association Council on High Blood Pressure Research. Circulation 2005; 111:697–716.

Indirect Methods

2. McKay DW, Campbell NR, Parab LS, et al. Clinical assessment of blood pressure. J Hum Hypertens 1990; 4:639–645.

3. Villegas I, Arias IC, Bortero A, Escobar A. Evaluation of the technique used by health-care workers for taking blood pressure. Hypertension 1995; 26:1204–1206.

4. Bur A, Hirschl M, Herkner H, et al. Accuracy of oscillometric blood pressure measurement according to the relation between cuff size and upper-arm circumference in critically ill patients. Crit Care Med 2000; 28:371–376.

5. Shevchenko YL, Tsitlik JE. 90th anniversary of the development by Nicolai S. Korotkoff of the auscultatory method of measuring blood pressure. Circulation 1996; 94:116–118.

6. Ellestad MH. Reliability of blood pressure recordings. Am J Cardiol 1989; 63:983–985.

7. van Montfrans GA. Oscillometric blood pressure measurement: progress and problems. Blood Press Monit 2001; 6:287–290.

8. Smulyan S, Safar ME. Blood pressure measurement: retrospective and prospective views. Am J Hypertens 2011; 24:628–634.

9. Cohn JN. Blood pressure measurement in shock. JAMA 1967; 199:118–122.

Direct Measurements

10. Augusto J-L, Teboul J-L, Radermacher P, Asfar P. Interpretation of blood pressure signal: physiological bases, clinical relevance, and objectives during shock states. Intens Care Med 2011; 37:411–419.

11. Nichols WW, O'Rourke MF. McDonald's blood flow in arteries. 3rd ed. Philadelphia: Lea & Febiger, 1990; 251–269.

12. Shapiro DS, Loiacono LA. Mean arterial pressure: therapeutic goals and pharmacologic support. Crit Care Clin 2010; 26:285–293.

13. Gardner RM. Direct blood pressure measurement dynamic response requirements. Anesthesiology 1981; 54:227–236.

14. Darovic GO, Vanriper S, Vanriper J. Fluid-filled monitoring systems. In Darovic GO, ed. Hemodynamic monitoring. 2nd ed. Philadelphia: WB Saunders, 1995; 149–175.

15. Kleinman B, Powell S, Kumar P, Gardner RM. The fast flush test measures the dynamic response of the entire blood pressure monitoring system. Anesthesiology 1992; 77:1215–1220.

16. Roger VL, Go AS, Lloyd-Jones DM, et al. Heart disease and stroke statistics — 2011 update. Circulation 2011; 123:e18–e209.

Chapter 8

THE PULMONARY ARTERY CATHETER

A searchlight cannot be used effectively without a fairly thorough knowledge of the territory to be searched.

Fergus Macartney, FRCP

The pulmonary artery catheter is a versatile monitoring device that provides a wealth of information on cardiac performance and systemic oxygen transport. Introduced in 1970 (1), the catheter rapidly gained in popularity and became a staple in critical care management in the latter part of the twentieth century. Unfortunately, the benefits of the pulmonary artery catheter as a monitoring device have not translated into a survival benefit in most patients (2–4). As a result, the popularity of the catheter has declined precipitously over the past decade, and use of the catheter is currently reserved for cases of refractory heart failure or life-threatening hemodynamic instability of uncertain etiology (5,6).

This chapter presents the spectrum of hemodynamic parameters that can be monitored with pulmonary artery catheters. The physiologic relationships and clinical applications of these parameters are described in Chapters 9 and 10.

THE CATHETER

The pulmonary artery (PA) catheter was conceived by a cardiologist named Jeremy Swan (1), who designed a catheter that is equipped with a small inflatable balloon. When inflated, the balloon allows the flow of venous blood to carry the catheter through the right side of the heart and into one of the pulmonary arteries (like floating down a river on an inflatable rubber raft). This *balloon flotation* principle allows a right heart catheterization to be performed at the bedside, without fluoroscopic guidance.

Features

The basic features of a PA catheter are shown in Figure 8.1. The catheter is 110 cm long and has an outside diameter of 2.3 mm (about 7 French). There are two internal channels: one channel emerges at the tip of the catheter (the distal or PA lumen), and the other channel emerges 30 cm proximal to the catheter tip, which should be situated in the right atrium (the proximal or RA lumen). The tip of the catheter has a small inflatable balloon (1.5 mL capacity) that helps to carry the catheter to its final destination (as just described). When the balloon is fully inflated, it creates a recess for the tip of the catheter that prevents the tip from damaging the vessel wall as the catheter is advanced. A small thermistor (a temperature-sensing transducer) is placed near the tip of the catheter. This device is involved in the measurement of cardiac output, as described later in the chapter.

Placement

The PA catheter is inserted through a large-bore (8–9 French) introducer sheath that has been placed in the subclavian vein or internal jugular vein (see Figure 8.1). The distal lumen of the catheter is attached to a

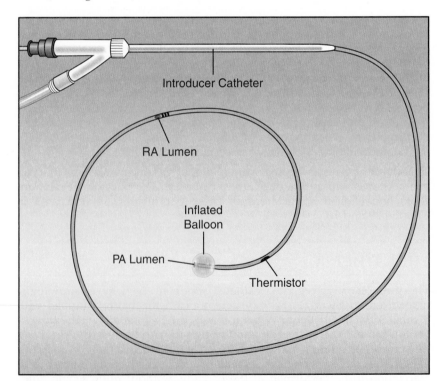

FIGURE 8.1 The basic features of a pulmonary artery (PA) catheter. Note that the PA catheter has been threaded through a large-bore introducer catheter that has a side-arm infusion port.

pressure transducer to monitor vascular pressures as the catheter is advanced. When the catheter is passed through the introducer sheath and enters the superior vena cava, a venous pressure waveform appears. When this occurs, the balloon is inflated with 1.5 mL of air, and the catheter is advanced with the balloon inflated. The location of the catheter tip is determined by the pressure tracings recorded from the distal lumen, as shown in Figure 8.2.

1. The superior vena cava pressure is identified by a venous pressure waveform, which appears as small amplitude oscillations. This pressure remains unchanged after the catheter tip is advanced into the right atrium.

2. When the catheter tip is advanced across the tricuspid valve and into the right ventricle, a pulsatile waveform appears. The peak (systolic) pressure is a function of the strength of right ventricular contraction, and the lowest (diastolic) pressure is equivalent to the right-atrial pressure.

3. When the catheter moves across the pulmonic valve and into a main pulmonary artery, the pressure waveform shows a sudden rise in diastolic pressure with no change in the systolic pressure. The rise in diastolic pressure is caused by resistance to flow in the pulmonary circulation.

4. As the catheter is advanced along the pulmonary artery, the pulsatile waveform disappears, leaving a nonpulsatile pressure that is typically at the same level as the diastolic pressure of the pulsatile waveform. This is the pulmonary artery wedge pressure, or simply the *wedge pressure*, and is a reflection of the filling pressure on the left side of the heart (see the next section).

5. When the wedge pressure tracing appears, the catheter is left in place (not advanced further). The balloon is then deflated, and the pulsatile pressure waveform should reappear. The catheter is then secured in place, and the balloon is left deflated.

On occasion, the pulsatile pressure in the pulmonary arteries never disappears despite advancing the catheter maximally (unexplained observation). If this occurs, the pulmonary artery diastolic pressure can be used as a surrogate measure of the wedge pressure (the two pressures should be equivalent in the absence of pulmonary hypertension).

THE WEDGE PRESSURE

The wedge pressure is obtained by slowly inflating the balloon at the tip of the PA catheter until the pulsatile pressure disappears, as shown in Figure 8.3. Note that the wedge pressure is at the same level as the diastolic pressure in the pulmonary artery. This relationship is altered in pulmonary hypertension, where the wedge pressure is lower than the pulmonary artery diastolic pressure.

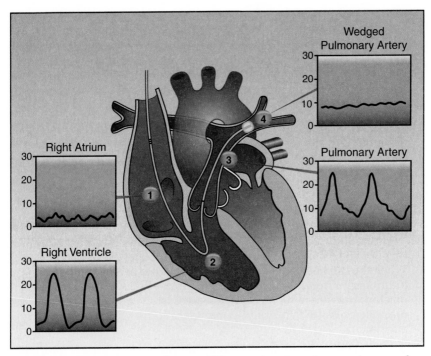

FIGURE 8.2 The pressure waveforms at different points along the normal course of a pulmonary artery catheter. These waveforms are used to identify the location of the catheter tip as it is advanced.

Wedge Pressure Tracing

The wedge pressure represents the venous pressure on the left side of the heart, and the magnified section of the wedge pressure in Figure 8.3 shows a typical venous contour that is similar to the venous pressure on the right side of the heart. The *a* wave is produced by left atrial contraction, the *c* wave is produced by closure of the mitral valve (during isometric contraction of the left ventricle), and the *v* wave is produced by systolic contraction of the left ventricle against a closed mitral valve. These components are often difficult to distinguish, but prominent *v* waves are readily apparent in patients with mitral regurgitation.

Principle of the Wedge Pressure

The principle of the wedge pressure is illustrated in Figure 8.4. When the balloon on the PA catheter is inflated to obstruct flow (Q=0), there is a static column of blood between the tip of the catheter and the left atrium, and the wedge pressure at the tip of the catheter (P_W) is equivalent to the pulmonary capillary pressure (P_c) and the pressure in the left atrium (P_{LA}). To summarize: if Q=0, then $P_W = P_c = P_{LA}$. If the mitral valve is behaving normally, the left atrial pressure (wedge pressure) will be equivalent to the end-diastolic pressure (the filling pressure) of the left

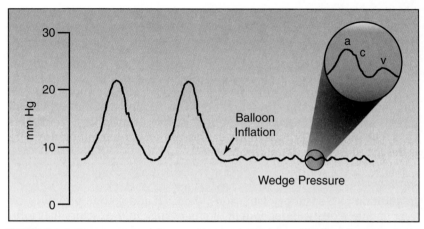

FIGURE 8.3 Pressure tracing showing the transition from a pulsatile pulmonary artery pressure to a balloon occlusion (wedge) pressure. The magnified area shows the components of the wedge pressure: *a* wave (atrial contraction), *c* wave (mitral valve closure), and *v* wave (ventricular contraction).

ventricle. Therefore, *in the absence of mitral valve disease, the wedge pressure is a measure of left ventricular filling pressure.*

Influence of Alveolar Pressure

The wedge pressure will reflect left atrial pressure only if the pulmonary capillary pressure is greater than the alveolar pressure ($P_c > P_A$ in Figure 8.4); otherwise the wedge pressure will reflect the alveolar pressure. Capillary pressure exceeds alveolar pressure when the tip of the PA

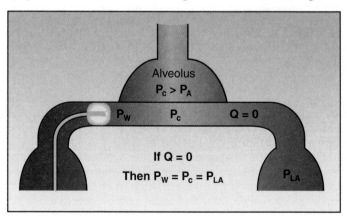

FIGURE 8.4 The principle of the wedge pressure measurement. When flow ceases because of balloon inflation (Q=0), the wedge pressure (P_W) is equivalent to the pulmonary capillary pressure (P_c) and the pressure in the left atrium (P_{LA}). This occurs only in the most dependent lung region, where the pulmonary capillary pressure (P_c) is greater than the alveolar pressure (P_A).

catheter is below the level of the left atrium, or posterior to the left atrium in the supine position. Most PA catheters enter dependent lung regions naturally (because the blood flow is highest in these regions), and lateral chest x-rays are rarely obtained to verify catheter tip position.

Respiratory variations in the wedge pressure suggest that the catheter tip is in a region where alveolar pressure exceeds capillary pressure (7). In this situation, the wedge pressure should be measured at the end of expiration, when the alveolar pressure is closest to atmospheric (zero) pressure. The influence of intrathoracic pressure on cardiac filling pressures is described in more detail in Chapter 9.

Spontaneous Variations

In addition to respiratory variations, the CVP and wedge pressures can vary spontaneously, independent of any change in the factors that influence these pressures. The spontaneous variation in wedge pressure is ≤4 mm Hg in 60% of patients, but it can be as high as 7 mm Hg (8). In general, *a change in the wedge pressure should exceed 4 mm Hg to be considered a clinically significant change.*

Wedge vs. Hydrostatic Pressure

The wedge pressure is often mistaken as the hydrostatic pressure in the pulmonary capillaries, but this is not the case (9,10). The wedge pressure is measured in the absence of blood flow. When the balloon is deflated and flow resumes, the pressure in the pulmonary capillaries (P_c) will be higher than the pressure in the left atrium (P_{LA}), and the difference in pressures will be dependent on the flow rate (Q) and the resistance to flow in the pulmonary veins (R_V); i.e.,

$$P_c - P_{LA} = Q \times R_V \qquad (8.1)$$

Since the wedge pressure is equivalent to left atrial pressure, Equation 8.1 can be restated using the wedge pressure (P_W) as a substitute for left atrial pressure (P_{LA}).

$$P_c - P_W = Q \times R_V \qquad (8.2)$$

Therefore *the wedge pressure and capillary hydrostatic pressure must be different to create a pressure gradient for venous flow to the left side of the heart.* The magnitude of this difference is unclear because it is not possible to determine R_V. However, the discrepancy between wedge and capillary hydrostatic pressures may be magnified in ICU patients because conditions that promote pulmonary venoconstriction (i.e., increase R_V), such as hypoxemia, endotoxemia, and the acute respiratory distress syndrome (11,12), are common in these patients.

Wedge Pressure in ARDS

The wedge pressure is used to differentiate hydrostatic pulmonary edema from the acute respiratory distress syndrome (ARDS); a normal wedge pressure is considered evidence of ARDS (13). However, since the capillary hydrostatic pressure is higher than the wedge pressure, *a normal wedge pressure measurement will not rule out the diagnosis of hydrostatic pulmonary edema.* Therefore, the use of a normal wedge pressure as a diagnostic criterion for ARDS should be abandoned.

THERMODILUTION CARDIAC OUTPUT

The ability to measure cardiac output increases the monitoring capacity of the PA catheter from 2 parameters (i.e., central venous pressure and wedge pressure) to at least 10 parameters (see Tables 8.1 and 8.2), and allows a physiologic evaluation of cardiac performance and systemic oxygen transport.

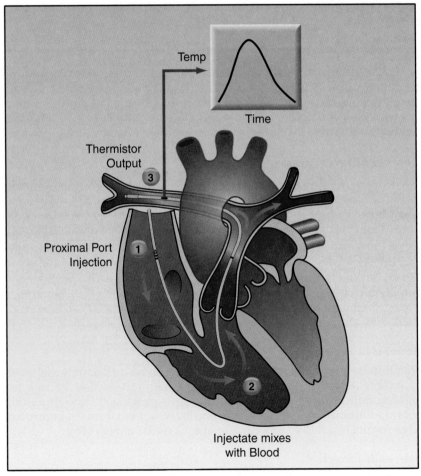

FIGURE 8.5 The thermodilution method of measuring cardiac output. See text for explanation.

The indicator-dilution method of measuring blood flow is based on the premise that, when an indicator substance is added to circulating blood, the rate of blood flow is inversely proportional to the change in concentration of the indicator over time. If the indicator is a temperature, the method is known as *thermodilution*.

The thermodilution method is illustrated in Figure 8.5. A dextrose or saline solution that is colder than blood is injected through the proximal port of the catheter in the right atrium. The cold fluid mixes with blood in the right heart chambers, and the cooled blood is ejected into the pulmonary artery and flows past the thermistor on the distal end of the catheter. The thermistor records the change in blood temperature with time; the area under this curve is inversely proportional to the flow rate in the pulmonary artery, which is equivalent to the cardiac output in the absence of intracardiac shunts. Electronic monitors integrate the area under the temperature–time curves and provide a digital display of the calculated cardiac output.

Thermodilution Curves

Examples of thermodilution curves are shown in Figure 8.6. The low cardiac output curve (upper panel) has a gradual rise and fall, whereas the high output curve (middle panel) has a rapid rise, an abbreviated peak, and a steep downslope. Note that the area under the low cardiac output curve is greater than the area under the high output curve (i.e., the area under the curves is inversely related to the flow rate).

Sources of Error

Serial measurements are recommended for each cardiac output determination. Three measurements are sufficient if they differ by 10% or less, and the cardiac output is taken as the average of all measurements. Serial measurements that differ by more than 10% are considered unreliable (14).

Variability

Thermodilution cardiac output can vary by as much as 10% without any apparent change in the clinical condition of the patient (15). Therefore, a change in thermodilution cardiac output should exceed 10% to be considered clinically significant.

Tricuspid Regurgitation

Regurgitant flow across the tricuspid valve can be common during positive-pressure mechanical ventilation. The regurgitant flow causes the indicator fluid to be recycled, producing a prolonged, low-amplitude thermodilution curve similar to the one in the bottom frame of Figure 8.6. This results in a falsely low cardiac output measurement (16).

Intracardiac Shunts

Intracardiac shunts produce falsely high thermodilution cardiac output measurements. In right-to-left shunts, a portion of the cold indicator

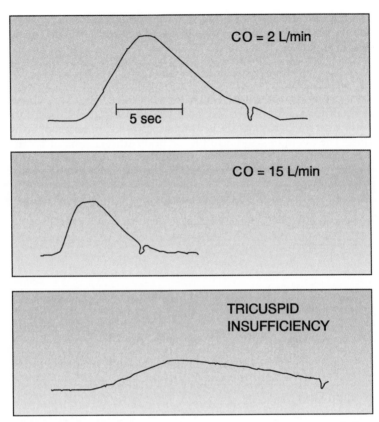

FIGURE 8.6 Thermodilution curves for a low cardiac output *(upper panel)*, a high cardiac output *(middle panel)*, and tricuspid insufficiency *(lower panel)*. The sharp inflection in each curve marks the end of the measurement period. CO = cardiac output.

fluid passes through the shunt, thereby creating an abbreviated thermodilution curve similar to the high-output curve in the middle panel of Figure 8.6. In left-to-right shunts, the thermodilution curve is abbreviated be-cause the shunted blood increases the blood volume in the right heart chambers, and this dilutes the indicator solution that is injected.

HEMODYNAMIC PARAMETERS

The PA catheter provides a wealth of information on cardiovascular function and systemic oxygen transport. This section provides a brief description of the hemodynamic parameters that can be measured or derived with the PA catheter. These parameters are included in Table 8.1.

Body Size

Hemodynamic parameters are often expressed in relation to body size, and the popular measure of body size for hemodynamic measurements is the body surface area (BSA), which can be determined with the following simple equation (17).

$$BSA (m^2) = Ht (cm) + Wt (kg) - 60/100 \qquad (8.3)$$

Why not use body weight to adjust for body size? BSA was chosen for hemodynamic measurements because cardiac output is linked to metabolic rate, and the basal metabolic rate is expressed in terms of body surface area. The average-sized adult has a body surface area of 1.7 m^2.

Table 8.1	Hemodynamic and Oxygen Transport Parameters	
Parameter	**Abbreviation**	**Normal Range**
Central Venous Pressure	CVP	0 – 5 mm Hg
Pulmonary Artery Wedge Pressure	PAWP	6 – 12 mm Hg
Cardiac Index	CI	2.4 – 4.0 L/min/m^2
Stroke Index	SI	20 – 40 mL/m^2
Systemic Vascular Resistance Index	SVRI	25–30 Wood Units[†]
Pulmonary Vascular Resistance Index	PVRI	1 – 2 Wood Units[†]
Oxygen Delivery (Index)	DO$_2$	520 – 570 mL/min/m^2
Oxygen Uptake (Index)	VO$_2$	110 – 160 mL/min/m^2
Oxygen Extraction Ratio	O$_2$ER	0.2 – 0.3

[†]mm Hg/L/min/m^2

Cardiovascular Parameters

The following parameters are used to evaluate cardiac performance and mean arterial pressure. The normal ranges for these parameters are included in Table 8.1. Parameters that are adjusted for body surface area are identified by the term *index*.

Central Venous Pressure

When the PA catheter is properly placed, the proximal port of the catheter should be situated in the right atrium, and the pressure recorded from this port should be the right atrial pressure (RAP). As mentioned previously, the pressure in the right atrium is the same as the pressure in the superior vena cava, and these pressures are collectively called the *central venous pressure* (CVP). In the absence of tricuspid valve dysfunction, the CVP should be equivalent to the right-ventricular end-diastolic pressure (RVEDP).

$$CVP = RAP = RVEDP \qquad (8.4)$$

The CVP is used as a measure of the right ventricular filling pressure. The normal range for the CVP is 0 – 5 mm Hg, and it can be a negative pressure in the sitting position. The CVP is a popular measurement in critical care, and is described in more detail in the next chapter.

Pulmonary Artery Wedge Pressure

The pulmonary artery wedge pressure (PAWP) is described earlier in the chapter. The PAWP is a measure of left-atrial pressure (LAP), which is equivalent to the left-ventricular end-diastolic pressure (LVEDP) when mitral valve function is normal.

$$\text{PAWP} = \text{LAP} = \text{LVEDP} \tag{8.5}$$

The wedge pressure is a measure of the left ventricular filling pressure. It is slightly higher than the CVP (to keep the foramen ovale closed), and the normal range is 6 – 12 mm Hg.

Cardiac Index

The thermodilution cardiac output (CO) is the average stroke output of the heart in one-minute periods. It is typically adjusted to body surface area (BSA), and is called the *cardiac index* (CI).

$$\text{CI} = \text{CO}/\text{BSA} \tag{8.6}$$

In the average-sized adult, the cardiac index is about 60% of the cardiac output, and the normal range is $2.4 - 4$ L/min/m^2.

Stroke Index

The heart is a stroke pump, and the stroke volume is the volume of blood ejected in one pumping cycle. The stroke volume is equivalent to the average stroke output of the heart per minute (the measured cardiac output) divided by the heart rate (HR). When cardiac index (CI) is used, the stroke volume is called the *stroke index* (SI).

$$\text{SI} = \text{CI}/\text{HR} \tag{8.7}$$

The stroke index is a measure of the systolic performance of the heart during one cardiac cycle. The normal range in adults is $20 - 40$ mL/m^2.

Systemic Vascular Resistance Index

The hydraulic resistance in the systemic circulation is not a measurable quantity for a variety of reasons (e.g., resistance is flow-dependent and varies in different regions). Instead, the systemic vascular resistance (SVR) is a global measure of the relationship between systemic pressure and flow. The SVR is directly related to the pressure drop from the aorta to the right atrium (MAP – CVP), and inversely related to the cardiac output (CI).

$$\text{SVRI} = (\text{MAP} - \text{CVP})/\text{CI} \tag{8.8}$$

The SVRI is expressed in Wood units (mm Hg/L/min/m^2), which can be multiplied by 80 to obtain more conventional units of resistance (dynes•sec^{-1}•cm^{-5}/m^2), but this conversion offers no advantage (18).

Pulmonary Vascular Resistance Index

The pulmonary vascular resistance (PVR) has the same limitations as mentioned for the systemic vascular resistance. The PVR is a global measure of the relationship between pressure and flow in the lungs, and is derived as the pressure drop from the pulmonary artery to the left atrium, divided by the cardiac output. Because the pulmonary artery wedge pressure (PAWP) is equivalent to the left atrial pressure, the pressure gradient across the lungs can be expressed as the difference between the mean pulmonary artery pressure and the wedge pressure (PAP – PAWP).

$$PVRI = (PAP - PAWP)/CI \qquad (8.9)$$

Like the SVRI, the PVRI is expressed in Wood units (mm Hg/L/min/m^2), which can be multiplied by 80 to obtain more conventional units of resistance (dynes•sec^{-1}•cm^{-5}/m^2).

Oxygen Transport Parameters

The oxygen transport parameters provide a global (whole body) measure of oxygen supply and oxygen consumption. These parameters are described in detail in Chapter 10 and are presented only briefly here.

Oxygen Delivery

The rate of oxygen transport in arterial blood is called the *oxygen delivery* (DO$_2$), and is the product of the cardiac output (or CI) and the oxygen concentration in arterial blood (CaO$_2$).

$$DO_2 = CI \times CaO_2 \qquad (8.10)$$

The O$_2$ concentration in arterial blood (CaO$_2$) is a function of the hemoglobin concentration (Hb) and the percent saturation of hemoglobin with oxygen (SaO$_2$): CaO$_2$ = 1.3 × Hb × SaO$_2$. Therefore, the DO$_2$ equation can be rewritten as:

$$DO_2 = CI \times (1.3 \times Hb \times SaO_2) \qquad (8.11)$$

DO$_2$ is expressed as mL/min/m^2 (if the cardiac index is used instead of the cardiac output), and the normal range is shown in table 8.1.

Oxygen Uptake

Oxygen uptake (VO$_2$), also called oxygen consumption, is the rate at which oxygen is taken up from the systemic capillaries into the tissues. The VO$_2$ is calculated as the product of the cardiac output (or CI) and the difference in oxygen concentration between arterial and venous blood (CaO$_2$ – CvO$_2$). The venous blood in this instance is "mixed" venous blood in the pulmonary artery.

$$VO_2 = CI \times (CaO_2 - CvO_2) \tag{8.12}$$

If the CaO_2 and CvO_2 are each broken down into their component parts, the VO_2 equation can be rewritten as:

$$VO_2 = CI \times 1.3 \times Hb \times (SaO_2 - SvO_2) \tag{8.13}$$

(where SaO_2 and SvO_2 are the oxyhemoglobin saturations in arterial and mixed venous blood, respectively). VO_2 is expressed as $mL/min/m^2$ (when the cardiac index is used instead of the cardiac output), and the normal range is shown in Table 8.1. An abnormally low VO_2 (< 100 $mL/min/m^2$) is evidence of impaired aerobic metabolism.

Oxygen Extraction Ratio

The oxygen extraction ratio (O_2ER) is the fractional uptake of oxygen from the systemic microcirculation, and is equivalent to the ratio of O_2 uptake to O_2 delivery. Multiplying the ratio by 100 expresses it as a percent.

$$O_2ER = VO_2 / DO_2 \ (\times 100) \tag{8.14}$$

The O_2ER is a measure of the balance between O_2 delivery and O_2 uptake. It is normally about 25%, which means that 25% of the oxygen delivered to the systemic capillaries is taken up into the tissues.

APPLICATIONS

Hemodynamic Patterns

Most hemodynamic problems can be identified by noting the pattern of changes in three hemodynamic parameters: cardiac filling pressure (CVP or PAWP), cardiac output, and systemic or pulmonary vascular resistance. This is demonstrated in Table 8.2 using the three classic forms of shock: hypovolemic, cardiogenic, and vasogenic. Each of these conditions produces a distinct pattern of changes in the three parameters. Since there are 3 parameters and 3 possible conditions (low, normal, or high), there are 3^3 or 27 possible hemodynamic patterns, each representing a distinct hemodynamic condition.

Table 8.2	Hemodynamic Patterns in Different Types of Shock		
Parameter	**Hypovolemic Shock**	**Cardiogenic Shock**	**Vasogenic Shock**
CVP or PAWP	Low	High	Low
Cardiac Output	Low	Low	High
Systemic Vascular Resistance	High	High	Low

Tissue Oxygenation

The hemodynamic patterns just described can identify a hemodynamic problem, but they provide no information about the impact of the problem on tissue oxygenation. The addition of the oxygen uptake (VO_2) will correct this shortcoming, and can help identify a state of clinical shock. Clinical shock can be defined as a condition where tissue oxygenation is inadequate for the needs of aerobic metabolism. Since a VO_2 that is below normal can be used as indirect evidence of oxygen-limited aerobic metabolism, a subnormal VO_2 can be used as indirect evidence of clinical shock. The following example shows how the VO_2 can add to the evaluation of a patient with cardiac pump failure.

Table 8.3	Compensated Heart Failure vs. Cardiogenic Shock
Heart Failure	**Cardiogenic Shock**
High CVP	High CVP
Low CI	Low CI
High SVRI	High SVRI
Normal VO_2	Low VO_2

Without the VO_2 measurement in Table 8.3, it is impossible to differentiate compensated heart failure from cardiogenic shock. This illustrates how oxygen transport monitoring can be used to determine the consequences of hemodynamic abnormalities on systemic oxygenation. Oxygen transport monitoring is described in more detail in Chapter 10.

A FINAL WORD

Despite the wealth of physiologically relevant information provided by the PA catheter, the catheter has been vilified and almost abandoned in recent years because clinical studies have shown added risk with little or no survival benefit, associated with use of the catheter (2–4). The following points are made in support of the PA catheter.

1. First and foremost, *the PA catheter is a monitoring device, not a therapy.* If a PA catheter is placed to evaluate a problem and it uncovers a disorder that is untreatable (e.g., cardiogenic shock), the problem is not the catheter, but a lack of effective therapy. Clinical outcomes should be used to evaluate therapies, not measurements.

2. In addition, surveys indicate that *physicians often don't understand the measurements provided by PA catheters* (19,20). Any tool can be a weapon in the wrong hands.

3. Finally, the incessant use of mortality rates to evaluate critical care interventions is problematic because *the presumption that every intervention has to save lives to be of value is flawed.* Interventions should (and

do) have more specific and immediate goals other than life or death. In the case of a monitoring device, the goal is to provide clinical information, and the PA catheter achieves this goal with distinction.

REFERENCES

1. Swan HJ. The pulmonary artery catheter. Dis Mon 1991; 37:473–543.

2. The ESCAPE Investigators. Evaluation study of congestive heart failure and pulmonary artery catheterization effectiveness: the ESCAPE trial. JAMA 2005; 294:1625–1633.

3. The NHLBI Acute Respiratory Distress Syndrome (ARDS) Clinical Trials Network. Pulmonary artery versus central venous catheter to guide treatment of acute lung injury. N Engl J Med 2006; 354:2213–2224.

4. Harvey S, Young D, Brampton W, et al. Pulmonary artery catheters for adult patients in intensive care. Cochrane Database Syst Rev 2006; 3:CD003408.

5. Chatterjee K. The Swan-Ganz catheters: past, present, and future. Circulation 2009; 119:147–152.

6. Kahwash R, Leier CV, Miller L. Role of pulmonary artery catheter in diagnosis and management of heart failure. Cardiol Clin 2011; 29:281–288.

7. O'Quin R, Marini JJ. Pulmonary artery occlusion pressure: clinical physiology, measurement, and interpretation. Am Rev Respir Dis 1983; 128:319–326.

8. Nemens EJ, Woods SL. Normal fluctuations in pulmonary artery and pulmonary capillary wedge pressures in acutely ill patients. Heart Lung 1982; 11:393–398.

9. Cope DK, Grimbert F, Downey JM, et al. Pulmonary capillary pressure: a review. Crit Care Med 1992; 20:1043–1056.

10. Pinsky MR. Hemodynamic monitoring in the intensive care unit. Clin Chest Med 2003; 24:549–560.

11. Tracey WR, Hamilton JT, Craig ID, Paterson NAM. Effect of endothelial injury on the responses of isolated guinea pig pulmonary venules to reduced oxygen tension. J Appl Physiol 1989; 67:2147–2153.

12. Kloess T, Birkenhauer U, Kottler B. Pulmonary pressure–flow relationship and peripheral oxygen supply in ARDS due to bacterial sepsis. Second Vienna Shock Forum, 1989:175–180.

13. Bernard GR, Artigas A, Brigham KL, et al. The American–European Consensus Conference on ARDS: definitions, mechanisms, relevant outcomes, and clinical trial coordination. Am Rev Respir Crit Care Med 1994; 149:818–824.

14. Nadeau S, Noble WH. Limitations of cardiac output measurement by thermodilution. Can J Anesth 1986; 33:780–784.

15. Sasse SA, Chen PA, Berry RB, et al. Variability of cardiac output over time in medical intensive care unit patients. Chest 1994; 22:225–232.

16. Konishi T, Nakamura Y, Morii I, et al. Comparison of thermodilution and Fick methods for measurement of cardiac output in tricuspid regurgitation. Am J Cardiol 1992; 70:538–540.

17. Mattar JA. A simple calculation to estimate body surface area in adults and its correlation with the Dubois formula. Crit Care Med 1989; 846–847.

18. Bartlett RH. Critical Care Physiology. New York: Little, Brown & Co, 1996:36.

19. Iberti TJ, Fischer EP, Liebowitz AB, et al. A multicenter study of physicians' knowledge of the pulmonary artery catheter. JAMA 1990; 264:2928–2932.

20. Gnaegi A, Feihl F, Perret C. Intensive care physicians' insufficient knowledge of right heart catheterization at the bedside: time to act? Crit Care Med 1997; 25:213–220.

Chapter 9

CARDIOVASCULAR PERFORMANCE

When is a piece of matter said to be alive?
When it goes on "doing something", moving,
exchanging material with its environment.

Erwin Schrodinger
What is Life? (1944)

The human organism has an estimated 100,000,000,000,000 cells that must go on exchanging material with the external environment to stay alive. This exchange is made possible by the human circulatory system: a closed hydraulic circuit with an automatic stroke pump that averages 100,000 strokes daily, a volumetric flow that averages 8,000 liters/day, and a network of conducting vessels that, if placed end-to-end, would stretch more than 60,000 miles (more than twice the circumference of the Earth!) (1). The design and performance of this circulatory system is a reminder of the following quote by Aristotle: *In all things of nature, there is something of the marvelous* (2).

This chapter describes the forces that govern blood flow through the circulatory system, both pulsatile flow (cardiac stroke output) and steady flow (peripheral blood flow), and the available methods for monitoring these forces in the clinical setting. Many of the concepts in this chapter are old friends from the physiology classroom.

VENTRICULAR PRELOAD

Definition of Preload

If one end of a muscle fiber is suspended from a rigid strut and a weight is attached to the free end of the muscle, the muscle will be stretched to a new length. The added weight in this situation represents a force called the *preload*. (The prefix *pre* indicates that the load is imposed prior to the onset of muscle contraction.) Preload is thus defined as the *force imposed on resting muscle that stretches the muscle to a new length.* According to the length-tension relationship of muscle, an increase in the length of a resting muscle will increase the strength of muscle contraction (because more cross-bridges are formed between contractile elements in the muscle) (3). Therefore, *the preload force acts to augment the strength of muscle contraction.*

Preload and Cardiac Performance

In the intact heart, the volume in the ventricles at the end of diastole is the force that stretches the resting muscle to a new length. Therefore, *the end-diastolic volume of the ventricles is the preload force of the intact heart* (3).

The influence of end-diastolic volume (preload) on cardiac performance is demonstrated in Figure 9.1. The lower curve shows the changes in end-diastolic pressure, which is a reflection of the distensibility of the ventricle , and the upper curve shows the peak pressure developed during systole. At any given end-diastolic volume, the increment from end-diastolic pressure to peak systolic pressure is a reflection of the strength of ventricular contraction. This increment in pressure increases as the end-diastolic volume increases, indicating that the preload force augments the strength of ventricular contraction. This relationship between preload and the strength of ventricular contraction was discovered independently by Otto Frank (a German engineer) and Ernest Starling (a British physiologist), and their discovery is commonly referred to as the *Frank-Starling relationship of the heart* (3). This relationship can be stated as follows: *In the normal heart, diastolic volume is the principal force that governs the strength of ventricular contraction* (3).

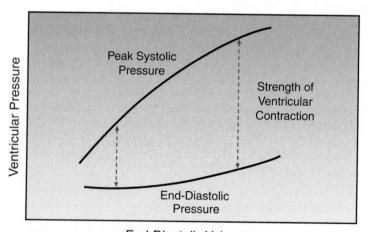

FIGURE 9.1 The influence of ventricular end-diastolic volume (preload) on end-diastolic pressure and peak systolic pressure. At any given end-diastolic volume, the increment from end-diastolic pressure to peak systolic pressure is a reflection of the strength of ventricular contraction during systole.

Clinical Measures

Ventricular end-diastolic volume is not easily measured at the bedside, and end-diastolic pressure is used as the clinical measure of ventricular preload. The end-diastolic pressure in the right and left ventricles is measured as follows:

1. The pressure in the superior vena cava, also called the central venous pressure (CVP), is equivalent to the right atrial pressure (RAP). In the absence of tricuspid valve dysfunction, the RAP is equivalent to the right ventricular end-diastolic pressure (RVEDP); i.e.,

$$CVP = RAP = RVEDP$$

Therefore, the CVP can be used as the filling pressure of the right ventricle when tricuspid valve function is normal.

2. The pulmonary artery wedge pressure (PAWP), which is described in the last chapter, is equivalent to the left atrial pressure (LAP). In the absence of mitral valve dysfunction, the LAP is equivalent to the left ventricular end-diastolic pressure (LVEDP); i.e.,

$$PAWP = LAP = LVEDP$$

Therefore, the wedge pressure can be used as the left ventricular filling pressure when mitral valve function is normal.

The reference ranges for the CVP and wedge pressures are shown in Table 9.1 (4,5). Note the very low pressure range for the CVP, which helps to promote venous return to the heart. Note also that the wedge pressure is slightly higher than the CVP; the higher pressure in the left atrium closes the flap over the foramen ovale and prevents right-to-left shunting in patients with a patent foramen ovale (about 30% of adults).

Table 9.1	Measures of Right and Left Ventricular Performance		
Parameter		**Abbreviation**	**Normal Range**
Right Ventricle			
End-Diastolic Pressure		RVEDP	0–5 mm Hg
End-Diastolic Volume		RVEDV	45–90 mL/m^2
Stroke Volume		SV	20–40 mL/m^2
Ejection Fraction		EF	≥44%
Left Ventricle			
End-Diastolic Pressure		LVEDP	6–12 mm Hg
End-Diastolic Volume		LVEDV	35–75 mL/m^2
Stroke Volume		SV	20–40 mL/m^2
Ejection Fraction		EF	≥55%

From Reference 4 and 5. End-diastolic volumes and stroke volumes are expressed relative to body surface area.

Ventricular Function Curves

The relationship between ventricular end-diastolic pressure and cardiac stroke output is described with *ventricular function curves* like the ones in Figure 9.2 (6). The principal feature of the normal curve is the steep slope, which results in a 2.5-fold increase in cardiac output over the normal range of right atrial pressure (0–5 mm Hg). This demonstrates the profound effect of ventricular filling on the strength of ventricular contraction, as predicted by the Frank-Starling relationship of the heart. The ventricular function curve is displaced downward in patients with heart failure, indicating that the strength of ventricular contraction is reduced at any given ventricular filling pressure in patients with heart failure.

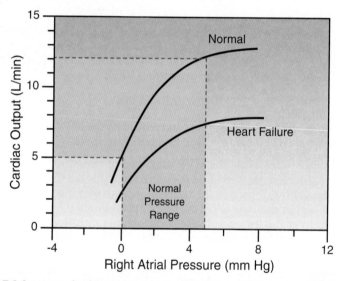

FIGURE 9.2 Ventricular function curves describing the relationship between right atrial pressure and cardiac output. Normal curve is redrawn from Reference 6.

End-Diastolic Pressure vs. Volume

Although the end-diastolic pressure is the clinical measure of preload, clinical studies have shown a poor correlation between end-diastolic pressure and end-diastolic volume (preload) (7–9). This is demonstrated in Figure 9.3, which shows the results of a study that compared measurements of right ventricular end-diastolic pressure (i.e., CVP) and right ventricular end-diastolic volume (RVEDV) before and after a volume challenge with isotonic saline (9). The graph on the left shows the corresponding measures of CVP and RVEDV prior to volume infusion, and the graph on the right shows the corresponding changes in CVP and RVEDV in response to the volume infusion. The distribution of data points in both graphs shows no relationship between CVP and RVEDV, or between changes in CVP and RVEDV. This is confirmed by the correlation coefficients (r) in the upper left corner of each graph. Similar results have been reported for the left ventricle (8,9). These studies indicate that *ventricular filling pressures (i.e., CVP and wedge pressures) are unreliable as surrogate measures of ventricular filling.*

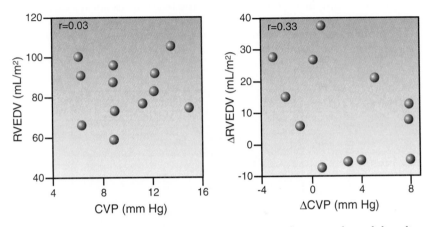

FIGURE 9.3 Graphs showing the relationships between right ventricular end-diastolic pressure (CVP) and right ventricular end-diastolic volume (RVEDV) in healthy adults who received a volume infusion with isotonic saline (3 liters over 3 hours). The graph on the left shows the baseline measurements of CVP and RVEDV, and the graph on the right shows the changes in CVP and RVEDV in response to the volume infusion. The correlation coefficients (r) are shown in the upper left corner of each graph. Graphs redrawn from Reference 9.

The poor correlation between end-diastolic pressures and volume in Figure 9.3 is particularly noteworthy because the subjects were healthy adults with normal cardiac function. When ventricular distensibility is impaired (i.e., diastolic dysfunction), which is common in critically ill patients (10), the discrepancy between end-diastolic pressures and volumes will be greater than usual. The influence of ventricular distensibility on diastolic pressure-volume relationships is described next.

Ventricular Compliance

Ventricular filling is influenced by the tendency of the ventricular walls to stretch during diastole (i.e., distensibility). The more popular term for distensibility is compliance. Ventricular compliance is derived as the ratio of associated changes in end-diastolic volume (ΔEDV) and end-diastolic pressure (ΔEDP):

$$\text{Compliance} = \Delta EDV / \Delta EDP \qquad (9.1)$$

A decrease in ventricular compliance will result in a greater change in EDP for a given change in EDV, or a smaller change in EDV for a given change in EDP.

The influence of compliance on diastolic pressure-volume relationships is shown in Figure 9.4 (11). The lower curve in this figure is from a control subject with no cardiac disease, and the upper curve is from a patient with hypertrophic cardiomyopathy. Note the increased slope of the curve for the hypertrophic cardiomyopathy, indicating a decrease in ventricular compliance. Comparing the position of the two curves shows that, at any given end-diastolic volume, the end-diastolic pressure is higher in the noncompliant ventricle. Therefore, *when ventricular compliance is reduced, the end-diastolic pressure will overestimate the end-diastolic volume.*

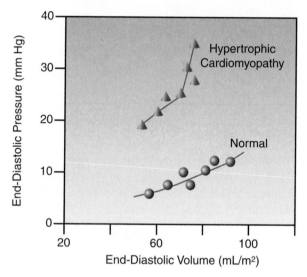

FIGURE 9.4 Diastolic pressure-volume curves for the left ventricle in a control subject and a patient with hypertrophic cardiomyopathy. Data from Reference 11.

Diastolic Heart Failure

In the early stages of cardiac disease where ventricular distensibility is impaired (i.e., diastolic dysfunction), ventricular end-diastolic volume is preserved but end-diastolic pressure rises. As the condition progresses, the progressive increase in end-diastolic pressure eventually results in a decrease in venous return, and this is accompanied by a decrease in ventricular filling and a subsequent decrease in cardiac output. When impaired ventricular distensibility compromises ventricular filling, the condition is known as *diastolic heart failure* (11,12).

Diastolic heart failure can be difficult to distinguish from heart failure due to contractile dysfunction (*systolic heart failure*) because both conditions are associated with increased end-diastolic pressures and a downward shift in the ventricular function curve. (In Figure 9.2, the lower "heart failure" curve could represent diastolic or systolic heart failure.) The changes in end-diastolic pressure (EDP), end-diastolic volume (EDV), and ventricular ejection fraction (EF) in the two types of heart failure are shown below (12):

Systolic Failure: High EDP / High EDV / Low EF

Diastolic Failure: High EDP / Low EDV / Normal EF

The EDV and EF can distinguish diastolic from systolic heart failure. (The EF, which is the ratio of stroke volume to end-diastolic volume, is the standard distinguishing feature. Table 9.1 includes the normal EF for the right and left ventricles). The fact that the EDP and EDV change in opposite directions in diastolic heart failure highlights the discrepancy be-tween EDP and ventricular preload (EDV) when ventricular compliance is reduced.

(Note: The terms "diastolic heart failure" and "systolic heart failure" have recently been abandoned. Diastolic failure is now called "heart failure with normal ejection fraction," and systolic failure is called "heart failure with a reduced ejection fraction." These two conditions will be described in more detail in Chapter 13.)

CENTRAL VENOUS PRESSURE

Despite the shortcomings of EDP as a measure of ventricular filling, CVP monitoring continues to be a popular practice in ICUs. However, errors in the CVP measurement are common (13), and this section highlights the potential sources of error.

The Catheter-Transducer Circuit

The catheters used for CVP monitoring are multilumen central venous catheters (15 to 20 cm in length) that are inserted in the subclavian or internal jugular veins and advanced into the superior vena cava. Peri-pherally inserted central catheters (PICCs) are not used for CVP monitoring because of concerns that the length of the catheters (up to 70 cm) will attenuate the pressure signal. However, there is a study showing that PICCs can provide accurate CVP measurements when a continuous infusion of saline (at rates comparable to those used for arterial catheters) is used to maintain catheter patency (14). Monitoring through PICCs is appealing because it eliminates the risks (i.e., arterial puncture and pneumothorax) associated with cannulation of the subclavian and internal jugular veins.

The Reference Level

The CVP is a hydrostatic pressure, so it is important that the fluid-filled transducer is at the same level as the right atrium. The traditional reference point for the right atrium is the intersection of the mid-axillary line (midway between the anterior and posterior axillary folds) and the fourth intercostal space, with the patient in the supine position. An alternative reference point that can be used in the semirecumbent position (up to 60°) is located 5 cm directly below the sternal angle (the angle of Louis), where the sternum meets the second rib (15).

Venous Pressures in the Thorax

The CVP and wedge pressure measurements can be misleading because the recorded pressure differs from the physiologically relevant pressure. This is demonstrated in the illustration in Figure 9.5. The pressure in the superior vena cava (the CVP) is recorded as an *intravascular pressure*; i.e., the pressure in the blood vessel relative to atmospheric (zero) pressure. However, the pressure that distends the ventricles to allow ventricular filling is the *transmural pressure*, which is the difference between the intravascular pressure and the surrounding intrathoracic pressure. Therefore, the recorded (intravascular) pressure will reflect the relevant (transmural) pressure only when the intrathoracic pressure is equivalent to atmospheric pressure. This normally occurs at the end of expiration. Therefore, the CVP and wedge pressure should be measured at the end of expiration.

Influence of Intrathoracic Pressure

When intrathoracic pressure changes (i.e., during spontaneous breathing or positive pressure ventilation), the pressure change can be transmitted into the lumen of the veins within the thorax, resulting in a change in the measured (intravascular) pressure without a change in the relevant

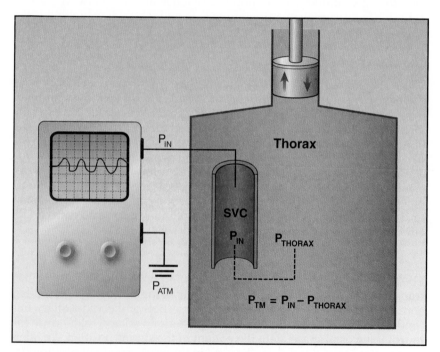

FIGURE 9.5 Illustration showing the difference between the intravascular pressure (P_{IN}) recorded electronically and the transmural pressure (P_{TM}) that is the responsible for distending the ventricles during diastole. P_{ATM} = atmospheric pressure; P_{THORAX} = intrathoracic pressure; SVC = superior vena cava.

(transmural) pressure. An example of this phenomenon is shown in the CVP tracing in Figure 9.6. The undulations in this tracing are the result of respiratory changes in intrathoracic pressure that are transmitted into the superior vena cava. Although the recorded (intravascular) pressure is changing, the relevant (transmural) pressure is unchanged. Therefore, *respiratory variations in the CVP (and wedge pressure) do not represent changes in ventricular filling pressure.* When respiratory variations are evident, the cardiac filling pressure should be measured at the end of expiration, when intrathoracic pressure is normally at atmospheric (zero) level. For the CVP tracing in Figure 9.6, which was recorded during positive-pressure ventilation, the end-expiratory pressure is the lowest pressure on the tracing, so the CVP is 0–3 mm Hg. When respiratory variations occur during spontaneous (negative pressure) breathing, the end-expiratory pressure will be the highest pressure in the tracing.

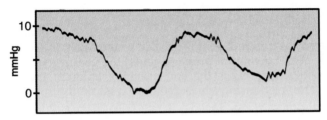

FIGURE 9.6 Respiratory variations in the central venous pressure (CVP).

Positive End-Expiratory Pressure (PEEP)

Positive end-expiratory pressure (PEEP) can falsely elevate the cardiac filling pressures at end-expiration because the intrathoracic pressure is higher than atmospheric pressure. When PEEP is applied during mechanical ventilation (which is a routine practice), the patient can be briefly disconnected from the ventilator to measure the CVP (16). For patients with "intrinsic PEEP" (caused by incomplete emptying of the lungs), accurate measurement of the cardiac filling pressures can be difficult (17). Chapter 28 includes a description of intrinsic PEEP, and a method for correcting the effect of intrinsic PEEP on the recorded filling pressures.

Variability

The CVP and wedge pressure can vary spontaneously by as much as 4 mm Hg (18), so changes in these pressures must exceed 4 mm Hg to be considered clinically significant.

VENTRICULAR AFTERLOAD

Definition of Afterload

When a weight is attached to one end of a contracting muscle, the force of muscle contraction must be enough to lift the weight before the muscle begins to shorten. The weight in this situation represents a force called the afterload, which is the load imposed on a muscle after the onset of muscle contraction. Unlike the preload force, which facilitates muscle contraction, the afterload force opposes muscle contraction. In the intact heart, *the afterload force is equivalent to the peak tension developed across the wall of the ventricles during systole* (3). Afterload is thus the wall stress associated with ejection of the stroke volume.

Law of Laplace

The determinants of ventricular wall tension are derived from observations on soap bubbles made by the Marquis de Laplace in 1820. His observations are expressed in the Law of Laplace, which states that the wall tension in a thin-walled sphere is directly related to the chamber pressure and the radius of the sphere: A modified version of the Laplace Law is shown below.

$$\text{Wall Tension} = (\text{pressure} \times \text{radius}) / (2 \times \text{wall thickness}) \qquad (9.2)$$

When the Laplace relationship is applied to the heart, the relevant pressure is the peak transmural pressure across the ventricle during systole, and the relevant radius is the end-diastolic radius of the ventricular chamber. The relationships in equation 9.2 allow the following statements:

1. The greater the peak transmural pressure during systole, the greater the wall stress.
2. The larger the ventricular chamber size, the greater the wall stress.
3. The greater the ventricular hypertrophy, the less the wall stress.

Components of Afterload

The forces that contribute to ventricular afterload can be identified by their relationship to the variables in the Laplace equation. This is demonstrated by the flow diagram in Figure 9.7. The component forces of ventricular afterload include end-diastolic volume (preload), pleural pressure, vascular impedance, and peripheral vascular resistance. Each of these forces is briefly described in this section.

Pleural Pressure

Since afterload is a transmural wall tension, it will be influenced by the pleural pressure surrounding the heart.

NEGATIVE PLEURAL PRESSURE: Negative pressure surrounding the heart will impede ventricular emptying by opposing the inward movement of the ventricular wall during systole (19,20). This effect is responsible for the transient decrease in systolic blood pressure that occurs during the inspiratory phase of spontaneous breathing. When the inspiratory drop

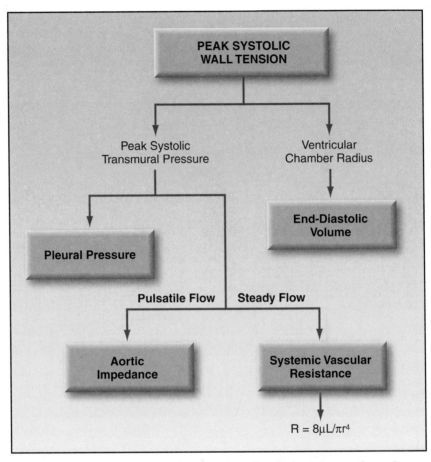

FIGURE 9.7 The forces that contribute to ventricular afterload. See text for explanation.

in systolic pressure is greater than 15 mm Hg, the condition is called "pulsus paradoxus" (which is a misnomer, since the response is not paradoxical, but is an exaggeration of the normal response).

POSITIVE PLEURAL PRESSURE: Positive pressures surrounding the heart will promote ventricular emptying by facilitating the inward movement of the ventricular wall during systole (19,21). This effect is responsible for the phenomenon shown in Figure 9.8. The tracings in this figure show the effect of a positive-pressure lung inflation on the arterial blood pressure. Note that when intrathoracic pressure rises during a positive-pressure breath, there is a transient rise in systolic blood pressure (reflecting an increase in the stroke output of the heart). The inspiratory rise in blood pressure during mechanical ventilation is known as "reverse pulsus paradoxus."

The "unloading" effect of positive intrathoracic pressure is the basis for the use of positive-pressure breathing as a "ventricular assist" maneuver for patients with advanced heart failure (21,22). The cardiovascular effects of mechanical ventilation are described in more detail in Chapter 25.

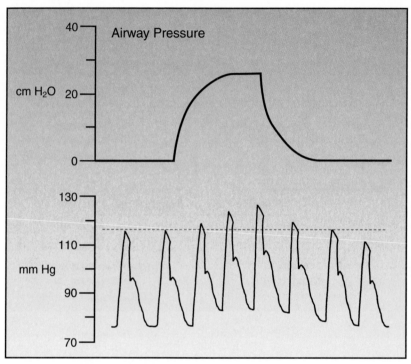

FIGURE 9.8 Changes in arterial blood pressure in response to a positive-pressure breath.

Vascular Components

The stroke output of the left ventricle produces pulsatile pressure and flow patterns in the aorta and major arteries, but the phasic changes in pressure and flow are progressively dampened as the blood moves peripherally, and by the time the blood reaches the small peripheral arterioles, pressure and flow are steady and non-pulsatile. The force that opposes pulsatile flow is known as *impedance,* and the force that opposes steady flow is *resistance.*

IMPEDANCE: Vascular impedance is the force that opposes the rate of change in pressure and flow, and it is expressed primarily in the large, proximal arteries, where pulsatile flow is predominant. Impedance in the ascending aorta is considered the principal afterload force for the left ventricle, and impedance in the main pulmonary arteries is considered the principal afterload force for the right ventricle (23). Vascular imped-ance is a dynamic force that changes frequently during a single cardiac cycle, and it is not easily measured in the clinical setting.

RESISTANCE: Vascular resistance is the force that opposes non-pulsatile or steady flow, and is expressed primarily in small, terminal blood vessels, where non-pulsatile flow is predominant. About 75% of the vascular resistance is in arterioles and capillaries (24). Vascular resistance is calcu-lated as described next, but the relevance of these calculations is ques-tioned.

Vascular Resistance

The resistance (R) to steady flow in a hydraulic circuit is directly related to the driving pressure across the circuit ($P_{in} - P_{out}$), and inversely relat-ed to the rate of steady flow (Q) through the circuit:

$$R = (\, P_{in} - P_{out}) \, / \, Q \qquad (9.3)$$

Applying these relationships to the systemic and pulmonary circulations yields the following equations for systemic vascular resistance (SVR) and pulmonary vascular resistance (PVR):

$$SVR = MAP - RAP \, / \, CO \qquad (9.4)$$

$$PVR = PAP - LAP \, / \, CO \qquad (9.5)$$

where MAP = mean arterial pressure, RAP = right atrial pressure, PAP = mean pulmonary artery pressure, LAP = left atrial pressure, and CO = cardiac output. The normal values for SVR and PVR are included in Table 8.1 in Chapter 8. As mentioned in that chapter, the PVR and SVR are not considered to be accurate representations of the resistance to flow in the pulmonary and systemic circulations (25). This is particularly the case in the systemic circulation, where the actual resistance to flow is an immeas-urable mix of flow resistances in multiple vascular beds.

Vascular Resistance and Afterload

Because vascular impedance is not easily measured, vascular resistance is often used as a clinical measure of ventricular afterload. However, ani-mal studies have shown a poor correlation between direct measures of ventricular wall tension (true afterload) and the calculated vascular resistance (26). This is consistent with the notion that vascular impedance (i.e., the force opposing pulsatile flow) is the principal afterload force for ventricular emptying (25). However, the contribution of vascular resist-ance to afterload cannot be determined with the SVR and PVR because these parameters do not represent the actual resistance to flow in the cir-culatory system. In the next section, the role of vascular resistance as a force that opposes cardiac output is described using the factors that determine vascular resistance.

PERIPHERAL BLOOD FLOW

As mentioned earlier, the design of the heart as an intermittent stroke pump results in a phasic or pulsatile pattern of pressure and flow in the large, proximal arteries. As the blood moves away from the heart, the arterial circuit acts to progressively dampen the pulsatile pattern of pressure and flow, culminating in a non-pulsatile or steady flow rate by the time the blood reaches the microcirculation. (Steady flow permits more efficient exchange in the microcirculation.) The pulsations in the proximal arteries represent wasted cardiac work (i.e., not involved in promoting capillary flow and exchange), whereas the maintenance of steady flow in peripheral blood vessels represents the energy-efficient portion of cardiac work.

Resistance to Steady Flow

Because flow in the peripheral circulation is predominantly non-pulsatile, it can be described with the Hagen-Poiseuille equation, which identifies the determinants of steady flow through small rigid tubes (27). This equation is shown below, and is also included in Chapter 1 to describe flow through vascular catheters.

$$Q = \Delta P \times (\pi\, r^4 / 8 \mu L) \tag{9.6}$$

According to this equation, steady flow (Q) through a rigid tube is directly related to the pressure gradient along the tube (ΔP) and the fourth power of the radius (r) of the tube, and is inversely related to the length (L) of the tube and the viscosity (μ) of the fluid. The final term in the equation is the reciprocal of resistance (1/R), so resistance to flow can be described as:

$$R = 8 \mu L / \pi r^4 \tag{9.7}$$

This equation identifies the radius of blood vessels as the single most important factor in determining the resistance to steady flow in the peripheral circulation; i.e., a two fold increase in vessel radius will result in a 16-fold increase in flow rate ($r^4 \times r^4 = r^{16}$). This highlights the importance of vasodilator therapy for promoting cardiac output in patients with heart failure.

Blood Viscosity

According to equations 9.6 and 9.7, steady flow will vary inversely with changes in the viscosity (μ) of blood. Viscosity is defined as the resistance of a fluid to changes in flow rate (28), and has also been called the "gooiness" of a fluid (29). The viscosity of whole blood is the result of cross-linking of erythrocytes by plasma fibrinogen, and the principal determinant of whole blood viscosity is the concentration of erythrocytes (the hematocrit). The influence of hematocrit on blood viscosity is shown in Table 9.2. Note that blood viscosity can be expressed in absolute or relative terms (relative to water). The viscosity of plasma (zero hematocrit) is only slightly higher than that of water, while the viscosity of whole blood at a normal hematocrit (45%) is about 3 times greater than plasma and about 4 times greater than water. The influence of hematocrit on blood viscosity is the single most important factor that determines the hemodynamic effects of anemia and blood transfusions (see later).

Table 9.2	Relationship Between Hematocrit and Blood Viscosity	
Hematocrit (%)	Relative Viscosity (water = 1)	Absolute Viscosity (centipoise)
0	1.4	—
10	1.8	1.2
20	2.1	1.5
30	2.8	1.8
40	3.7	2.3
50	4.8	2.9
60	5.8	3.8

From Documenta Geigy Scientific Tables. 7th Ed. Basel: Documenta Geigy, 1966:557–8.

Shear Thinning

The viscosity of some fluids varies inversely with changes in the velocity of flow (28). Blood is one of these fluids. (Another is ketchup, which is thick and difficult to get out of the bottle, but once it starts to flow, it thins out and flows more easily.) The velocity of blood flow increases as the blood vessels narrow (like the nozzle on a garden hose works), and the velocity of plasma increases more than the velocity of erythrocytes. This results in a relative increase in plasma volume (and a decrease in blood viscosity) in the small, peripheral blood vessels. This process is called *shear thinning* (shear is a tangential force that influences flow rate), and it facilitates flow through small vessels.

Influence on Cardiac Output

The influence of blood viscosity on cardiac output is shown in Figure 9.9. The data in this graph is from a patient with polycythemia who was treated with phlebotomy to achieve a therapeutic reduction in hematocrit and blood viscosity (30). The progressive decrease in hematocrit is associated with a steady rise in cardiac output, and the change in cardiac output is proportionally greater than the change in hematocrit. The disproportionate increase in cardiac output can be explained by the inverse relationship between blood viscosity and flow velocity; i.e., as cardiac output is increased in response to hemodilution, the increase in flow velocity will result in a further reduction in viscosity, which will then lead to a further increase in cardiac output, and so one. This process magnifies the influence of blood viscosity on cardiac output.

Clinical Relevance

Viscosity is rarely measured in the clinical setting because of the concern that in vitro measurements of viscosity do not take into account in vivo conditions like shear thinning that influence viscosity and blood flow. Despite the lack of meaningful measurements, viscosity is an important consideration for understanding the hemodynamic effects of conditions like anemia, blood transfusions, and dehydration.

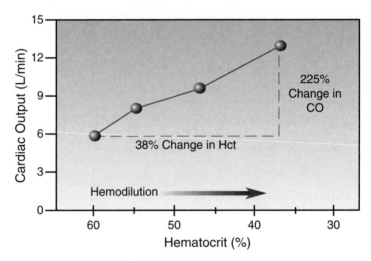

FIGURE 9.9 The influence of progressive hemodilution on cardiac output in a patient with polycythemia. CO = cardiac output. Data from Reference 30.

A FINAL WORD

One of the distinguishing features of critical care medicine is the opportunity to apply basic principles of cardiovascular and respiratory physiology to bedside patient care. This, of course, requires a working knowledge of the concepts in this chapter (and the ones in Chapters 10, 20, and 25). Some of the salient points in this chapter are summarized below.

1. The heart is a volume-regulated stroke pump, and the ventricular end-diastolic volume (preload) is the major determinant of the strength of ventricular contraction.

2. Ventricular filling pressures (i.e., the CVP and wedge pressure) are used as a surrogate measure of ventricular filling volumes, but are unreliable.

3. When ventricular compliance is reduced, which is common in critically ill patients, ventricular filling pressures will overestimate ventricular filling volumes.

4. Pleural pressure can have a significant effect on ventricular empty-ing. Negative pleural pressure impedes ventricular emptying, and positive pleural pressure promotes ventricular emptying.

5. Ventricular afterload has several component forces, and is not measurable.

REFERENCES

1. Vogel S. Vital circuits. New York: Oxford University Press, 1992:1–17.

2. Aristotle. De Partibus Animalum. circa 350 B.C.: p 645, first column, line 16.

Ventricular Preload

3. Opie LH. Mechanisms of cardiac contraction and relaxation. In Libby P, Bonow RO, Mann DL, Zipes DP (eds). Braunwald's Heart Disease: A Text-book of Cardiovascular Medicine. 8th ed., Philadelphia: Saunders Elsevier, 2008:509–539.

4. Rudski LG, Lai WW, Afilalo J, et al. Guidelines for the echocardiographic assessment of the right heart in adults: A report from the American Society of Echocardiography. J Am Soc Echocardiogr 2010; 23:685–713.

5. Lang RM, Bierig M, Devereux RB, et al. Recommendations for chamber quantification: A report from the American Society of Echocardiography's Guidelines and Standards Committee and the Chamber Quantification Working Group, in conjunction with the European Association of Echocar-diography. J Am Soc Echocardiogr 2005; 18:1440–1463.

6. Guyton AC, Jones CE, Coleman TH. Patterns of cardiac output curves. In Circulatory Physiology: Cardiac Output and its Regulation. 2nd ed., Philadelphia: W.B. Saunders, 1973:158–172.

7. Nahouraii RA, Rowell SE. Static measures of preload assessment. Crit Care Clin 2010; 26:295–305.

8. Hansen RM, Viquerat CE, Matthay MA, et al. Poor correlation between pul-monary arterial wedge pressure and left ventricular end-diastolic volume after coronary artery bypass graft surgery. Anesthesiology 1986; 64:764–770.

9. Kumar A, Anel R, Bunnell E, et al. Pulmonary artery occlusion pressure and central venous pressure fail to predict ventricular filling volume, cardiac per-formance, or the response to volume infusion in normal subjects. Crit Care Med 2004; 32:691–699.

10. Saleh M, Viellard-Baron A. On the role of left ventricular diastolic dysfunc-tion in the critically ill patient. Intensive Care Med 2012; 38:189–191.

11. Mandinov L, Eberli FR, Seiler C, Hess OM. Diastolic heart failure. Cardiovasc Res 2000; 45:813–825.

12. Paulus WJ, Tschope C, Sanderson JE, et al. How to diagnose diastolic heart failure: a consensus statement on the diagnosis of heart failure with normal left ventricular ejection fraction by the Heart Failure and Echocardiography Association of the European Society of Cardiology. Europ Heart J 2007; 28:2539–2550.

Central Venous Pressure

13. Figg KK, Nemergut EC. Error in central venous pressure measurement. Anesth Analg 2009; 108:1209–1211.

14. Black IH, Blosser SA, Murray WB. Central venous pressure measurements: peripherally inserted catheters versus centrally inserted catheters. Crit Care Med 2000; 28:3833–3836.

15. Magder S. Central venous pressure: A useful but not so simple measurement. Crit Care Med 2006; 34:2224–2227.

16. Pinsky M, Vincent J-L, De Smet J-M. Estimating left ventricular filling pressure during positive end-expiratory pressure in humans. Am Rev Respir Dis 1991; 143:25–31.

17. Teboul J-L, Pinsky MR, Mercat A, et al. Estimating cardiac filling pressure in mechanically ventilated patients with hyperinflation. Crit Care Med 2000; 28:3631–3636.

18. Nemens EJ, Woods SL. Normal fluctuations in pulmonary artery and pulmonary capillary wedge pressures in acutely ill patients. Heart Lung 1982; 11:393–398.

Ventricular Afterload

19. Pinsky MR. Cardiopulmonary interactions: the effects of negative and positive changes in pleural pressures on cardiac output. In Dantzger DR (ed). Cardiopulmonary critical care. 2nd ed. Philadelphia: WB Saunders, 1991:87–120.

20. Hausnecht N, Brin K, Weisfeldt M, Permutt s, Yin F. Effects of left ventricular loading by negative intrathoracic pressure in dogs. Circ Res 1988; 62:620–631.

21. Yan AT, Bradley TD, Liu PP. The role of continuous positive airway pressure in the treatment of congestive heart failure. Chest 2001; 120:1675–1685.

22. Boehmer JP, Popjes E. Cardiac failure: Mechanical support strategies. Crit Care Med 2006; 34(Suppl):S268–S277.

23. Nichols WW, O'Rourke MF. Input impedance as ventricular load. In: McDonald's Blood Flow in Arteries, 3rd ed. Philadelphia: Lea & Febiger, 1990:330–342.

24. Nichols WW, O'Rourke MF. The nature of flow of a fluid. In: McDonald's Blood Flow in Arteries, 3rd ed. Philadelphia: Lea & Febiger, 1990:27.

25. Pinsky MR. Hemodynamic monitoring in the intensive care unit. Clin Chest Med 2003; 24:549–560.

26. Lang RM, Borrow KM, Neumann A, et al. Systemic vascular resistance: an unreliable index of left ventricular afterload. Circulation 1986; 74:1114–1123.

Peripheral Blood Flow

27. Chien S, Usami S, Skalak R. Blood flow in small tubes. In Renkin EM, Michel CC (eds). Handbook of Physiology. Section 2: The cardiovascular system. Volume IV. The microcirculation. Bethesda: American Physiological Society, 1984:217–249.

28. Merrill EW. Rheology of blood. Physiol Rev 1969; 49:863–888.

29. Vogel S. Life in Moving Fluids. Princeton: Princeton University Press, 1981:11–24.

30. LeVeen HH, Ahmed N, Mascardo T, et al. Lowering blood viscosity to overcome vascular resistance. Surg Gynecol Obstet 1980; 150:139–149.

31. Lowe GOD. Blood rheology in vitro and in vivo. Bailleres Clin Hematol 1987; 1:597.

32. Reggiori G, Occhipinti G, de Gasperi A, et al. Early alterations of red blood cell rheology in critically ill patients. Crit Care Med 2009; 37:3041–3046.

Chapter 10

SYSTEMIC OXYGENATION

Oxygen may be necessary for life, but it doesn't prevent death.

P.L.M.

Critical care management is dominated by interventions that promote tissue oxygenation, yet there are no direct measurements of the oxygen tension in tissues. Instead, a variety of global, indirect measures of tissue oxygenation are used to guide aerobic support. This chapter describes these indirect measures, and how they are obtained. Because of the global nature of these measurements, the term *systemic oxygenation* seems more suitable for what is measured.

OXYGEN IN BLOOD

The oxygenation of arterial and venous blood is frequently involved in the evaluation of systemic oxygenation. The relevant measures of oxygen (O_2) in blood include the partial pressure of O_2 (PO_2), the O_2 saturation of hemoglobin (SO_2), the concentrations of hemoglobin-bound O_2 and dissolved O_2, and the total O_2 concentration (also called O_2 content). The normal values of these measures in arterial and venous blood are shown in Table 10.1.

Oxygenation of Hemoglobin

The oxygenation of hemoglobin is evaluated by the fraction of the hemoglobin in blood that is fully saturated with O_2. This is called the O_2 *saturation* (SO_2), and is the ratio of fully oxygenated hemoglobin to the total hemoglobin in blood.

$$SO_2 = \text{Oxygenated Hb/Total Hb} \qquad (10.1)$$

This ratio is typically reported as a percentage (the *percent saturation* of hemoglobin). The SO_2 can be measured using spectrophotometry (which is called oximetry, and is described in Chapter 21), or it can be estimated using the PO_2 of blood, as described next.

Table 10.1	Normal Measures of Oxygen in Arterial and Venous Blood	
Measure	**Arterial Blood**	**Venous Blood**
Partial Pressure of O_2	90 mm Hg	40 mm Hg
O_2 Saturation of Hb	98%	73%
Hb-Bound O_2	19.7 mL/dL	14.7 mL/dL
Dissolved O_2	0.3 mL/dL	0.1 mL/dL
Total O_2 Content	20 mL/dL	14.8 mL/dL
Blood Volume†	1.25 L	3.75 L
Total Volume of O_2	250 mL	555 mL

Values shown are for a body temperature of 37° C and a hemoglobin concentration of 15 g/dL.

†Volume estimates based on a total blood volume (TBV) of 5 Liters, arterial blood volume = 25% of TBV, and venous blood volume = 75% of TBV.

Abbreviations: Hb = hemoglobin; dL = deciliter (100 mL).

Oxyhemoglobin Dissociation Curve

The SO_2 is determined by the PO_2 in blood and the tendency of the iron moieties in hemoglobin to bind O_2. The relationship between SO_2 and PO_2 is described by the *oxyhemoglobin dissociation curve* like the one shown in Figure 10.1. The "S" shape of the curve offers two advantages. First, the arterial PO_2 (PaO_2) is normally on the upper, flat part of the curve, which means that a large drop in PaO_2 (down to 60 mm Hg) results in only minor changes in the arterial O_2 saturation (SaO_2). Secondly, the capillary PO_2 (which is equivalent to the venous PO_2 or PvO_2 after equilibration with the tissues) is on the steep portion of the curve, which facilitates the exchange of O_2 in both the pulmonary and systemic capillaries.

SHIFTS IN THE CURVE: A number of conditions can alter the affinity of hemoglobin for O_2 and shift the position of the oxyhemoglobin dissociation curve. These are listed in the boxes in Figure 10.1. A shift of the curve to the right facilitates oxygen release in the systemic capillaries, while a shift to the left facilitates oxygen uptake in the pulmonary capillaries. The position of the curve is indicated by the P_{50}, which is the PO_2 that corresponds to an O_2 saturation of 50%. The P_{50} is normally about 27 mm Hg (1), and it increases when the curve shifts to the right, and decreases when the curve shifts to the left. A decrease in the P_{50} to 15 mm Hg has been reported in blood that is stored in acid-citrate-dextrose (ACD) preservative for 3 weeks, due to a leftward shift in the oxyhemoglobin dissociation curve from depletion of 2,3 diphosphoglycerate (2,3-DPG) in the red blood cells (2).

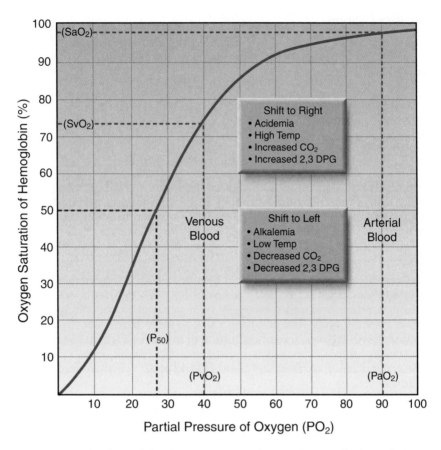

FIGURE 10.1 Oxyhemoglobin dissociation curve showing the normal relationship between the PO_2 in blood and the O_2 saturation of hemoglobin. The P_{50} is the PO_2 that corresponds to 50% saturation of hemoglobin with O_2. Abbreviations: PaO_2 = arterial PO_2; PvO_2 = venous PO_2; SaO_2 = arterial SO_2; SvO_2 = venous SO_2.

Shifts in the oxyhemoglobin dissociation curve have opposing effects in the pulmonary and systemic capillaries that seem to cancel each other. For example, a rightward shift of the curve caused by acidemia (the Bohr effect) will facilitate O_2 release in the systemic capillaries but will hinder O_2 uptake in the pulmonary capillaries. So what is the net effect of acidemia on tissue oxygenation? The answer is based on the influence of shifts in the oxyhemoglobin dissociation curve on different portions of the curve; i.e., shifts in the curve cause less of a change in the flat portion of the curve (where the arterial PO_2 and SO_2 reside) than in the steep portion of the curve (where the capillary PO_2 and SO_2 reside). Therefore, a rightward shift of the curve from acidemia will facilitate O_2 release in the systemic capillaries more than it hinders O_2 uptake in the pulmonary capillaries, and the overall effect benefits tissue oxygenation.

Oxygen Content

The concentration of O_2 in blood (called the O_2 *content*) is the summed contribution of the O_2 that is bound to hemoglobin and the O_2 that is dissolved in plasma.

Hemoglobin-Bound Oxygen

The concentration of hemoglobin-bound O_2 (HbO_2) is described by the following equation (3):

$$HbO_2 = 1.34 \times [Hb] \times SO_2 \ (mL/dL) \tag{10.2}$$

where: [Hb] is the concentration of hemoglobin in g/dL (grams per 100 mL), 1.34 is the O_2 binding capacity of hemoglobin, in mL/g (i.e., one gram of hemoglobin will bind 1.34 mL of O_2 when fully saturated), and SO_2 is the O_2 saturation, expressed as a ratio.

Dissolved Oxygen

Oxygen does not dissolve readily in plasma (which is why hemoglobin is needed as a carrier molecule). The solubility of O_2 in plasma is temperature-dependent, and varies inversely with a change in body temperature. At a normal body temperature (37°C), each increment in PO_2 of 1 mm Hg will increase the concentration of dissolved O_2 by 0.03 mL/L (4). This relationship is expressed as a *solubility coefficient* of 0.03 mL/L/mm Hg. The concentration of dissolved O_2 in plasma at 37° C is then described as follows:

$$\text{Dissolved } O_2 = 0.003 \times PO_2 \ (mL/dL) \tag{10.3}$$

(Note that the solubility coefficient is reduced by a factor of 10 so the units of dissolved O_2 are the same as those for hemoglobin-bound O_2.) This equation highlights the limited solubility of oxygen in plasma (see next).

Arterial O_2 Content

The O_2 content in arterial blood (CaO_2) is determined by combining equations 10.2 and 10.3 and inserting the SO_2 and PO_2 of arterial blood (SaO_2 and PaO_2).

$$CaO_2 = (1.34 \times [Hb] \times SaO_2) + (0.003 \times PaO_2) \tag{10.4}$$

As shown in Table 10.1, the normal arterial O_2 content is 20 mL/dL (or 200 mL/L), and only 1.5% (0.3 mL/dL) represents dissolved O_2. Note also that the total volume of O_2 in arterial blood is less than half the volume of O_2 in venous blood (!). This is a reflection of the uneven distribution of blood volume in the circulatory system, with 75% of the volume in the veins.

Venous O_2 Content

The venous O_2 content (CvO_2) represents the O_2 content in "mixed" venous blood (from the right heart or pulmonary artery). The equation describing CvO_2 is similar in format to equation 10.4, but the SO_2 and PO_2 are for mixed venous blood (SvO_2 and PvO_2).

$$CvO_2 = (1.34 \times [Hb] \times SvO_2) + (0.003 \times PvO_2) \qquad (10.5)$$

As shown in Table 10.1, the normal mixed venous O_2 content is about 15 mL/dL, and less than 1% (0.1 mL/dL) represents dissolved O_2. Note also that the difference between the arterial and venous O_2 content ($CaO_2 - CvO_2$) is 5 ml/dL, or 50 mL/L, which means that 50 mL of O_2 is extracted from each liter of blood flowing through the capillaries. At a normal cardiac output of 5 L/min, the O_2 extracted from capillary blood would be $5 \times 50 = 250$ mL/min, which is the normal O_2 consumption in an adult at rest. This demonstrates how *the oxygenation of blood can provide information about tissue oxygenation.*

Simplified O_2 Content Equation

The dissolved O_2 is such a small fraction of the total O_2 content that it is usually eliminated from the equation describing O_2 content, as shown below.

$$O_2 \text{ Content} = 1.34 \times [Hb] \times SO_2 \qquad (10.6)$$

The O_2 content of blood is thus equivalent to the Hb-bound O_2, as described in Equation 10.2.

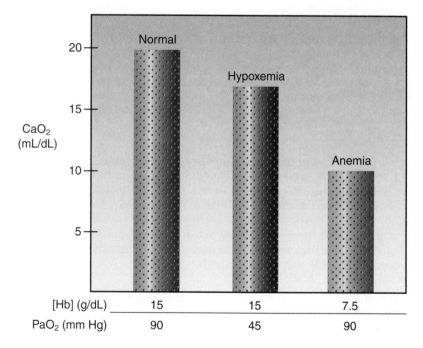

FIGURE 10.2 The effects of equivalent (50%) reductions in hemoglobin concentration [Hb] and arterial PO_2 (PaO_2) on the oxygen content in arterial blood (CaO_2).

Anemia vs. Hypoxemia

There is a tendency to use the arterial PO_2 (PaO_2) as an indication of how much O_2 is in the blood. However, the O_2 content of blood is determined primarily by [Hb], as shown in equation 10.6. The influence of proportional decreases in [Hb] and PaO_2 on the arterial O_2 content is shown in Figure 10.2. A 50% reduction in [Hb] (from 15 to 7.5 g/dL) results in an equivalent 50% reduction in CaO_2 (from 20 to 10 mL/dL), while a 50% reduction in the PaO_2 (from 90 to 45 mm Hg, which corresponds to a decrease in SaO_2 from 98% to 78%) results in only a 20% decrease in CaO_2 (from 20 to 16 mL/dL). This demonstrates that *anemia has a much greater influence on arterial oxygenation than hypoxemia*. The PaO_2 measurement is useful for evaluating gas exchange in the lungs (as described in Chapter 20), not for evaluating the oxygenation of blood.

SYSTEMIC OXYGEN BALANCE

Oxygen Transport & Energy Metabolism

The business of nutrient metabolism is to extract the energy stored in nutrient fuels (which is accomplished by disrupting high-energy carbon bonds) and transfer the energy to storage molecules like adenosine triphosphate (ATP). The energy yield from this process is determined by the balance between rate of O_2 transport to metabolizing tissues and the rate of metabolism. This balance is illustrated in Figure 10.3. Oxygen transport has two components: the rate of O_2 delivery to the microcirculation (DO_2), and the rate of O_2 uptake into the tissues (VO_2). When the VO_2 matches the metabolic rate (MR), glucose is completely oxidized to yield 36 ATP molecules (673 kcal) per mole. When VO_2 is less than the metabolic rate (i.e., when $VO_2 < MR$), some of the glucose is diverted to form lactate, and the energy yield falls to 2 ATP molecules (47 kcal) per mole.

Types of Hypoxia

The condition where the energy yield of nutrient metabolism is limited by the availability of oxygen is called *dysoxia* (5), and the clinical expression of this condition is multiorgan dysfunction progressing to multiorgan failure. Dysoxia can be the result of an inadequate supply of O_2, which results in tissue *hypoxia*, or it can be caused by a defect in oxygen utilization in the mitochondria, which is called *cytopathic hypoxia* (6,7). Tissue hypoxia is the mechanism of organ injury in hypovolemic and cardiogenic shock (6), whereas cytopathic hypoxia is operative in severe sepsis and septic shock (7).

As demonstrated in Figure 10.3, the DO_2 and VO_2 play an important role in determining the energy yield from nutrient metabolism. The remainder of this section will describe how the DO_2 and VO_2 are derived, and how the relationship between DO_2 and VO_2 can be used to evaluate the state of tissue oxygenation. These parameters require a measurement of cardiac output, which can be obtained using the thermodilution technique

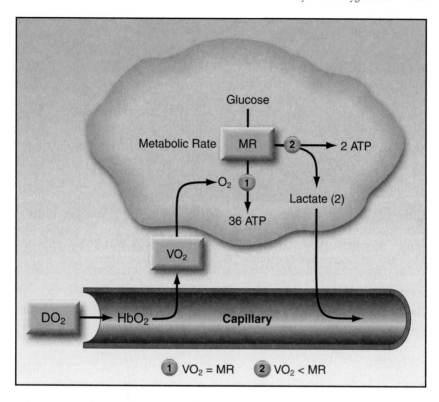

FIGURE 10.3 Illustration of the factors that determine the energy yield from glucose metabolism. When the rate of oxygen uptake (VO_2) into the tissues is unable to match the metabolic rate (MR), glucose metabolism is diverted to lactate production, and the energy yield drops dramatically. Abbreviations: DO_2 = rate of O_2 delivery; HbO_2 = oxygenated hemoglobin; ATP = adenosine triphosphate.

(described in Chapter 8) or a variety of noninvasive techniques (described in Reference 8). The normal range of values for the O_2 transport parameters are shown in Table 10.2.

Table 10.2	Oxygen Transport Parameters and Normal Range of Values	
Parameter	**Absolute Range**	**Size-Adjusted Range†**
Cardiac Output	5–6 L/min	2.4–4.0 L/min/m²
O_2 Delivery	900–1100 mL/min	520–600 mL/min/m²
O_2 Uptake	200–270 mL/min	110–160 mL/min/m²
O_2 Extraction Ratio	0.20–0.30	

†Size-adjusted values are the absolute values divided by the patient's body surface area in square meters (m²).

Oxygen Delivery (DO_2)

The rate of O_2 transport from the heart to the systemic capillaries is called the *oxygen delivery* (DO_2), and is a function of the cardiac output (CO) and the O_2 content of arterial blood (CaO_2) (9).

$$DO_2 = CO \times CaO_2 \times 10 \; (mL/min) \qquad (10.7)$$

(The multiplier of 10 is used to convert the CaO_2 from mL/dL to mL/L.) If the CaO_2 is broken down into its components ($1.34 \times$ [Hb] $\times SaO_2$), equation 10.7 can be rewritten as:

$$DO_2 = CO \times (1.34 \times [Hb] \times SaO_2) \times 10 \qquad (10.8)$$

Three measurements are needed to calculate the DO_2: cardiac output, hemoglobin concentration, and arterial O_2 saturation. The DO_2 in healthy adults at rest is 900–1100 mL/min, or 500–600 mL/min/m² when adjusted for body size (see Table 10.2).

Oxygen Uptake

The rate of O_2 transport from the systemic capillaries into the tissues is called the *oxygen uptake* (VO_2). Since oxygen is not stored in tissues, the VO_2 is also a global measure of the *oxygen consumption* of metabolizing tissues. The VO_2 can be described as the product of the cardiac output (CO) and the difference between arterial and venous O_2 content ($CaO_2 - CvO_2$).

$$VO_2 = CO \times (CaO_2 - CvO_2) \times 10 \; (mL/min) \qquad (10.9)$$

(The multiplier of 10 is included for the same reason as explained for the DO_2.) This equation is a modified version of the Fick equation for cardiac output (CO = $VO_2/CaO_2 - CvO_2$); using this equation to calculate the VO_2 is called the *reverse Fick method* (10). The CaO_2 and CvO_2 in equation 10.9 share a common term ($1.34 \times$ [Hb]), so the equation can be restated as:

$$VO_2 = CO \times 1.34 \times [Hb] \times (SaO_2 - SvO_2) \times 10 \qquad (10.10)$$

Four measurements are required to calculate the VO_2: the 3 measurements used for the DO_2 calculation, plus the O_2 saturation in "mixed" venous blood (SvO_2) in the pulmonary artery, which requires a pulmonary artery catheter. The VO_2 in healthy adults at rest is 200–300 mL/min, or 110–160 mL/min/m² when adjusted for body size (see Table 10.2).

Variability

Each of the 4 measurements used to derive the VO_2 has an inherent variability, and these are shown in Table 10.3 (10–12). The variability of the calculated VO_2 is ±18%, which is the summed variability of the component measurements. Therefore, *the VO_2 that is calculated from the modified Fick equation must change by at least 18% for the change to be considered significant.*

Fick Method vs. Whole Body VO$_2$

The calculated VO$_2$ from the modified Fick equation is not the whole body VO$_2$ because it *does not include the O$_2$ consumption of the lungs* (10,13,14). Normally, the VO$_2$ of the lungs accounts for less than 5% of the whole body VO$_2$ (13), but it can make up 20% of the whole body VO$_2$ when there is inflammation in the lungs (which is common in ICU patients) (14).

WHOLE BODY VO$_2$: The whole body VO$_2$ is measured by monitoring the O$_2$ concentration in inhaled and exhaled gas. This requires a specialized instrument equipped with an oxygen analyzer (such as the metabolic carts used by nutrition support services). The instrument is connected to the proximal airway (usually in intubated patients), and it records the VO$_2$ as the product of minute ventilation (VE) and the fractional concentration of O$_2$ in inhaled and exhaled gas (FiO$_2$ and FeO$_2$).

$$VO_2 = VE \times (FiO_2 - FeO_2) \qquad (10.11)$$

The measured (whole body) VO$_2$ has a variability of $\pm 5\%$ (10,12), which is much less than the variability of the calculated VO$_2$, as shown in Table 10.3. The major drawback of the measured VO$_2$ is the need for specialized equipment and trained personnel, which is costly and limits the availability of the measurement.

Table 10.3	Variability of Measurements Related to VO$_2$
Measurement	**Variability**
Thermodilution	$\pm 10\%$
Hemoglobin Concentration	$\pm 2\%$
O$_2$ Saturation of Hemoglobin	$\pm 2\%$
O$_2$ Content of Blood	$\pm 4\%$
CaO$_2$ – CvO$_2$	$\pm 8\%$
Calculated VO$_2$	$\pm 18\%$
Measured VO$_2$	$\pm 5\%$

From References 10–12.

Using the VO$_2$

The two conditions associated with a low VO$_2$ are a decreased metabolic rate (hypometabolism) and inadequate tissue oxygenation resulting in anaerobic metabolism. Since hypometabolism is uncommon in ICU patients, *an abnormally low VO$_2$ (< 200 mL/min or < 110 mL/min/m^2) can be used as evidence of inadequate tissue oxygenation.* An example of this is shown in Figure 10.4, which shows serial measurements of cardiac index (CI), systemic O$_2$ uptake (VO$_2$), and serum lactate levels during the first postoperative day in a patient who underwent an abdominal aortic aneurysm repair. Note that the VO_2 is abnormally low throughout the study period, while the serum lactate began to rise above normal (> 4 mM/L) at the 8th postoperative hour. The abnormally low VO_2 represents inadequate tissue oxygenation, as confirmed by the eventual rise in blood lactate levels. However, there is a lag time of 6 hours from the first evidence of a low VO_2 to the first evidence of an elevated lactate level. This indicates that *the VO_2 may be a more sensitive marker of inadequate tissue oxygenation than the serum lactate level.* Note that the cardiac index remains in the normal range despite the evidence of impaired tissue oxygenation, demonstrating the nonvalue of cardiac output monitoring for evaluating tissue oxygenation.

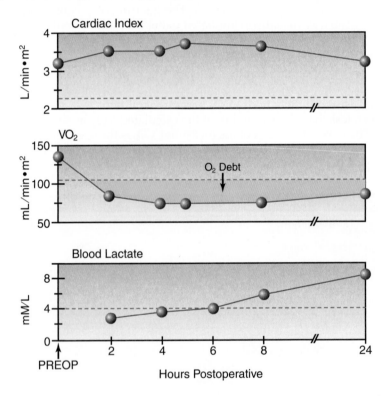

FIGURE 10.4 Serial measurements of cardiac index, systemic O_2 uptake (VO_2), and blood lactate levels in the postoperative period following an abdominal aortic aneurysm repair. The dotted lines indicate the upper or lower limits of normal for each measurement. The shaded area represents the oxygen debt.

OXYGEN DEBT: The shaded area in the VO_2 curve in Figure 10.4 shows the magnitude of the VO_2 deficit over time. The cumulative deficit in tissue oxygenation is called the *oxygen debt*, and clinical studies have shown a direct relationship between the size of the oxygen debt and the risk of multiorgan failure (15,16).

Oxygen Extraction

The fractional uptake of O_2 into tissues is determined with the oxygen extraction ratio (O_2ER), which is the ratio of O_2 uptake (VO_2) to O_2 delivery (DO_2).

$$O_2ER = VO_2/DO_2 \tag{10.12}$$

This ratio can be multiplied by 100 and expressed as a percentage. The VO_2 and DO_2 share common terms ($Q \times 1.34 \times [Hb] \times 10$), which allows equation 10.12 to be restated as follows:

$$O_2ER = (SaO_2 - SvO_2)/SaO_2 \tag{10.13}$$

Maintaining an SaO_2 above 0.9 (90%) is a standard practice, so the denominator in equation 10.13 can be eliminated; i.e.,

$$O_2ER = (SaO_2 - SvO_2) \tag{10.14}$$

When arterial blood is fully oxygenated ($SaO_2 = 1$), the O_2ER is determined by a single variable, as shown below:

$$O_2ER = 1 - SvO_2. \tag{10.15}$$

The VO_2 is normally about 25% of the DO_2, so the normal O_2ER is 0.25 (range = 0.2–0.3, as shown in Table 10.2). Thus, only 25% of the O_2 delivered to the capillaries is taken up into the tissues when conditions are normal. This changes when O_2 delivery is reduced, as described next.

Control of VO_2

The oxygen transport system operates to maintain a constant VO_2 in the face of variations in O_2 delivery (DO_2), and this is accomplished by compensatory changes in the O_2 extraction (17). This control system is described by rearranging the terms in equation 10.12 so that VO_2 is the dependent variable:

$$VO_2 = DO_2 \times O_2ER \tag{10.16}$$

This equation predicts that the VO_2 will remain constant when DO_2 is decreased if there is an equivalent increase in O_2 extraction. However, if O_2 extraction is fixed, a decrease in DO_2 will result in an equivalent decrease in VO_2.

The control of VO_2 is demonstrated by the relationship between DO_2 and VO_2 in Figure 10.5 (17). O_2 extraction is represented by the ($SaO_2 - SvO_2$) difference because the SaO2 is above 90%. At the normal point on the curve, the ($SaO_2 - SvO_2$) is 25%. As the DO_2 decreases below normal (moving to the left along the curve), the VO_2 initially remains unchanged, indicating that the O_2 extraction is increasing. However, a point is eventually reached where the VO_2 begins to decrease; at this point, the SvO_2 has dropped to 50%, resulting in an increase in ($SaO_2 - SvO_2$) to almost 50%. The point where the VO_2 begins to decrease is the point where O_2 extraction is maximal (about 50%) and is unable to increase further.

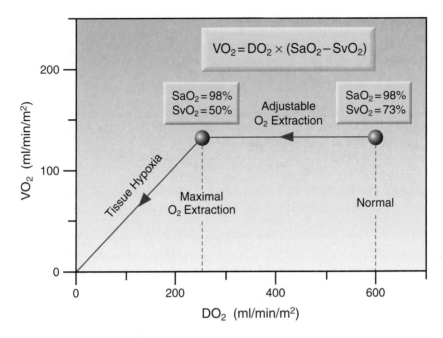

FIGURE 10.5 Graph showing the relationship between O_2 delivery (DO_2) and O_2 uptake (VO_2). O_2 extraction is represented by ($SaO_2 - SvO_2$). See text for explanation.

Beyond this point, decreases in DO_2 are accompanied by similar decreases in VO_2, indicating the onset of tissue hypoxia. Thus, *the point where O_2 extraction is maximal is the anaerobic threshold.*

Monitoring O_2 Extraction

The O_2 extraction can be monitored as the ($SaO_2 - SvO_2$) as long as the SaO_2 is above 90%. The SaO_2 is monitored by pulse oximetry (described in Chapter 21) and the SvO_2 is monitored with pulmonary artery catheters (or central venous catheters, as described later). The following general rules can be applied to the interpretation of ($SaO_2 - SvO_2$). These interpretations are based on the assumption that the metabolic rate is normal or unchanging.

1. The normal ($SaO_2 - SvO_2$) is 20% to 30%.

2. An increase in ($SaO_2 - SvO_2$) above 30% indicates a decrease in O_2 delivery (i.e., usually anemia or a low cardiac output).

3. An increase in ($SaO_2 - SvO_2$) that approaches 50% indicates either threatened or inadequate tissue oxygenation.

4. A decrease in ($SaO_2 - SvO_2$) below 20% indicates a defect in O_2 utilization in tissues, which is usually the result of inflammatory cell injury in severe sepsis or septic shock.

When the SaO_2 approaches 100%, O_2 extraction can be monitored using only the SvO_2, as described next.

Venous Oxygen Saturation

The modified Fick equation for VO_2 (i.e., equation 10.10) can be modified again so the derived variable is the mixed venous O_2 saturation (SvO_2). This results in the following equation, which identifies the determinants of SvO_2.

$$SvO_2 = SaO_2 - (VO_2/CO \times 1.34 \times [Hb]) \tag{10.17}$$

If arterial blood is fully oxygenated ($SaO_2 = 1$), the denominator in the parentheses is equivalent to the DO_2, and the equation can be rewritten as:

$$SvO_2 = 1 - VO_2/DO_2 \tag{10.18}$$

This equation predicts that the SvO_2 will vary inversely (i.e., in the opposite direction) with changes in O_2 extraction (VO_2/DO_2).

Monitoring the SvO_2

The SvO_2 is ideally measured in mixed venous blood in the pulmonary arteries, which requires a pulmonary artery catheter. The SvO_2 can be measured periodically in blood samples withdrawn through the PA catheter, or it can be monitored continuously using fiberoptic PA catheters. (The measurement of SvO_2 with fiberoptic catheters is described in Chapter 21). The normal range for SvO_2 in pulmonary artery blood is 65% to 75% (18). Continuous SvO_2 monitoring is associated with spontaneous fluctuations that average 5% but can be as high as 20% (19). A change in SvO_2 must exceed 5% and persist for longer than 10 minutes to be considered a significant change (20).

The following rules for interpreting the SvO_2 are based on the relationships in equations 10.16 and 10.18, and are similar in principle to the rules for interpreting the ($SaO_2 - SvO_2$) described earlier.

1. The normal SvO_2 is 65–75%.

2. A decrease in SvO_2 below 65% indicates a decrease in O_2 delivery (i.e., usually anemia or a low cardiac output).

3. A decrease in SvO_2 that approaches 50% indicates either threatened or inadequate tissue oxygenation.

4. An increase in SvO_2 above 75% indicates a defect in O_2 utilization in tissues, which is usually the result of inflammatory cell injury in severe sepsis or septic shock.

Central Venous O_2 Saturation

The O_2 saturation in the superior vena cava, known as the "central venous" O_2 saturation ($ScvO_2$), has been proposed as an alternative to the mixed venous O_2 saturation (SvO_2) because it eliminates the need for a PA catheter. However, the $ScvO_2$ is higher than the SvO_2 by an average of $7\pm4\%$ (absolute difference) in critically ill patients (18,21). Discrepancies in the two measurements are greatest in patients with heart failure, cardiogenic shock, and sepsis. The higher $ScvO_2$ in low output states is attributed to peripheral vasoconstriction with preservation of cerebral blood flow, and the higher $ScvO_2$ in sepsis is attributed to an increase in splanchnic O_2 consumption (21).

Despite this discrepancy, changes in $ScvO_2$ generally mirror those in the SvO_2 (21), and trends in the $ScvO_2$ are considered more informative than individual measurements (22). The normal range of $ScvO_2$ in one study was preselected at 70% to 89% (23), which is consistent with the use of an $ScvO_2 > 70\%$ as one of the early goals of management in patients with severe sepsis or septic shock (24).

The $ScvO_2$ is monitored with central venous catheters, but the tip of the catheter must be in the superior vena cava. Periodic measurements of $ScvO_2$ can be obtained in blood samples withdrawn through the catheter, or the $ScvO_2$ can be monitored continuously using specially designed fiberoptic catheters (PreSep Catheters, Edwards Life Sciences, Irvine, CA). The criteria for a significant change in $ScvO_2$ are the same as those mentioned for SvO_2.

A summary of the oxygen-related measurements that can be used as markers of impaired tissue oxygenation is shown in Table 10.4. The value of the O_2-related markers is enhanced if they are used in combination with the chemical markers described next.

Table 10.4	Markers of Inadequate Tissue Oxygenation

I. Oxygen Markers

    1. $VO_2 < 200$ mL/min or <110 mL/min/m^2

    2. $(SaO_2 - SvO_2) \geq 50\%$

    3. $SvO_2 \leq 50\%$

II. Chemical Markers

    1. Serum Lactate >2 mM/L (or ≥ 4 mM/L)

    2. Arterial Base Deficit >2 mM/L

CHEMICAL MARKERS

The serum lactate level and arterial base deficit are readily available measurements that have both diagnostic and prognostic value. The lactate level is the superior measurement, as will be shown.

Lactate

(Note: There are several conditions that elevate blood lactate levels without an associated derangement in tissue oxygenation, and these are described in Chapter 32. The following description pertains only to conditions where elevated lactate levels are associated with abnormalities in O_2 availability or O_2 utilization in tissues.)

Lactate is well suited for the detection of anaerobic conditions because it is the end-product of anaerobic glycolysis. (The end-product is actually lactic acid, a weak acid that promptly dissociates to form lactate.) One possible drawback is the negative charge of the lactate molecule, which will hinder movement through cell membranes and could delay the appearance of lactate in the blood. This is consistent with the observations in Figure 10.4, which shows a delay of several hours from the first evidence of anaerobic metabolism (low VO_2) to the first evidence of an elevated blood lactate level.

Lactate in Blood

Lactate production is the major end-point of metabolism in erythrocytes (because they have no mitochondria), and circulating erythrocytes are second only to skeletal muscle in the daily production of lactate (25). Lactate production in erythrocytes does not, however, create a difference in lactate concentration between whole blood and plasma (26). Activated neutrophils are a significant source of lactate production in inflammatory conditions like the acute respiratory distress syndrome (described in Chapter 23), but lactate release from lung inflammation does not create a difference in lactate levels between venous and arterial blood (25). Therefore, lactate levels can be measured in plasma, whole blood, venous blood, or arterial blood, with similar results. The normal lactate concentration in blood is ≤2 mmol/L, but lactate levels above 4 mM/L have more prognostic value, as described next.

Prognostic Value

The serum lactate level is more than a diagnostic tool because it has prognostic implications as well. Studies in critically ill patients have shown that the probability of survival is related to the initial lactate level (prior to treatment), and to the time required for an elevated lactate to return to normal (lactate clearance). This is shown in Figure 10.6.

INITIAL LACTATE LEVEL: The graph on the left in Figure 10.6 is from a study involving septic patients (28) that shows an increase in the in-hospital mortality rate as the initial serum lactate level increases to above 2 mmol/L. Also shown is a dramatic increase in mortality rate in the first 3 days (as indicated by the horizontal lines in each column) when the initial lactate level is ≥ 4 mM/L. This is consistent with other studies (25,26) showing that *an initial lactate level ≥ 4 mM/L indicates a significant risk of a fatal outcome during the ICU stay.*

LACTATE CLEARANCE: The graph on the right in Figure 10.6 is from a study that included serial measurements of serum lactate in a group of hemodynamically unstable patients with elevated lactate levels (29). The lowest mortality rate occurred when lactate levels normalized within 24 hours, and the mortality rate increased dramatically when lactate levels did not normalize within 48 hours . This relationship between the rate of lactate clearance and the mortality rate has been observed in several

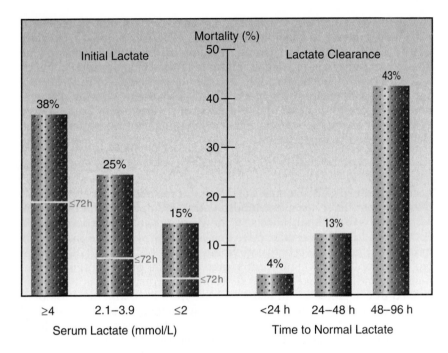

FIGURE 10.6 Graphs showing the prognostic value of monitoring serum lactate levels. Graph on the left (from Reference 28) shows the association between initial lactate levels and in-hospital mortality rate, including the mortality rate in the first 3 days after the initial lactate. Graph on the right (from Reference 29) shows the association between the time for lactate levels to normalize (lactate clearance) and in-hospital mortality rate.

studies (25,27,29,30), and occurs predominantly in patients with severe sepsis and septic shock. The rate of lactate clearance in these patients has greater prognostic value than the initial lactate level (25, 30). Lactate clearance can be incorporated into the early goals of management in patients with severe sepsis and septic shock (which are described in Chapter 14) because of the observation that a lactate clearance > 10% in the first 6 hours after diagnosis is associated with improved survival (30).

Lactate in Sepsis

Lactate accumulation in sepsis is *not the result of an inadequate supply of O_2*, but instead appears to be related to the accumulation of pyruvate as a result of inhibition of pyruvate dehydrogenase (the enzyme that converts pyruvate to acetyl coenzyme A and moves glycolysis from the cytoplasm to the Krebs cycle in mitochondria) (31). Endotoxin and other components of bacterial cell walls have been implicated in the inhibition of this enzyme (31). This mechanism of lactate accumulation is consistent with the notion that a defect in O_2 utilization in mitochondria (i.e., cytopathic hypoxia) is the cause of cell injury in severe sepsis and septic shock (7), as mentioned earlier. The notion that tissue O_2 levels are not deficient in patients with severe sepsis and septic shock has important implications for the management of these patients (which is described in Chapter 14).

Lactate as an Adaptive Fuel

The association of elevated serum lactate levels with poor outcomes has created a perception that the lactate molecule has deleterious effects. This is unproven, and it is possible that lactate may have a beneficial role as an "adaptive fuel" in critically ill patients (32). The energy yield from the oxidative metabolism of lactate is equivalent to that of glucose, as shown in Table 10.5. The caloric density (kcal/g) of lactate and glucose are equivalent and, since one glucose molecule produces 2 lactate molecules, the energy yield from the complete oxidation (kcal/mole) of lactate and glucose are equivalent. There is evidence that lactate oxidation in the heart is increased in patients with septic shock (33), and evidence that lactate oxidation is an important source of energy in neuronal tissue subjected to hypoxia and ischemia (34). Therefore, it is possible that lactate is more friend than foe in critically ill patients.

Table 10.5	Glucose vs. Lactate as Oxidative Fuels		
Substrate	Molecular Weight	Heat of Combustion	Caloric Value
Glucose	180	673 kcal/mole	3.74 kcal/g
Lactate	90	326 kcal/mole	3.62 kcal/g
Lactate × 2	180	673 kcal/mole	3.62 kcal/g

Arterial Base Deficit

The "base deficit" is considered a more specific marker of metabolic acidosis than the serum bicarbonate (35), and is defined as the amount (in millimoles) of base that must be added to one liter of blood to raise the pH to 7.40 (at a PCO_2 of 40 mm Hg). Most blood gas analyzers determine the base deficit routinely using a PCO_2/HCO_3 nomogram, and the results are included in the blood gas report. The normal arterial base deficit is ≤2 mmol/L; increases above 2 mmol/L are classified as mild (2 to 5 mmol/L), moderate (6 to 14 mmol/L), and severe (≥ 15 mmol/L).

Arterial base deficit has been a popular marker of impaired tissue oxygenation in acute surgical emergencies, especially trauma. Studies in trauma victims show a correlation between the magnitude of acute blood loss and the magnitude of elevation in arterial base deficit (36), and acute trauma resuscitation that normalizes the arterial base deficit within hours is associated with a favorable outcome (36). Based on these observations, normalization of the arterial base deficit is one of the end-points of trauma resuscitation (37).

Base Excess vs. Lactate

When used as a marker of tissue oxygenation, the arterial base deficit is a surrogate measure of serum lactate levels. However, base deficit is not specific for lactate because it is influenced by other causes of metabolic acidosis (e.g., ketosis, renal insufficiency). In one study comparing base deficit and lactate levels in patients admitted to a surgical ICU (38), both were similar in predictive value on admission, but lactate was superior to base deficit for predicting outcome when serial measurements of both were followed after ICU admission. This observation, combined with the lack of specificity of arterial base deficit as a measure of lactate, indicates that the *arterial base deficit offers no advantages over blood lactate levels in the evaluation of tissue oxygenation.*

NEAR INFRARED SPECTROSCOPY

Near infrared spectroscopy (NIRS) is a noninvasive method of measuring the venous O_2 saturation in tissues using the optical properties of hemoglobin in the oxygenated (HbO_2) and dexoxygenated (Hb) state. This is described in Chapter 21 in relation to pulse oximetry. NIRS is essentially tissue oximetry without the "pulse" component. A light source is placed on the skin that emits light with wavelengths specific for HbO_2 (990 nm) and Hb (660 nm), and the light of each wavelength that is reflected back from the underlying tissues (subcutaneous tissue and muscle) is picked up by a photodetector and processed to display the *tissue O_2 saturation* (StO_2):

$$StO_2 = HbO_2 / HbO_2 + Hb \qquad (10.19)$$

The StO_2 includes the O_2 saturation in arteries, capillaries, and veins within the tissue, but most of the blood in tissues (70–75%) is in veins, so the StO_2 is assumed to be a measure of the venous O_2 saturation in the underlying tissue, which is then used as a measure of the balance between O_2 delivery and O_2 consumption in that tissue (i.e., equation 10.18 for tissues instead of the whole body). It has been used mostly in the brain and skeletal muscle (39), and is not without problems; e.g., several other factors can influence StO_2, such as skin color, tissue thickness and composition, and myoglobin (for muscle), and a few studies indicate 50% to 100% of the NIRS signal from skeletal muscle is from myoglobin (40). This is one of the problems with NIRS; i.e., you are not sure what is being measured.

Cytochrome Oxidase

The most exciting feature of NIRS is the potential to monitor mitochondrial O_2 consumption (41). This is possible because of the optical properties of cytochrome oxidase, the enzyme responsible for converting O_2 to water at the end of the electron transport chain. Cytocrome oxidase (CytOx) is the "waste disposal unit" of the electron transport chain; i.e., it receives electrons that have been "spent" producing ATP, and disposes of these electrons by donating them to oxygen (4 electrons per O_2 molecule). This reduces O_2 to water, and is responsible for about 90% of cellular O_2 consumption.

$$O_2 + 4e^- + 4H^+ \rightarrow 2H_2O \tag{10.20}$$

The loss of electrons converts CytOx from a reduced to an oxidized state. In a steady state condition, CytOx is a balance of oxidized and reduced forms, and it absorbs light at 830 nm in this balanced redox state. This absorption band is lost when CytOx is in the reduced form, which occurs when CytOx is no longer donating electrons to O_2 (and mitochondrial O_2 consumption therefore ceases). Thus, the presence or absence of the 830 nm absorption band is a potential marker for the presence or absence of mitochondrial ATP production.

Unfortunately, cytochrome oxidase is present in miniscule amounts compared to hemoglobin, and this makes it difficult to detect the absorption band. The absence of an 830 nm absorption band could mean either CytOx is in the reduced state (and metabolism is anaerobic) or you can't pick up the signal from CytOx in a balanced redox state (and metabolism is aerobic). Once again, understanding what you are monitoring can be problematic with NIRS.

I was first introduced to NIRS in the mid-1970s (in the laboratory of Britton Chance, who discovered cytochrome oxidase), and in the almost-40 years since that time, NIRS has always been an exciting but unrealized technology. The next few years will probably be more of the same.

A FINAL WORD

The importance of monitoring systemic or tissue oxygenation is based on the premise that inadequate tissue oxygenation is responsible for cell injury, multiorgan failure, and fatal outcomes in critically ill patients. This premise is difficult to evaluate because of the inability to directly measure tissue O_2 levels. Increased serum lactate levels have been used as evidence of inadequate tissue oxygenation in critically ill patients, but the elevated lactate levels in septic shock are not the result of limited O_2 availability in tissues (31), as described earlier in the chapter. In fact, the consensus opinion is that *inflammatory cell injury* is the culprit responsible for multiorgan failure and fatal outcomes in septic shock (see Chapter 14). Since septic shock is the leading cause of death in ICUs, it seems that inadequate tissue oxygenation is not as important as we think it is in critically ill patients. This, of course, has obvious implications for the current emphasis on promoting tissue oxygenation in critical care management.

REFERENCES

Oxygen in Blood

1. Nunn JF. Oxygen. In Nunn's Applied Respiratory Physiology. 4th ed. London: Butterworth-Heinemann Ltd, 1993:247–305.

2. McConn R, Derrick JB. The respiratory function of blood: transfusion and blood storage. Anesthesiology 1972; 36:119–127.

3. Zander R. Calculation of oxygen concentration. In: Zander R, Mertzlufft F, eds. The oxygen status of arterial blood. Basel: S. Karger, 1991:203–209.

4. Christoforides C, Laasberg L, Hedley-Whyte J. Effect of temperature on solubility of O_2 in plasma. J. Appl Physiol 1969; 26:56–60.

Systemic Oxygen Balance

5. Connett RJ, Honig CR, Gayeski TEJ, Brooks GA. Defining hypoxia: a systems view of VO_2, glycolysis, energetics, and intracellular PO_2. J Appl Physiol 1990; 68:833–842.

6. Loiacono LA, Shapiro DS. Detection of hypoxia at the cellular level. Crit Care Clin 2010; 26:409–421.

7. Fink MP. Cytopathic hypoxia. Mitochondrial dysfunction as a mechanism contributing to organ dysfunction in sepsis. Crit Care Clin 2001; 17:219–237.

8. Mohammed I, Phillips C. Techniques for determining cardiac output in the intensive care unit. Crit Care Clin 2010; 26:353–364.

9. Hameed SM, Aird WC, Cohn SM. Oxygen delivery. Crit Care Med 2003; 31(Suppl): S658–S667.

10. Schneeweiss B, Druml W, Graninger W, et al. Assessment of oxygen-consumption by use of reverse Fick-principle and indirect calorimetry in critically ill patients. Clin Nutr 1989; 8:89–93.

11. Sasse SA, Chen PA, Berry RB, et al. Variability of cardiac output over time in medical intensive care unit patients. Chest 1994; 22:225–232.

12. Bartlett RH, Dechert RE. Oxygen kinetics: Pitfalls in clinical research. J Crit Care 1990; 5:77–80.

13. Nunn JF. Non respiratory functions of the lung. In: Nunn JF (ed). Applied Respiratory Physiology. Butterworth, London, 1993:306–317.

14. Jolliet P, Thorens JB, Nicod L, et al. Relationship between pulmonary oxygen consumption, lung inflammation, and calculated venous admixture in patients with acute lung injury. Intensive Care Med 1996; 22:277–285.

15. Dunham CM, Seigel JH, Weireter L, et al. Oxygen debt and metabolic acidemia as quantitative predictors of mortality and the severity of the ischemic insult in hemorrhagic shock. Crit Care Med 1991; 19:231–243.

16. Shoemaker WC, Appel PL, Krom HB. Role of oxygen debt in the development of organ failure, sepsis, and death in high-risk surgical patients. Chest 1992; 102:208–215.

17. Leach RM, Treacher DF. The relationship between oxygen delivery and consumption. Disease-a-Month 1994; 30:301–368.

18. Maddirala S, Khan A. Optimizing hemodynamic support in septic shock using central venous and mixed venous oxygen saturation. Crit Care Clin 2010; 26:323–333.

19. Noll ML, Fountain RL, Duncan CA, et al. Fluctuations in mixed venous oxygen saturation in critically ill medical patients: a pilot study. Am J Crit Care 1992; 3:102–106.

20. Krafft P, Stelzer H, Heismay M, et al. Mixed venous oxygen saturation in critically ill septic shock patients. Chest 1993; 103:900–906.

21. Reinhart K, Kuhn H-J, Hartog C, Bredle DL. Continuous central venous and pulmonary artery oxygen saturation monitoring in the critically ill. Intensive Care Med 2004; 30:1572–1578.

22. Dueck MH, Kilmek M, Appenrodt S, et al. Trends but not individual values of central venous oxygen saturation agree with mixed venous oxygen saturation during varying hemodynamic conditions. Anesthesiology 2005; 103:249–257.

23. Pope JV, Jones AE, Gaieski DF, et al. Multicenter study of central venous oxygen saturation ($ScvO_2$) as a predictor of mortality in patients with sepsis. Ann Emerg Med 2010; 55:40–46.

24. Dellinger RP, Levy MM, Carlet JM, et al. Surviving sepsis campaign: international guidelines for management of severe sepsis and septic shock: 2008. Crit Care Med 2008; 36:296–327.

Chemical Markers

25. Okorie ON, Dellinger P. Lactate: biomarker and potential therapeutic target. Crit Care Clin 2011; 27:299–326.

26. Aduen J, Bernstein WK, Khastgir T, et al. The use and clinical importance of a substrate-specific electrode for rapid determination of blood lactate concentrations. JAMA 1994; 272:1678–1685.

27. Vernon C, LeTourneau JL. Lactic acidosis: recognition, kinetics, and associated prognosis. Crit Care Clin 2010; 26:255–283.

28. Trzeciak S, Dellinger RP, Chansky ME, et al. Serum lactate as a predictor of mortality in patients with infection. Intensive Care Med 2007; 33:970–977.

29. McNelis J, Marini CP, Jurkiewicz A, et al. Prolonged lactate clearance is associated with increased mortality in the surgical intensive care unit. Am J Surg 2001; 182:481–485.

30. Nguyen HB, Rivers EP, Knoblich BP, et al. Early lactate clearance is associated with improved outcome in severe sepsis and septic shock. Crit Care Med 2004; 32:1637–1642.

31. Thomas GW, Mains CW, Slone DS, et al. Potential dysregulation of the pyruvate dehydrogenase complex by bacterial toxins and insulin. J Trauma 2009; 67:628–633.

32. Gladden LB. Lactate metabolism: a new paradigm for the third millenium. J Physiol 2004; 558.1:5–30.

33. Dhainaut J-F, Huyghebaert M-F, Monsallier JF, et al. Coronary hemodynamics and myocardial metabolism of lactate, free fatty acids, glucose, and ketones in patients with septic shock. Circulation 1987; 75:533–541.

34. Schurr A. Lactate, glucose, and energy metabolism in the ischemic brain. Int J Mol Med 2002; 10:131–136.

35. Severinghaus JW. Case for standard-base excess as the measure of non-respiratory acid-base imbalance. J Clin Monit 1991; 7:276–277.

36. Davis JW, Shackford SR, Mackersie RC, Hoyt DB. Base deficit as a guide to volume resuscitation. J Trauma 1998; 28:1464–1467.

37. Tisherman SA, Barie P, Bokhari F, et al. Clinical practice guideline: endpoints of resuscitation. J Trauma 57:898–912.

38. Martin MJ, Fitzsullivan E, Salim A, et al. Discordance between lactate and base deficit in the surgical intensive care unit: which one do you trust? Am J Surg 2006; 191:625–630.

Near Infrared Spectroscopy

39. Boushel R, Piantadosi CA. Near-infrared spectroscopy for monitoring muscle oxygenation. Acta Physiol Scandinav 2000; 168:615–622.

40. Ward KR, Ivatury RR, Barbee RW, et al. Near infrared spectroscopy for evaluation of the trauma patient: a technological review. Resuscitation 2006; 27–64.

41. Cooper CE, Springett R. Measurement of cytochrome oxidase and mitochondrial energetics by near-infrared spectroscopy. Phil Trans R Soc Lond 1997; 352:669–676.

DISORDERS OF CIRCULATORY FLOW

Variability is the law of life...no two individuals react alike or behave alike under the abnormal conditions which we know as disease.

Sir William Osler
*On the Educational Value of
the Medical Society*
1903

Chapter 11

HEMORRHAGE AND HYPOVOLEMIA

It is a bad sign in acute illnesses when the extremities become cold.

Hippocrates

The human circulatory system operates with a small volume and a volume-responsive stroke pump. This is an energy-efficient design that limits the workload of the heart, but the system quickly falters when volume is removed. While most internal organs like the lungs, liver, and kidneys can lose as much as 75% of their functional mass without life-threatening organ failure, loss of only 35% to 40% of the blood volume can be fatal. This *intolerance of the circulatory system to loss of blood volume is the dominant concern in the bleeding patient.*

This chapter describes the evaluation and management of hypovolemia, with emphasis on acute blood loss, and includes a section on damage-control resuscitation for the severely injured patient.

BODY FLUIDS & BLOOD LOSS

Distribution of Body Fluids

The volume of selected body fluids in adults is shown in Table 11.1. Total body fluid accounts for about 60% of the lean body weight in males (600 mL/kg) and 50% of the lean body weight in females (500 mL/kg). An average sized adult male who weighs 75 kg (165 lbs) will thus have $0.6 \times 75 = 45$ liters of total body fluid, and an average sized adult female who weighs 60 kg (132 lbs) will have $0.5 \times 60 = 30$ liters of total body fluid. The volume of blood accounts for 6% to 7% of body weight (66 mL/kg in males, and 60 mL/kg in females) (1). As shown in Table 11.1, the blood volume is 5 liters in an average sized male, and only 3.6 liters in an average sized female. Comparing the volumes of blood and total body fluid indicates that *blood represents only 11–12% of total body fluid.* The meager distribution of total body fluid in the vascular compartment is an important factor in the intolerance to blood loss.

Table 11.1	Volume of Body Fluids in Adults			
Body Fluid	**Men**		**Women**	
	mL/kg	75 kg†	mL/kg	60 kg†
Total Body Fluid	600	45 L	500	30 L
Interstitial Fluid	150	11.3 L	125	7.5 L
Blood	66	5 L	60	3.6 L
Red Cell	26	2 L	24	1.4 L
Plasma	40	3 L	36	2.2 L

†Lean body weight for an average sized adult male and female.
Volume of blood, red cells, and plasma (in mL/kg) are from Reference 1.

Plasma vs. Interstitial Fluid

Extracellular fluid accounts for about 40% of the total body fluid, and is composed of extravascular (interstitial) and intravascular (plasma) fluid compartments. Comparison of interstitial fluid and plasma volumes in Table 11.1 shows that *plasma volume is about 25% of interstitial fluid volume*. This relationship is important for understanding the volume effects of sodium-based (saline) fluids; i.e., since sodium equilibrates throughout the extracellular fluid, 75% of infused saline solutions will distribute in the interstitial fluid, and 25% will distribute in the plasma. Thus, the principal effect of saline solutions is to enhance the interstitial fluid volume, not the plasma volume (2).

Blood Loss

Compensatory Responses

Acute blood loss triggers two compensatory responses aimed at restoring volume deficits (3). The earliest response involves movement of interstitial fluid into the bloodstream. This *transcapillary refill* can add as much as one liter to the plasma volume, but it leaves an interstitial fluid deficit. The second response involves activation of the renin–angiotensin–aldosterone system (from decreased renal perfusion), which results in sodium conservation by the kidneys. The retained sodium will primarily enhance the interstitial volume, and thus will help to replace the interstitial fluid deficits created by transcapillary refill. These two responses can fully compensate for the loss of 15% to 20% of the blood volume (3).

Severity of Blood Loss

The American College of Surgeons has proposed the following classification system for acute blood loss (4).

CLASS I. Loss of ≤15% of the blood volume (or ≤10 mL/kg). This degree of blood loss is usually fully compensated by transcapillary refill. Because blood volume is maintained, clinical findings are minimal or absent, and volume resuscitation is not necessary (3).

CLASS II. Loss of 15–30% of the blood volume (or 10–20 mL/kg). This represents the compensated phase of hypovolemia, where blood pressure is maintained by systemic vasoconstriction (5). Postural changes in pulse rate and blood pressure may be evident, but these findings are inconsistent (see later), and the hypovolemia can be clinically silent. The vasoconstrictor response to hypovolemia is most intense in the splanchnic circulation, and splanchnic hypoperfusion can lead to disruption of the intestinal mucosa and invasion of the bloodstream with enteric pathogens (6).

CLASS III. Loss of 30–45% of the blood volume (or 20–30 mL/kg). This marks the onset of decompensated blood loss or *hemorrhagic shock*, where the vasoconstrictor response is no longer able to sustain blood pressure and organ perfusion. The clinical consequences can include supine hypotension, evidence of impaired organ perfusion (e.g., cool extremities, oliguria, depressed consciousness), and evidence of anaerobic metabolism (i.e., lactate accumulation in blood).

CLASS IV. Loss of > 45% of blood volume (or > 30 mL/kg). This degree of blood loss results in profound hemorrhagic shock, which may be irreversible. Clinical manifestations include multiorgan failure and severe metabolic (lactic) acidosis. This category includes *massive blood loss,* which is described later in the chapter.

ASSESSMENT OF BLOOD VOLUME

The importance of an accurate assessment of the intravascular volume is matched by the difficulties encountered, and the clinical evaluation of intravascular volume is so flawed that it has been called a "comedy of errors" (7).

Vital Signs

The changes in pulse rate and blood pressure that occur in acute hypovolemia are listed in Table 11.2, along with the reported sensitivities and specificities at two levels of blood loss (8,9). Supine tachycardia and hypotension are absent in a large majority of patients with blood volume deficits up to 1.1 liters (up to a 25% loss of blood volume in average sized males). The absence of tachycardia is contrary to traditional beliefs, yet bradycardia may be more prevalent in patients with acute blood loss (8).

Table 11.2	Operating Characteristics of Vital Signs in the Detection of Hypovolemia	
Abnormal Finding	**Sensitivity/Specificity**	
	Moderate Blood Loss (450–630 mL)†	**Severe Blood Loss (630–1150 mL)§**
Supine Tachycardia[1]	0 / 96%	12% / 96%
Supine Hypotension[2]	13% / 97%	33% / 97%
Postural Pulse Increment[3]	22% / 98%	97% / 98%
Postural Hypotension[4] Age <65 yrs Age ≥65 yrs	9% / 94% 27% / 86%	Not studied Not studied

[1]Pulse rate >100 beats/min; [2]Systolic pressure <95 mm Hg; [3]Increase in pulse rate ≥ 30 beats/min; [4]Decrease in systolic pressure >20 mm Hg.
†Equivalent to a 10–12.5% loss of blood volume in an average sized adult male.
§Equivalent to a 12.5–25% loss of blood in an average sized adult male.
From References 8 and 9.

Postural Changes

Moving from the supine to the standing position causes a shift of 7 to 8 mL/kg of blood to the lower extremities (8). In healthy subjects, this change in body position is associated with a small increase in heart rate (about 10 beats/min) and a small decrease in systolic blood pressure (about 3 to 4 mm Hg). These changes can be exaggerated in hypovolemia. The expected postural changes in hypovolemia include an increment in pulse rate of at least 30 beats/minute, and a decrease in systolic blood pressure that exceeds 20 mm Hg. As shown in Table 11.2, these postural changes are uncommon when blood loss is less than 630 mL (≤12% decrease in blood volume), but above this level, the postural pulse increment is a sensitive and specific marker of acute blood loss (as indicated by the boxed numbers in Table 11.2).

In summary, vital signs provide little benefit in the evaluation of hypovolemia, particularly in excluding the diagnosis. Supine hypotension may suggest the presence of profound hypovolemia, but this condition should be accompanied by other more reliable markers of severe volume loss (e.g., diminished urine output, elevated serum lactate levels).

Hematocrit

The use of the hematocrit (and hemoglobin concentration) to evaluate the presence and severity of acute blood loss is both common and inappropriate. Changes in hematocrit show a poor correlation with blood volume deficits and erythrocyte deficits in acute hemorrhage (10), and the reason for this discrepancy is demonstrated in Figure 11.1. Acute blood loss involves the loss of whole blood, which results in proportional decreases in the volume of plasma and erythrocytes. As a result, acute blood loss results in a decrease in blood volume, but not a decrease in hematocrit. (There is a small dilutional effect from transcapillary refill in acute blood loss, but this is usually not enough to cause a significant decrease in hematocrit.) In the absence of volume resuscitation, the hematocrit will eventually decrease because hypovolemia activates the renin-angiotensin-aldosterone system, and the renal retention of sodium and water that follows will have a dilutional effect on the hematocrit. This process begins 8 to 12 hours after acute blood loss, and can take a few days to become fully established.

Influence of Fluid Resuscitation

The influence of fluid resuscitation on the hematocrit is demonstrated in Figure 11.1. Infusion of isotonic saline augments the plasma volume but not the red cell volume, resulting in a dilutional decrease in the hematocrit. All asanguinous fluids (i.e., colloid and crystalloid fluids) have a similar dilutional effect on the hematocrit (11), and the volume of fluid infused will determine the magnitude of the decrease in hematocrit. Resuscitation with erythrocyte-containing fluids will have a different effect. This is demonstrated in Figure 11.1 using whole blood as the resuscitation fluid. In this situation, erythrocyte and plasma volumes are increased proportionately, so there is no change in hematocrit. This demonstrates how, *in the early hours after acute blood loss, the hematocrit is a*

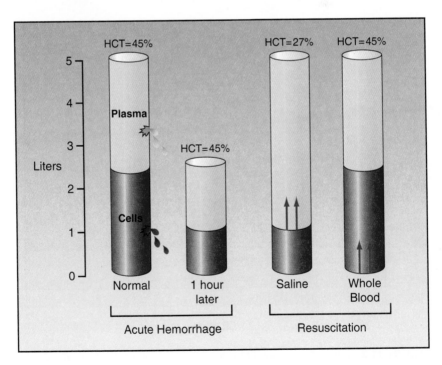

FIGURE 11.1 Influence of acute hemorrhage and fluid resuscitation on blood volume and hematocrit. See text for explanation

reflection of the resuscitation effort (the type and volume of fluids infused), *and not the extent of blood loss.*

Invasive Measures

Cardiac Filling Pressures

Cardiac filling pressures (i.e., central venous pressure and pulmonary artery occlusion pressure) have traditionally played a prominent role in the evaluation of ventricular volume and circulating blood volume. However, neither role is justified because experimental studies have shown a poor correlation between cardiac filling pressures and ventricular end-diastolic volume (see Figure 9.3 in Chapter 9) (12), and even less of a correlation between cardiac filling pressures and circulating blood volume (13–15). The latter observation is demonstrated in Figure 11.2, which shows the relationship between paired measurements of central venous pressure (CVP) and circulating blood volume in a group of post-operative patients. The scattered distribution of the data points illustrates the lack of a significant relationship between the two measurements, which is confirmed by the correlation coefficient (r) and p value in the upper left corner of the graph. Similar results have been reported in other clinical studies (13,15). The consistent lack of correlation between CVP and blood volume measurements has prompted the recommendation

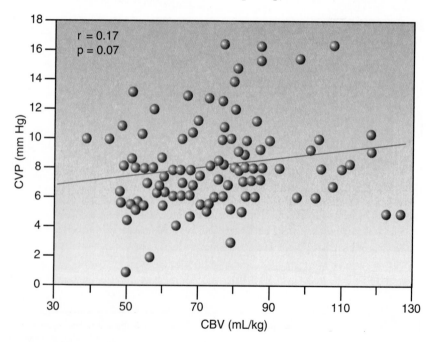

FIGURE 11.2 Scatter plot showing 112 paired measurements of circulating blood volume (CBV) and central venous pressure (CVP) in a group of postoperative patients. Correlation coefficient (R) and p value indicate no significant relationship between CVP and blood volume. Redrawn from Reference 14.

that *the CVP should never be used to make decisions regarding fluid management* (13).

Systemic O_2 Transport

The systemic O_2 transport parameters are described in detail in Chapter 10. The typical pattern with hemorrhage or hypovolemia is a decrease in systemic O_2 delivery (DO_2) with an increase in O_2 extraction ($SaO_2 - SvO_2$). Systemic O_2 consumption (VO_2) is normal in cases of compensated hypovolemia (when the increase in O_2 extraction fully compensates for the decrease in DO_2, as shown in Figure 10.5), and the VO_2 is abnormally low in cases of hypovolemic shock. It is usually not possible to monitor these parameters in cases of acute hemorrhage, and chemical markers of tissue dysoxia are used to determine if acute blood loss results in hemorrhagic shock.

Chemical Markers of Dysoxia

Active hemorrhage can reduce systemic O_2 delivery to levels that are unable to sustain aerobic energy metabolism. The resulting oxygen-limited energy metabolism, also known as *dysoxia*, is accompanied by enhanced production of lactic acid via anaerobic glycolysis. The clinical expression of this condition is hemorrhagic shock, which is characterized by an elevated lactate concentration in blood. Since this condition can appear after loss of only 30% of the blood volume (1.5 liters in an average sized male), cases of active hemorrhage are monitored routinely for evidence of hemorrhagic shock using serum lactate concentrations or arterial base deficit. These two markers of impaired tissue oxygenation are described in detail in Chapter 10, and are mentioned only briefly here.

Serum Lactate

As just mentioned, an elevated serum lactate level in the setting of acute blood loss is presumptive evidence of hemorrhagic shock. The possibility that lactate accumulation in low flow states is the result of reduced lactate clearance is not supported by clinical studies showing equivalent rates of lactate removal in healthy adults and patients with cardiogenic shock (16). Although the threshold for an elevated serum lactate level is 2 mM/L, lactate levels ≥ 4 mM/L are more predictive of increased mortality (17), so *a threshold of 4 mM/L is often used to identify life-threatening elevations of serum lactate.*

LACTATE CLEARANCE: According to the bar graphs in Figure 10.6 (Chapter 10), the mortality rate in critically ill patients is not only related to the initial lactate level, but is also a function of the rate of decline in lactate levels after treatment is initiated (lactate clearance). The panel on the right in Figure 10.6 indicates that mortality is lowest when lactate levels return to normal within 24 hours. In one study of trauma victims with hemorrhagic shock, there were no deaths when lactate levels returned to normal within 24 hours, while 86% of the patients died when lactate levels remained elevated after 48 hours (18). Therefore, normalization of lactate levels within 24 hours can be used as an end-point of resuscitation for hemorrhagic shock (see later).

Arterial Base Deficit

Arterial base deficit is a non-specific marker of metabolic acidosis that was adopted as a surrogate measure of lactic acidosis because of its availability in blood gas reports. However, lactate-specific analyzers are now routinely available that provide lactate measurements within a few minutes, and this obviates the need for arterial base deficit in the evaluation and management of hemorrhagic shock.

Fluid Responsiveness

Concern about the liberal use of fluids in critical care management (which creates risks without apparent rewards) led to the practice of evaluating patients for fluid responsiveness before infusing fluids empirically. This practice is not aimed at uncovering occult hypovolemia, but is an attempt to limit volume therapy to those who are likely to respond. It is primarily intended for patients who have an uncertain intravascular volume and are hemodynamically unstable. Mechanical methods of modulating cardiac preload have been proposed for evaluating fluid responsiveness (19), but these methods can be problematic, and fluid challenges remain the recommended method for evaluating fluid responsiveness (20).

Fluid Challenges

There is no standard protocol for fluid challenges. The principal concern is to ensure that the fluid challenge will increase ventricular preload (i.e., end-diastolic volume), and the rate of infusion is more important than the volume infused for achieving this goal (21). The fluid challenge favored in clinical studies is *500 mL of isotonic saline infused over 10–15 minutes* (22). Fluid responsiveness is evaluated by the response of the cardiac output (which can be measured noninvasively using Doppler ultrasound techniques). An increase in cardiac output of at least 12–15% after a fluid challenge is used as evidence of fluid responsiveness (23). About 50% of critically ill patients are fluid responsive when tested in this manner (21,23). This percentage is much lower than expected, and may indicate that fluid challenges often fall short of augmenting ventricular preload.

PASSIVE LEG RAISING: Elevating the legs to 45° above the horizontal plane while in the supine position will move 150 mL to 750 mL of blood out of the legs and towards the heart (19), thereby serving as a "built-in" fluid challenge. This maneuver augments aortic blood flow within 30 seconds (22), and an increase in flow rate of 10–15% predicts fluid responsiveness with a sensitivity and specificity of 90% (23). Passive leg raising is recommended as an alternative to fluid challenges when volume restriction is desirable. It is not advised in patients with increased intra-abdominal pressure because the hemodynamic effects are attenuated or lost (24).

Measuring Blood Volume

Blood volume measurements have traditionally required too much time to perform to be clinically useful in an ICU setting, but this has changed with

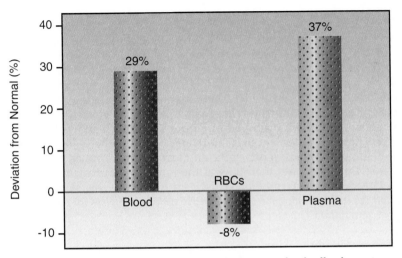

FIGURE 11.3 Deviations from normal for blood, plasma, and red cell volumes in patients with circulatory shock being managed with pulmonary artery catheters. Data from Reference 25.

the introduction of a semiautomated blood volume analyzer (Daxor Corporation, New York, NY) that provides blood volume measurements is less than an hour. The information in Figure 11.3 was provided by measurements obtained with this device in a surgical ICU (25). In this case, blinded measurements of blood, red cell, and plasma volumes were performed in patients with circulatory shock who were managed with pulmonary artery catheters, and the results show that blood and plasma volumes were considerably higher than normal. When blood volume measurements were made available for patient care, 53% of the measurements led to a change in fluid management, and this was associated with a significant decrease in mortality rate (from 24% to 8%) (25). These results will require corroboration, but they highlight the limitations of the clinical assessment of blood volume, and the potential for improved outcomes when blood volume measurements are utilized for fluid management.

INFUSING FLUIDS

The steady flow of fluids through small, rigid tubes is described by the *Hagen-Poiseuille equation* shown below (26).

$$Q = \Delta P \, (\pi r^4 / 8\mu L) \tag{11.1}$$

This equation states that steady flow (Q) through a rigid tube is directly related to the driving pressure (ΔP) for flow and the fourth power of the inner radius (r) of the tube, and is inversely related to the length (L) of the tube and the viscosity (μ) of the infusate. These relationships also describe fluid flow through vascular catheters, as presented next.

Central vs. Peripheral Catheters

There is a tendency to cannulate the large central veins for volume resuscitation because of the perception that larger veins allow more rapid infusion of fluids. However, *infusion rates are determined by the dimensions of the catheter, not the size of the vein.* The influence of catheter dimensions on flow rates is described in detail in Chapter 1. According to the Hagen Poiseuille equation, infusion rates will be higher in shorter or larger bore catheters. This is demonstrated in Figure 11.4, which shows the gravity-driven flow of water through short, peripheral catheters and a longer, triple-lumen central venous catheter. Flow in the peripheral catheters is at least 4 times greater than flow in the lumen of equivalent diameter in the central venous catheter. This demonstrates why *short, large-bore peripheral catheters are preferred to central venous catheters for aggressive volume resuscitation.*

Introducer Sheaths

The resuscitation of trauma victims sometimes requires infusion of more than 5 liters in the first hour (> 83 mL/min) (27), and resuscitation using more than 50 liters in one hour has been reported (28). Because flow increases with the fourth power of the radius of a catheter, very rapid flow rates are best achieved with large-bore introducer sheaths used as conduits for pulmonary artery catheters (see Figure 8.1). These sheaths

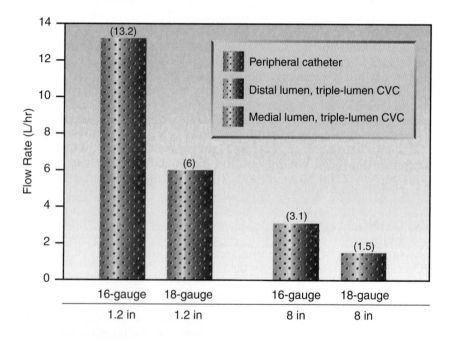

FIGURE 11.4 The influence of catheter dimensions on the gravity-driven infusion rate of water. The triple-lumen central venous catheter (CVC) is a popular size (7 French, 20 cm in length). Flow rates from Table 1.2 and Table 1.3 in Chapter 1.

can be used as stand-alone infusion catheters, and are available in sizes of 8.5 French (2.7 mm outside diameter) or 9 French (3 mm outside diameter). Flow through introducer sheaths can reach 15 mL/sec (900 mL/min or 54 L/hr), which is only slightly less than the maximum flow (18 mL/sec) through standard (3 mm diameter) intravenous tubing (29). Some introducer sheaths have an additional side infusion port on the hub (see Figure 8.1), but the flow capacity of this port is only 25% of the flow capacity of the introducer sheath (29), so it should be bypassed for rapid infusion rates. Introducer sheaths are available without side infusion ports (e.g., Cook Access Plus, Cook Critical care), and these are preferred for rapid infusion rates.

Infusing Packed Red Blood Cells

Whole blood is not available for replacement of blood loss, and erythrocyte losses are replaced with stored units of concentrated erythrocytes called *packed red blood cells*. Each unit of packed RBCs has a hematocrit of 55% to 60%, which imparts a high viscosity (see Table 9.2 for the relationship between hematocrit and blood viscosity). As a result, packed RBCs can flow sluggishly unless diluted with saline (as predicted in the Hagen-Poiseuille equation).

The influence of dilution with isotonic saline on the infusion rate of packed RBCs is shown in Figure 11.5 (30). When infused alone, the flow rate of packed RBCs through average sized (18-gauge or 20-gauge) peripheral catheters is 3–5 mL/min, which means that one unit of undiluted packed RBCs (which has a volume of about 350 mL) can be infused over 70–117 minutes (about 1–2 hours). This is sufficient for replacing erythrocyte losses in hemodynamically stable patients, but more rapid flow rates may be needed for patients with active bleeding. Figure 11.5 shows that dilution of packed RBCs with 100 mL of isotonic saline results in 7-fold to 8-fold increases in infusion rates, while dilution with 250 mL saline increases flow rates over 10-fold. At the highest infusion rate of 96 mL/min in the 16- gauge catheter, one unit of packed RBCs (350 mL plus 250 mL saline) can be infused in 6–7 minutes. More rapid rates require pressurized infusions, which can increase infusion rates to 120 mL/min using a 16-gauge catheter (30).

RESUSCITATION STRATEGIES

The immediate goal of resuscitation for acute blood loss is to support oxygen delivery (DO_2) to vital organs. The determinants of DO_2 are identified in the following equation (the derivation of this equation is described in Chapter 10):

$$DO_2 = CO \times (1.34 \times [Hb] \times SaO_2) \times 10 \qquad (11.2)$$

Acute blood loss affects two components of this equation: cardiac output (CO) and hemoglobin concentration in blood, [Hb]. Therefore, the immediate goals of resuscitation are to promote cardiac output and maintain an adequate [Hb]. (Other goals will emerge as we proceed.)

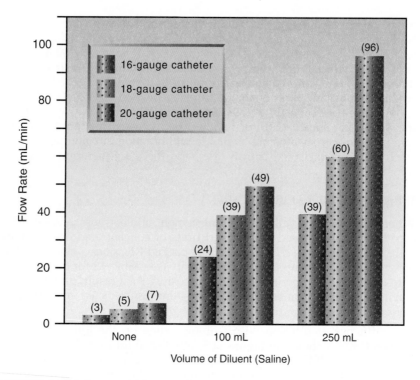

FIGURE 11.5 Influence of dilution with isotonic saline on the gravity-driven infusion rate of erythrocyte concentrates (packed red blood cells) through peripheral catheters. Data from Reference 30.

Promoting Cardiac Output

The consequences of a low cardiac output are far more threatening than the consequences of anemia, so *the first priority in the bleeding patient is to support cardiac output.*

Resuscitation Fluids

The different types of resuscitation fluids are shown in Table 11.3. The fluids used to promote cardiac output are crystalloid fluids and colloid fluids. Plasma is used to provide clotting factors, and is not used as a volume expander. The distinction between crystalloid and colloid fluids is briefly described below.

1. Crystalloid fluids are sodium-rich electrolyte solutions that distribute throughout the extracellular space, and these fluids expand the extracellular volume.

2. Colloid fluids are sodium-rich electrolyte solutions that contain large molecules that do not pass readily out of the bloodstream. The retained molecules hold water in the intravascular compartment; as a result, colloid fluids primarily expand the intravascular (plasma) volume.

Table 11.3	Different Types of Resuscitation Fluid	
Type of Fluid	**Products**	**Principal Use or Result**
Colloid Fluid	Albumin (5%, 25%) Hetastarch (6%) Dextrans	Expands the plasma volume
Crystalloid Fluid	Isotonic Saline Ringer's lactate Normosol	Expands the extracellular volume
RBC Concentrate	Packed RBC's	Increases O_2 content of blood
Stored Plasma	Fresh Frozen Plasma	Provides coagulation factors
Procoagulant Mixture	Cryoprecipitate	Low-volume source of fibrinogen
Platelet Concentrate	Pooled platelets Apharesis platelets	Restores circulating platelet pool

The influence of different types of resuscitation fluids on cardiac output is shown in Figure 11.6 (31). The infusion volume of each fluid (except Ringer's lactate) is roughly the same. The colloid fluid (dextran-40) is clearly the most effective fluid for augmenting cardiac output, while the crystalloid fluid (Ringer's lactate) is only about 25% as effective, despite having twice the infusion volume. Packed RBCs are the least effective in promoting cardiac output, and have actually been shown to *decrease* cardiac output (32). This is due to the viscosity effect of the concentrated erythrocytes in packed RBCs, and this viscosity effect also explains why whole blood is less effective than the colloid fluid for augmenting cardiac output.

Figure 11.6 thus demonstrates that *colloid fluids are much more effective than crystalloid fluids for promoting cardiac output.*

Distribution of Infused Fluids

The superiority of colloid fluids over crystalloid fluids for augmenting cardiac output is explained by the distribution of each fluid. Crystalloid fluids are primarily sodium chloride solutions, and sodium is distributed uniformly in the extracellular fluid. Because plasma represents only 25% of the extracellular fluid, *only 25% of the infused volume of crystalloid fluids will remain in the vascular space and add to the plasma volume*, while the remaining 75% will add to the interstitial fluid volume (33). Colloid fluids, on the other hand, have large molecules that do not readily escape from the bloodstream, and these retained molecules hold water in the intravascular compartment. As a result, *as much as 100% of the infused volume of colloid fluids will remain in the vascular space and add to the plasma volume* (33), at least in the first few hours after infusion. The increase in plasma volume augments cardiac output not only by increasing ventricular

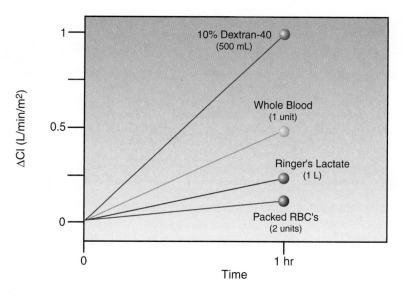

FIGURE 11.6 Change in cardiac index after a one-hour infusion of different resuscitation fluids. The infusion volumes are roughly equivalent (500 mL), except for Ringers lactate (1 liter). From Reference 31.

preload (volume effect) but also by decreasing ventricular afterload (dilutional effect on blood viscosity).

The Preferred Fluid

Despite the superiority of colloid fluids for increasing plasma volume and promoting cardiac output, crystalloid fluids have been the preferred resuscitation fluid for hemorrhagic shock for the past 50 years. The origins of this preference will be described in the next chapter; the principal reasons for the crystalloid preference are the low cost of crystalloid fluids and the lack of a documented survival benefit with colloid resuscitation (34). The favored crystalloid fluid is *Ringer's lactate*, which does not produce the metabolic acidosis that accompanies high-volume resuscitation with isotonic saline (see Figure 12.3).

Colloid fluids remain a reasonable choice in hypovolemia that is not associated with acute blood loss, particularly since ICU patients often have a low plasma oncotic pressure, which will be lowered further by crystalloid resuscitation. There is also much concern about the deleterious effects of high-volume crystalloid resuscitation, including edema formation in the lungs, heart, and intestinal tract, and the abdominal compartment syndrome (34). Chapter 12 has a more detailed comparison of colloid and crystalloid fluid resuscitation.

Standard Resuscitation Regimen

The standard practice for managing a trauma victim who presents with active bleeding or hypotension is to infuse 2 liters of crystalloid fluid over 15 minutes (35). If hypotension or bleeding continue, packed RBCs are infused along with crystalloid fluids to maintain a mean blood pressure ≥ 65 mm Hg. The volume of crystalloid resuscitation will be about 3 times the estimated volume of plasma loss, as shown in Table 11.4 (assume a $\geq 30\%$ loss of blood volume in hemorrhagic shock). When bleeding is controlled and the patient is stable hemodynamically, the threshold for further RBC transfusions is a hemoglobin of 7 g/dL, or ≥ 9 g/dL in patients with active coronary artery disease (36).

Table 11.4	Estimating Resuscitation Volumes for Asanguinous Fluids
Steps	**Methods**
1. Estimate normal blood volume (BV)	BV = 66 mL/kg (M) = 60 mL/kg (F)
2. Estimate % loss of blood volume	Class I: <15% Class II: 15–30% Class III: 30–45% Class IV: >45%
3. Calculate blood volume defect (BVD)	BVD = BV × % loss BV
4. Calculate plasma volume deficit (PVD)	PVD = 0.6 × BVD
6. Estimate resuscitation volume (RV)	RV = PVD × 1 (colloids) = PVD × 3 (crystalloids)

Damage Control Resuscitation

Because uncontrolled exsanguinating hemorrhage is the leading cause of death in hemorrhagic shock, the following practices are being adopted to limit the extent of bleeding in cases of massive blood loss (defined as the loss of one blood volume in 24 hours). These practices are part of an overall approach known as *damage control resuscitation* (37).

Hypotensive Resuscitation

Observations with combat injuries and penetrating trauma have shown that aggressive volume replacement can exacerbate bleeding before the hemorrhage is controlled (34,37). This has led to an emphasis on permitting low blood pressures (i.e., systolic BP = 90 mm Hg or mean BP = 50 mm Hg) in trauma patients with hemorrhagic shock until the bleeding is controlled. This strategy has been shown to reduce resuscitation volumes (38,39), and increase survival rates (38). Low blood pressures are allowed only if there is evidence of adequate organ perfusion (e.g., patient is awake and follows commands).

Hemostatic Resuscitation

FRESH FROZEN PLASMA: For the resuscitation of massive blood loss, the traditional practice has been to give one unit of fresh frozen plasma (FFP) for every 6 units of packed RBCs (34). However, the discovery that severely injured trauma victims often have a coagulopathy on presentation (40) has led to the practice of giving one unit of FFP for every one or two units of packed RBCs, and several studies have shown improved survival rates with this practice (34,37,41). Transfusion of FFP is aimed at maintaining an INR <1.5 and an activated PTT <1.5 times normal (42).

CRYOPRECIPITATE: Although FFP is a good source of fibrinogen (2–5 g/L), cryoprecipitate provides equivalent amounts of fibrinogen in a much smaller volume (3.2–4 grams in 150–200 mL, which is 2 "pools" of cryoprecipitate) (42). Therefore, cryoprecipitate can be used to maintain serum fibrinogen levels (>1 g/L) if volume control is desirable.

PLATELETS: The standard practice of giving one unit of platelets for every 10 units of packed RBCs has also been questioned, and improved survival rates have been recorded when one unit of platelets is given for every 2 to 5 units of packed RBCs (34). The optimal ratio of platelets to packed RBCs has yet to be determined, and platelet transfusions can be guided by the platelet count. The standard goal is to maintain a platelet count >50,000/µL when bleeding is active, but some advocate a platelet count >75,000/µL until bleeding is controlled (42).

Avoiding Hypothermia

Severe trauma is accompanied by loss of thermoregulation, and trauma-related hypothermia (body temp <32° C) is associated with increased mortality, possibly from reduced activity of coagulation factors and platelets (37). Since hypothermia is a risk with infusion of room- temperature fluids and cold blood products (stored at 4° C), in-line fluid warmers are used routinely for the resuscitation of massive blood loss (28). The use of warming blankets and in-line fluid warmers has reduced the incidence of hypothermia to <1% in combat support hospitals (37).

End-Points of Resuscitation

A summary of the general goals and associated end-points of resuscitation for hemorrhagic shock are shown in Figure 11.7. (Some of these end-points, such as the cardiac output and the O_2 transport parameters, are not routinely available.) Limiting blood loss and prompt reversal of tissue ischemia are the most important considerations, and normalization of serum lactate levels within 24 hours is one of the most important end-points.

POSTRESUSCITATION INJURY

The restoration of blood pressure and hemoglobin levels in hemorrhagic shock does not ensure a satisfactory outcome because it can be followed in 48–72 hours by progressive multiorgan failure (43). The earliest manifestation of postresuscitation injury is progressive respiratory dysfunction from the acute respiratory distress syndrome (described in Chapter 23), and this can be followed within 5–6 days by progressive dysfunction involving the kidneys, liver, heart, and central nervous system. The mortality rate is determined by the number of organs involved, and averages 50–60% (43).

Pathophysiology

Postresuscitation injury is a form of *reperfusion injury* (44) that is believed to originate in the splanchnic circulation, where reperfusion of ischemic bowel releases proinflammatory cytokines that gain access to the systemic circulation and activate circulating neutrophils, which adhere to the walls of capillaries and migrate into the parenchyma of vital organs to incite inflammatory injury (43). (This is the underlying mechanism for the multiorgan failure associated with sepsis, as described in Chapter 14.)

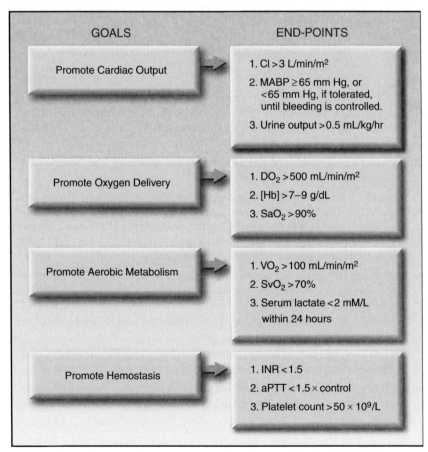

FIGURE 11.7 The general goals and associated end-points of resuscitation for hemorrhagic shock. CI = cardiac index; MABP = mean arterial blood pressure; DO_2 = systemic O_2 delivery; [Hb] = hemoglobin concentration in blood; VO_2 = systemic O_2 consumption; SvO_2 = mixed venous O_2 saturation; INR = international normalized ratio; aPTT = activated partial thromboplastin time.

Several factors predispose to postresuscitation injury, including the time required to reverse tissue ischemia (e.g., lactate clearance > 24 hours), the volume of crystalloid resuscitation (i.e., predisposes to the abdominal compartment syndrome), the number of units of RBCs transfused (> 6 units in 12 hrs), and the age of the transfused blood (stored > 3 weeks) (43). Infection may be involved if the onset of multiorgan failure is more than 3 days after the resuscitation effort (43).

Management

There is no specific therapy for postresuscitation injury, and preventive measures such as rapid reversal of ischemia, limiting the resuscitation volume (both crystalloid fluids and RBC products) and avoiding the transfusion of old blood, if possible, are advised. In late-onset multiorgan failure (onset > 72 hrs after resuscitation), recognition and prompt treatment of underlying sepsis is crucial.

A FINAL WORD

The following points in this chapter deserve emphasis:

1. The clinical evaluation of intravascular volume, including the use of central venous pressure (CVP) measurements, is so flawed it has been called a "comedy of errors" (7).

2. Direct measurements of blood volume are clinically feasible, but are underutilized .

3. Colloid fluids are much more effective than crystalloid fluids for expanding the plasma volume and promoting cardiac output, yet crystalloid fluids are preferred for the resuscitation of hemorrhagic shock because of cost considerations and the lack of a survival benefit with colloid resuscitation.

4. In the severely injured patient, *damage control resuscitation* incorporates alternative strategies like *hypotensive resuscitation* (maintaining a lower-than-usual blood pressure until bleeding is controlled) and *hemostatic resuscitation* (giving fresh frozen plasma and platelets more frequently than usual).

5. Return of serum lactate levels to normal within 24 hours is the end-point of resuscitation that is the most predictive of a satisfactory outcome.

6. Multiorgan failure can appear 48 – 72 hours after resuscitation of hemorrhagic shock as a result of reperfusion-induced systemic inflammation.

REFERENCES

Body Fluids and Blood Loss

1. Walker RH (ed). Technical Manual of the American Association of Blood Banks. 10th ed., Arlington, VA: American Association of Blood Banks, 1990:650.

2. Moore FD, Dagher FJ, Boyden CM, et al. Hemorrhage in normal man: I. Distribution and dispersal of saline infusions following acute blood loss. Ann Surg 2966; 163:485–504.

3. Moore FD. Effects of hemorrhage on body composition. New Engl J Med 1965; 273:567–577.

4. American College of Surgeons. Advanced Trauma Life Support Manual, 7th ed. Chicago, IL: American College of Surgeons, 2004.

5. Schadt JC, Ludbrook J. Hemodynamic and neurohumoral responses to acute hypovolemia in conscious animals. Am J Physiol 1991; 260:H305–H318.

6. Fiddian-Green RG. Studies in splanchnic ischemia and multiple organ failure. In Marston A, Bulkley GB, Fiddian-Green RG, Haglund UH, eds. Splanchnic ischemia and multiple organ failure. St. Louis, CV Mosby, 1989:349–364.

Assessment of Blood Volume

7. Marik PE. Assessment of intravascular volume: A comedy of errors. Crit Care Med 2001; 29:1635.

8. McGee S, Abernathy WB, Simel DL. Is this patient hypovolemic. JAMA 1999; 281:1022–1029.

9. Sinert R, Spektor M. Clinical assessment of hypovolemia. Ann Emerg Med 2005; 45:327–329.

10. Cordts PR, LaMorte WW, Fisher JB, et al. Poor predictive value of hematocrit and hemodynamic parameters for erythrocyte deficits after extensive vascular operations. Surg Gynecol Obstet 1992; 175:243–248.

11. Stamler KD. Effect of crystalloid infusion on hematocrit in nonbleeding patients, with applications to clinical traumatology. Ann Emerg Med 1989; 18:747–749.

12. Kumar A, Anel R, Bunnell E, et al. Pulmonary artery occlusion pressure and central venous pressure fail to predict ventricular filling volumes, cardiac performance, or the response to volume infusion in normal subjects. Crit Care Med 2004; 32:691–699.

13. Marik PE, Baram M, Vahid B. Does central venous pressure predict fluid responsiveness? Chest 2008; 134:172-178.

14. Oohashi S, Endoh H. Does central venous pressure or pulmonary capillary wedge pressure reflect the status of circulating blood volume in patients after extended transthoracic esophagectomy? J Anesth 2005; 19:21–25.

15. Kuntscher MV, Germann G, Hartmann B. Correlations between cardiac output, stroke volume, central venous pressure, intra-abdominal pressure and total circulating blood volume in resuscitation of major burns. Resuscitation 2006; 70:37–43.

16. Revelly JP, Tappy L, Martinez A, et al. Lactate and glucose metabolism in severe sepsis and cardiogenic shock. Crit Care Med 2005; 33:2235–2240.

17. Okorie ON, Dellinger P. Lactate: biomarker and potential therapeutic agent. Crit Care Clin 2011; 27:299–326.

18. Abramson D, Scalea TM, Hitchcock R, et al. Lactate clearance and survival following injury. J Trauma 1993; 35:584–589.

19. Enomoto TM, Harder L. Dynamic indices of preload. Crit Care Clin 2010; 26:307–321.

20. Antonelli M, Levy M, Andrews PJD, et al. Hemodynamic monitoring in shock and implications for management. International Consensus Conference, Paris France, 2006. Intensive Care Med 2007; 33:575–590.

21. Cecconi M, Parsons A, Rhodes A. What is a fluid challenge? Curr Opin Crit Care 2011; 17:290–295.

22. Monnet X, Rienzo M, Osman D, et al. Passive leg raising predicts fluid responsiveness in the critically ill. Crit Care Med 2006; 34:1402–1407.

23. Cavallaro F, Sandroni C, Marano C, et al. Diagnostic accuracy of passive leg raising for prediction of fluid responsiveness in adults: systematic review and meta-analysis of clinical studies. Intensive Care Med 2010; 36:1475–1483.

24. Mahjoub Y, Touzeau J, Airapetian N, et al. The passive leg-raising maneuver cannot accurately predict fluid responsiveness in patients with intra-abdominal hypertension. Crit Care Med 2010; 36:1824–1829.

25. Yu M, Pei K, Moran S, et al. A prospective randomized trial using blood volume analysis in addition to pulmonary artery catheter, compared with pulmonary artery catheter alone to guide shock resuscitation in critically ill surgical patients. Shock 2011; 35:220–228.

Infusing Fluids

26. Chien S, Usami S, Skalak R. Blood flow in small tubes. In Renkin EM, Michel CC (eds). Handbook of Physiology. Section 2: The cardiovascular system. Volume IV. The microcirculation. Bethesda: American Physiological Society, 1984:217–249.

27. Buchman TG, Menker JB, Lipsett PA. Strategies for trauma resuscitation. Surg Gynecol Obstet 1991; 172:8–12.

28. Barcelona SL, Vilich F, Cote CJ. A comparison of flow rates and warming capabilities of the Level 1 and Rapid Infusion Systems with various-size intravenous catheters. Aneth Analg 2003; 97:358–363.

29. Hyman SA, Smith DW, England R, et al. Pulmonary artery catheter introducers: Do the component parts affect flow rate? Anesth Analg 1991; 73:573–575.

30. de la Roche MRP, Gauthier L. Rapid transfusion of packed red blood cells: effects of dilution, pressure, and catheter size. Ann Emerg Med 1993; 22:1551–1555.

Resuscitation Strategies

31. Shoemaker WC. Relationship of oxygen transport patterns to the pathophysiology and therapy of shock states. Intensive Care Med 1987; 213:230–243.

32. Marik PE, Sibbald WJ. Effect of stored-blood transfusion on oxygen delivery in patients with sepsis. JAMA 1993; 269:3024–3029.

33. Imm A, Carlson RW. Fluid resuscitation in circulatory shock. Crit Care Clin 1993; 9:313–333.

34. Dantry HP, Alam HB. Fluid resuscitation: past, present, and future. Shock 2010; 33:229–241.

35. American College of Surgeons. Shock. In Advanced Trauma Life Support Manual, 7th ed. Chicago: American College of Surgeons, 2004:87–107.

36. Napolitano LM, Kurek S, Luchette FA, et al. Clinical practice guideline: red blood cell transfusion in adult trauma and critical care. Crit Care Med 2009; 37:3124–3157.

37. Beekley AC. Damage control resuscitation: a sensible approach to the exanguinating surgical patient. Crit Care Med 2008; 36:S267–S274.

38. Bickell WH, Wall MJ Jr, Pepe PE, et al. Immediate versus delayed fluid resuscitation for hypotensive patients with penetrating torso injuries. N Engl J Med 1994; 331:1105–1109.

39. Morrison CA, Carrick M, Norman MA, et al. Hypotensive resuscitation strategy reduces transfusion requirements and severe postoperative coagulopathy in trauma patients with hemorrhagic shock: preliminary results of a randomized controlled trial. J Trauma 2011; 70:652–663.

40. Brohi K, Singh J, Heron M, Coats T. Acute traumatic coagulopathy. J Trauma 2003; 54:1127–1130.

41. Magnotti LJ, Zarzaur BL, Fischer PE, et al. Improved survival after hemostatic resuscitation: does the emperor have no clothes? J Trauma 2011; 70:97–°102.

42. Stainsby D, MacLennan S, Thomas D, et al, for the British Committee for Standards in Hematology. Guidelines on the management of massive blood loss. Br J Haematol 2006; 135:634–641.

Postresuscitation Injury

43. Dewar D, Moore FA, Moore EE, Balogh Z. Postinjury multiorgan failure. Injury 2009; 40:912–918.

44. Eltzschig HK, Collard CD. Vascular ischaemia and reperfusion injury. Br Med Bull 2004; 70:71–86.

Chapter 12

COLLOID & CRYSTALLOID RESUSCITATION

The secret of science is to ask the right question.

Sir Henry Tizard

In 1861, Thomas Graham's investigations on diffusion led him to classify substances as crystalloids or colloids based on their ability to diffuse through a parchment membrane. Crystalloids passed readily through the membrane, whereas colloids (from the Greek word for glue) did not. Intravenous fluids are similarly classified based on their ability to pass through capillary walls that separate the intravascular and interstitial fluid compartments (see Figure 12.1). This chapter presents the variety of crystalloid and colloid fluids available for use, and describes the salient features of these fluids, both individually and as a group.

CRYSTALLOID FLUIDS

Volume Distribution

Crystalloid fluids are electrolyte solutions with small molecules that can diffuse freely from intravascular to interstitial fluid compartments. The principal component of crystalloid fluids is sodium chloride. Sodium is the principal determinant of extracellular volume, and is distributed uniformly in the extracellular fluid. The sodium in crystalloid fluids also distributes uniformly in the extracellular fluid. Because the plasma volume is only 25% of the interstitial fluid volume (see Table 11.1), only 25% of an infused crystalloid fluid will expand the plasma volume, while 75% of the infused volume will expand the interstitial fluid. Thus, *the predominant effect of crystalloid fluids is to expand the interstitial volume, not the plasma volume.*

217

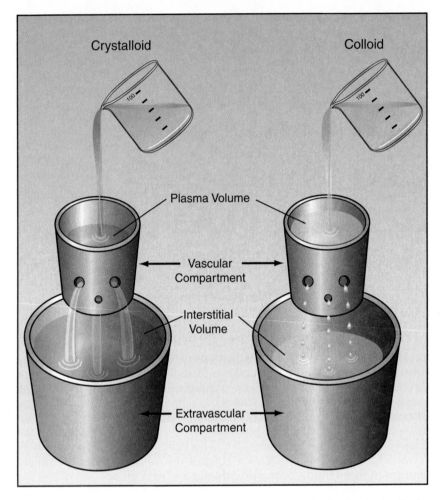

FIGURE 12.1 Illustration depicting the different tendencies of colloid and crystalloid fluids to expand the plasma volume and the interstitial fluid volume. See text for further explanation.

Isotonic Saline

One of the most widely used crystalloid fluids is 0.9% sodium chloride (1), with annual sales of 200 *million* liters in the United States (data from Baxter Healthcare). This solution has a variety of names, including normal saline, physiologic saline, and isotonic saline, none of which is appropriate (see next). The term used for 0.9% NaCL in this text is *isotonic saline*, to distinguish it from hypertonic saline (described later).

Normal Saline is Not Normal

The most popular term for 0.9% NaCL is *normal saline*, but this solution is neither chemically nor physiologically normal. It is not normal chemically because the concentration of a one-normal (1 N) NaCL solution is 58 grams per liter (the combined molecular weights of sodium and chloride), while 0.9% NaCL contains only 9 grams of NaCL per liter. It is not normal physiologically because the composition of 0.9% NaCL differs from the composition of extracellular fluid. This is shown in Table 12.1. When compared to plasma (extracellular fluid), 0.9% NaCL has a higher sodium concentration (154 vs. 140 mEq/L), a much higher chloride concentration (154 vs. 103 mEq/L), a higher osmolality (308 vs. 290 mOsm/L), and a lower pH (5.7 vs. 7.4). These differences can have deleterious effects on fluid and acid-base balance, as described next.

Table 12.1	Comparison of Plasma and Crystalloid Resuscitation Fluids							
Fluid	**mEq/L**							**Osmolality**
	Na	**CL**	**K**	**Ca**[§]	**Mg**	**Buffers**	**pH**	**(mOsm/L)**
Plasma	140	103	4	4	2	HCO_3^-(25)	7.4	290
0.9% NaCL	154	154	–	–	–	–	5.7	308
7.5% NaCL[†]	1283	1283	–	–	–	–	5.7	2567
Ringer's Injection	147	156	4	4	–	–	5.8	309
Ringer's Lactate	130	109	4	3	–	Lactate (28)	6.5	273
Ringer's Acetate	131	109	4	3	–	Acetate (28)	6.7	275
Normosol Plasma-Lyte A	140	98	5	–	3	Acetate (27) Gluconate (23)	7.4	295

[§]Concentration of ionized calcium in mg/dL.
[†]Not commercially available.

Volume Effects

The effects of 0.9% NaCL on expanding the plasma volume and interstitial fluid volume are shown in Figure 12.2. Infusion of one liter of 0.9% NaCL adds 275 mL to the plasma volume and 825 mL to the interstitial volume (2). This is the distribution expected of a crystalloid fluid. However, there is one unexpected finding; i.e., the total increase in extracellular volume (1,100 mL) is slightly greater than the infused volume. This is the result of a fluid shift from the intracellular to extracellular fluid, which occurs because 0.9% NaCL is slightly hypertonic in relation to extracellular fluid, as shown in Table 12.1.

INTERSTITIAL EDEMA: Infusions of 0.9% NaCL promote interstitial edema more than crystalloid fluids with a lower sodium content (e.g., Ringer's lactate, Plasma-Lyte) (3). This is related to the increased sodium load from 0.9% NaCL, which increases the "tonicity" of the interstitial fluid (as just described) and promotes sodium retention by suppressing the renin-angiotensin-aldosterone axis (4). Decreases in renal perfusion have also been observed after infusion of 0.9% NaCL (3), presumably as a

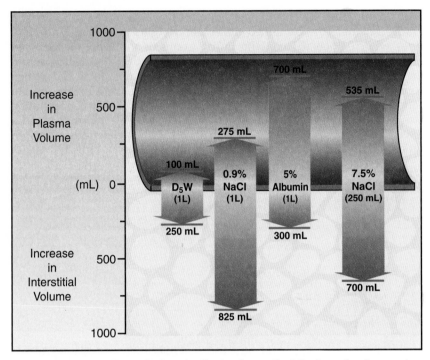

FIGURE 12.2 The effects of selected colloid and crystalloid fluids on the plasma volume and interstitial fluid volume. The infusion volume of each fluid is shown in parentheses. Data from Reference 2.

result of chloride-mediated renal vasoconstriction. The increase in interstitial edema with 0.9% NaCL can have a negative influence on clinical outcomes (5).

Acid-Base Effect

Large-volume infusions of 0.9% NaCL produce a *metabolic acidosis* (6,7), as demonstrated in Figure 12.3. In this clinical study (6), infusion of isotonic saline (0.9% NaCL) at a rate of 30 mL/kg/h was accompanied by a progressive decline in the pH of blood (from 7.41 to 7.28) over two hours, while the pH was unchanged when Ringer's lactate solution was infused at a similar rate. The saline-induced metabolic acidosis is a *hyperchloremic acidosis*, and is *caused by the high concentration of chloride in 0.9% saline relative to plasma* (154 versus 103 mEq/L). The close match between the chloride concentration in Ringer's lactate solution and plasma (see Table 12.1) explains the lack of a pH effect associated with large-volume infusion of Ringer's lactate solution.

STRONG ION DIFFERENCE: The influence of crystalloid fluids on acid-base balance can also be explained using the *strong ion difference* (SID), which is the difference between readily dissociated (strong) cations and anions

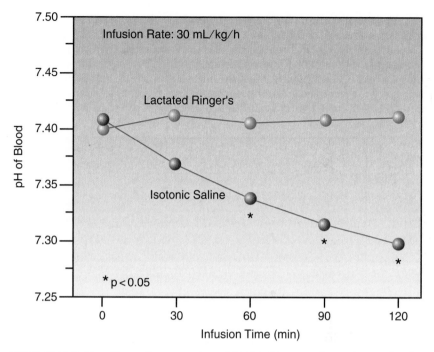

FIGURE 12.3 The effects of isotonic saline (0.9% NaCL) versus lactated Ringer's solution on the pH of blood in patients undergoing elective surgery. Total volume infused after 2 hours was 5 to 6 liters for each fluid. Data from Reference 6.

in extracellular fluid (8). (The SID of plasma is roughly equivalent to the plasma [Na] – plasma [CL] since these are the most prevalent strong ions in extracellular fluid. Plasma HCO_3 is not included in the SID because HCO_3 is not a strong ion.) The principle of electrical neutrality requires an equal concentration of cations and anions in the extracellular fluid, so the relationship between SID and the ions that dissociate from water (H^+ and OH^-) can be described as follows:

$$SID + [H^+] - [OH^-] = 0 \qquad (12.1)$$

Since the $[OH^-]$ is negligible in the physiologic pH range, equation 12.1 can be rewritten as:

$$SID + [H^+] = 0 \qquad (12.2)$$

According to this relationship, a change in SID must be accompanied by a reciprocal change in $[H^+]$ (or a proportional change in pH) to maintain electrical neutrality. The relationship between the SID and pH of plasma is shown in Figure 12.4 (9). Note that the SID and pH change in the same direction (because pH is used instead of $[H^+]$). The normal SID of plasma is 40 mEq/L (as indicated by the dotted line), which is roughly equivalent to the normal plasma $[Na^+]$ – $[CL^-]$ difference (140 – 103 mEq/L).

The SID of intravenous fluids determines their ability to influence the pH of plasma. The SID of 0.9% NaCL is zero (Na – CL = 154 – 154 = 0) , so infusions of 0.9% NaCL will reduce the SID of plasma and thereby reduce the plasma pH. The SID of Ringer's lactate fluid is 28 mEq/L (Na + K + Ca – CL = 130 + 4 + 3 – 109 = 28) if all the infused lactate is metabolized. This SID is not far removed from the normal SID of plasma, so Ringer's lactate infusions will have less of an influence on plasma pH than 0.9% NaCL.

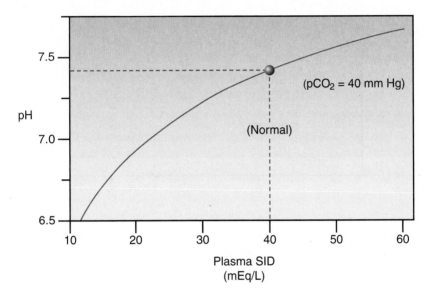

FIGURE 12.4 The relationship between the strong ion difference (SID) and the pH of extracellular fluid (plasma). The normal SID of plasma is about 40 mEq/L. The SID of a crystalloid fluid relative to plasma determines the tendency of the fluid to influence acid-base status. See text for further explanation. Graph redrawn from Reference 9.

Ringer's Fluids

Sydney Ringer, a British physician who studied the contraction of isolated frog hearts, introduced a sodium chloride solution in 1880 that contained calcium and potassium to promote cardiac contraction and cell viability (10). This solution is shown as *Ringer's injection* in Table 12.1, and is essentially 0.9% NaCL with potassium and ionized calcium added.

Ringer's Lactate

In the early 1930's, an American pediatrician named Alexis Hartmann added sodium lactate to Ringer's solution to provide a buffer for the treatment of metabolic acidosis (10). This solution was originally called Hartmann's solution, and is now known as *Ringer's lactate* solution. The composition of this solution is shown in Table 12.1. The sodium concentration in Ringer's lactate is reduced to compensate for the sodium released from sodium lactate, and the chloride concentration is reduced to compensate for the negatively-charged lactate molecule; both changes result in an electrically neutral salt solution.

Ringer's Acetate

Because of concerns that large-volume infusions of Ringer's lactate solution could increase plasma lactate levels in patients with impaired lactate clearance (e.g., from liver disease), the lactate buffer was replaced by acetate to create *Ringer's acetate* solution. Acetate is metabolized in muscle rather than liver (10), which makes Ringer's acetate a reasonable alternative to Ringer's lactate in patients with liver failure. (The influence of Ringer's lactate on serum lactate levels is described below). As shown in Table 12.1, the composition of Ringer's acetate and Ringer's lactate solutions is almost identical with the exception of the added buffer.

Advantages & Disadvantages

The principal advantage of Ringer's lactate and Ringer's acetate over isotonic saline (0.9% NaCL) is the lack of a significant effect on acid-base balance. The principal disadvantage of Ringer's solutions is the calcium content; i.e., the ionized calcium in Ringer's solutions can bind to the citrated anticoagulant in stored RBCs and promote clot formation. For this reason, *Ringer's solutions are contraindicated as diluent fluids for the transfusion of erythrocyte concentrates (packed red blood cells)* (11). However, clot formation does not occur if the volume of Ringer's solution does not exceed 50% of the volume of packed RBCs (12).

LACTATE CONSIDERATIONS: As mentioned above, the lactate content in Ringer's lactate solution (28 mM/L) creates concern about the risk of spurious hyperlactatemia with large-volume infusions of the fluid. In healthy subjects, infusion of one liter of lactated Ringer's over one hour does not raise serum lactate levels (8). In critically ill patients, who may have impaired lactate clearance from circulatory shock or hepatic insufficiency, the impact of lactated Ringer's infusions on serum lactate levels is not known. However, if lactate clearance is zero, the addition of one liter of lactated Ringer's to a blood volume of 5 liters (which would require infusion of 3–4 liters of fluid) would raise the serum lactate level by 4.6 mM/L (13). Therefore, lactated Ringer's infusions are unlikely to have a considerable impact on serum lactate levels unless large volumes are infused in patients with virtually no capacity for clearing lactate from the bloodstream.

Blood samples obtained from intravenous catheters that are being used for lactated Ringer's infusions can yield spuriously high serum lactate determinations (14). Therefore, in patients receiving lactated Ringer's infusions, blood samples for lactate measurements should be obtained from sites other than the infusion catheter.

Other Balanced Salt Solutions

Two of the crystalloid fluids in Table 12.1 (i.e., Normosol and Plasma-Lyte) contain magnesium instead of calcium, and contain both acetate

and gluconate buffers to achieve a pH of 7.4 These fluids are not as popular as isotonic saline or Ringer's lactate, but the absence of calcium
makes them suitable as diluents for RBC transfusions, and Plasma-Lyte
has shown less of a tendency to promote interstitial edema when compared with isotonic saline (3,5).

Hypertonic Saline

Hypertonic saline solutions like 7.5% NaCL (which has an osmolality
8–9 times greater than plasma) are much more effective at expanding the
extracellular volume than isotonic crystalloid fluids. This is demonstrated in Figure 12.2, which shows that infusion of 250 mL of 7.5% NaCL
results in a 1,235 mL increase in extracellular fluid, which is about 5 times
greater than the infusion volume. (The added volume comes from the
intracellular fluid.) Animal studies have shown that hypertonic saline is
effective for limited-volume resuscitation of hemorrhagic shock. This is
demonstrated in Figure 12.5, which shows that hypertonic saline can
restore and maintain cardiac output with $1/5$ the volume required with
isotonic saline (15).

Observations like the one in Figure 12.5 suggested that hypertonic saline
would be well suited for situations where small volumes of resuscitation
fluid are advantageous; e.g., the prehospital resuscitation of trauma vic-

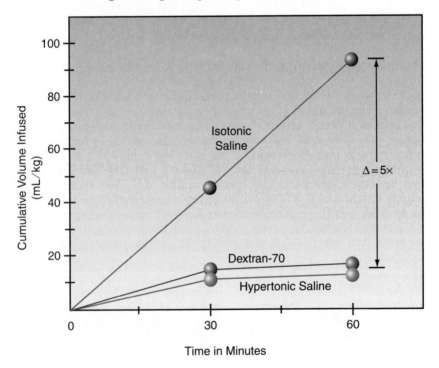

FIGURE 12.5 A comparison of the cumulative volume of three intravenous fluids
needed to maintain a normal rate of aortic blood flow in an animal model of hemorrhagic shock. Data from Reference 15.

tims, particularly those with traumatic brain injury (16). Unfortunately, the accumulated evidence shows *no apparent survival benefit from hypertonic saline compared to isotonic crystalloids for the management of traumatic shock* (17) *or traumatic brain injury* (18). The addition of 6% dextran-70 to hypertonic saline to make a hyperoncotic-hypertonic fluid has not improved the results (16.18,19). As a result, hypertonic resuscitation is currently in the graveyard of resuscitation strategies.

5% DEXTROSE SOLUTIONS

The once-popular use of 5% dextrose solutions (D_5 solutions) has fallen out of favor, as explained in this section.

Protein-Sparing Effect

Prior to the standard use of enteral tube feedings and total parenteral nutrition (TPN), 5% dextrose solutions were used to provide calories in patients who were unable to eat. Dextrose provides 3.4 kilocalories (kcal) per gram when fully metabolized, so a 5% dextrose solution (50 grams dextrose per liter) provides 170 kcal per liter. Infusion of 3 liters of a D_5 solution daily (125 mL/min) provides 3 x 170 = 510 kcal/day, which is enough nonprotein calories to limit the breakdown of endogenous proteins to provide calories (i.e., *protein-sparing effect*). This is no longer necessary, as most patients can tolerate enteral tube feedings, and those who cannot will receive TPN.

Volume Effects

The addition of dextrose to intravenous fluids increases osmolality (50 g of dextrose adds 278 mOsm/L to an intravenous fluid). For a 5% dextrose-in-water solution (D_5W), the added dextrose brings the osmolality close to that of plasma. However, since the dextrose is taken up by cells and metabolized, this osmolality effect rapidly wanes, and the added water then moves into cells. This is shown in Figure 12.2. The infusion of one liter of D_5W results in an increase in extracellular fluid (plasma plus interstitial fluid) of about 350 mL, which means the remaining 650 mL (two-thirds of the infused volume) has moved intracellularly. Therefore, *the predominant effect of D_5W is cellular swelling*.

An effect opposite to that of D_5W can occur when dextrose is added to 0.9% NaCL. As described previously, the osmolality of 0.9% NaCL is slightly higher than extracellular fluid (308 vs. 290 mOsm/L), and this results in some movement of water out of cells. When 50 grams of dextrose is added to make D_5-normal saline, the osmolality of the fluid increases to 560 mOsm/L, which is almost twice the normal osmolality of the extracellular fluid. *If glucose utilization is impaired (as is common in critically ill patients), large-volume infusions of D_5W can result in cellular dehydration*.

Enhanced Lactate Production

In healthy subjects, only 5% of an infused glucose load will result in lactate formation, but in critically ill patients with tissue hypoperfusion, as much as 85% of glucose metabolism is diverted to lactate production (20). This latter effect is demonstrated in Figure 12.6. In this case, tissue hypoperfusion was induced by aortic clamping during abdominal aortic aneurysm surgery (21). Patients received intraoperative fluids to maintain normal cardiac filling pressures using either a Ringer's solution or a 5% dextrose solution. When the dextrose-containing fluid was infused, the serum lactate levels began to rise after the aorta was cross-clamped, and the increase in circulating lactate levels persisted throughout the remainder of the surgery. These results indicate that, *when circulatory flow is compromised, infusion of 5% dextrose solutions can result in lactic acid production and significant elevations of serum lactate.*

Hyperglycemia

About 20% of patients admitted to ICUs are diabetic (22), and as many as 90% of patients will develop hyperglycemia at some time during their ICU stay (23). Hyperglycemia has several deleterious effects in critically ill patients, including immune suppression (22), increased risk of infection (23), aggravation of ischemic brain injury (24), and increased mortality, particularly following cardiac surgery (23). Because of the association between hyperglycemia and increased morbidity and mortality, blood glucose levels are typically not allowed to remain above 180 mg/dL in ICU patients (25).

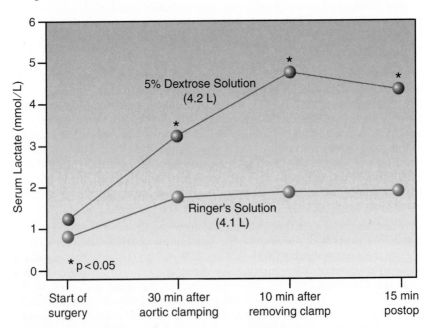

FIGURE 12.6 The effect of intravenous fluid therapy with and without dextrose on blood lactate levels in patients undergoing abdominal aortic aneurysm repair. Each point represents the mean lactate level in 10 study patients. The average infusion volume for each fluid is indicated in parentheses. Data from Reference 21.

Considering the high risk of hyperglycemia in ICU patients, and the numerous adverse consequences of hyperglycemia, infusion of dextrose-containing fluids should be avoided whenever possible. In fact, considering the potential for harm, it seems that *the routine use of 5% dextrose solutions should be abandoned in critically ill patients.*

COLLOID FLUIDS

In chemical terms, a colloidal solution is a particulate solution with particles that do not dissolve completely. (These solutions are also called *suspensions*). In clinical terms, a colloid fluid is a saline solution with large solute molecules that do not pass readily from plasma to interstitial fluid. The retained molecules in a colloid fluid create an osmotic force called the *colloid osmotic pressure* or *oncotic pressure* that holds water in the vascular compartment, as reviewed next.

Capillary Fluid Exchange

The direction and rate of fluid exchange (Q) between capillary blood and interstitial fluid is determined, in part, by the balance between the hydrostatic pressure in the capillaries (P_c), which promotes the movement of fluid out of capillaries, and the colloid osmotic pressure of plasma (COP), which favors the movement of fluid into capillaries.

$$Q \approx P_C - COP \qquad\qquad (12.3)$$

In the supine position, the normal P_c averages about 20 mm Hg (30 mm Hg at the arterial end of the capillaries and 10 mm Hg at the venous end of the capillaries); the normal COP of plasma is about 28 mm Hg (26), so the net forces normally favor the movement of fluid into capillaries (which preserves the plasma volume). About 80% of the plasma COP is due to the albumin fraction of plasma proteins (26), so a reduction in the plasma albumin concentration (hypoalbuminemia) favors the movement of fluid out of the capillaries and promotes interstitial edema.

Resuscitation Fluids

The volume distribution of colloid and crystalloid fluids can be explained by their influence on the plasma COP. Crystalloid fluids reduce the plasma COP (dilutional effect), which favors the movement of these fluids out of the bloodstream. Colloid fluids can preserve the normal COP (iso-oncotic fluids), which holds these fluids in the bloodstream, or they can increase the plasma COP (hyperoncotic colloid fluids), which pulls interstitial fluid into the bloodstream.

Volume Effects

The volume distribution of a (nearly iso-oncotic) colloid fluid is demonstrated in Figure 12.2. The colloid fluid in this case is a 5% albumin solution, which has a COP of 20 mm Hg. Infusion of one liter of this solution results in a 700 mL increment in the plasma volume and a 300 mL increment in the interstitial fluid volume. When compared with the increment in plasma volume after one liter of 0.9% NaCL (275 mL), the colloid fluid is about 3 times more effective in expanding the plasma volume than the crystalloid fluid. Most observations indicate that, *in equivalent volumes, colloid fluids are at least three times more effective than crystalloid fluids for expanding the plasma volume* (2, 27–29).

As expected from Figure 12.2, colloid fluids promote cardiac output at much lower infusate volumes than required with crystalloid fluids. This is demonstrated in Figure 12.5 (described earlier), which shows that restoring the cardiac output in hemorrhagic shock requires five times more volume when a crystalloid fluid (isotonic saline) is infused instead of a colloid fluid (dextran-70).

Colloid Fluid Comparisons

As mentioned earlier, the ability of a colloid fluid to augment the plasma volume is determined by the COP of the fluid relative to the plasma COP. This is demonstrated in Table 12.2, which includes the commonly used colloid fluids in the United States, along with the oncotic pressure (COP) of each fluid and the increment in plasma volume produced by a given infusate volume. Note that the higher the COP of the fluid, the greater the increment in plasma volume relative to the infusate volume. Fluids with a COP of 20–30 mm Hg are considered to be iso-oncotic fluids (i.e., fluid COP equivalent to plasma COP); these fluids produce increments in plasma volume that are roughly equivalent to the infusate volume (range = 70–130% of infusate volume). Colloid fluids with a COP > 30 mm Hg are hyperoncotic fluids (fluid COP > plasma COP); these fluids produce increments in plasma volume that are usually greater than the infusate volume. This is most apparent with 25% albumin, which has a COP of 70 mm Hg, and produces an increment in plasma volume that is 3 to 4 times greater than the infusate volume.

Table 12.2	Characteristics of Individual Colloid Fluids			
Fluid	**Average Molecular Wt (kilodaltons)**	**Oncotic Pressure (mm Hg)**	**ΔPlasma Volume / Infusate Volume**	**Duration of Effect**
25% Albumin	69	70	3.0 – 4.0	12 h
10% Dextran-40	26	40	1.0 – 1.5	6 h
6% Hetastarch	450	30	1.0 – 1.3	24 h
5% Albumin	69	20	0.7 – 1.3	12 h

Data from References 2, 27–29, 38.

Albumin Solutions

Albumin is a versatile plasma protein with several functions. It is the principal determinant of plasma COP (26), the principal transport protein in blood (see Table 12.3), has significant antioxidant activity (30), and helps maintain the fluidity of blood by inhibiting platelet aggregation (31). As much as $2/3$ of the albumin in the body is located outside blood vessels (32); the role of the extravascular albumin pool is unclear.

Features

Albumin solutions are heat-treated preparations of human serum albumin that are available as a 5% solution (50 g/L) and a 25% solution (250 g/L) in 0.9% NaCL. The 5% albumin solution is usually given in aliquots of 250 mL; the colloid osmotic pressure is 20 mm Hg, and the plasma volume increment averages 100% of the infused volume. The volume effect begins to dissipate at 6 hours, and can be lost after 12 hours (2,27).

Table 12.3	Substances Transported by Albumin	
Drugs	**Others**	
Benzodiazepines	Bilirubin	
Cephalosporine	Copper	
Furosemide		
NSAIDS	Estrogen	
Phenytoin	Fatty Acids	
Quinidine	Progesterone	
Salicylates		
Sulfonamides	Prostaglandins	
Valproic Acid	Testosterone	
Warfarin	Zinc	

The 25% albumin solution is a hyperoncotic fluid with a colloid osmotic pressure of 70 mm Hg (more than twice that of plasma). It is given in aliquots of 50–100 mL, and the plasma volume increment is 3 to 4 times the infusate volume. The effect is produced by fluid shifts from the interstitial space, so interstitial fluid volume decreases as plasma volume increases. Because it does not replace lost volume, but instead shifts fluid from one compartment to another, *25% albumin should not be used for volume resuscitation in patients with blood loss*. This fluid should be reserved for instances where hypovolemia is the result of hypoalbuminemia, which promotes fluid shifts from plasma to interstitial fluid.

Safety

Albumin's reputation was sullied in 1998 when a clinical review suggested that one of every 17 patients who received albumin infusions died as a result of the fluid (33). This has been refuted in subsequent studies showing that albumin poses no greater risk of death than other volume expanders (34,35). The consensus opinion at the present time is that 5% albumin is safe to use as a resuscitation fluid (32), except possibly in traumatic head injury, where one large study has shown a higher mortality rate in patients who received albumin instead of isotonic saline (36). Hyperoncotic (25%) albumin has been associated with an increased risk of renal injury and death in patients with circulatory shock (37), which is similar to the renal injury reported with other hyperoncotic colloid fluids (see next).

Hydroxyethyl Starch

Hydroxyethyl starch (HES) is a chemically modified polysaccharide composed of long chains of branched glucose polymers substituted periodically by hydroxyl radicals (OH), which resist enzymatic degradation. HES elimination involves hydrolysis by amylase enzymes in the bloodstream, which cleave the parent molecule until it is small enough to be cleared by the kidneys. The following is a summary of the important features of HES preparations (32,38).

Features

MOLECULAR WEIGHT: HES preparations have different molecular weights, and are classified as high MW (450 kilodaltons or kD), medium MW (200 kD), and low MW (70 kD). High MW preparations have a prolonged duration of action because amylase cleavage results in progressively smaller molecules that are osmotically active. When the cleavage products reach a molecular weight of 50 kD, they can be cleared by the kidneys (32).

MOLAR SUBSTITUTION RATIO: HES preparations are also classified by the ratio of hydroxyl radical substitutions per glucose polymer (OH/glucose), which is called the *molar substitution ratio* and ranges from zero to one (32). Since hydroxyl radicals resist enzymatic degradation, higher OH/glucose ratios are associated with prolonged activity. Higher molar substitution ratios increase the risk of HES-associated coagulopathy (see later).

INDIVIDUAL PREPARATIONS: Individual HES preparations are described by their concentration, MW, and molar substitution ratio, as shown in Table 12.4. Most preparations are available as 6% solutions in 0.9% NaCL. The prefix of the HES preparation indicates the molar substitution ratio (e.g., *penta*starch = 0.5, *tetra*starch = 0.4). Hetastarch is the most commonly used HES preparation in the United States, and has a high MW(450 kD) and a high molar substitution ratio (0.7). Tetrastarch is the most recent HES preparation introduced for use in the United States, and has the lowest MW (130 kD) and the lowest molar substitution ratio (0.4). Tetrastarch is available as Voluven (Hospira).

Volume Effects

The performance of 6% HES solutions as plasma volume expanders is very similar to 5% albumin. The oncotic pressure is higher than 5% albumin, and the increment in plasma volume can be higher as well (see Table 12.2). The effect on plasma volume can last up to 24 hours with high MW preparations such as hetastarch (38). The duration of action of the lower

MW preparations is at least 6 hours, but effects begin to dissipate within one hour (4).

Table 12.4	Characteristics of Hydroxyethylstarch Preparations		
Name	Concentration	MW	(OH/Glucoss)
Hetastarch	6%	450 kD	0.7
Hexastarch	6%	200 kD	0.6
Pentastarch	6%, 10%	200 kD	0.5
Tetrastarch	6%	130 kD	0.4

Altered Hemostasis

HES can impair hemostasis by inhibition of Factor VII and von Wille-brand factor, and impaired platelet adhesiveness (32,39). This effect was originally attributed to high MW preparations, but high (OH/glucose) ratios are now considered more important in determining the risk of altered hemostasis (32). Clinically significant coagulopathies are uncommon unless large volumes of HES are infused (e.g., > 50 mL/kg for tetrastarch) (28).

Nephrotoxicity

Several studies have shown an association between HES infusions and an increased risk of renal injury and death; this association has been reported with hetastarch (40), pentastarch (41), and tetrastarch (42). The colloid osmotic pressure of HES preparations (30 mm Hg for hetastarch and 36 mm Hg for tetrastarch) has been implicated in renal injury, although the precise mechanism is not clear. HES-associated renal injury has been reported mostly in patients with life-threatening conditions such as severe sepsis and circulatory shock (32,41,42). In patients who are less severely ill, there is no association between HES and renal injury (32), and some studies show a favorable responses to HES in such patients (43).

Hyperamylasemia

The amylase enzymes involved in the hydrolysis of HES attach to the HES molecules, and this reduces amylase clearance by the kidneys. This can result is an increase in serum amylase levels to 2–3 times above normal (38,44). Levels usually return to normal within one week after HES is discontinued. Serum lipase levels are unaffected by HES infusions (44).

The Dextrans

The dextrans are glucose polymers produced by a bacterium (*Leuconostoc*) incubated in a sucrose medium. First introduced in the 1940s, these colloids are not popular (at least in the United States) because of the perceived risk of adverse reactions. The two most common dextran preparations are 10% dextran-40 and 6% dextran-70, each preparation using 0.9% NaCL as a diluent. The features of 10% dextran-40 are shown in Table 12.2.

Features

Both dextran preparations have a colloid osmotic pressure of 40 mm Hg, and cause a greater increase in plasma volume than either 5% albumin or 6% hetastarch (see Table 12.2). Dextran-70 may be preferred because the duration of action (12 hours) is longer than that of dextran-40 (6 hours) (27).

Disadvantages

1. Dextrans produce a dose-related bleeding tendency that involves impaired platelet aggregation, decreased levels of Factor VIII and von Willebrand factor, and enhanced fibrinolysis (39,44). The hemostatic defects are minimized by limiting the daily dextran dose to 20 mL/kg.

2. Dextrans coat the surface of red blood cells and can interfere with the ability to cross-match blood. Red cell preparations must be washed to eliminate this problem. Dextrans also increase the erythrocyte sedimentation rate as a result of their interactions with red blood cells (44).

3. Dextrans have been associated with an osmotically-mediated renal injury similar to that observed with HES preparations (44,45). However, this complication occurs only rarely with dextran infusions. Anaphylactic reactions, once common with dextrans, are now reported in only .03% of infusions (44).

COLLOID–CRYSTALLOID CONUNDRUM

There is a longstanding debate concerning the type of fluid that is most appropriate for volume resuscitation, and each type of fluid has its loyalists who passionately defend the merits of their chosen fluid. The following is a brief description of the issues involved in this debate, and a suggested compromise.

Early Focus on Crystalloids

Early studies of acute blood loss in the 1960s showed that hemorrhagic shock was associated with an interstitial fluid deficit, partly as a result of a fluid shift from the interstitial fluid into the bloodstream (46). In an animal model of hemorrhagic shock, replacement of the shed blood was almost universally fatal, while survival improved significantly if Ringer's lactate fluid was added to the replacement of shed blood (47). These results were interpreted as indicating that replacement of the interstitial fluid deficit (with Ringer's lactate) was the critical factor in the successful resuscitation of hemorrhagic shock. This led to the popularity of crystalloid fluids for the resuscitation of blood loss. Therefore, *crystalloid fluids were popularized for volume resuscitation because of their ability to resuscitate the interstitial volume, not the plasma volume.*

More Recent Concerns

Since those early studies, the importance of promoting cardiac output and systemic O_2 delivery have emerged as the primary focus of volume resuscitation. To this end, colloid fluids have proven superior to crystalloid fluids, as demonstrated in Figure 11.6 (Chapter 11). Despite this superiority, crystalloid fluids remain the popular choice for volume resuscitation (at least in the United States). The principal argument in favor of crystalloid resuscitation is the lack of proven survival benefit with colloid resuscitation (48,49), and the lower cost of crystalloid fluids (see Table 12.5). The problem with crystalloid resuscitation is the relatively large volumes needed to expand the plasma volume (at least 3 times greater than the volume of colloid fluids), which promotes edema formation and a positive fluid balance, both of which are associated with increased morbidity and mortality in critically ill patients (5,50).

Table 12.5	Relative Cost of Intravenous Fluids		
Fluid	**Manufacturer**	**Unit Size**	**Unit Cost†**
Crystalloid Fluids			
0.9% NaCL	Baxter	1,000 mL	$1.95
Ringer's Lactate	Baxter	1,000 mL	$2.06
Colloid Fluids			
5% Albumin	Grifols	250 mL	$43.92
25% Albumin	Grifols	50 mL	$43.92
6% Hetastarch	Hospira	500 mL	$41.72
6% Tetrastarch§	Hospira	500 mL	$60.27

†Hospital cost in 2012. §Available as Voluven.

A Problem-Based Approach

The colloid-crystalloid controversy is fueled by the premise that one type of fluid is optimal in all cases of hypovolemia. This seems unreasonable, since no single resuscitation fluid will perform optimally in all conditions associated with hypovolemia. The following are some examples of hypovolemia where different resuscitation fluids would be most effective.

1. In cases of life-threatening hypovolemia from blood loss (where a prompt increase in plasma volume is necessary), an iso-oncotic colloid fluid (e.g., 5% albumin) would be most effective.

2. In cases of hypovolemia secondary to dehydration (where there is a uniform loss of extracellular fluid), a crystalloid fluid (e.g., Ringer's lactate) is appropriate.

3. In cases of hypovolemia where hypoalbuminemia is implicated (causing fluid shifts from plasma to interstitial fluid) a hyperoncotic colloid fluid (e.g., 25% albumin) is an appropriate choice.

As demonstrated in these examples, tailoring the type of resuscitation fluid to the specific cause and severity of hypovolemia is a more reasoned approach than using the same type of fluid for all cases of hypovolemia. Thus, to apply Sir Henry Tizard's introductory quote to resuscitation fluids, one could say that *the secret to selecting the appropriate resuscitation fluid is to ask the question — what is the cause and severity of the hypovolemia in this patient?*

A FINAL WORD

The following information in this chapters deserves emphasis:

1. Normal saline (0.9% NaCL) is not normal, either chemically or physiologically, and infusions of this fluid often results in a metabolic acidosis. This does not occur with Ringer's lactate or Ringer's acetate solutions.

2. Isotonic crystalloid fluids expand the interstitial fluid volume more than the plasma volume, and large-volume infusion of crystalloid fluids can lead to troublesome edema formation.

3. Colloid fluids are superior to crystalloid fluids for expanding the plasma volume.

4. Hyperoncotic colloid fluids, particularly the hydroxyethyl starches, are associated with an increased risk of renal injury in patients with acute, life-threatening conditions (e.g., severe sepsis and septic shock). This complication is not usually observed in less severely ill patients (e.g., postoperative patients).

5. The colloid-crystalloid debate is misguided because there is no single resuscitation fluid that is optimal for all cases of hypovolemia.

REFERENCES

Crystalloid Fluids

1. Awad S, Allison S, Lobo DN. The history of 0.9% saline. Clin Nutr 2008; 27:179–188.

2. Imm A, Carlson RW. Fluid resuscitation in circulatory shock. Crit Care Clin 1993; 9:313–333.

3. Chowdhury AH, Cox EF, Francis ST, Lobo DN. A randomized, controlled, double-blind crossover study on the effects of 2-L infusions of 0.9% saline and Plasma-Lyte 148 on renal blood flow and renal cortical tissue perfusion in healthy volunteers. Ann Surg 2012; 256:18–24.

4. Lobo DN, Stanga Z, Aloysius MM, et al. Effect of volume loading 1 liter intravenous infusions of 0.9% NaCL, 4% succinated gelatine (Gelofusine), and hydroxyethyl starch (Voluven) on blood volume and endocrine responses: a randomized three-way crossover study in healthy volunteers. Crit Care Med 2010; 38:464–470.

5. Shaw AD, Bagshaw SM, Goldstein SL, et al. Major complications, mortality, and resource utilization after open abdominal surgery: 0.9% saline compared to Plasma-Lyte. Ann Surg 2012; 255:821–829.

6. Scheingraber S, Rehm M, Schmisch C, Finsterer U. Rapid saline infusion produces hyperchloremic acidosis in patients undergoing gynecologic surgery. Anesthesiology 1999; 90:1265–1270.

7. Prough DS, Bidani A. Hyperchloremic metabolic acidosis is a predictable consequence of intraoperative infusion of 0.9% saline. Anesthesiology 1999; 90:1247–1249.

8. Stewart PA. Modern quantitative acid-base chemistry. Can J Physiol Pharmacol 1983; 61:1444–1461.

9. Kellum JA, Elbers PWG, eds. Stewart's Textbook of Acid Base, 2nd ed. Amsterdam: Acidbase.org, 2009, pg 140.

10. Griffith CA. The family of Ringer's solutions. J Natl Intravenous Ther Assoc 1986; 9:480–483.

11. American Association of Blood Banks Technical Manual. 10th ed. Arlington, VA: American Association of Blood Banks, 1990:368.

12. King WH, Patten ED, Bee DE. An in vitro evaluation of ionized calcium levels and clotting in red blood cells diluted with lactated Ringer's solution. Anesthesiology 1988; 68:115–121.

13. Didwania A, Miller J, Kassel; D, et al. Effect of intravenous lactated Ringer's solution infusion on the circulating lactate concentration: Part 3. Result of a prospective, randomized, double-blind, placebo-controlled trial. Crit Care Med 1997; 25:1851–1854.

14. Jackson EV Jr, Wiese J, Sigal B, et al. Effects of crystalloid solutions on circulating lactate concentrations. Part 1. Implications for the proper handling of blood specimens obtained from critically ill patients. Crit Care Med 1997; 25:1840–1846.

15. Chiara O, Pelosi P, Brazzi L, et al. Resuscitation from hemorrhagic shock: Experimental model comparing normal saline, dextran, and hypertonic saline solutions. Crit Care Med 2003; 31:1915–1922.

16. Patanwala AE, Amini A, Erstad BL. Use of hypertonic saline injection in trauma. Am J Health Sys Pharm 2010; 67:1920–1928.

17. Bunn F, Roberts I, Tasker R, et al. Hypertonic versus near isotonic crystalloid for fluid resuscitation in critically ill patients. Cochrane Database Syst Rev 2004; 3:CD002045.

18. Bulger EM, May S, Brasel KJ, et al. Out-of-hospital hypertonic resuscitation following severe traumatic brain injury. JAMA 2010; 304:1455–1464.

19. Santy HP, Alam HB. Fluid resuscitation: past, present, and future. Shock 2010; 33:229–241.

5% Dextrose Solutions

20. Gunther B, Jauch W, Hartl W, et al. Low-dose glucose infusion in patients who have undergone surgery. Arch Surg 1987; 122:765–771.

21. DeGoute CS, Ray MJ, Manchon M, et al. Intraoperative glucose infusion and blood lactate: endocrine and metabolic relationships during abdominal aortic surgery. Anesthesiology 1989; 71;355–361.

22. Turina M, Fry D, Polk HC, Jr. Acute hyperglycemia and the innate immune system: Clinical, cellular, and molecular aspects. Crit Care Med 2005; 33:1624–1633.

23. Van Den Berghe G, Wouters P, Weekers F, et al. Intensive insulin therapy in critically ill patients. New Engl J Med 2001;345:1359–1367.

24. Sieber FE, Traystman RJ. Special issues: glucose and the brain. Crit Care Med 1992; 20:104–114.

25. Kavanagh BP, McCowen KC. Glycemic control in the ICU. N Engl J Med 2010; 363:25402546.

Colloid Fluids

26. Guyton AC, Hall JE. Textbook of Medical Physiology. 10th ed., Philadelphia: W.B. Saunders, Co, 2000, pp. 169–170.

27. Griffel MI, Kaufman BS. Pharmacology of colloids and crystalloids. Crit Care Clin 1992; 8:235–254.

28. Kaminski MV, Haase TJ. Albumin and colloid osmotic pressure: implications for fluid resuscitation. Crit Care Clin 1992; 8:311–322.

29. Sutin KM, Ruskin KJ, Kaufman BS. Intravenous fluid therapy in neurologic injury. Crit Care Clin 1992; 8:367–408.

30. Halliwell B. Albumin — an important extracellular antioxidant? Biochem Pharmacol 1988; 37:569–571.

31. Soni N, Margarson M. Albumin, where are we now? Curr Anesthes & Crit Care 2004; 15:61–68.

32. Muller M, Lefrant J-Y. Metabolic effects of plasma expanders. Transfusion Alter Transfusion Med 2010; 11:10–21.

33. Cochrane injuries Group Albumin Reviewers: Human albumin administration in critically ill patients: Systematic review of randomized, controlled trials. Br Med J 1998; 317:235–240.

34. Wilkes MN, Navickis RJ. Patient survival after human albumin administration: A meta-analysis of randomized, controlled trials. Ann Intern Med 2001; 135:149–164.

35. SAFE Study Investigators. A comparison of albumin and saline for fluid resuscitation in the Intensive Care Unit. N Engl J Med 2004; 350:2247–2256.

36. The SAFE Study Investigators. Saline or albumin for fluid resuscitation in patients with severe head injury. N Engl J Med 2007; 357:874–884.

37. Schortgen F, Girou E, Deve N, et al. The risk associated with hyperoncotic colloids in patients with shock. Intensive Care Med 2008; 34:2157–2168.

38. Treib J, Baron JF, Grauer MT, Strauss RG. An international view of hydroxyethyl starches. Intensive Care Med 1999; 25:258–268.

39. de Jonge E, Levi M. Effects of different plasma substitutes on blood coagulation: A comparative review. Crit Care Med 2001; 29:1261–1267.

40. Lissauer ME, Chi A, Kramer ME. et al. Association of 6% hetastarch resuscitation with adverse outcomes in critically ill trauma patients. Am J Surg 2011; 202:53–58.

41. Brunkhorst FM, Engel C, Bloos F, et al. Intensive insulin therapy and pentastarch resuscitation in severe sepsis. N Engl J Med 2008; 358:125–139.

42. Perner A, Haase N, Guttormsen AB, et al. Hydroxyethyl starch 130/0.4 versus Ringer's acetate in severe sepsis. N Engl J Med 2012; 367:124–134.

43. Magder S, Potter BJ, De Varennes B, et al. Fluids after cardiac surgery: A pilot study of the use of colloids versus crystalloids. Crit Care Med 2010; 38:2117–2124.

44. Nearman HS, Herman ML. Toxic effects of colloids in the intensive care unit. Crit Care Clin 1991; 7:713–723.

45. Drumi W, Polzleitner D, Laggner AN, et al. Dextran-40, acute renal failure, and elevated plasma oncotic pressure. N Engl J Med 1988; 318:252–254.

Colloid-Crystalloid Conundrum

46. Moore FD. The effects of hemorrhage on body composition. N Engl J Med 1965; 273:567–577.

47. Shires T, Carrico J, Lightfoot S. Fluid therapy in hemorrhagic shock. Arch Surg 1964; 88:688–693.

48. Roberts I, Blackhall K, Alderson P, et al. Human albumin solution for resuscitation and volume expansion in critically ill patients. Cochrane Database Syst Rev 2011; 10:CD001208.

49. Perel P, Roberts I. Colloids versus crystalloids for fluid resuscitation in critically ill patients. Cochrane Database Syst Rev 2012; 6:CD000567.

50. Boyd JH, Forbes J, Nakada T-a, et al. Fluid resuscitation in septic shock: A positive fluid balance and elevated central venous pressure are associated with increased mortality. Crit Care Med 2011; 39:259–265.

Chapter 13

ACUTE HEART FAILURE IN THE ICU

Movement is the cause of all life.

Leonardo da Vinci

Notebooks, Vol. I

Acute heart failure is responsible for about one million hospital admissions each year in the United States (1), and about 80% of the admissions involve the elderly (age ≥ 65 yrs) (2). The first appearance of acute, decompensated heart failure often marks the beginning of a progressive decline in clinical status. Although most patients (> 95%) survive the initial hospitalization for heart failure (5), 50% of patients are readmitted within 6 months (2), and 25–35% of patients die within 12 months after hospital discharge (2).

Heart failure is not a single entity, but is classified according to the portion of the cardiac cycle that is affected (systolic or diastolic dysfunction) and the side of the heart that is involved (right-sided or left-sided heart failure). This chapter describes each of these heart failure syndromes, and focuses on the advanced stages of heart failure that require management in an intensive care unit. Many of the recommendations in this chapter are derived from the clinical practice guidelines listed in the bibliography at the end of the chapter (2–5).

PATHOPHYSIOLOGY

Heart failure can originate from pathologic disorders involving the pericardium, myocardium, endocardium, or great vessels, as indicated in Figure 13.1. Most cases of heart failure originate in the myocardium, and are the result of ischemic injury or hypertrophy (2).

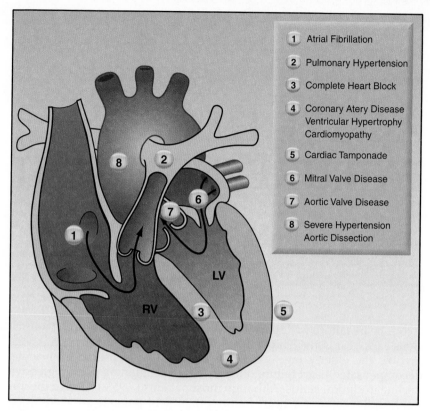

FIGURE 13.1 Possible causes of acute heart failure, indicated by the anatomic region involved. *RV* = right ventricle, *LV* = left ventricle.

Progressive Heart Failure

The changes in cardiac performance that occur in progressive stages of heart failure are shown in Figure 13.2. Three distinct stages are identified, and each is summarized below (using the corresponding numbers in Figure 13.2).

1. The earliest sign of ventricular dysfunction is an increase in cardiac filling pressure (i.e., the pulmonary artery wedge pressure). The stroke volume is maintained, but at the expense of the elevated filling pressure, which produces venous congestion in the lungs and the resulting sensation of dyspnea.

2. The next stage is marked by a decrease in stroke volume and an increase in heart rate. The tachycardia offsets the reduction in stroke volume, so the minute output of the heart (the cardiac output) is preserved.

3. The final stage is characterized by a decrease in cardiac output. and a further increase in the filling pressure. The point at which the cardiac output begins to fall marks the transition from compensated to decompensated heart failure.

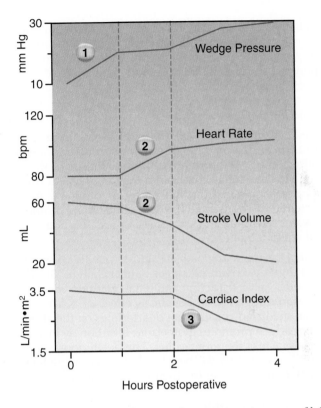

FIGURE 13.2 Changes in cardiac performance during progressive stages of left-sided heart failure in a postoperative patient. See text for further explanation.

Neurohumoral Responses

Heart failure triggers a multitude of endogenous responses, some beneficial and some counterproductive. The responses described here have the most clinical relevance (6).

Natriuretic Peptides

Increases in atrial and ventricular wall tension are accompanied by the release of four structurally similar *natriuretic peptides* from cardiac myocytes. These peptides "unload" the ventricles by promoting sodium excretion in the urine (which reduces ventricular preload) and dilating systemic blood vessels (which reduces ventricular preload and afterload). Natriuretic peptides also stimulate lipolysis in adipose tissue (7), but the relevance of this action is unclear. Natriuretic peptides play an important role in the evaluation of suspected heart failure, as described later in this section.

Sympathetic Nervous System

Decreases in stroke volume are sensed by baroreceptors in the carotid and pulmonary arteries, and activation of these receptors (through complex mechanisms) results in brainstem activation of the sympathetic nervous system. This occurs in the early stages of heart failure, and the principal results are positive inotropic and chronotropic effects in the heart, peripheral vasoconstriction, and activation of the renin-aldos-terone-angiotensin system.

Renin-Angiotensin-Aldosterone System

Specialized cells in the renal arterioles release renin in response to renal hypoperfusion and adrenergic β-receptor stimulation. Renin release has three consequences: the formation of angiotensin II, the production of aldosterone in the adrenal cortex, and the (angiotensin-triggered) release of arginine vasopressin from the posterior pituitary. Angiotensin produces systemic vasoconstriction, while aldosterone promotes renal sodium and water retention, and vasopressin promotes both vasoconstriction and renal water retention.

Activation of the renin-angiotensin-aldosterone (RAA) system is not fully developed until the advanced stages of heart failure (8), when the principal effects (i.e., vasoconstriction and renal retention of sodium and water) are counterproductive. One beneficial effect of RAA activation is the angiotensin-mediated constriction of arterioles on the efferent side of the glomerulus, which promotes glomerular filtration by increasing the filtration pressure across the glomerulus. The deleterious effects of the RAA system are confirmed by the beneficial effects of angiotensin converting enzyme (ACE) inhibitors in the treatment of heart failure (2).

B-Type Natriuretic Peptide

One of the natriuretic peptides described earlier, brain-type or *B-type natriuretic peptide* (BNP), is released as a precursor or prohormone (proBNP) from both ventricles in response to increased wall tension. The prohormone is cleaved to form BNP (the active hormone) and N-terminal (NT)-proBNP, which is metabolically inactive. The clearance of BNP and NT-proBNP is primarily via the kidneys. Peptide receptors in adipose tissue also contribute to BNP clearance (7), which might explain why plasma BNP levels are inversely related to body mass index (BMI) (8). NT-proBNP has a longer half-life than BNP, resulting in plasma levels that are 3–5 times higher than BNP levels.

Clinical Use

Plasma levels of both BNP and NT-proBNP are used as biomarkers for evaluating the presence and severity of heart failure (4). The predictive value of BNP and NT-proBNP levels for detecting heart failure is shown in Table 13.1 (9–11). As indicated, advancing age and renal insufficiency can also elevate natriuretic peptide levels. Severe sepsis also elevates natriuretic peptide levels, and the magnitude of the elevation can be as great as in heart failure (12). Because elevated peptide levels lack specificity, *natriuretic peptide levels are better suited for excluding the presence of heart failure* (4).

Table 13.1	Predictive Value of Natriuretic Peptide in the Evaluation of Suspected Acute Heart Failure		
Peptide Assay and Conditions	**Likelihood of Acute Heart Failure**		
	Unlikely	**Uncertain**	**Likely**
BNP (pg/mL):			
Age ≥18 yrs	< 100	100 – 500	> 500
GFR < 60 mL/min	< 200	200 – 500	> 500
NT-proBNP (pg/mL):			
Age 18 – 49 yrs	< 300	300 – 450	> 450
Age 50 – 75 yrs	< 300	300 – 900	> 900
Age > 75 yrs	< 300	300 – 1800	> 1800

From References 9–11.

Role in the ICU

Natriuretic peptide levels are most useful in the emergency department, for evaluating patients with suspected heart failure. For patients with heart failure that are admitted to the ICU, the use of serial measurements of natriuretic peptide levels to evaluate the response to therapy has not been studied. However, spurious elevations in natriuretic peptide levels from renal insufficiency and severe sepsis are likely to be commonplace in critically ill patients, and thus it seems unlikely that natriuretic peptide levels will have a clinical role in the ICU setting.

TYPES OF HEART FAILURE

As mentioned earlier, heart failure can be classified by the portion of the cardiac cycle that is affected (systolic and diastolic heart failure) and the side of the heart that is involved (left-sided and right-sided heart failure). These distinctions are the focus of this section of the chapter.

Systolic vs. Diastolic Heart Failure

Early descriptions of heart failure attributed most cases to contractile failure during systole (i.e., *systolic heart failure*). However, observations over the past 30 years indicate that *diastolic dysfunction is responsible for up to 60% of cases of heart failure* (2). The hallmark of *diastolic heart failure* is a decrease in ventricular distensibility with impaired ventricular filling during diastole (13). Common causes of diastolic heart failure include ventricular hypertrophy, myocardial ischemia (stunned myocardium), restrictive or fibrotic cardiomyopathy, and pericardial tamponade. Additional sources of impaired diastolic filling in ICU patients are positive-pressure ventilation and positive end-expiratory pressure (PEEP).

Cardiac Performance

The graphs in Figure 13.3 show the influence of systolic and diastolic dysfunction on measures of cardiac performance in decompensated heart failure. The upper graph shows the relationship between end-diastolic pressure and stroke volume (similar to the graph in Figure 9.2) The curve representing heart failure has a decreased slope, and the point on the curve indicates that heart failure is associated with an increase in end-diastolic pressure and a decrease in stroke volume (similar to stage 2 and stage 3 in Figure 13.2). The lower graph shows the relationship between end-diastolic pressure and end-diastolic volume. The curve representing diastolic dysfunction has a decreased slope, which reflects a decrease in ventricular compliance (distensibility) according to the following relationship:

$$\text{Compliance} = \Delta \text{ EDV} / \Delta \text{ EDP} \qquad (13.1)$$

The points on the ventricular compliance curves indicate that the increase in end-diastolic pressure in heart failure is associated with differ-

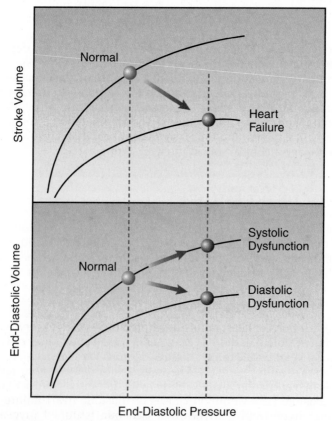

FIGURE 13.3 Graphs showing the influence of systolic and diastolic dysfunction on measures of cardiac performance in decompensated heart failure. Lower panel shows diastolic pressure-volume curves, and upper panel shows ventricular function curves. See text for further explanation

ent end-diastolic volumes with systolic and diastolic dysfunction; i.e., systolic dysfunction results in an increase in end-diastolic volume, and diastolic dysfunction results in a decrease in end-diastolic volume. Therefore, *the end-diastolic volume (not the end-diastolic pressure) can distinguish between systolic and diastolic dysfunction in patients with heart failure.* This is evident in the diagnostic criteria shown in Table 13.2, where a left ventricular end-diastolic volume of 97 mL/m² (measured relative to body surface area in m²) is the threshold value for identifying systolic vs. diastolic dysfunction as the cause of heart failure (14).

Table 13.2	Measures of Left Ventricular (LV) Performance in Systolic and Diastolic Heart Failure	
LV Performance Measure	**Systolic Heart Failure**	**Diastolic Heart Failure**
End-Diastolic Pressure	>16 mm Hg	>16 mm Hg
End-Diastolic Volume	> 97 mL/m²	≤ 97 mL/m²
Ejection Fraction	< 45%	> 50%

From References 14 and 16.

Ejection Fraction

The fraction of the end-diastolic volume that is ejected during systole, known as the *ejection fraction* (EF), is equivalent to the ratio of stroke volume to end-diastolic volume (EDV):

$$EF = SV/EDV \qquad (13.2)$$

The EF is directly related to the strength of ventricular contraction, and is used a measure of systolic function. The normal EF of the left ventricle is ≥ 55% (15,16), but lower values of 45–50% are used as normal in the evaluation of heart failure because increases in afterload can reduce EF by 5 to 10% (16). As shown in Table 13.2, an EF > 50% is used as evidence of normal systolic function, and an EF < 45% is used as evidence of abnormal systolic function (14,16). Transthoracic ultrasound is an accepted method for measuring EF, and can be performed at the bedside in the ICU.

TERMINOLOGY: Because many cases of heart failure have some degree of systolic and diastolic dysfunction, the terms "diastolic heart failure" and "systolic heart failure" have been replaced by the following terminology:

1. Heart failure that is predominantly the result of systolic dysfunction is called *heart failure with reduced ejection fraction*.

2. Heart failure that is predominantly the result of diastolic dysfunction is called *heart failure with normal ejection fraction*.

Because this newer terminology is lengthy and probably not necessary, the terms "diastolic heart failure" and "systolic heart failure" are used in this chapter, and throughout the book.

Right Heart Failure

Right-sided heart failure is more prevalent than suspected in ICU patients (17), and can be difficult to detect in the early stages. Most cases are the result of pulmonary hypertension (e.g., from pulmonary emboli or chronic lung disease) and inferior wall myocardial infarction.

Cardiac Filling Pressures

Acute right heart failure is a contractile (systolic) failure that results in an increase in right ventricular end-diastolic volume (RVEDV). However, the central venous pressure (CVP) does not rise until the increase in RVEDV is restricted by the pericardium (*pericardial constraint*) (17). The delayed rise in the CVP is one of the reasons that the early stages of right heart failure are often undetected. The following hemodynamic criteria have been proposed for the diagnosis of right heart failure (18): CVP > 10 mm Hg and CVP = PAWP or CVP within 5 mm Hg of PAWP. (PAWP is the pulmonary artery wedge pressure.) Equalization of right and left ventricular filling pressures is also characteristic of cardiac tamponade, and this similarity shows the importance of pericardial constraint in right heart failure.

INTERVENTRICULAR INTERDEPENDENCE: Because of pericardial constraint, progressive distension of the right ventricle pushes the interventricular septum towards the left ventricle and reduces the size of the left ventricular chamber, as shown in Figure 13.4. This septal displacement impairs left ventricular filling and increases the left ventricular end-diastolic pressure. In this situation, the filling pressures of both ventricles "equilibrate" to produce equalization of pressures, as indicated by the diastolic pressures in the right and left ventricle in Figure 13.4. This mechanism whereby *right-sided heart failure can produce diastolic dysfunction in the left ventricle* is known as *interventricular interdependence*.

Echocardiography

Cardiac ultrasound is an invaluable tool for detecting right heart failure in the ICU. The variety of measurements used to evaluate the right heart is beyond the scope of this chapter, and the most recent guidelines on this subject are included in the bibliography at the end of the chapter (Reference 19). The diameter of the right ventricular chamber is a popular measurement to identify right heart dilatation. Measurements of right ventricular end-diastolic volume and ejection fraction require 3-dimensional echocardiography, and validation studies are currently ongoing to determine reliable reference ranges (19). The lower limit of normal for right ventricular ejection fraction is currently set at 44% (19).

MANAGEMENT STRATEGIES

The management of acute heart failure described here is limited to the advanced stages of heart failure, where cardiac output is impaired and

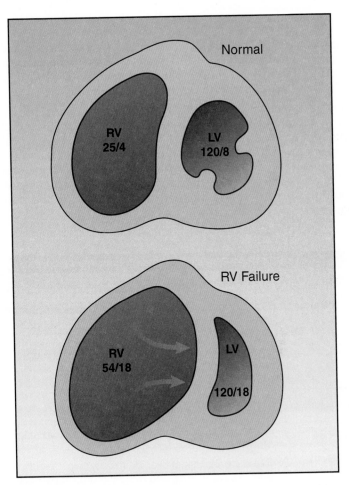

FIGURE 13.4 Interventricular interdependence: i.e., the mechanism whereby right heart failure can impair left ventricular filling and produce diastolic left-heart failure. The numbers in each chamber represent the peak systolic and end-diastolic pressures. *RV* = right ventricle; *LV* = left ventricle.

the perfusion of vital organs is threatened. The management is described using measures of cardiac performance rather than symptomatology, and most of the drugs are administered by continuous intravenous infusion.

Left Heart Failure

The following management pertains to non-valvular heart failure resulting from systolic or diastolic dysfunction, where the hemodynamic changes are characterized by an increased pulmonary artery wedge pressure (PAWP), a decreased cardiac output (CO), and an increased systemic vascular resistance (SVR). Three approaches are described, based on the blood pressure (i.e., high, normal, and low).

Profile: High PAWP / Low CO / High SVR / High BP.

Management: Vasodilator therapy with nitroglycerin, nitroprusside, or nesiritide, followed by diuretic therapy with furosemide if there is evidence of volume overload, or if the PAWP remains above 20 mm Hg despite vasodilator therapy.

The dosing regimens for continuous-infusion vasodilator therapy are shown in Table 13.3 (21). The vasodilators in this table are capable of dilating both arteries and veins, and will decrease both ventricular preload and afterload. The decrease in preload reduces venous congestion in the lungs, and the decrease in afterload promotes cardiac output. The overall effect is a decrease in arterial blood pressure, an increase in cardiac output, and a decrease in hydrostatic pressure in the pulmonary capillaries.

Table 13.3	Dosing Regimens for Continuous-Infusion Vasodilator Therapy
Vasodilator	**Dosing Regimens and Precautions**
Nitroglycerin	1. Do NOT infuse through polyvinylchloride (PVC) tubing (drug binds to PVC).
	2. Start infusion at 5 μg/min, and increase by 5 μg/min every 5 min to achieve the desired effect. The effective dose is 5–100 μg/min in most cases, and doses above 200 μg/min are not advised.
Nitroprusside	1. Start infusion at 0.2 μg/kg/min and titrate upward every 5 min to achieve the desired effect. The effective dose is 2–5 μg/kg/min in most cases, and the maximum dose allowed is 10 μg/kg/min.
	2. To reduce the risk of cyanide toxicity, avoid prolonged infusions >3 μg/kg/min, and avoid the drug in patients with renal failure. Thiosulfate (500 mg) can be added to the infusate to bind the cyanide released from nitroprusside.
Nesiritide	1. Do NOT infuse through heparin-bonded catheters (drug binds to heparin).
	2. Start with a bolus dose of 2 μg/kg, and infuse at 0.01 μg/kg/min. If necessary, a second bolus dose of 1 μg/kg can be given, followed by an increase in infusion rate of 0.005 μg/kg/min, and this can be repeated every 3 hrs to a maximum rate of 0.03 μg/kg/min.

NITROPRUSSIDE: The vasodilating effects of nitroprusside are the result of nitric oxide release from the nitroprusside molecule. Unfortunately, cyanide ions are also released (5 atoms per molecule) and accumulation of these ions can produce life-threatening cyanide intoxication (22,23). Both the liver and kidneys participate in cyanide clearance, and thus *nitroprusside is not recommended in patients with renal or hepatic insufficiency.*

Thiosulfate binds cyanide and reduces the risk of cyanide toxicity (23), and sodium thiosulfate can be added to nitroprusside infusions as a preventive measure (see Table 13.3). A detailed description of nitroprusside-induced cyanide intoxication is included in Chapter 53.

Nitroprusside has an additional risk in patients with ischemic heart disease because it can produce a *coronary steal syndrome* by diverting blood flow away from non-dilating blood vessels in ischemic regions of the myocardium (24). Because of this risk, *nitroprusside is not recommended in patients with ischemic heart disease.*

NITROGLYCERIN: Nitroglycerin is a "nitric oxide" vasodilator like nitroprusside, but is a much safer drug to use. Nitrate ions released during nitroglycerin metabolism can oxidize hemoglobin to form methemoglobin, but clinically significant methemoglobinemia is rare during therapeutic nitroglycerin infusions (25). The major drawback with nitroglycerin infusions is *tachyphylaxis*, which can appear after 16 to 24 hours of continuous drug administration (24). (See Chapter 53 for more information on nitroglycerin.)

NESIRITIDE: Nesiritide (Natrecor) is a recombinant human B-type natriuretic peptide with the same natriuretic and vasodilator effects as the endogenous BNP described earlier in the chapter. Although nesiritide has a potential advantage over other vasodilators by promoting diuresis as well as vasodilation, clinical studies have shown no benefit associated with nesiritide treatment of acute, decompensated heart failure (26). Early concerns about worsening renal function with nesiritide have not been confirmed in more recent studies (26).

WHICH AGENT IS PREFERRED?: Nitroglycerin should be the preferred vasodilator, particularly in patients with coronary artery disease. Nitroprusside is contraindicated in the presence of myocardial ischemia, and is not advised in patients with hepatic or renal insufficiency. Nitroprusside is most suited for the short-term management of hypertensive crisis, but infusion rates should not exceed $3\mu g/kg/min$ to limit the risk of cyanide toxicity. Nesiritide is not currently recommended for the routine management of acute heart failure.

DIURETICS: Diuretic therapy with intravenous furosemide is indicated only if vasodilator therapy does not reduce the wedge pressure to the desired level, or there is evidence of volume overload (e.g., recent weight gain). *Intravenous furosemide produces an acute vasoconstrictor response* (27) by stimulating renin release and promoting the formation of angiotensin II, a potent vasoconstrictor. Because this response is counterproductive in the setting of hypertension, furosemide administration should be delayed until the blood pressure is controlled with vasodilator therapy.

The desired wedge pressure in left heart failure is the highest pressure that will augment cardiac output without producing pulmonary edema. This pressure usually corresponds to a wedge pressure of 18 to 20 mm Hg (28). Therefore, diuretic therapy can be added if the wedge pressure remains above 20 mm Hg during vasodilator therapy. The features of diuretic therapy for decompensated heart failure are described later.

Normal Blood Pressure

Decompensated heart failure with a normal blood pressure is a common presentation of acute exacerbation of chronic heart failure, and can involve diastolic and/or systolic dysfunction.

Profile: High PAWP /Low CO /High SVR /Normal BP.

Treatment: Vasodilator therapy, if tolerated, or inodilator therapy with dobutamine, milrinone, or levosimendan. Add diuretic therapy with furosemide for volume overload, or for a persistent PAWP above 20 mm Hg.

Vasodilator therapy (usually with nitroglycerin) is preferred for treating normotensive heart failure because it avoids unwanted cardiac stimulation, but vasodilator use is limited by the risk of hypotension. When vasodilator therapy is not feasible, the next choice is the use of *inodilators;* i.e., drugs with positive inotropic and vasodilator actions. These drugs also have positive *lusitropic* actions; i.e., they promote myocardial relaxation and improve diastolic filling. The inodilators given by continuous infusion are shown in Table 13.4, along with the dosing recommendations for each drug.

DOBUTAMINE: Dobutamine is a potent β_1-receptor agonist and a weak β_2-receptor agonist: the β_1 stimulation produces positive inotropic, lusitropic and chronotropic effects, and the β_2 stimulation produces peripheral vasodilatation. The effect of dobutamine on cardiac performance is described in Chapter 53 (see Figure 53.1). Adverse effects of dobutamine include tachycardia and an increase in myocardial O_2 consumption (29); this latter effect is deleterious in the ischemic myocardium (where oxygen supply is impaired) and in the failing myocardium (where O_2 consumption is already increased).

MILRINONE: Milrinone is a phosphodiesterase inhibitor that enhances myocardial contractility and relaxation via the same mechanism as dobutamine (i.e., cyclic AMP-mediated calcium influx into cardiac myocytes). Milrinone has similar effects on cardiac performance as dobutamine, but is more likely to produce hypotension (29). The dosage of milrinone requires adjustment in renal insufficiency, as indicated in Table 13.4 (30).

LEVOSIMENDAN: Levosimendan (Simdax, Abbot Pharmaceuticals) increases cardiac contractility by sensitizing cardiac myofilaments to calcium (31), and promotes vasodilation by facilitating potassium influx into vascular smooth muscle (32). This drug is particularly appealing in patients with coronary artery disease because it dilates coronary arteries and *does not stimulate myocardial O_2 consumption;* animal studies have confirmed the drug's ability to protect the myocardium from ischemic injury (32). Infusions of levosimendan are usually limited to 24 hours, but long-acting active metabolites (which peak at 72 hours after the onset of therapy) produce salutary effects that last for at least 7 days (see Figure 13.5) (33).

Table 13.4	Dosing Regimens for Continuous-Infusion Inodilator Therapy
Inodilator	**Dosing Regimens and Precautions**
Dobutamine	1. Do NOT infuse with alkaline solutions. 2. Start at infusion rate of 5 µg/kg/min, and increase in increments of 3–5 µg/kg/min, if necessary. Usual dose range is 5–20 µg/kg/min.
Levosimendan	1. Initial dose is 12 µg/kg (over 10 min), followed by an infusion rate of 0.1 µg/kg/min. Rate can be increased to 0.2 µg/kg/min, if necessary. 2. Infusions are usually limited to 24 hrs, but long-acting active metabolites produce salutary effects for at least 7 days.
Milrinone	1. Initial dose is 50 µg/kg (over 10 min), followed by an infusion rate of 0.375–0.75 µg/kg/min. Daily dose should not exceed 1.13 mg/kg. 2. The following dose adjustments are recommended for patients with renal insufficiency: **Creatinine Clearance** **Infusion Rate** 50 mL/min 0.43 µg/kg/min 40 0.38 30 0.33 20 0.28 10 0.23 5 0.20

WHICH INODILATOR IS PREFERRED?: Levosimendan is emerging as the preferred inodilator, particularly in the setting of myocardial ischemia or infarction, and is the only inodilator that is associated with improved survival (34). The benefit of levosimendan over dobutamine in reducing plasma BNP levels is demonstrated in Figure 13.5 (36). Dobutamine is the least favored inodilator because of the deleterious effects of adrenergic stimulation in the failing heart.

DIURETICS: The indications for diuretic therapy with furosemide are the same as those described for heart failure with high blood pressure.

Low Blood Pressure

Acute heart failure accompanied by hypotension is a life-threatening condition that often represents cardiogenic shock (when accompanied by an elevated serum lactate level). This condition is most often the result of acute myocardial infarction.

Profile: High PAWP /Low CO/High SVR /Low BP.

Treatment: Dobutamine or vasoconstrictor therapy with dopamine, combined with mechanical cardiac support.

Dobutamine can sometimes increase blood pressure (when the increase in stroke volume is greater than the decrease in systemic vascular resistance); otherwise a vasoconstrictor drug is required to raise the blood pressure. Since systemic vasoconstriction is a prominent feature of cardiogenic shock, drug-induced vasoconstriction can further aggravate tissue hypoperfusion. To limit this risk, a vasoconstrictor drug that also promotes cardiac output is the favored choice in cardiogenic shock. Dopamine is such a drug, when given in the appropriate dose range.

DOPAMINE: Dopamine stimulates both cardiac β-receptors (which promotes cardiac output) and peripheral α-receptors (which promotes systemic vasoconstriction). In moderate doses (3–10 μg/kg/min), the β-receptor effect predominates, while in higher doses (> 10 μg/kg/min), α-receptor stimulation predominates. At dose rates of 5–15 μg/kg/min, dopamine can promote cardiac output and produce systemic vasoconstriction (29). Therefore *dopamine infusion at a rate of 5–15 μg/kg/min is a reasonable choice in the management of cardiogenic shock.* (See Chapter 53 for a more detailed description of dopamine.)

The mortality rate in cardiogenic shock remains high (about 80%) with the use of hemodynamic drugs alone, and other measures, such as mechanical cardiac support and coronary revascularization, are required to improve outcomes. Mechanical cardiac support using intra-aortic balloon counterpulsation is described later in the chapter.

Diuretic Therapy

Diuretic therapy is a cornerstone of management for chronic heart failure. However, the following observations indicate that diuretic therapy

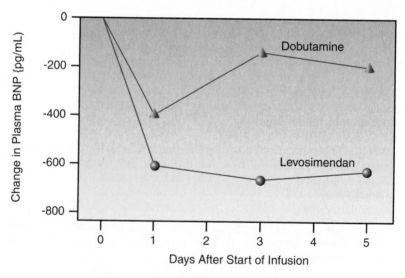

FIGURE 13.5 Changes in plasma BNP levels associated with short-term (24 hr) infusions of dobutamine and levosimendan in patients with acute decompensated heart failure. Graph redrawn from Reference 35.

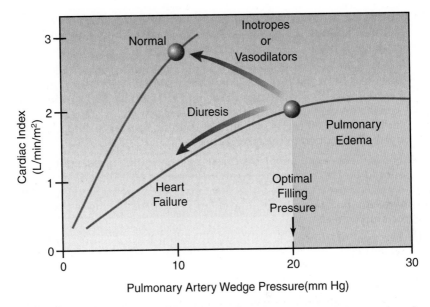

FIGURE 13.6 Ventricular function curves for the normal and failing left ventricle with arrows indicating the expected changes associated with each type of drug therapy. The shaded area indicates the high-risk region for pulmonary edema.

with intravenous furosemide should be used cautiously in patients with acute, decompensated heart failure.

1. Intravenous furosemide causes a decrease in cardiac output in acute heart failure (36–38), as indicated in Figure 13.6. This effect is the result of a decrease in venous return and an increase in left ventricular afterload; the latter effect is due to the acute vasoconstrictor response to furosemide mentioned earlier (31).

2. The presence of pulmonary edema in acute heart failure is NOT evidence of excess extracellular volume, and could be the result of an acute increase in PAWP from diastolic dysfunction (as seen in the "flash pulmonary edema" produced by ischemic myocardial "stunning").

In light of these observations, diuretic therapy with intravenous furosemide should only be used when there is evidence of hypervolemia (such as recent weight gain or peripheral edema), or when the PAWP remains elevated (> 20 mm Hg) despite vasodilator or inodilator therapy. Furthermore, intravenous furosemide should never be used alone in the treatment of heart failure associated with a low cardiac output, and should always be combined with vasodilator or inodilator therapy.

Furosemide Dosing

The salient features of conventional furosemide dosing are summarized below.

1. Furosemide is a sulfonamide, but can be used safely in patients with an allergy to sulfonamide antibiotics (39).

2. Following an intravenous bolus dose of furosemide, diuresis begins within 15 minutes, peaks at one hour, and lasts 2 hours (when renal function is normal) (40).

3. For patients with normal renal function, the initial furosemide dose is 40 mg IV. If the diuresis is not adequate (at least 1 liter) after 2 hours, the dose is increased to 80 mg IV. The dose that produces a satisfactory response is then given twice daily. Failure to respond to an IV dose of 80 mg is evidence of diuretic resistance, and is managed as described in the next section.

4. For patients with renal insufficiency, the initial furosemide dose should be 100 mg IV, which can be increased to 200 mg IV if necessary. The dose that produces a satisfactory response is then given twice daily. Failure to respond to an IV dose of 200 mg is evidence of diuretic resistance.

5. The goal of diuresis is a minimum weight loss of 5–10% of body weight (41).

Diuretic Resistance

Critically ill patients can have an attenuated response to loop diuretics like furosemide, particularly with continued use. Several factors may be involved, including rebound sodium retention, reduced renal blood flow, and "diuretic braking" (i.e., decreased responsiveness as hypervolemia resolves) (42). When the diuretic response to furosemide is inadequate, responsiveness can be enhanced as follows.

ADD A THIAZIDE: Thiazide diuretics block sodium reabsorption in the distal renal tubules, and can enhance the diuretic response to furosemide (which blocks sodium reabsorption in the loop of Henle). The thiazide most favored in furosemide resistance is *metolazone* because it retains its efficacy in renal insufficiency (42). The dose of metolazone is 2.5–10 mg daily in a single oral dose (the drug is only available as an oral preparation). The response to metolazone begins at one hour and peaks at 9 hours, so a single dose of metolazone should be given hours before furosemide, to allow time for effective blockade of sodium reabsorption in the distal tubules.

CONTINUOUS INFUSION FUROSEMIDE: Because the diuretic effect of furosemide is a function of the urinary excretion rate and not the plasma concentration (43), continuous infusions of the drug often (but not always) produce a more vigorous diuresis than bolus injection. The dosing regimen for continuous-infusion furosemide is influenced by renal function, as shown below (41,42):

Creatinine Clearance	Loading Dose	Initial Infusion Rate
> 75 mL/min	100 mg	10 mg/hr
25–75 mL/min	100–200 mg	10–20 mg/hr
< 25 mL/min	200 mg	20–40 mg/hr

The infusion rate can be increased as needed to achieve the desired urine output (e.g., ≥ 100 mL/hr). The maximum recommended infusion rate is 240–360 mg/hr (42), or 170 mg/hr in elderly patients (44).

Right Heart Failure

The following recommendations pertain to the management of infarction-related right heart failure associated with hemodynamic instability. These recommendations are based on measurements of the pulmonary artery wedge pressure (PAWP) or the right ventricular end-diastolic volume (RVEDV).

1. If the PAWP is below 15 mm Hg, infuse volume until the PAWP or CVP increases by 5 mm Hg or either one reaches 20 mm Hg (45).

2. If the PAWP or CVP is above 15 mm Hg, start inodilator therapy with dobutamine (47) or levosimendan (48).

4. For AV dissociation or complete heart block, use sequential A-V pacing and avoid ventricular pacing (45).

Volume infusion is the mainstay of therapy for right-sided heart failure with hemodynamic instability, but it must be carefully monitored to avoid septal displacement and compromised left ventricular filling, as described earlier (see Fig. 13.4). An increase in either the PAWP (indicating septal displacement) or the CVP (indicating pericardial constraint) can therefore be used as end-points of volume infusion in right heart failure. If volume infusion is not feasible or does not correct the hemodynamic instability, inodilator therapy (with dobutamine or levosimendan) is preferred to vasodilator infusions(47).

MECHANICAL CARDIAC SUPPORT

Intra-Aortic Balloon Counterpulsation

Intra-aortic balloon counterpulsation is used for temporary cardiac support in cases of unstable angina or cardiogenic shock where cardiac pump function is expected to improve as a result of some intervention; i.e., coronary angioplasty or coronary artery bypass surgery (49). This technique is contraindicated in patients with aortic valve insufficiency and aortic dissection.

Methodology

The intra-aortic balloon is an elongated polyurethane balloon that is inserted percutaneously into the femoral artery and advanced up the aorta until the tip lies just below the origin of the left subclavian artery (see Figure 13.7). A pump attached to the balloon uses helium, a low density gas, to rapidly inflate and deflate the balloon (inflation volume is generally 35 to 40 mL). Inflation begins at the onset of diastole, just after the aortic valve closes (the R wave on the ECG is a common trigger). The balloon is then deflated at the onset of ventricular systole, just before the

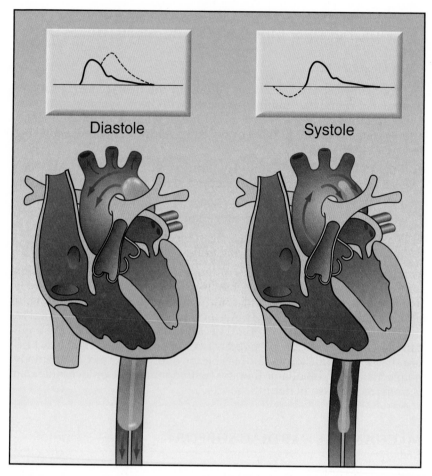

FIGURE 13.7 Intra-aortic balloon counterpulsation showing balloon inflation during diastole (left panel), and balloon deflation during systole (right panel). The arrows indicate the direction of blood flow. The effects on the aortic pressure waveform are indicated by the dotted lines on the waveforms at the top of each panel.

aortic valve opens (during isovolumic contraction). This pattern of balloon inflation and deflation produces two changes in the aortic pressure waveform, which are illustrated in Figure 13.7.

1. Inflation of the balloon during diastole increases the peak diastolic pressure and thereby increases the mean arterial pressure (which is equivalent to the integrated pressure under the aortic pressure curve). The increase in mean arterial pressure increases systemic blood flow, while the increase in diastolic pressure augments coronary blood flow (which occurs predominantly during diastole).

2. Deflation of the balloon creates a suction effect that reduces pressure in the aorta when the aortic valve opens, and this reduces the impedance to flow and augments ventricular stroke output.

The intra-aortic balloon pump (IABP) therefore promotes systemic blood flow by increasing mean arterial pressure and reducing ventricular afterload, while also increasing coronary blood flow. This latter effect, combined with the reduced ventricular afterload, improves the balance between O_2 delivery and O_2 consumption in the myocardium (50).

Complications

The principal concern with IABP support is vascular injury. Limb ischemia is reported in 3% to 20% of patients (49,51), and can appear while the balloon is in place or shortly after balloon removal. Most cases are the result of in-situ thrombosis at the catheter insertion site, but aortic dissection and aortoiliac injury may also be responsible.

The risk of limb ischemia mandates close monitoring of distal pulses and sensorimotor function in the legs. Loss of distal pulses alone does not warrant removal of the balloon as long as sensorimotor function in the legs is intact (52). Loss of sensorimotor function in the legs should always prompt immediate removal of the device. Surgical intervention is required in 30 to 50% of cases of limb ischemia (52).

Other complications of IABP support include catheter-related infection, balloon rupture, peripheral neuropathy, and pseudoaneurysm. Fever is reported in 50% of patients during IABP support, but bacteremia is reported in only 15% of patients (53).

Positive Pressure Breathing

As described in Chapter 9, positive intrathoracic pressure reduces left ventricular afterload by decreasing the transmural wall pressure developed by the ventricle during systole. This promotes ventricular emptying by facilitating the inward movement of the ventricular wall during systole. As a result, positive pressure breathing can augment the stroke output of the left ventricle (see Figure 9.8).

Clinical studies have demonstrated that breathing with continuous positive airway pressure (CPAP) reduces left ventricular transmural pressure (54) and, increases cardiac output (55) in patients with left-sided heart failure. Furthermore, in patients with cardiogenic pulmonary edema, CPAP hastens clinical improvement when added to conventional therapy for acute heart failure (56,57). As a result of these observations, CPAP (along with non-invasive pressure support ventilation) has emerged as a treatment modality for acute heart failure associated with pulmonary edema.

A FINAL WORD

The management of acute heart failure suffers from the following shortcomings:

1. Despite the increasing prevalence and poor prognosis associated with acute, decompensated heart failure, the management of this condition has changed very little in the last 10 to 15 years.

2. The treatment of heart failure is actually treating the *consequences* of heart failure (e.g., pulmonary venous congestion) and has little impact on the functional derangements in the myocytes. (Coronary revascularization is an exception to this rule.)

3. Many of the drug therapies for acute heart failure produce effects that are counterproductive (e.g., diuretics reduce cardiac output, which promotes sodium retention, vasodilators stimulate renin release, which results in vasoconstriction).

While these shortcomings are not unique to heart failure, they are more evident because of the prominence of cardiovascular disease as the leading cause of death in this country.

REFERENCES

Guidelines and Reviews

1. Roger V, Go AS, Lloyd-Jones D, et al. Heart disease and stroke statistics – 2012 update: a report from the American Heart Association. Circulation 2012; 125:e2–e220.

2. Hunt SA, Abraham WT, Chin MH, Feldman AM, et al. 2009 focused update incorporated into the ACC/AHA 2005 guidelines for the diagnosis and management of heart failure in adults: a report of the American College of Cardiology Foundation/ American Heart Association Task Force on Practice Guidelines. Circulation 2009; 119:e391–e479.

3. Gheorghiade M, Pang PS. Acute heart failure syndromes. J Am Coll Cardiol 2009; 53:557–573.

4. Weintraub NL, Collins SP, Pang PS, et al. Acute heart failure syndromes: emergency department presentation, treatment, and disposition: current approaches and future aims: a scientific statement from the American Heart Association. Circulation 2010; 122:1975–1996.

5. Task Force for the Diagnosis and Treatment of Acute and Chronic Heart Failure 2012 of the European Society of Cardiology. ESC guidelines for the diagnosis and treatment of acute and chronic heart failure 2012. Eur Heart J 2012; 33:1787–1847.

Pathophysiology

6. Mann DL. Pathophysiology of heart failure. In: Libby P, Bonow RO, Mann DL, Zipes DP, eds. Braunwald's Heart Disease. 8th ed. Philadelphia: Saunders Elsevier, 2008:541–560.

7. Wang TJ. The natriuretic peptides and fat metabolism. N Engl J Med 2012; 367:377–378.

8. McCord J, Mundy BJ, Hudson MP, et al. Relationship between obesity and B-type natriuretic peptide levels. Arch Intern Med 2004; 164:2247–2252.

9. Maisel AS, Krishnaswamy P, Nomak RM, et al. Rapid measurement of B-type natriuretic peptide in the emergency diagnosis of heart failure. New Engl J Med 2002; 347:161–167.

10. Maisel AS, McCord J, Nowak J, et al. Bedside B-type natriuretic peptide in the emergency diagnosis of heart failure with reduced or preserved ejection fraction. Results from the Breathing Not Properly Multinational Study. J Am Coll Cardiol 2003; 41:2010–2017.

11. Januzzi JL, van Kimmenade R, Lainchbury J, et al. NT-proBNP testing for diagnosis and short-term prognosis in acute destabilized heart failure: an international pooled analysis of 1256 patients. Europ Heart J 2006; 27:330–337.

12. Rudiger A, Gasser S, Fischler M, et al. Comparable increase of B-type natriuretic peptide and amino-terminal pro-B-type natriuretic peptide levels in patients with severe sepsis, septic shock, and acute heart failure. Crit Care Med 2006; 34:2140–2144.

Types of Heart Failure

13. Zile MR, Baicu CF, Gaasch WH. Diastolic heart failure – Abnormalities in active relaxation and passive stiffness of the left ventricle. New Engl J Med 2004; 350:1953–1959.

14. Paulus WJ, Tschope C, Sanderson JE, et al. How to diagnose diastolic heart failure: a consensus statement on the diagnosis of heart failure with normal left ventricular ejection fraction by the Heart Failure and Echocardiography Associations of the European Society of Cardiology. Europ Heart J 2007; 28:2539–2550.

15. Lang RM, Bierig M, Devereux RB, et al. Recommendations for chamber quantification: a report from the American Society of Echocardiography and the European Association of Echocardiography. J Am Soc Echocardiogr 2005; 18:1440–1463.

16. Hess OM, Carroll JD. Clinical assessment of heart failure. In: Libby P, Bonow RO, Mann DL, Zipes DP, eds. Braunwald's Heart Disease. 8th ed. Philadelphia: Saunders Elsevier, 2008:561–581.

17. Hurford WE, Zapol WM. The right ventricle and critical illness: a review of anatomy, physiology, and clinical evaluation of its function. Intensive Care Med 1988; 14:448–457.

18. Lopez-Sendon J, Coma-Canella I, Gamello C. Sensitivity and specificity of hemodynamic criteria in the diagnosis of right ventricular infarction. Circulation 1981; 64:515–525.

19. Rudski LG, Lai WW, Afilalo J, et al. Guidelines for the echocardiographic assessment of the right heart in adults: A report from the American Society of Echocardiography. J Am Soc Echocardiogr 2010; 23:685–713.

Management Strategies

20. Flaherty JT, Magee PA, Gardner TL, et al. Comparison of intravenous nitroglycerin and sodium nitroprusside for treatment of acute hypertension developing after coronary artery bypass surgery. Circulation 1982; 65:1072–1077

21. Rhoney D, Peacock WF. Intravenous therapy for hypertensive emergencies, part 1. Am J Health Syst Pharm 2009; 66:1343–1352.

22. Sodium Nitroprusside. In: McEvoy GK, ed. AHFS Drug Information, 2012. Bethesda, MD: American Society of Health System Pharmacists, 2012:1811–1814.

23. Hall VA, Guest JM. Sodium nitroprusside-induced cyanide intoxication and prevention with sodium thiosulfate prophylaxis. Am J Crit Care 1992; 2:19–27.

24. Mann T, Cohn PF, Holman LB, et al. Effect of nitroprusside on regional myocardial blood flow in coronary artery disease. Results in 25 patients and comparison with nitroglycerin. Circulation 1978; 57:732–738.

25. Curry SC, Arnold-Cappell P. Nitroprusside, nitroglycerin, and angiotensin-converting enzyme inhibitors. Crit Care Clin 1991; 7:555–582.

26. O'Connor CM, Starling RC, Hernanadez PW, et al. Effect of nesiritide in patients with acute decompensated heart failure. N Engl J Med 2011; 365:32–43.

27. Francis GS, Siegel RM, Goldsmith SR, et al. Acute vasoconstrictor response to intravenous furosemide in patients with chronic congestive heart failure. Ann Intern Med 1986; 103:1–6.

28. Franciosa JA. Optimal left heart filling pressure during nitroprusside infusion for congestive heart failure. Am J Med 1983; 74:457–464.

29. Bayram M, De Luca L, Massie B, Gheorghiade M. Reassessment of dobutamine, dopamine, and milrinone in the management of acute heart failure syndromes. Am J Cardiol 2005; 96(Suppl): 47G–58G.

30. Milrinone Lactate. In: McEvoy GK, ed. AHFS Drug Information, 2012. Bethesda, MD: American Society of Health System Pharmacists, 2012:1724–1726.

31. Gheorghiade M, Teerlionk JR, Mebazaa A. Pharmacology of new agents for acute heart failure syndromes. Am J Cardiol 2005; 96(Suppl):68G–73G.

32. Kersten JR, Montgomery MW, Pagel PL, Waltier DC. Levosimendan, a new positive inotropic drug, decreases myocardial infarct size via activation of K(ATP) channels. Anesth Analg 2000; 90:5–11.

33. Antila S, Sundberg S, Lehtonen LA. Clinical pharmacology of levosimendan. Clin Pharmacokinet 2007; 46:535–552.

34. Landoni G, Biondi-Zoccai G, Greco M, et al. Effects of levosimendan on mortality and hospitalization: a meta-analysis of randomized, controlled studies. Crit Care Med 2012; 40:634–636.

35. Mebazza A, Niemenen MS, Packer M, et al. Levosimendan vs dobutamine for patients with acute decompensated heart failure: the SURVIVE randomized trial. JAMA 2007; 297:1883–1891.

Diuretic Therapy

36. Kiely J, Kelly DT, Taylor DR, Pitt B. The role of furosemide in the treatment of left ventricular dysfunction associated with acute myocardial infarction. Circulation 1973; 58:581–587.

37. Mond H, Hunt D, Sloman G. Haemodynamic effects of frusemide in patients suspected of having acute myocardial infarction. Br Heart J 1974; 36:44–53.

38. Nelson GIC, Ahuja RC, Silke B, et al. Haemodynamic advantages of isosorbide dinitrate over frusemide in acute heart failure following myocardial infarction. Lancet 1983a; i:730–733.

39. Strom BL, Schinnar R, Apter AJ, et al. Absence of cross-reactivity between sulfonamide antibiotics and sulfonamide nonantibiotics. N Engl J Med 2003; 349:1628–1635.

40. Furosemide. In: McEvoy GK, ed. AHFS Drug Information, 2012. Bethesda, MD: American Society of Health System Pharmacists, 2012:2792–2796.

41. Jenkins PG. Diuretic strategies in acute heart failure. N Engl J Med 2011; 364:21.

42. Asare K, Lindsey K. Management of loop diuretic resistance in the intensive care unit. Am J Health Syst Pharm 2009; 66:1635–1640.

43. van Meyel JJM, Smits P, Russell FGM, et al. Diuretic efficiency of furosemide during continuous administration versus bolus injection in healthy volunteers. Clin Pharmacol Ther 1992; 51:440–444.

44. Howard PA, Dunn MI. Aggressive diuresis for severe heart failure in the elderly. Chest 2001; 119:807–810.

Right Heart Failure

45. Isner JM. Right ventricular myocardial infarction. JAMA 1988; 259:712–718.

46. Reuse C, Vincent JL, Pinsky MR. Measurement of right ventricular volumes during fluid challenge. Chest 1990; 98:1450–1454.

47. Dell'Italia LJ, Starling MR, Blumhardt R, et al. Comparative effects of volume loading, dobutamine and nitroprusside in patients with predominant right ventricular infarction. Circulation 1986; 72:1327–1335.

48. Russ MA, Prondzinsky R, Carter JM, et al. Right ventricular function in myocardial infarction complicated by cardiogenic shock: improvement with levosimendan. Crit Care Med 2009; 37:3017–3023.

Mechanical Cardiac Support

49. Boehner JP, Popjes E. Cardiac failure: mechanical support strategies. Crit Care Med 2006; 34(Suppl):S268–S277.

50. Williams DO, Korr KS, Gewirtz H, Most AS. The effect of intra-aortic balloon counterpulsation on regional myocardial blood flow and oxygen consumption in the presence of coronary artery stenosis with unstable angina. Circulation 1982; 66:593–597.

51. Arafa OE, Pedersen TH, Svennevig JL, et al. Vascular complications of the intra-aortic balloon pump in patients undergoing open heart operations: 15-year experience. Ann Thorac Surg 1999; 67:645–651.

52. Baldyga AP. Complications of intra-aortic balloon pump therapy. In Maccioli GA, ed. Intra-aortic balloon pump therapy. Philadelphia: Williams & Wilkins, 1997, 127–162.

53. Crystal E, Borer A, Gilad J, et al. Incidence and clinical significance of bacteremia and sepsis among cardiac patients treated with intra-aortic balloon counterpulsation pump. Am J Cardiol 2000; 86:1281–1284.

54. Naughton MT, Raman MK, Hara K, et al. Effect of continuous positive airway pressure on intrathoracic and left ventricular transmural pressures in patients with congestive heart failure. Circulation 1995; 91:1725–1731.

55. Bradley TD, Holloway BM, McLaughlin PR, et al. Cardiac output response to continuous positive airway pressure in congestive heart failure. Am Rev Respir Crit Care Med 1992; 145:377–382.

56. Nouira S, Boukef R, Bouida W, et al. Non-invasive pressure support ventilation and CPAP in cardiogenic pulmonary edema: a multicenter randomized study in the emrgency department. Intensive Care Med 2011; 37:249–256.

57. Ducros L, Logeart D, Vicaut E, et al. CPAP for acute cardiogenic pulmonary edema from out-of-hospital to cardiac intensive care unit: a randomized multicenter study. Intensive Care Med 2011; 37:150.

Chapter 14

INFLAMMATORY SHOCK SYNDROMES

Inflammation is not itself considered a disease but a salutary operation . . .
but when it cannot accomplish that salutary purpose . . . it does mischief.

John Hunter, MD

(1728–1793)

The introductory quote is from a distinguished 18th century Scottish surgeon who is most remembered for a reckless self-experiment where he intentionally injected himself with a purulent discharge from a patient with venereal disease, and subsequently developed both gonorrhea and syphilis (I). On the brighter side, John Hunter was a skilled observer, and his observations on inflammation revealed a tendency to produce harm, as indicated in his statement. A quarter of a millennium later, the harmful effects of inflammation are recognized as a leading source of morbidity and mortality in critically ill patients.

This chapter describes the features of inflammatory injury, and presents the manifestations and management of two *inflammatory shock* syndromes: i.e., septic shock and anaphylactic shock. These conditions will demonstrate the widespread damage that occurs when inflammation "does mischief."

INFLAMMATORY INJURY

The inflammatory response is a complex process that is triggered by conditions that threaten the functional integrity of the host (e.g., physical injury or microbial invasion). Once activated, the inflammatory response generates a variety of noxious substances that are designed to control or eliminate the threat, while the host organism is not adversely affected. However, persistent or widespread inflammation can produce tissue

263

damage in any or all of the vital organs. Inflammatory injury is problematic because it tends to become a self-sustaining process; i.e., the inflammatory tissue damage triggers more inflammation, which produces more tissue damage, and so on. This condition of self-sustaining and progressive inflammatory injury is known as *malignant inflammation*, and it is characterized by progressive multiorgan dysfunction and multiorgan failure (1,2).

Oxidant Injury

One of the principal sources of inflammatory injury is the release of toxic oxygen metabolites from activated neutrophils (3,4). The purpose of neutrophil activation is to generate these metabolites, as described next.

Neutrophil Activation

Activation of neutrophils, which occurs in the early stages of the inflammatory response, is associated with a 20- to 50-fold increase in O_2 consumption. This is called the *respiratory burst* (4), which is a misleading term because it is not associated with increased energy production, but *is designed to generate toxic metabolites of oxygen* (6). This is illustrated in Figure 14.1. When neutrophils are activated, a specialized oxidase enzyme on the inner surface of the cell membrane is activated; this triggers the metabolic reduction of oxygen to water, which generates a series of highly-reactive metabolites that include the superoxide radical, hydrogen peroxide, and the hydroxyl radical. Neutrophils also have a myeloperoxidase enzyme that converts hydrogen peroxide to hypochlorite, a powerful germicidal agent that is the active ingredient in household bleach (5). The oxygen metabolites generated during the respiratory burst are stored in cytoplasmic granules, and are released during neutrophil degranulation.

Oxidant Stress

Oxygen metabolites are powerful oxidizing agents or *oxidants* that can disrupt cell membranes, denature proteins, and fracture DNA molecules. Once released, these metabolites are capable or producing lethal damage in invading microorganisms, while the cells of the host are normally protected by endogenous antioxidants. However, when oxidant activity exceeds antioxidant protection (a condition known as *oxidant stress*), the cells of the host are also damaged by the oxygen metabolites. This *oxidant cell injury* is the major source of damage produced by the inflammatory response, and the spectrum of organ damage than can occur is shown in Table 14.1.

Chain Reactions

Free radicals such as the superoxide radical and the hydroxyl radical are highly reactive because they have an unpaired electron in their outer orbitals. When a free radical reacts with a non-radical, the non-radical loses an electron and is transformed into a free radical. Such radical-regenerating reactions become repetitive, creating a series of self-sustain-

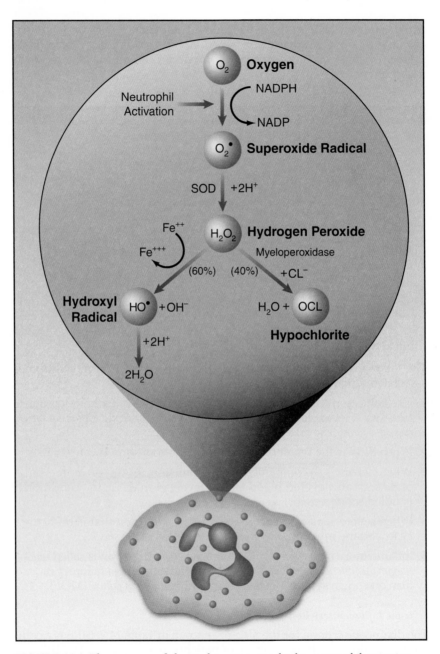

FIGURE 14.1 The sequence of chemical reactions involved in neutrophil activation, which generates a series of highly reactive oxygen metabolites that are stored in cytoplasmic granules. SOD = superoxide dismutase. See text for further explanation.

ing reactions known as a *chain reaction* (6). These self-sustaining reactions are troublesome because they continue after the inciting event is eliminated, and tend to produce widespread damage. Fires are a familiar example of an oxidative chain reaction. The oxidation of membrane lipids, which is a major component of oxidant cell injury, also proceeds as a chain reaction (7).

Table 14.1	Clinical Conditions Attributed to Inflammatory Injury
Organ or System	**Condition**
Brain	Septic encephalopathy
Bone Marrow	Anemia of critical illness
Cardiovascular	Septic shock
Kidneys	Acute kidney injury
Lungs	Acute respiratory distress syndrome
Peripheral Nerves	Critical illness polyneuropathy
Skeletal Muscle	Critical illness myopathy

Clinical Syndromes

The following definitions have been adopted for the clinical syndromes associated with systemic inflammation (8,9):

1. The condition that is characterized by signs of systemic inflammation (e.g., fever, leukocytosis) is called the *systemic inflammatory response syndrome* (SIRS).

2. When SIRS is the result of an infection, the condition is called *sepsis*.

3. When sepsis is accompanied by dysfunction in one or more vital organs, or an elevated blood lactate level (>4 mM/L), the condition is called *severe sepsis*.

4. When severe sepsis is accompanied by hypotension that is refractory to volume infusion, the condition is called *septic shock*.

5. Inflammatory injury involving more than one vital organ is called *multiorgan dysfunction syndrome* (MODS), and the subsequent failure of more than one organ system is called (surprise!) *multiorgan failure* (MOF).

Systemic Inflammatory Response Syndrome (SIRS)

The diagnostic criteria for the SIRS are shown in Table 14.2. SIRS is a common condition; i.e., in one survey of patients in a surgical ICU, SIRS was identified in 93% of the patients (10). *The presence of SIRS does not imply the presence of infection.* Infection is identified in only 25 to 50% of patients with SIRS (10,11). The distinction between inflammation and infection is an essential ingredient in the rational approach to patients with fever and leukocytosis.

Table 14.2	Diagnostic Criteria for SIRS

The diagnosis of SIRS requires at least 2 of the following:

1. Temperature > 38°C or < 36°C
2. Heart rate > 90 beats/min
3. Respiratory rate > 20 breaths/min, or arterial PCO_2 < 32 mm Hg
4. WBC count > 12,000/mm³ or < 4000/mm³, or > 10% immature neutrophils (band forms)

From Reference 8.

Inflammatory Organ Failure

The organs most often damaged by systemic inflammation are the lungs, kidneys, cardiovascular system, and central nervous system (see Table 14.1). The most common manifestation of inflammatory organ injury is the *acute respiratory distress syndrome* (ARDS), which has been reported in 40% of patients with severe sepsis (12), and is one of the leading causes of acute respiratory failure in critically ill patients (see Chapter 23).

The number of organs that are damaged by inflammatory injury has important prognostic implications. This is shown in Figure 14.2, which includes surveys from the United States (12) and Europe (13) showing a direct relationship between the mortality rate and the number of organ

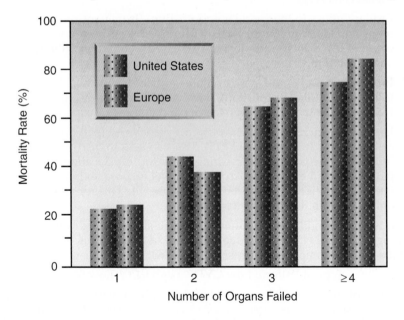

FIGURE 14.2 The relationship between mortality rate and the number of inflammation-related organ failures. Data from References 12 and 13.

failures related to inflammation. This demonstrates the lethal potential of uncontrolled systemic inflammation.

SEPTIC SHOCK

Severe sepsis and septic shock (which are essentially the same condition with different blood pressures) have been implicated in one of every four deaths worldwide (9), and the incidence of these conditions is steadily rising. The mortality rate averages about 30–50% (12,14), and varies with age and the number of associated organ failures (as just described). *The mortality rate is not related to the site of infection or the causative organism, including multidrug-resistant organisms* (14). This observation is evidence that inflammation, not infection, is the principal determinant of outcome in severe sepsis and septic shock.

Hemodynamic Alterations

The hemodynamic alterations in septic shock are summarized below:

1. The principal hemodynamic problem is systemic *vasodilatation* (involving both arteries and veins), which reduces ventricular pre-load (cardiac filling pressures) and ventricular afterload (systemic vascular resistance). The vascular changes are attributed to the enhanced production of nitric oxide (a free radical) in vascular endothelial cells (15).

2. Oxidant injury in the vascular endothelium (from neutrophil attachment and degranulation) leads to fluid extravasation and hypovolemia (15), which adds to the decreased ventricular filling from venodilatation.

3. Proinflammatory cytokines promote cardiac dysfunction (both systolic and diastolic dysfunction); however, the cardiac output is usually increased as a result of tachycardia and volume resuscitation (16).

4. Despite the increased cardiac output, splanchnic blood flow is typically reduced in septic shock (15). This can lead to disruption of the intestinal mucosa, thereby creating a risk for translocation of enteric pathogens and endotoxin across the bowel mucosa and into the systemic circulation (as described in Chapter 5). This, of course, will only aggravate the inciting condition.

The typical hemodynamic pattern in septic shock includes low cardiac filling pressures (CVP or wedge pressure), a high cardiac output (CO), and a low systemic vascular resistance (SVR); i.e.,

Typical Pattern: Low CVP / High CO / Low SVR

Because of the high cardiac output and peripheral vasodilatation, septic shock is also known as *hyperdynamic shock* or *warm shock*. In the advanced stages of septic shock, cardiac dysfunction is more prominent and the cardiac output is reduced, resulting in a hemodynamic pattern that resembles cardiogenic shock (i.e., high CVP, low CO, high SVR). A declining cardiac output in septic shock usually indicates a poor prognosis.

Tissue Oxygenation

As mentioned in Chapter 10, the impaired energy metabolism in septic shock is not the result of inadequate tissue oxygenation, but is caused by a defect in oxygen utilization in mitochondria (17,18). This condition is known as *cytopathic hypoxia* (17), and the culprit is oxidant-induced inhibition of cytochrome oxidase and other proteins in the electron transport chain (19). A decrease in oxygen utilization would explain the observation shown in Figure 14.3, where the PO_2 in skeletal muscle is *increased* in patients with severe sepsis (19).

The proposed decrease in oxygen utilization in sepsis is not consistent with the increase in whole-body O_2 consumption that is often observed in sepsis. This discrepancy can be resolved by proposing that the increased O_2 consumption in sepsis is not a reflection of aerobic metabolism, but is a manifestation of the increased O_2 consumption that occurs during neutrophil activation (i.e., the respiratory burst) (21).

Clinical Implications

The discovery that tissue oxygenation is (more than) adequate in severe sepsis and septic shock has important implications because it means that *efforts to improve tissue oxygenation* in these conditions (e.g., with blood transfusions) *are not justified.*

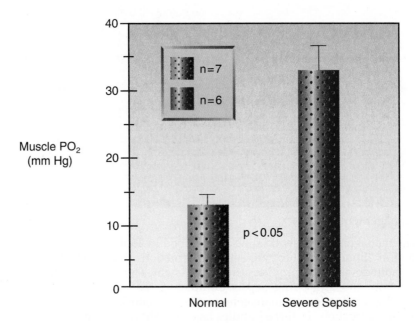

FIGURE 14.3 Direct measurements of tissue PO_2 in the forearm muscles of healthy volunteers and patients with severe sepsis. The height of the columns represents the mean value for each group, and the crossbars represent the standard error of the mean. Data from Reference 20.

Serum Lactate Levels

As mentioned in Chapter 10, the increase in serum lactate levels in severe sepsis and septic shock is not the result of inadequate tissue oxygenation, but instead appears to be the result of enhanced production of pyruvate and inhibition of pyruvate dehydrogenase (22,23), the enzyme that converts pyruvate to acetyl coenzyme A in mitochondria. Endotoxin and other bacterial cell wall components have been implicated in the inhibition of this enzyme (22). This mechanism of lactate accumulation is consistent with the notion that tissue oxygenation is not impaired in severe sepsis and septic shock.

Table 14.3	The Management of Septic Shock Using Bundles
Bundle	**Components**
Acute Sepsis Bundle: Complete within 6 hrs of diagnosis	1. Obtain appropriate cultures.
	2. Obtain plasma lactate level.
	3. Administer appropriate antibiotics.
	4. Achieve the following goals:
	a. CVP = 8–12 mm Hg
	b. MAP ≥ 65 mm Hg
	c. Urine output ≥0.5 mL/kg/hr
	d. $SvO_2 \geq 65\%$ or $ScvO_2 \geq 70\%$
Sepsis Management Bundle: Complete within 24 hrs of diagnosis	1. Administer low-dose steroid if indicated.
	2. Maintain blood glucose levels at 120–150 mg/dL.
	3. Maintain plateau airway pressure at ≤30 cm H_2O in ventilator-dependent patients (see Chapter 23).

From References 9 and 24. CVP = central venous pressure; MAP = mean arterial pressure; SvO_2 = mixed venous O_2 saturation; $ScvO_2$ = central venous O_2 saturation.

Management

The management of septic shock is outlined in Table 14.3, and is organized in "bundles," which are sets of instructions that must be followed without deviation to provide a survival benefit. The bundles in Table 14.3 are from the "Surviving Sepsis Campaign" (an internationally recognized guideline for the management of septic shock) (9), and adherence to the instructions in these bundles has been shown to improve survival in patients with septic shock (24). The acute sepsis bundle is considered the most important, and must be completed within 6 hours after the diagnosis of septic shock.

Volume Resuscitation

Volume resuscitation is often necessary in septic shock because cardiac filling pressures are reduced from venodilatation and fluid extravasation. The following recommendation for volume resuscitation is taken from the Surviving Sepsis Campaign guidelines (9), and it requires the insertion of a central venous catheter to monitor the central venous pressure (CVP).

1. Infuse 500–1,000 mL of crystalloid fluid or 300–500 mL of colloid fluid over 30 minutes.

2. Repeat as needed until the CVP reaches 8 mm Hg, or 12 mm Hg in ventilator-dependent patients.

THE CVP: The use of the CVP in the above protocol is problematic for two reasons. First, volume resuscitation will be delayed by the time required to insert the central line and obtain a chest x-ray to check for proper catheter placement. Secondly, the consensus opinion is that the CVP should NOT be used to guide fluid management because it is not an accurate reflection of the circulating blood volume. The discrepancy between the CVP and circulating blood volume is demonstrated in Figure 11.2 (Chapter 11). If CVP measurements are not available, a volume of at least 20 mL/kg (crystalloid fluid) can be used for the volume resuscitation (25).

After the initial period of volume resuscitation, the infusion rate of intravenous fluids should be reduced to avoid unnecessary fluid accumulation. A positive fluid balance is associated with increased mortality in septic shock (26), so attention to avoiding fluid accumulation will improve the chances of a favorable outcome.

Vasopressors

If hypotension persists after the initial volume resuscitation, infusion of a vasoconstrictor drug (vasopressor) like norepinephrine or dopamine should begin (9). Vasoconstrictor drugs must be infused through a central venous catheter, and the goal is to achieve a mean arterial pressure (MAP) ≥ 65 mm Hg (9).

1. For norepinephrine, start with a dose rate of 0.1 µg/kg/min and titrate upward as needed. Dose rates up to 3.3 µg/kg/min are successful in raising the blood pressure in a majority of patients with septic shock (27). If the desired MAP is not achieved at a dose rate of 3–3.5 µg/kg/min, add dopamine as a second vasopressor.

2. For dopamine, start at a dose rate of 5 µg/kg/min and titrate upward as needed. Vasoconstriction is the predominant effect at dose rates above 10 µg/kg/min (27). If the desired MAP is not achieved with a dose rate of 20 µg/kg/min, add norepinephrine as a second vasopressor.

Norepinephrine is favored by many because it is more likely to raise the blood pressure than dopamine, and is less likely to promote arrhythmias (27).

However, neither agent has proven superior to the other for improving the outcome in septic shock (26). (Norepinephrine and dopamine are described in more detail in Chapter 53.)

VASOPRESSIN: When hypotension is refractory to norepinephrine and dopamine, vasopressin may be effective in raising the blood pressure. (Vasopressin is used as an additional pressor rather than a replacement for norepinephrine or dopamine.) The dose range for vasopressin is 0.01–0.04 units/min, but the popular dose rate in septic shock is 0.03 units/min (9). Vasopressin is a pure vasoconstrictor that can promote splanchnic and digital ischemia, especially at high dose rates. Although vasopressin may help in raising the blood pressure, the accumulated experience with vasopressin shows no influence on outcomes in septic shock (28).

Corticosteroids

Corticosteroids have two actions that are potentially beneficial in septic shock: they have antiinflammatory activity, and they magnify the vaso-constrictor response to catecholamines. Unfortunately, after more than 50 years of investigations, there is no convincing evidence that steroids provide any benefit in the treatment of septic shock (29,30). Yet steroid therapy continues to be popular in septic shock. The following comments reflect the current recommendations regarding steroid therapy in septic shock (9).

1. Steroid therapy should be considered in cases of septic shock where the blood pressure is poorly responsive to intravenous fluids and vasopressor therapy. Evidence of adrenal insufficiency (by the rapid ACTH stimulation test) is not required.

2. Intravenous hydrocortisone is preferred to dexamethasone (because of the mineralocorticoid effects of hydrocortisone), and the dose should not exceed 300 mg daily (to limit the risk of infection).

3. Steroid therapy should be continued as long as vasopressor therapy is required.

Despite the persistent use of steroids in septic shock, it seems that if a drug effect is not apparent after 50 years of investigation (!), then it's time to conclude that the drug does not produce the effect.

Antimicrobial Therapy

Delays in initiating appropriate antibiotic therapy are associated with an increased mortality rate in severe sepsis and septic shock (31), and this has prompted the recommendation that *antibiotic therapy should be started within one hour of the diagnosis of severe sepsis or septic shock* (9). This leaves little time to identify potential pathogens, so the initial antibiotic(s) should have a broad spectrum of activity. See Chapter 43 for recommendations concerning empiric antibiotic coverage for patients with suspected sepsis.

BLOOD CULTURES: One dose of an intravenous antibiotic can sterilize blood cultures within a few hours, so blood cultures should be obtained prior to administering antibiotics. At least 2 sets of blood cultures are recommended (9). Two sets of blood cultures will detect about 90% of bloodstream infections, while 3 sets of blood cultures will detect close to 98% of bloodstream infections (32). The yield from blood cultures is influenced by the volume of blood that is cultured, and a volume of at least 20 mL is recommended for each set of blood cultures (33).

Table 14.4	Clinical Manifestations of Anaphylaxis
Manifestation	**Frequency of Occurrence**
Urticaria	85–90%
Subcutaneous angioedema	85–90%
Upper airway angioedema	50–60%
Bronchospasm and wheezing	45–50%
Hypotension	30–35%
Abdominal cramping, diarrhea	25–30%
Substernal chest pain	4–6%
Pruritis without rash	2–5%

From Reference 35.

ANAPHYLAXIS

Anaphylaxis is an acute multiorgan dysfunction syndrome produced by the immunogenic release of inflammatory mediators from basophils and mast cells. The characteristic feature is an exaggerated immunoglobulin E (IgE) response to an external antigen; i.e., a *hypersensitivity reaction*. The manifestations of anaphylaxis typically involve the skin, lungs, gastrointestinal tract, and cardiovascular system (35). Identical manifestations can occur without the involvement of IgE; these are called *anaphylactoid* reactions, and are not immunogenic in origin (36). Common triggers for anaphylactic reactions include food, antimicrobial agents, and insect bites, while common triggers for anaphylactoid reactions include opiates and radiocontrast dyes. Anaphylaxis can also appear without an identifiable external trigger.

Clinical Features

Anaphylactic reactions are typically abrupt in onset, and appear within minutes of exposure to the external trigger. Some reactions are delayed, and can appear as late as 72 hours after exposure (35). A characteristic feature of anaphylactic reactions is edema and swelling in the involved organ, caused by increased vascular permeability with extravasation of fluid. As much as *35% of the intravascular volume can be lost within 10 minutes* in severe anaphylactic reactions (35).

The clinical manifestations of anaphylaxis are shown in Table 14.4, and are listed by their frequency of occurrence. The most common manifestations are urticaria and subcutaneous angioedema (typically involving the face), and the most concerning manifestations are angioedema of the upper airway (e.g., laryngeal edema), bronchospasm, and hypotension. The most feared manifestation of anaphylaxis is profound hypotension with evidence of systemic hypoperfusion, which represents *anaphylactic shock*.

Management

The management of anaphylaxis includes drugs that halt the progress of anaphylactic reactions (i.e., epinephrine), and drugs that alleviate signs and symptoms (e.g., bronchodilators).

Epinephrine

Epinephrine is the most effective drug available for treating anaphylaxis, and is capable of blocking the release of inflammatory mediators from sensitized basophils and mast cells. The drug is available in a (confusing) variety of aqueous solutions, and these are shown in Table 14.5. The usual treatment for anaphylactic reactions is 0.3–0.5 mg of epinephrine (0.3–0.5 mL of 1:1000 epinephrine solution) administered by deep intramuscular (IM) injection in the lateral thigh, and repeated every 5 minutes if necessary (35). Drug absorption is slower with subcutaneous injection (36), and with drug injection in the deltoid muscle instead of the thigh (35). Epinephrine can be nebulized for patients with laryngeal edema using the dosing regimen shown in Table 14.5; however, the efficacy of nebulized epinephrine is unclear.

GLUCAGON: The actions of epinephrine to inhibit degranulation of mast cells and basophils is mediated by β-adrenergic receptors, and ongoing therapy with β-receptor antagonists can attenuate or eliminate the response to epinephrine. When anaphylactic reactions are refractory to epinephrine in patients receiving β-blocker drugs, glucagon can be effective (for reasons described in Chapter 54). The dose of glucagon is 1–5 mg by slow intravenous injection (over 5 min), followed by a continuous infusion at 5–15 μg/min, titrated to the desired response (35). Glucagon can trigger vomiting, and patients with depressed consciousness should be placed on their side to limit the risk of aspiration when glucagon is administered.

Second-Line Agents

The following drugs can be given after epinephrine is administered, and should never be used as a replacement for epinephrine.

ANTIHISTAMINES: Histamine receptor antagonists are often used for cutaneous anaphylactic reactions, and can help in alleviating pruritis. The histamine H_1 blocker *diphenhydramine* (25–50 mg PO, IM, or IV) and the histamine-H_2 blocker *ranitidine* (50 mg IV or 150 mg PO) should be given together because they are more effective in combination.

Table 14.5	Aqueous Epinephrine Solutions and Their Clinical Uses	
Aqueous Dilution	**Condition**	**Dosing Regimen**
1:100 (10 mg/mL)	Laryngeal Edema	0.25 mL (2.5 mg) in 2 mL saline, administered by nebulizer.
1:1,000 (1 mg/mL)	Anaphylaxis	0.3–0.5 mL (mg) by deep IM injection in the thigh every 5 min as needed.
1:10,000 (0.1 mg/mL)	Asystole or PEA	10 mL (1 mg) IV every 3–5 min as needed
1:100,000 (10μg/mL)	Anaphylactic Shock	Add 1 mL of 1:1,000 solution to 100 mL of saline (1 mg/100 mL or 10 μg/mL) and infuse at 30–100 mL/hr (5–15 μg/min).

From Reference 35. PEA = Pulseless Electrical Activity.

ANTIHISTAMINES: Histamine receptor antagonists are often used for cutaneous anaphylactic reactions, and can help in alleviating pruritis. The histamine H_1 blocker *diphenhydramine* (25–50 mg PO, IM, or IV) and the histamine-H_2 blocker *ranitidine* (50 mg IV or 150 mg PO) should be given together because they are more effective in combination.

BRONCHODILATORS: Inhaled β_2-receptor agonists like *albuterol* are used to relieve bronchospasm, and are administered by nebulizer (2.5 mL or a 0.5% solution) or by metered-dose inhaler.

CORTICOSTEROIDS: Despite the popularity of steroids for treating hypersensitivity reactions, there is no evidence that steroids are effective in reversing, slowing, or preventing the recurrence of anaphylactic reactions (35). As a result, the most recent practice guideline on treating anaphylaxis does not include a recommendation for steroid therapy (35).

Anaphylactic Shock

Anaphylactic shock is an immediate threat to life, with profound hypotension from systemic vasodilatation and massive fluid loss through leaky capillaries (35). The hemodynamic alterations in anaphylactic shock are similar to those in septic shock, but are often more pronounced. Because of the potential for rapid deterioration, anaphylactic shock requires prompt and aggressive management using the measures described next.

Epinephrine

There is no standardized dosing regimen for epinephrine in anaphylactic shock, but the epinephrine infusion regimen in Table 14.5, which uses dose rates of 5–15 µg/min, has been cited for its efficacy (35). An intravenous bolus dose of epinephrine (5–10 µg) can precede the continuous drug infusion (37).

Volume Resuscitation

Aggressive volume resuscitation is essential in anaphylactic shock because at least 35% of the intravascular volume can be lost through leaky capillaries (35), which is enough to produce hypovolemic shock (see Chapter 11). Volume resuscitation can begin by infusing 1–2 liters of crystalloid fluid (or 20 mL/kg), or 500 mL of iso-oncotic colloid fluid (e.g., 5% albumin), over the first 5 minutes (35). Thereafter, the infusion rate of fluids should be tailored to the clinical condition of the patient.

Refractory Hypotension

Persistent hypotension despite epinephrine infusion and volume resuscitation can be managed by adding glucagon or another vasopressor such as norepinephrine or dopamine (the dosing regimens for these drugs have been described earlier).

A FINAL WORD

Another Look at Inflammatory Injury

The discovery that inflammation is the source of multiorgan failure and fatal outcomes in septic shock has created interest in therapies aimed at inhibiting the inflammatory response in septic shock. So far, these therapies have failed to produce the anticipated benefits. This is not unexpected, because *the problem with inflammatory injury is not the inflammation, but the inability of the host to protect itself from inflammatory injury.* Since the damage inflicted by inflammation is largely due to oxidation (i.e., oxidant cell injury), inflammatory injury is a manifestation of oxidant stress, where the production of oxidants (like the reactive oxygen metabolites in Figure 14.1) overwhelms the body's endogenous antioxidant defenses. Therefore, *inflammatory injury can be the result of inadequate antioxidant protection.*

Conditions like severe sepsis and septic shock create an oxidation-rich environment in tissues, which requires an antioxidant-rich defense system. However, antioxidant support is never provided for critically ill patients. It seems likely that persistent oxidation will eventually deplete endogenous antioxidants like glutathione (the major intracellular antioxidant) and vitamin E (which protects cell membranes from oxidant injury), ensuring the progressive march of inflammatory injury and multiorgan failure. There is some evidence that daily administration of endogenous antioxidants improves outcomes in septic shock (38), and the promise of this approach deserves much more attention.

REFERENCES

Moore W. The Knife Man: Blood, Body Snatching, and the Birth of Modern Surgery. New York: Broadway Books, 2005.

Inflammatory Injury

1. Pinsky MR, Matuschak GM. Multiple systems organ failure: failure of host defense mechanisms. Crit Care Clin 1989; 5:199–220.

2. Pinsky MR, Vincent J-L, Deviere J, et al. Serum cytokine levels in human septic shock: Relation to multiple-system organ failure and mortality. Chest 1993; 103:565–575.

3. Fujishima S, Aikawa N. Neutrophil-mediated tissue injury and its modulation. Intensive Care Med 1995; 21:277–285.

4. Babior BM. The respiratory burst of phagocytes. J Clin Invest 1984; 73:599–601.

5. Bernovsky C. Nucleotide chloramines and neutrophil-mediated cytotoxicity. FASEB Journal 1991; 5:295–300.

6. Halliwell B, Gutteridge JMC. The chemistry of free radicals and related 'reactive species'. In: Free Radicals in Biology and Medicine. 4th ed. New York: Oxford University Press, 2007:30–79.

7. Niki E, Yamamoto Y, Komura E, Sato K. Membrane damage due to lipid oxidation. Am J Clin Nutr 1991; 53:201S–205S.

8. American College of Chest Physicians/Society of Critical Care Medicine Consensus Conference Committee. Definitions of sepsis and organ failure and guidelines for the use of innovative therapies in sepsis. Chest 1992; 101:1644–1655.

9. Dellinger RP, Levy MM, Carlet JM, et al. Surviving Sepsis Campaign: international guidelines for management of severe sepsis and septic shock. Intensive Care Med 2008; 34:17–60.

10. Pittet D, Rangel-Frausto S, Li N, et al. Systemic inflammatory response syndrome, sepsis, severe sepsis, and septic shock: incidence, morbidities and outcomes in surgical ICU patients. Intensive Care Med 1995; 21:302–309.

11. Rangel-Frausto MS, Pittet D, Costigan M, et al. Natural history of the systemic inflammatory response syndrome (SIRS). JAMA 1995; 273:117–123.

12. Angus DC, Linde-Zwirble WT, Lidicker J, et al. Epidemiology of severe sepsis in the United States: Analysis of incidence, outcome, and associated costs of care. Crit Care Med 2001; 29:1303–1310.

13. Vincent J-L, de Mendonca A, Cantraine F, et al. Use of the SOFA score to assess the incidence of organ dysfunction/failure in intensive care units: Results of a multicenter, prospective study. Crit Care Med 1998; 26:1793–1800.

Severe Sepsis and Septic Shock

14. Zahar J-R, Timsit J-F, Garrouste-Orgeas M, et al. Outcomes in severe sepsis and patients with septic shock: pathogen species and infection sites are not associated with mortality. Crit Care Med 2011; 39:1886–1895.

15. Abraham E, Singer M. Mechanisms of sepsis-induced organ dysfunction. Crit Care Med 2007; 35:2409–2416.

16. Snell RJ, Parillo JE. Cardiovascular dysfunction in septic shock. Chest 1991; 99:1000–1009.

17. Fink MP. Cytopathic hypoxia. Mitochondrial dysfunction as mechanism contributing to organ dysfunction in sepsis. Crit Care Clin 2001; 17:219–237.

18. Ruggieri AJ, Levy RJ, Deutschman CS. Mitochondrial dysfunction and resuscitation in sepsis. Crit Care Clin 2010; 26:567–575.

19. Muravchick S, Levy RJ. Clinical implications of mitochondrial dysfunction. Anesthesiology 2006; 105:819–837.

20. Sair M, Etherington PJ, Winlove CP, Evans TW. Tissue oxygenation and perfusion in patients with systemic sepsis. Crit Care Med 2001; 29:1343–1349.

21. Vlessis AA, Goldman RK, Trunkey DD. New concepts in the pathophysiology of oxygen metabolism during sepsis. Br J Surg 1995; 82:870–876.

22. Thomas GW, Mains CW, Slone DS, et al. Potential dysregulation of the pyruvate dehydrogenase complex by bacterial toxins and insulin. J Trauma 2009; 67:628–633.

23. Loiacono LA, Shapiro DS. Detection of hypoxia at the cellular level. Crit Care Clin 2010; 26:409–421.

24. Barochia AV, Cui X, Vitberg D, et al. Bundled care for septic shock: an analysis of clinical trials. Crit Care Med 2010; 38:668–678.

25. The Surviving Sepsis Campaign website (www.survivingsepsis.org); accessed Sept 15, 2012.

26. Boyd JH, Forbes J, Nakada T-a, et al. Fluid resuscitation in septic shock: a positive fluid balance and elevated central venous pressure are associated with increased mortality. Crit Care Med 2011; 39:259–265.

27. Hollenberg SM. Inotropes and vasopressor therapy of septic shock. Crit Care Clin 2009; 25:781–802.

28. Polito A, Parisini E, Ricci Z, et al. Vasopressin for treatment of vasodilatory shock: an ESICM systematic review and meta-analysis. Intensive Care Med 2012; 38:9–19.

29. Sprung CL, Annane D, Keh D, et al. Hydrocortisone therapy for patients with septic shock. N Engl J Med 2008; 358:111–124.

30. Sherwin RL, Garcia AJ, Bilkovski R. Do low-dose corticosteroids improve mortality or shock reversal in patients with septic shock? J Emerg Med 2012; 43:7–12.

31. Gaieski DF, Mikkelsen ME, Band RA, et al. Impact of time to antibiotics on survival in patients with severe sepsis or septic shock in whom early goal-directed therapy was initiated in the emergency department. Crit Care Med 2010; 38:1045–1053.

32. Lee A, Mirrett S, Reller B, Weinstein MP. Detection of bloodstream infections in adults: how many blood cultures are needed? J Clin Microbiol 2007; 45:3546–3548.

33. Cockerill FR III, Wilson JW, Vetter EA, et al. Optimal testing parameters for blood cultures. Clin Infect Dis 2004; 38:1724–1730.

34. Marik PE, Preiser J-C. Toward understanding tight glycemic control in the ICU. Chest 2010; 137:544–551.

Anaphylaxis

35. Lieberman P, Nicklas RA, Oppenheimer J, et al. The diagnosis and management of anaphylaxis practice parameter: 2010 update. J Allergy Clin Immunol 2010; 126:480.e1–480.e42.

36. Simons FER, Gu X, Simons KJ. Epinephrine absorption in adults: intramuscular versus subcutaneous injection. J Allergy Clin Immunol 2001; 108(5):871–873.

37. Sampson HA, Munoz-Furlong A, Campbell RL, et al. Second symposium on the definition and management of anaphylaxis: summary report – second National Institute of Allergy and Infectious Disease/Food Allergy and Anaphylaxis Network symposium. Ann Emerg Med 2006; 47:373–380.

A Final Word

38. Angstwurm MWA, Engelmann L, Zimmermann T, et al. Selenium in intensive care (SIC): results of a prospective randomized placebo-controlled study in patients with severe systemic inflammatory response syndrome, sepsis, and septic shock. Crit Care Med 2007; 35:118–126.

CARDIAC EMERGENCIES

Nothing is so firmly believed as that which is least known.

Francis Jeffrey
(1773-1850)

Chapter 15

TACHYARRHYTHMIAS

A rapid heart rate or *tachycardia* while at rest is usually evidence of a problem, but the tachycardia may not be the problem. This chapter describes tachycardias that *are* a problem (i.e., *tachyarrhythmias*), and require prompt evaluation and management. Most of the recommendations in this chapter are borrowed from the clinical practice guidelines listed at the end of the chapter (1–4).

RECOGNITION

The evaluation of tachycardias (heart rate > 100 beats/min) is based on 3 ECG findings: i.e., the duration of the QRS complex, the uniformity of the R-R intervals, and the characteristics of the atrial activity. The results of this evaluation are demonstrated in Figure 15.1. The duration of the QRS complex is used to distinguish *narrow-QRS-complex tachycardias* (QRS duration ≤ 0.12 sec) from *wide-QRS-complex tachycardias* (QRS duration > 0.12 sec). This helps to identify the point of origin of the tachycardia, as described next.

Narrow-QRS-Complex Tachycardias

Tachycardias with a narrow QRS complex (≤ 0.12 sec) originate from a site above the AV conduction system. These *supraventricular tachycardias* include sinus tachycardia, atrial tachycardia, AV nodal re-entrant tachycardia (also called paroxysmal supraventricular tachycardia), atrial flutter, and atrial fibrillation. The specific arrhythmia can be identified using the uniformity of the R-R interval (i.e., the regularity of the rhythm), and the characteristics of the atrial activity, as described next.

Regular Rhythm

If the R-R intervals are uniform in length (indicating a regular rhythm), the possible arrhythmias include sinus tachycardia, AV nodal re-entrant tachycardia, or atrial flutter with a fixed (2:1, 3:1) AV block. The atrial activity on the ECG can identify each of these rhythms using the following criteria:

1. Uniform P waves and P–R intervals indicate a sinus tachycardia.

2. The absence of P waves suggests an AV nodal re-entrant tachycardia (see Figure 15.2).

3. Sawtooth waves are evidence of atrial flutter.

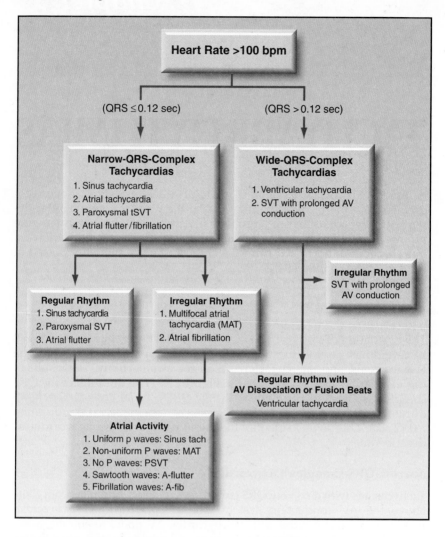

FIGURE 15.1 Flow diagram for the evaluation of tachycardias.

Irregular Rhythm

If the R-R intervals are not uniform in length (indicating an irregular rhythm), the most likely arrhythmias are multifocal atrial tachycardia and atrial fibrillation. Once again, the atrial activity on the ECG helps to identify each of these rhythms; i.e.,

1. Multiple P wave morphologies with variable P-R intervals is evidence of multifocal atrial tachycardia (see Panel A, Figure 15.3).

2. The absence of P waves with highly disorganized atrial activity (fibrillation waves) is evidence of atrial fibrillation (see Panel B, Figure 15.3).

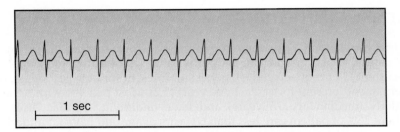

1 sec

FIGURE 15.2 Narrow-QRS-complex tachycardia with a regular rhythm. Note the absence of P waves, which are hidden in the QRS complexes. This is an AV nodal re-entrant tachycardia.

Wide-QRS-Complex Tachycardias

Tachycardias with a wide QRS complex (> 0.12 sec) can originate from a site below the AV conduction system (i.e., ventricular tachycardia), or they can represent a supraventricular tachycardia (SVT) with prolonged AV conduction (e.g., from a bundle branch block). These two arrhythmias can be difficult to distinguish. An irregular rhythm is evidence of an SVT with aberrant AV conduction, while certain ECG abnormalities (e.g., AV dissociation) provide evidence of VT. The distinction between VT and SVT with aberrant conduction is described in more detail later in the chapter.

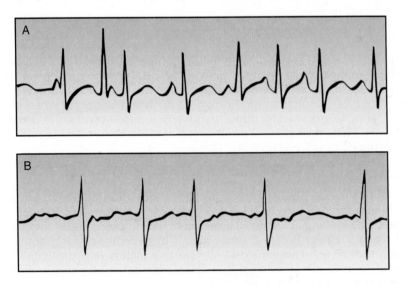

A

B

FIGURE 15.3 Narrow-QRS-complex tachycardias with an irregular rhythm. Panel A shows a multifocal atrial tachycardia (MAT), identified by multiple P wave morphologies and variable PR intervals. Panel B is atrial fibrillation, identified by the absence of P waves and the highly disorganized atrial activity (fibrillation waves).

ATRIAL FIBRILLATION

Atrial fibrillation (AF) is the most common cardiac rhythm disturbance in clinical practice, and can be paroxysmal (resolves spontaneously), recurrent (2 or more episodes), persistent (present for at least 7 days), or permanent (present for at least one year) (1,2). Most patients with AF are elderly (median age 75 years) and have underlying cardiac disease. About 25% of patients are less than 60 years of age and have no underlying cardiac disease (1): a condition known as *lone atrial fibrillation*.

Postoperative AF

Postoperative AF is reported in up to 45% of cardiac surgeries, up to 30% of non-cardiac thoracic surgeries, and up to 8% of other major surgeries (5). It usually appears in the first 5 postoperative days (6), and is associated with longer hospital stays and increased mortality (5,6). Several predisposing factors have been implicated, including heightened adrenergic activity, magnesium depletion, and oxidant stress. Prophylaxis with β-blockers and magnesium is currently popular (5,7), and there is evidence that the antioxidant N-acetylcysteine (a glutathione surrogate) provides effective prophylaxis following cardiac surgery (7). Most cases of postoperative AF resolve within a few months.

Adverse Consequences

The adverse consequences of AF include impaired cardiac performance and thromboembolism.

Cardiac Performance

Atrial contraction is responsible for 25% of the ventricular end-diastolic volume in the normal heart (8). Loss of the atrial contribution to ventricular filling in AF has little noticeable effect when cardiac function is normal, but it can result in a significant decrease in stroke output when diastolic filling is impaired by mitral stenosis or reduced ventricular compliance (1). This effect is more pronounced at rapid heart rates (because of the reduced time for ventricular filling).

Thromboembolism

Atrial fibrillation predisposes to thrombus formation in the left atrium, and these thrombi can dislodge and embolize in the cerebral circulation, thereby producing an acute *ischemic stroke*. The average yearly incidence of ischemic stroke is 3 to 5 times higher in patients with AF, but only when the AF is accompanied by certain risk factors (e.g., heart failure, mitral stenosis, advanced age) (1,2). Recommendations for antithrombotic therapy are presented later.

Management Strategies

The acute management of AF can be divided into 3 components: i.e., control of the heart rate, cardioversion (electrical and pharmacological), and thromboprophylaxis.

Heart Rate Control

The typical strategy for uncomplicated AF is to slow the ventricular response with drugs that prolong AV conduction. A variety of drugs are available for this purpose, and the popular ones are included in Table 15.1. The following is a brief description of these drugs.

Table 15.1	Drug Regimens for Acute Rate Control in Atrial Fibrillation
Drug	**Dosing Regimen and Comments**
Diltiazem	Dosing: 0.25 mg/kg IV over 2 min, then infuse at 5–15 mg/hr. If heart rate >90 bpm after 15 min, give second bolus of 0.35 mg/kg.
	Comment: Has negative inotropic effects, but has been used safely in patients with heart failure.
Amiodarone	Dosing: 150 mg IV over 10 min, and repeat if needed, then infuse at 1 mg/min for 6 hr, followed by 0.5 mg/min for 18 hr. Total dose should not exceed 2.2 grams in 24 hrs.
	Comment: Can convert AF to sinus rhythm, which can be risky without adequate thromboprophylaxis. Preferred for AF with heart failure.
Metoprolol	Dosing: 2.5–5 mg IV over 2 min, and repeat every 5–10 min if needed to a total of 3 doses.
	Comment: Effective in AF associated with hyperadrenergic states. Bolus dosing is not optimal for strict rate control.
Esmolol	Dosing: 500 µg/kg IV bolus, then infuse at 50 µg/kg/min. Increase dose in increments of 25 µg/kg/min every 5 min if needed to a maximum rate of 200 µg/kg/min.
	Comment: An ultra-short-acting β-blocker that permits rapid dose titration. Effective in AF associated with hyperadrenergic states.
Digoxin	Dosing: 0.25 mg IV every 2 hr to a total dose of 1.5 mg, then 0.125–0.375 mg IV daily.
	Comment: Slow-acting drug that should not be used alone for acute rate control. Preferred for AF with heart failure.

From the clinical practice guidelines in References 1 and 4.

DILTIAZEM: Diltiazem is a calcium channel blocker that achieves *satisfactory rate reduction in up to 90% of cases of uncomplicated AF* (9). The acute response to diltiazem is shown in Figure 15.4: note the superiority of diltiazem over amiodarone and digoxin after the first hour of therapy. Adverse effects of diltiazem include hypotension and cardiac depression.

Although diltiazem has negative inotropic effects, it has been used safely in patients with moderate to severe heart failure (10).

β-RECEPTOR ANTAGONISTS: β-blockers achieve *successful rate control in 70% of cases of acute AF* (11), and they are the preferred agents for rate control when AF is associated with hyperadrenergic states (such as acute MI and post-cardiac surgery) (1,5). Two β-blockers with proven efficacy in AF are *esmolol* (Brevibloc) and *metoprolol* (Lopressor). Both are cardioselective agents that preferentially block β-1 receptors in the heart. Esmolol is more attractive than metoprolol because it is an ultra short-acting drug (with a serum half-life of 9 minutes), which allows rapid dose titration to the desired effect (12).

AMIODARONE: Amiodarone prolongs conduction in the AV node, but is less effective for acute rate control than diltiazem, as shown in Figure 15.4. However, amiodarone produces less cardiac depression than diltiazem (13), and it is favored by some for AF with heart failure (1). Amiodarone is also an antiarrhythmic agent (Class III), and is *capable of converting AF to a sinus rhythm*. The success rate for converting recent-onset AF is 55% to 95% when a loading dose and continuous infusion are

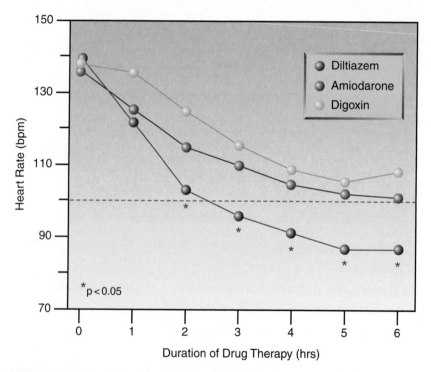

FIGURE 15.4 Comparison of acute rate control with intravenous diltiazem, amiodarone, and digoxin in patients with uncomplicated atrial fibrillation. Data points marked with a star indicate a significant difference with diltiazem compared to the other two drugs. Data from Reference 10.

used, and the daily dose exceeds 1500 mg (1,14). However, unanticipated cardioversion with amiodarone can be a problem when patients are not adequately anticoagulated (see later).

The adverse effects of short-term intravenous amiodarone include hypotension (15%), infusion phlebitis (15%), bradycardia (5%), and elevated liver enzymes (3%) (15,16). Hypotension is the most common side effect, and is related to the combined vasodilator actions of amiodarone and the solvent (polysorbate 80 surfactant) used to enhance water solubility of injectable amiodarone (17). Amiodarone also has several drug interactions by virtue of its metabolism by the cytochrome P450 enzyme system in the liver (16). The most relevant interactions in the ICU setting are inhibition of digoxin and warfarin metabolism, which requires attention if amiodarone is continued orally for long-term management.

DIGOXIN: Digoxin prolongs conduction in the AV node, and is a popular drug for long-term rate control in AF. However, the response to intravenous digoxin is slow to develop; i.e., it is usually not apparent for at least one hour, and the peak response can take longer than 6 hours to develop (1). In comparison, the response to an intravenous dose of diltiazem is apparent in 3–5 minutes, and the peak response occurs at 5–7 minutes (17). The superiority of diltiazem over digoxin for acute rate control in AF is demonstrated in Figure 15.4. Note that the heart rate remains above 100 beats/min (the threshold for tachycardia) at 6 hours after the start of rate-control therapy with digoxin. Digoxin may have a role in treating AF associated with heart failure, but it should not be used alone for acute rate control in AF (1,4).

Electrical Cardioversion

More than 50% of episodes of recent-onset AF will spontaneously revert to sinus rhythm within the first 72 hours (18). For the remaining cases of AF that are complicated by hypotension, pulmonary edema, or myocardial ischemia, direct-current cardioversion is the appropriate intervention. Biphasic shocks have replaced monophasic shocks as the standard of care for cardioversion because they require less energy for a successful result. An energy of 100 J is usually enough for successful cardioversion using biphasic shocks, but 200 J is recommended for the initial cardioversion attempt in the most recent guidelines on AF (1). If additional shocks are needed, the energy level is increased in increments of 100 J to a maximum energy level of 400 J. Success may be fleeting when AF has persisted for more than a year (1).

Pharmacological Cardioversion

Drug-induced cardioversion is used in cases of uncomplicated AF that are refractory to rate control, or for first episodes of uncomplicated AF that are less than 48 hours in duration, to eliminate the need for anticoagulation (see later). Several antiarrhythmic agents can be effective in terminating AF, including *amiodarone* and *ibutilide*. The success rate of amiodarone in recent-onset AF has been mentioned previously. Ibutilide (at a dose of 1 mg IV over 10 minutes, repeated once if necessary) has a reported success rate of about 50% in recent-onset AF (15). Ibutilide prolongs the QT interval, and is one of the high-risk drugs for promoting polymorphic ventricular tachycardia (torsade de pointes) (15), as shown later in Table 15.4

Thromboprophylaxis

Recommendations for antithrombotic therapy in AF are shown in Table 15.2. To summarize, anticoagulation is recommended for any patient with AF and one or more of the following risk factors: mitral stenosis, coronary artery disease, congestive heart failure, hypertension, age ≥ 75 yrs, diabetes mellitus, and prior stroke or TIA (1,2). This, of course, excludes patients who have a contraindication to anticoagulation.

Table 15.2	Antithrombotic Therapy in Atrial Fibrillation (AF)
Conditions	**Recommendations**
†CHADS$_2$ Score = 0	No anticoagulation
†CHADS$_2$ Score ≥ 1	Long-term R$_x$ with dabigatran, 150 mg BID$^\alpha$
Mitral Stenosis, Stable Coronary Disease	Long-term R$_x$ with warfarin to INR of 2–3
Elective Cardioversion: AF > 48 hr or unknown	Therapeutic anticoagulation from 3 weeks before to 4 weeks after the procedure
Urgent Cardioversion	Therapeutic anticoagulation during, and for 4 weeks after the procedure

†CHADS$_2$: Congestive heart failure (1 point), history of Hypertension (1 point), Age ≥75 yrs, (1 point), Diabetes mellitus (1 point), prior Stroke or TIA (2 points).

$^\alpha$Decrease dose to 75 mg BID for creatinine clearance of 15–30 mL/min, and do NOT use if creatinine clearance <15 mL/min.

Recommendations from the ACCP guidelines in Reference 2.

DABIGATRAN: The ACCP guidelines (2) recommend the use of dabigatran (150 mg BID), a direct thrombin inhibitor, for patients with AF and one or more risk factors in the CHADS$_2$ score. This is based on one study showing that dabigatran in a dose of 150 mg BID (but not lower) was associated with fewer strokes than warfarin (19). This study excluded patients with renal insufficiency because dabigatran is cleared by the kidneys. In fact, it is important to note that *a dose reduction of 50% (to 75 mg BID) is required for patients with renal impairment* (i.e., creatinine clearance of 15–30 mL/min), while the drug is *contraindicated in patients with renal failure* (i.e., creatinine clearance < 15 mL/min) (2).

Since the degree of anticoagulation is not routinely monitored when using thrombin inhibitors, and there is no antidote to reverse dabigatran in cases of drug-associated bleeding, it is probably wise to avoid this drug in patients with any degree of renal impairment.

CARDIOVERSION: Thromboembolic events following cardioversion have been reported in 1% to 7% of patients who were not anticoagulated at the time of the procedure (1,2). This is the basis for the recommendation to begin anticoagulation 3 weeks prior to an elective cardioversion, and continue anticoagulation for 4 weeks after the procedure (2). For emergent cardioversion, anticoagulation with heparin should be initiated as soon as possible prior to the procedure, followed by four weeks of anticoagulation after the procedure. When AF is less than 48 hours in duration, cardioversion has a low risk of thromboembolism (<1%), and periprocedural anticoagulation is not necessary (1).

Wolff-Parkinson-White Syndrome

The Wolff-Parkinson-White (WPW) syndrome (short P–R interval and delta waves before the QRS) is characterized by recurrent supraventricular tachycardias that originate from an accessory pathway in the AV node. (The mechanism for these tachycardias is explained in the section on re-entrant tachycardias.) When atrial fibrillation occurs in a patient with an accessory pathway, drugs that block conduction in the AV node (e.g., calcium channel blockers, β-blockers, digoxin) are unlikely to slow the ventricular rate because the accessory pathway is not blocked (1,4). Furthermore, selective block of the AV node can precipitate ventricular fibrillation (4). Therefore, *drugs that block the AV node* (e.g., calcium channel blockers, β-blockers, and digoxin) *should NOT be used when AF is associated with the WPW syndrome* (1,4). The preferred management in this situation is electrical cardioversion or antiarrhythmic drugs such as amiodarone or procainamide.

MULTIFOCAL ATRIAL TACHYCARDIA

Multifocal atrial tachycardia or MAT (see Panel A in Figure 15.3) is a disorder of the elderly (average age = 70), and over half of the cases occur in patients with chronic lung disease (20). Other associated conditions include magnesium and potassium depletion, and coronary artery disease (21).

Acute Management

The following measures are recommended for the acute management of MAT, but this is a stubborn arrhythmia that is often refractory to medical management.

1. Identify and correct hypomagnesemia and hypokalemia if necessary. If both disorders co-exist, the magnesium deficiency must be corrected before potassium deficits can be replaced. This is explained in Chapter 37.
2. Since serum magnesium levels can be normal when total body magnesium is depleted (also explained in Chapter 37), intravenous mag-

nesium can be given as an empiric measure when serum magnesium levels are normal. The following regimen can be used:

> Start with 2 grams $MgSO_4$ (in 50 mL saline) IV over 15 minutes,
>
> then infuse 6 grams $MgSO_4$ (in 500 mL saline) over 6 hours.

In one study, this regimen had a remarkable 88% success rate in converting MAT to a sinus rhythm, and the effect was independent of serum magnesium levels (21). This success may be explained by the membrane-stabilizing effect of magnesium (22), and by the actions of magnesium as "nature's calcium channel blocker" (see Chapter 37). There is no risk of magnesium overload from this empiric regimen.

3. If the prior measures fail, and COPD is not the cause of the MAT, *metoprolol* in the doses shown in Table 15.1 has a reported *80% success rate in converting MAT to sinus rhythm* (20). If metoprolol is a concern in patients with COPD, the calcium channel blocker *verapamil* can be effective. Verapamil converts MAT to sinus rhythm in less than 50% of cases (20), but it can also slow the ventricular rate. The dose is 0.25–5 mg IV over 2 min, which can be repeated every 15–30 min, if necessary, to a total dose of 20 mg (4). Verapamil is a potent negative inotropic agent, and hypotension is a frequent side effect. The drug is not recommended for patients with heart failure (4).

PAROXYSMAL SUPRAVENTRICULAR TACHYCARDIA

Paroxysmal supraventricular tachycardias (PSVT) are narrow-QRS-complex tachycardias that are second only to atrial fibrillation as the most prevalent rhythm disturbances in the general populace.

Mechanism

These arrhythmias occur when impulse transmission in one pathway of the AV conduction system is slowed. This creates a difference in the refractory period for impulse transmission in the abnormal and normal conduction pathways, and this allows impulses travelling down one pathway to travel back through the other pathway. The retrograde transmission of impulses is called *re-entry*, and it results in a circular pattern of impulse transmission that is self-sustaining; i.e., a *re-entrant tachycardia*. Re-entry is triggered by an ectopic atrial impulse in one of the two conduction pathways, which results in the abrupt onset that is characteristic of re-entrant tachycardias.

There are 5 different types of PSVT, based on the location of the re-entrant pathway. The most common PSVT is *AV nodal re-entrant tachycardia*, where the re-entrant pathway is located in the AV node.

AV Nodal Re-Entrant Tachycardia

AV nodal re-entrant tachycardia (AVNRT) accounts for 50 to 60% of cases of PSVT (23). It typically appears in patients who have no history of heart disease, and is more common in women than men. The onset is abrupt, and the predominant complaints are palpitations and lightheadedness. There is no evidence of heart failure or myocardial ischemia, and significant hemodynamic compromise is uncommon. The ECG shows a narrow-QRS-complex tachycardia with a regular rhythm and a heart rate between 140 and 250 bpm (23). There are often no visible P waves on the ECG, as shown in Figure 15.2.

AVNRT is frequently mistaken for sinus tachycardia, but the onset is different (abrupt onset vs. gradual onset for sinus tachycardia), the heart rate is often different (usually higher than 140 beats/min in AVNRT and rarely higher than 150 beats/min in sinus tachycardia), and the ECG appearance is different (no visible P waves in AVNRT and P waves before each QRS complex in sinus tachycardia).

Vagal Maneuvers

Maneuvers that increase vagal tone are recommended as an initial attempt to terminate AVNRT. A variety of maneuvers have been identified, including carotid sinus massage and the Valsalva maneuver (maximal expiratory effort with a closed glottis). The success of these maneuvers has not been adequately studied; one study of 148 patients with paroxysmal SVT showed a success rate of 18% with the Valsalva maneuver and 12% with carotid sinus massage (24).

Adenosine

When vagal maneuvers are ineffective, *adenosine is the drug of choice for terminating re-entrant tachycardias involving the AV node* (25,26). Adenosine is an endogenous nucleotide (the backbone of the ATP molecule) that relaxes vascular smooth muscle and slows conduction in the AV node. When given by rapid intravenous injection, adenosine has a rapid onset of action (< 30 sec) and produces a transient AV block that can terminate AV nodal re-entrant tachycardias. Adenosine is quickly cleared from the bloodstream (by receptors on RBCs and endothelial cells), and the effects last only 1–2 minutes.

Dosing Considerations

The dosing regimen for adenosine is shown in Table 15.3. The initial dose is 6 mg, which is injected rapidly into a peripheral vein and followed by a saline flush. Optimal results are obtained if the drug is injected at the hub of the catheter. If conversion to sinus rhythm does not occur after 2 minutes, a second 12 mg dose is given, and this can be repeated once if necessary. This regimen *terminates re-entrant tachycardias in over 90% of cases* (24–26). The effective dose of adenosine was determined using drug injection into peripheral veins, and ventricular asystole has been reported when standard doses of adenosine are injected through central venous catheters (27). As a result, *a dose reduction of 50% has been recommended* by some (including the manufacturer) *when adenosine is injected through a central venous catheter* (27).

Table 15.3	Intravenous Adenosine for Paroxysmal SVT	
Feature	**Drug Characteristics**	
Dosing Regimen	1. Deliver through a peripheral vein.	
	2. Give 6 mg by rapid IV injection and flush catheter with saline.	
	3. If response inadequate after 2 min, give 12 mg by rapid IV injection and flush catheter with saline.	
	4. If response still inadequate after 2 min, another 12 mg can be given by rapid IV injection.	
Dose Adjustments	Decrease dose by 50% for:	
	• Drug injection into the superior vena cava	
	• Patient receiving calcium antagonist, β-blocker, or dipyridamole	
Drug Interactions	• Dipyridamole (blocks adenosine uptake)	
	• Theophylline (blocks adenosine receptors)	
Contraindications	• Asthma	
	• 2nd or 3rd degree AV block	
	• Sick sinus syndrome	
Adverse Effects	• Bradycardia, AV block (50%)	
	• Facial flushing (20%)	
	• Dyspnea (12%)	
	• Chest pressure (7%)	

From References 4, 25, 26.

Adverse Effects

The adverse effects of adenosine are short-lived because of the drug's ultra-short duration of action. The most frequent adverse effect is post-conversion bradycardia, including various degrees of AV block. The AV block is refractory to atropine, but resolves spontaneously within 60 seconds (26). Dipyridamole enhances the AV block produced by adenosine (26). Adenosine is contraindicated in patients with asthma because of reports of adenosine-induced bronchospasm (28), but more recent studies indicate that adenosine produces a sense of dyspnea, but not bronchospasm, in asthmatic subjects (29).

Refractory Tachycardias

Methylxanthines like theophylline block adenosine receptors and reduce the effectiveness of adenosine in terminating re-entrant tachycardias (26). This interaction has been minimized by the diminished use of theophylline as a bronchodilator. *When PSVT does not respond to adenosine, the calcium channel blockers diltiazem or verapamil can be effective.* (The dosing regimen for diltiazem is shown in Table 15.1, and the dosing regimen for verapamil was presented in the section on paroxysmal SVTs).

VENTRICULAR TACHYCARDIA

Ventricular tachycardia (VT) is a wide-QRS-complex tachycardia that has an abrupt onset, a regular rhythm, and a rate above 100 bpm (usually 140–200 bpm). The appearance can be *monomorphic* (uniform QRS complexes) or *polymorphic* (multiple QRS morphologies). VT rarely occurs in the absence of structural heart disease (30), and when it is sustained (i.e., lasts longer than 30 seconds), it can be an immediate threat to life.

VT versus SVT

Monomorphic VT can be difficult to distinguish from an SVT with prolonged AV conduction. This is demonstrated in Figure 15.5. The tracing in the upper panel shows a wide-QRS-complex tachycardia that looks like monomorphic VT. The tracing in the lower panel shows spontaneous conversion to sinus rhythm. Note that the QRS complex remains unchanged after the arrhythmia is terminated, revealing an underlying bundle branch block. Thus, the apparent VT in the upper panel is actually an SVT with a preexisting bundle branch block.

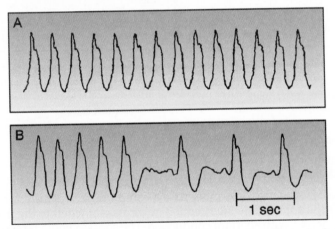

FIGURE 15.5 Upper panel shows a wide-QRS-complex tachycardia that looks like monomorphic VT. However, the lower panel shows spontaneous conversion to a sinus rhythm, which reveals an underlying bundle branch block, indicating that the rhythm in the upper panel is an SVT with a preexisting bundle branch block. Tracings courtesy of Richard M. Greenberg, M.D.

Clues

There are two abnormalities on an ECG that will identify VT as the cause of a wide-QRS-complex tachycardia.

1. The atria and ventricles beat independently in VT, and this results in *AV dissociation* on the ECG, where there is no fixed relationship between P waves and QRS complexes. This may not be evident on a single-lead tracing, and is more likely to be discovered on a 12-lead ECG. (P waves are most visible in the inferior limb leads and the anterior precordial leads.)

2. The presence of fusion beats like the one in Figure 15.6 is indirect evidence of VT. A fusion beat is produced by the retrograde transmission of a ventricular ectopic impulse that collides with a supraventricular (e.g., sinus node) impulse. The result is a hybrid QRS complex that is a mixture of the normal QRS complex and the ventricular ectopic impulse. The presence of a fusion beat (which should be evident on a single-lead ECG tracing) is indirect evidence of ventricular ectopic activity.

If there is no definitive evidence of VT on the ECG, the presence or absence of heart disease can be useful; i.e., *VT is the cause of 95% of wide-QRS-complex tachycardias in patients with underlying heart disease* (31). Therefore, a wide-QRS-complex tachycardia should be treated as probable VT in any patient with underlying heart disease.

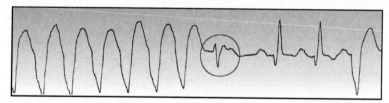

FIGURE 15.6 An example of a fusion beat (circled in red), which is a hybrid QRS complex produced by the collision of a ventricular ectopic impulse and a supraventricular (e.g., sinus node) impulse. The presence of fusion beats is evidence of ventricular ectopic activity.

Management

The management of patients with a wide-QRS-complex tachycardia can proceed as follows. This approach is organized in a flow diagram in Figure 15.7.

1. If there is evidence of hemodynamic compromise, *electrical cardioversion* is the appropriate intervention, regardless of whether the rhythm is VT or SVT with aberrant conduction. The shocks should be synchronized (timed with the QRS complex), with an initial shock of 100 J (biphasic or monophasic shocks) (30). This should terminate most cases of monomorphic VT, but shocks of 200 J (biphasic shocks) and up to 360 J (monophasic shocks) may be necessary.

2. If there is no hemodynamic compromise and the diagnosis of VT is certain, intravenous amiodarone should be used to terminate the arrhythmia. *Amiodarone is the favored drug for suppression of monomorphic VT* (4).

3. If there is no hemodynamic compromise and the diagnosis of VT is uncertain, the response to adenosine can be helpful because adenosine will abruptly terminate most cases of paroxysmal SVT, but will

not terminate VT. If a wide-QRS-complex tachycardia is refractory to adenosine, the likely diagnosis is VT, and intravenous amiodarone is indicated for arrhythmia suppression.

Torsade de Pointes

Torsade de pointes ("twisting around the points") is a polymorphic VT with QRS complexes that appear to be twisting around the isoelectric line of the ECG, as shown in Figure 15.8. This arrhythmia is associated with a prolonged QT interval, and it can be congenital or acquired. The acquired form is much more prevalent, and is caused by a variety of drugs and electrolyte abnormalities that prolong the QT interval (32,33). There is also a polymorphic VT that is associated with a normal QT interval, and the predisposing condition in this arrhythmia is myocardial ischemia (4).

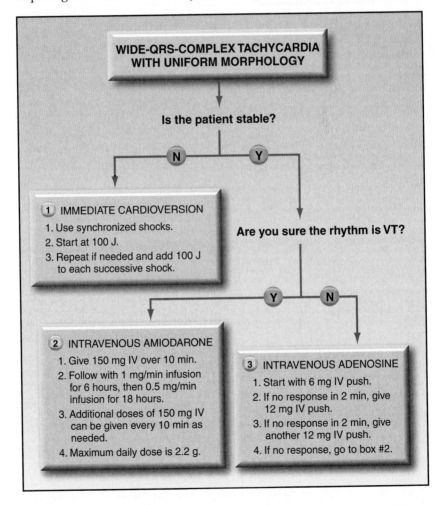

FIGURE 15.7 Flow diagram for the acute management of patients with wide-QRS-complex tachycardia. Based on recommendations in Reference 4.

Predisposing Factors

The drugs most frequently implicated in torsade de pointes are listed in Table 15.4 (33). The prominent offenders are antiarrhythmic agents (Class IA and III), macrolide antibiotics, neuroleptic agents, cisapride (a pro-motility drug), and methadone. The electrolyte disorders that prolong the QT interval include hypokalemia, hypocalcemia, and hypomagnesemia.

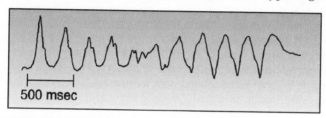

FIGURE 15.8 Torsade de pointes, a polymorphic ventricular tachycardia described as "twisting around the (isoelectric) points." Tracing courtesy of Richard M. Greenberg, M.D.

Table 15.4	Drugs That Can Induce Torsade de Pointes		
Antiarrhythmics	**Antimicrobials**	**Neuroleptics**	**Others**
IA { Quinidine	Clarithromycin	Chlorpromazine	Cisapride
Disopyramide	Erythromycin	Thioridazine	Methadone
Procainamide	Pentamidine	Droperidol	
III { Ibutilide		Haloperidol	
Sotalol			

From Reference 33. For a complete list of drugs, go to www.torsades.org.

Measuring the QT Interval:

The QT interval is the ECG manifestation of ventricular depolarization and repolarization, and is measured from the onset of the QRS complex to the end of the T wave. The longest QT intervals are usually in precordial leads V3 and V4, and these leads are most reliable for assessing QT prolongation. The QT interval varies inversely with heart rate (e.g., an increase in heart rate shortens the QT interval), and therefore a rate-corrected QT interval (QTc) provides a more accurate assessment of QT prolongation. The accepted method for determining the QTc is to divide the QT interval by the square root of the R-R interval (33-35); i.e.,

$$QTc = QT / \sqrt{R\text{-}R}$$

A normal QT interval corresponds to a QTc ≤ 0.44 seconds, and a QTc > 0.5 seconds represents an increased risk of torsade de pointes (35). The risk of torsade de points when the QTc = 0.45 – 0.5 seconds is not clear (33,35). There is no consensus on how to measure the QTc in highly irregular rhythms like atrial fibrillation.

Management

The management of polymorphic VT is summarized as follows:

1. Sustained polymorphic VT requires *nonsynchronized* electric cardioversion (i.e., defibrillation) (4).

2. For torsade de pointes, intravenous *magnesium* is used for pharmacological management (and can be combined with electrical cardioversion). There is no universal dosing regimen for magnesium in this setting. The ACLS guidelines recommend 1–2 grams magnesium sulfate (MgSO$_4$) IV over 15 minutes (4), while another recommended regimen is 2 grams MgSO$_4$ as an IV bolus, followed by a continuous magnesium infusion at 2–4 mg/min (33). Aggressive magnesium loading has no reported adverse consequences (even in patients with renal insufficiency), so the more aggressive magnesium regimen (33) should be the favored one.

3. Other measures for torsade de pointes include correcting high-risk electrolyte abnormalities and discontinuing high-risk drugs, to prevent recurrence.

4. For polymorphic VT with a normal QT interval, amiodarone or β-blockers (for myocardial ischemia) can help to prevent recurrences (4).

A FINAL WORD

The tachyarrhythmia that will dominate your time more than all the others combined is atrial fibrillation (AF). This is rarely a primary problem (in a non-coronary ICU), but it can require more attention than the primary problem. This arrhythmia is like an annoying person you meet who demands a lot of attention but is not threatening (not life-threatening, in the case of the arrhythmia).

The tachyarrhythmias that *are* an immediate threat to life (i.e., ventricular tachycardia) are not prevalent in non-coronary ICUs, even in patients with circulatory shock and multiorgan failure. In fact, in patients who are near death and are not resuscitated, the progression to ventricular asystole is usually populated by *brady*arrhythmias (e.g. AV blocks). This paucity of troublesome ventricular tachycardia outside the coronary care unit may be explained by the trigger for ventricular tachycardia (i.e., focal, rather than global, myocardial ischemia), which is not a common occurrence in critical illness when coronary artery disease is not the dominant problem.

REFERENCES

Clinical Practice Guidelines

1. Fuster V, Ryden LE, Cannom DS, et al. 2011 ACCF/AHA/ESC focused updates incorporated into the ACC/AHA/ESC 2006 guidelines for the management of patients with atrial fibrillation. J Am Coll Cardiol 2011; 57:e101–e198.

2. You JJ, Singer DE, Howard PA, et al. Antithrombotic therapy for atrial fibrillation. Antithrombotic Therapy and Prevention of Thrombosis, 9th ed. American College of Chest Physicians Evidence-Based Clinical Practice Guidelines. Chest 2012; 141(Suppl):e531S–e575S.

3. The Task Force for the Management of Atrial Fibrillation of the European Society of Cardiology (ESC). Guidelines for the management of atrial fibrillation. Europace 2010; 12:1360–1420.

4. Neumar RW, Otto CW, Link MS, et al. Part 8: adult advanced cardiovascular life support. 2010 American Heart Association Guidelines for Cardiopulmonary Resuscitation and Emergency Cardiovascular Care. Circulation 2010; 122(Suppl):S729–S767.

Atrial Fibrillation

5. Mayson SE, Greenspon AJ, Adams S, et al. The changing face of postoperative atrial fibrillation: a review of current medical therapy. Cardiol Rev 2007; 15:231–241.

6. Davis EM, Packard KA, Hilleman DE. Pharmacologic prophylaxis of postoperative atrial fibrillation in patients undergoing cardiac surgery: beyond beta blockers. Pharmacotherapy 2010; 30:274e–318e.

7. Ozaydin M, Peker O, Erdogan D, et al. N-acetylcysteine for the prevention of postoperative atrial fibrillation: a prospective, randomized, placebo-controlled pilot study. Eur Heart J 2008; 29:625–631.

8 Guyton AC. The relationship of cardiac output and arterial pressure control. Circulation 1981; 64:1079–1088.

9. Siu C-W, Lau C-P, Lee W-L, et al. Intravenous diltiazem is superior to intravenous amiodarone or digoxin for achieving ventricular rate control in patients with acute uncomplicated atrial fibrillation. Crit Care Med 2009; 37:2174–2179.

10. Goldenberg IF, Lewis WR, Dias VC, et al. Intravenous diltiazem for the treatment of patients with atrial fibrillation or flutter and moderate to severe congestive heart failure. Am J Cardiol 1994; 74:884–889.

11. Olshansky B, RosenfeldLE, Warner AI, et al. The Atrial Fibrillation Follow-up Investigation of Rhythm Management (AFFIRM) study: approaches to control rate in atrial fibrillation. J Am Coll Cardiol 2004; 43:1201–1208.

12. Gray RJ. Managing critically ill patients with esmolol. An ultra-short-acting β-adrenergic blocker. Chest 1988;93:398–404.

13. Karth GD, Geppert A, Neunteufl T, et al. Amiodarone versus diltiazem for rate control in critically ill patients with atrial tachyarrhythmias. Crit Care Med 2001; 29:1149–1153.

14. Khan IA, Mehta NJ, Gowda RM. Amiodarone for pharmacological cardioversion of recent-onset atrial fibrillation. Int J Cardiol 2003; 89:239–248.

15. VerNooy RA, Mounsey P. Antiarrhythmic drug therapy in atrial fibrillation. Cardiol Clin 2004; 22:21–34.

16. Chow MSS. Intravenous amiodarone: pharmacology, pharmacokinetics, and clinical use. Ann Pharmacother 1996; 30:637–643.

17. Diltiazem hydrochloride. In: McEvoy GK (ed). AHFS Drug Information: 2012. Bethesda, MD: American Society of Health System Pharmacists, 2012:1961-1969.

18. Danias PG, Caulfield TA, Weigner MJ, et al. Likelihood of spontaneous conversion of atrial fibrillation to sinus rhythm. J Am Coll Cardiol 1998; 31:588–592.

19. Connolly SJ, Ezekowitz MD, Yusuf S, et al. Dabigatran versus warfarin in patients with atrial fibrillation. N Engl J Med 2009; 361:1139–1151.

Multifocal Atrial Tachycardia

20. Kastor J. Multifocal atrial tachycardia. N Engl J Med 1990; 322:1713–1720.

21. Iseri LT, Fairshter RD, Hardeman JL, Brodsky MA. Magnesium and potassium therapy in multifocal atrial tachycardia. Am Heart J 1985; 312:21–26.

22. McLean RM. Magnesium and its therapeutic uses: a review. Am J Med 1994; 96:63–76.

Paroxysmal Supraventricular Tachycardias

23. Trohman RG. Supraventricular tachycardia: implications for the internist. Crit Care Med 2000; 28(Suppl):N129–N135.

24. Lim SH, Anantharaman V, Teo WS, et al. Comparison of treatment of supraventricular tachycardia by Valsalva maneuver and carotid sinus massage. Ann Emerg Med 1998; 31:30–35.

25. Rankin AC, Brooks R, Ruskin JM, McGovern BA. Adenosine and the treatment of supraventricular tachycardia. Am J Med 1992; 92:655–664.

26. Chronister C. Clinical management of supraventricular tachycardia with adenosine. Am J Crit Care 1993; 2:41–47.

27. McCollam PL, Uber W, Van Bakel AB. Adenosine-related ventricular asystole. Ann Intern Med 1993; 118:315–316.

28. Cushley MJ, Tattersfield AE, Holgate ST. Adenosine-induced bronchoconstriction in asthma. Am Rev Respir Dis 1984; 129:380–384.

29. Burki NK, Alam M, Lee L-Y. The pulmonary effects of intravenous adenosine in asthmatic subjects. Respir Res 2006; 7:139-146.

Ventricular Tachycardia

30. Gupta AK, Thakur RK. Wide QRS complex tachycardias. Med Clin N Am 2001; 85:245–266.

31. Akhtar M, Shenasa M, Jazayeri M, et al. Wide QRS complex tachycardia. Ann Intern Med 1988; 109:905–912.

32. Vukmir RB. Torsades de pointes: a review. Am J Emerg Med 1991; 9:250–262.

33. Gupta A, Lawrence AT, Krishnan K, et al. Current concepts in the mechanism and management of drug-induced QT prolongation and torsade de pointes. Am Heart J 2007; 153:891–899.

34. Sadanaga T, Sadanaga F, Yoo H, et al. An evaluation of ECG leads used to assess QT prolongation. Cardiology 2006; 105:149–154.

35. Al-Khatib SM, LaPointe NM, Kramer JM, Califf RM. What clinicians should know about the QT interval. JAMA 2003; 289:2120–2127.

Chapter 16

ACUTE CORONARY SYNDROMES

*The study of the causes of things must be preceded
by the study of things caused.*

John Hughlings Jackson
(1835–1911)

The dominance of coronary artery disease in the Western world is highlighted by a recent claim that fatal coronary events occur once every minute in the United States (1). Despite this dismal estimate, appropriate early intervention in patients with acute myocardial infarction can save lives. This survival benefit, however, is time-dependent, and steadily declines in the hours that follow the first signs of ischemic injury. This is the famous *time is muscle* axiom that drives the early management of acute myocardial infarction.

This chapter describes the early interventions that provide a clinical benefit in acute myocardial infarction, using the recommendations in the clinical practice guidelines listed at the end of the chapter (2–8).

CORONARY THROMBOSIS

Ischemic myocardial injury is the result of an occlusive thrombus in one or more coronary arteries. The trigger for thrombus formation is rupture of an atherosclerotic plaque (9), which releases thrombogenic lipids and activates platelets and clotting factors (see Figure 16.1). Plaque disruption may be the result of liquefaction caused by local inflammation (10). Hydraulic stress may also play a role, because ruptured plaques are typically located at branch points in the coronary circulation (11).

Clinical Syndromes

Coronary artery thrombosis is responsible for three clinical conditions: ST-segment elevation myocardial infarction (STEMI), non-ST-segment elevation myocardial infarction (NSTEMI), and unstable angina (UA). The first

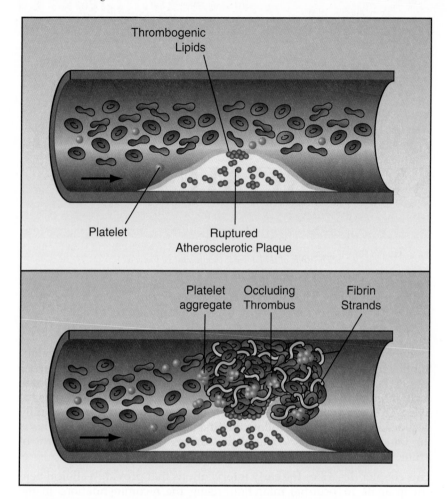

FIGURE 16.1 Illustration showing the pathogenesis of acute coronary syndromes. Rupture of an atherosclerotic plaque leads to activation of platelets and clotting factors (upper panel), and results in the formation of an occlusive thrombus (lower panel).

condition (STEMI) is the result of complete thrombotic occlusion of the involved artery, while the other two conditions (NSTEMI and UA) are the result of either partial thrombotic occlusion or transient complete occlusion with spontaneous revascularization (2–6). These 3 clinical conditions are called *acute coronary syndromes* (ACS).

Thrombocentric Management

The discovery that coronary thrombosis is the culprit in acute coronary syndromes has resulted in a number of therapeutic measures aimed at alleviating the thrombotic obstruction and preventing recurrences. These measures include the following:

1. Therapy with fibrinolytic drugs to promote clot dissolution.

2. Balloon catheter angioplasty to restore patency in obstructed coronary arteries, and vascular stenting to maintain patency.

3. Antiplatelet therapy (with aspirin, clopidogrel, and glycoprotein IIb/IIIa inhibitors) and anticoagulation therapy (with heparin) to prevent reocclusion in infarct-related arteries after flow is restored by thrombolysis or angioplasty.

Each of these measures is described in this chapter, along with other measures designed to prevent unwanted cardiac stimulation in the setting of compromised coronary blood flow.

ROUTINE MEASURES

The following measures are used when ACS is first suspected, often before the diagnostic evaluation is completed. Some of these interventions, which are summarized in Table 16.1, are used in the pre-hospital setting.

Table 16.1	Routine Measures in Acute Coronary Syndromes	
Drug	**Dosing Regimen and Comments**	
Oxygen	Dosing:	O_2 by nasal prongs or face mask to maintain $SaO_2 \geq 94\%$
	Comment:	O_2 therapy should be used cautiously because it promotes coronary vasoconstriction and generates toxic O_2 metabolites.
Nitroglycerin	Dosing:	For chest pain, 0.4 mg SL or by mouth spray, and repeat every 5 min x 2 if needed. For recurrent pain, CHF, or high BP, infuse at 5 µg/min and increase by 5–10 µg/min every 5 min to desired effect or to dose rate of 200 µg/min.
	Comment:	Avoid in patients with RV infarction and for 24 hr following R_x for erectile dysfunction.
Morphine	Dosing:	2–4 mg IV with increments of 2–8 mg IV every 5–15 min as needed.
	Comment:	Morphine-induced respiratory depression is uncommon in acute coronary syndromes.
Aspirin	Dosing:	162–325 mg (chewable form) initially, then 75–162 mg (enteric-coated tablets) daily.
	Comment:	Initial dose should be chewed to enhance buccal absorption.
β-Blockers	Dosing:	*Atenolol:* 10 mg IV, then 100 mg PO daily, or *Metoprolol:* 5 mg IV every 5 min for 3 doses, then 50 mg PO q 6 h for 48 hr, then 100 mg PO BID.
	Comment:	Do NOT use in cocaine-induced chest pain or MI.

Dosing regimens from the clinical practice guidelines in References 2, 3, and 5.

Oxygen Therapy

Providing supplemental O_2 has been a standard practice in patients with ACS (3,5), even when arterial oxygenation is normal. This practice has been questioned in recent years (12) because *oxygen promotes coronary vasoconstriction* (oxygen is a vasoconstrictor in all organs except the lungs, where it acts as a vasodilator), and because oxygen is the source of *toxic oxygen metabolites* (see Figure 14.1), which *have been implicated in reperfusion injury* (13). The deleterious effects of oxygen are emphasized in a recent study showing an increased risk of unfavorable outcomes associated with O_2 therapy in acute MI (14).

Concern about the potential for harm from unregulated O_2 breathing is evident in the most recent guidelines on acute coronary syndromes from the American Heart Association (2), which recommends supplemental O_2 only when the arterial O_2 saturation (SaO_2) falls below 94% (2). This is higher than the standard threshold for O_2 breathing ($SaO_2 < 90\%$), but it is still a significant step in the realization that oxygen can be a toxic gas.

Relieving Chest Pain

Relieving chest pain not only promotes a sense of well-being, it also helps to alleviate unwanted cardiac stimulation from anxiety-induced adrenergic hyperactivity.

Nitroglycerin

Nitroglycerin (0.4 mg) is given as a sublingual tablet or aerosol spray to relieve chest pain, and a total of 3 doses can be given in 5-minute intervals if necessary. (The mechanism of pain relief with nitroglycerin is unclear. It has been attributed to the coronary vasodilator effects of nitroglycerin, but other coronary vasodilators, such as, nitroprusside, do not relieve ischemic chest pain.) If the pain subsides, an intravenous infusion of nitroglycerin can be started for continued pain relief using the dosing regimen in Table 16.1. Intravenous nitroglycerin can also be used as a systemic vasodilator when ACS is accompanied by hypertension or decompensated heart failure (2). Chest pain that is not relieved by nitroglycerin should prompt the immediate administration of morphine.

CAVEATS: Nitroglycerin is not advised when right ventricular infarction is suspected (because the venodilator effects of nitroglycerin are counterproductive in this condition), and in patients who have taken a phosphodiesterase inhibitor for erectile dysfunction within the past 24 hours (because of the risk of hypotension) (3,5,8).

Morphine

Morphine is the drug of choice for chest pain that is refractory to nitroglycerin. The initial dose is 2 to 4 mg by slow intravenous push, and this can be followed by repeat doses of 2 to 8 mg every 5 or 10 minutes if needed (3).

Morphine administration is often followed by a modest decrease in heart rate and blood pressure, which is an expression of the decreased adrenergic system activity that accompanies pain relief. A drop in blood pressure to hypotensive levels often indicates hypovolemia, and can be corrected with fluid challenges (5). Morphine occasionally produces bradycardia and hypotension (vagomimetic effect), which can be managed with atropine (0.5–1.5 mg IV) if necessary (3). Morphine-induced respiratory depression is uncommon in ACS (3,5).

Aspirin

Aspirin is a well-known antiplatelet agent that produces an irreversible inhibition of platelet aggregation by inhibiting thromboxane production (15). When started within 24 hours of symptom onset in ACS, aspirin has been shown to reduce the mortality rate (absolute decrease is 2 to 3%) and the rate of re-infarction (16,17). As a result, aspirin is recommended for all patients with suspected ACS or a history of ACS (2–6).

In patients who are not taking aspirin regularly, the first dose of aspirin should be given as soon as possible after ACS is suspected. The initial dose is 162–325 mg, which should be given as chewable aspirin to enhance buccal absorption. This is followed by a daily aspirin dose of 75–162 mg, given as enteric-coated tablets. For patients with an aspirin allergy, clopidogrel (Plavix) is a suitable alternative (2–6). The dosing regimens for clopidogrel are presented later in the chapter.

β-Receptor Antagonists

The benefit of β-receptor antagonists in ACS is based on their ability to reduce cardiac work and decrease myocardial energy requirements. Early institution of beta-blocker therapy is recommended for all patients with ACS who do not have a contraindication to β-receptor blockade (2,3,5,7,8). These contraindications include high-grade AV block, systolic heart failure, hypotension, and reactive airway disease. In addition, β-receptor antagonists should not be used for cocaine-induced chest pain or myocardial infarction because there is a risk of aggravated coronary vasospasm from unopposed α-adrenergic receptor activity (3).

Oral β-blocker therapy is suitable for most cases of ACS, while intravenous therapy is reserved for patients with persistent chest pain, tachycardia, and hypertension (2,3,7). The β-blockers used most often in clinical trials of ACS are atenolol (Tenormin) and metoprolol (Lopressor), and the dosing regimens for these drugs is shown in Table 16.1.

REPERFUSION THERAPY

The principal determinant of outcomes in acute coronary syndromes is the ability to restore patency in occluded coronary arteries using *thrombolytic therapy* or *percutaneous coronary intervention* (PCI), which includes coronary angioplasty and stent placement, when indicated.

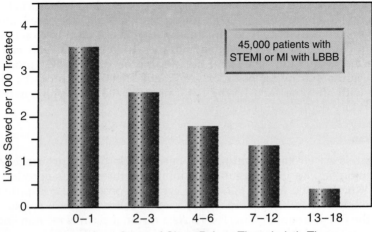

FIGURE 16.2 The survival benefit of thrombolytic therapy in relation to the time elapsed from the onset of chest pain to the start of therapy. STEMI = ST-segment elevation myocardial infarction, LBB = left bundle branch block. Data from Reference 19.

Thrombolytic Therapy

The evaluation of drugs that stimulate fibrinolysis began immediately after the discovery (in 1980) that transmural myocardial infarction was the result of occlusive coronary thrombosis. In 1986, the first clinical trial of thrombolytic therapy was published, and showed a time-dependent survival benefit in patients with ST-elevation MI (STEMI) (18).

Summary of Benefits

The following statements summarize the clinical experience with thrombolytic therapy in acute coronary syndromes.

1. Thrombolytic therapy provides a survival benefit in the following conditions (2,3,8):

   a. Acute MI associated with ST-segment elevation of at least 0.1 mV or 1 mm in two contiguous leads (STEMI).

   b. Acute MI associated with a new left bundle branch block.

   c. Acute, posterior-wall MI, which is characterized by ST-depression in the anterior precordial leads and ST-elevation in extreme lateral precordial leads V7–V9 (20).

3. The *survival benefit* of thrombolytic therapy is time-dependent; i.e., it is greatest in the first few hours after the onset of chest pain, and is *lost if more than 12 hours have elapsed from the onset of chest pain* (2,3,8,19). This is demonstrated in Figure 16.2. Note the steady decline in survival benefit over the first 12 hours after the onset of chest pain. This data highlights the most important feature of reperfusion therapy: i.e., *time lost is lives lost.*

4. To ensure optimal benefit from thrombolytic therapy, the American Heart Association recommends that *thrombolytic therapy should be started within 30 minutes after the initial presentation* (2,3). Since most presentations occur in the emergency department, this is known as the *door-to-needle time.*

5. In addition to time constraints, the use of thrombolytic therapy is restricted by a number of contraindications, which are listed in Table 16.2.

Table 16.2	Contraindications to Thrombolytic Therapy	
Absolute Contraindications	**Relative Contraindications**	
Active bleeding other than menses	Systolic BP >180 mm Hg or diastolic BP >110 mm Hg	
Malignant intracranial neoplasm (primary or metastatic)	Active bleeding in past 4 weeks	
Cardiovascular anomaly (e.g. AV malformation)	Noncompressible vascular punctures	
	Major surgery in past 3 weeks	
Suspected aortic dissection	Traumatic or prolonged (>10 min) CPR	
Ischemic stroke within 3 months (but not within 3 hrs)	Ischemic stroke over 3 months ago	
	Dementia	
Prior history of intracranial hemorrhage	Active peptic ulcer disease	
	Pregnancy	
Significant closed-head or facial trauma in past 3 months	Ongoing therapy with warfarin	

From Reference 2.

Thrombolytic Agents

Thrombolytic agents act by converting plasminogen to plasmin, which then breaks fibrin strands into smaller subunits. The fibrinolytic drugs used in ACS are shown in Table 16.3 These drugs act primarily on the plasminogen that is bound to fibrin (clot-specific fibrinolysis), and this limits the extent of systemic fibrinolysis and thereby limits the risk of unwanted hemorrhage.

ALTEPLASE (Activase) is a recombinant tissue plasminogen activator (tPA) that was popularized in 1993 by the GUSTO trial (21), which showed superior clinical outcomes with alteplase compared to streptokinase (the original fibrinolytic agent used in ACS). Alteplase is given as a fixed IV bolus dose followed by a 90-minute weight-based drug infusion (see Table 16.3). It has largely been replaced by the more rapid-acting fibrinolyitc agents, but there is no evidence of inferior clinical outcomes with alteplase compared to the more rapidly-acting fibrinolyitc agents (see next).

RETEPLASE (Retavase) is a recombinant variant of tPA that is given as an IV bolus (10 Units), which is repeated in 30 minutes. It produces more rapid clot lysis than alteplase (22), but clinical trials have shown no survival advantage with reteplase when compared to alteplase (23). Reteplase is the only fibrinolytic agent that is given in fixed (not weight-based) doses, and this has created some popularity for the drug.

TENECTEPLASE (TNK-ase) is another variant of tPA that is given as a single IV bolus using a weight-based dosing regimen (see Table 16.3). It produces more rapid clot lysis than reteplase (24), but clinical trials have shown no survival advantage with tenecteplase compared to alteplase (25).

Table 16.3	Thrombolytic Agents and Dosing Regimens for MI	
Drug	**Dosing Regimen and Comments**	
Alteplase	Dosing:	15 mg IV bolus, then 0.75 mg/kg (not to exceed 50 mg) over 30 min, then 0.5 mg/kg (not to exceed 35 mg) over 60 min. Maximum dose is 100 mg over 90 min.
	Comment:	The original (and slowest-acting) clot-specific thrombolytic agent.
Reteplase	Dosing:	10 Units as IV bolus and repeat in 30 min.
	Comment:	Produces more rapid clot lysis than alteplase, but clinical outcomes are no different.
Tenecteplase	Dosing:	Given as a single IV bolus using weight-based dosing: 30 mg for < 60 kg, 35 mg for 60–69 kg, 45 mg for 80–89 kg, and 50 mg for ≥ 90 kg.
	Comment:	Produces the most rapid clot lysis, but clinical outcomes are not superior to other thrombolytic agents.

Dosing regimens are manufacturer's recommendations.

Major Bleeding

Clot-specific fibrinolytic agents produce some degree of systemic fibrinolysis, which can deplete circulating fibrinogen and create an increased risk of bleeding. The risk of major bleeding such as intracerebral hemorrhage (0.5–1%) and extracranial bleeding that requires blood transfusions (5–15%) is equivalent with alteplase, reteplase, and tenecteplase (24,26). Major bleeding from thrombolysis can be treated with cryoprecipitate (10 to 15 bags) followed by fresh frozen plasma (up to 6 units) if necessary (the goal is a serum fibrinogen ≥1 mg/ml). The use of antifibrinolytic agents such as epsilon-aminocaproic acid (5 grams IV over 15–30 min) is discouraged because of the risk for thrombosis (26).

Summary

Despite differences in pharmacokinetic properties, the fibrinolytic agents in Table 16.3 are equivalent in terms of survival benefit and risk of bleeding. The clinical experience with thrombolytic therapy then leads to the following summation: *the important issue in thrombolytic therapy is not which agent to use, but how quickly to use it.*

Percutaneous Coronary Intervention

In 1977, a Swiss cardiologist named Andreas Gruntzig used a homemade balloon-tipped catheter to reopen an occluded left main coronary artery. This "Gruntzig procedure" (coronary angioplasty) was promptly sanctioned by the American Heart Association, and was introduced in the 1980s as an alternative to thrombolytic therapy. (Unfortunately, Dr. Gruntzig died in a plane crash in 1985, just as his procedure was gaining widespread use.) In the late 1990s, the placement of stents was introduced to maintain vascular patency after coronary angioplasty. The combination of coronary arteriography, angioplasty, and stent placement is known as *percutaneous coronary intervention* (PCI).

PCI in STEMI

Several clinical trials have shown that *PCI is superior to thrombolytic therapy* for restoring flow in occluded arteries and reducing the incidence of unfavorable outcomes (1–3, 27–29). This is shown in Figure 16.3. The bar graphs on the left (depicting vascular events) show superior results with PCI for restoring normal flow in infarct-related arteries and preventing reocclusion. The bar graphs on the right (depicting clinical outcomes) show superior results with PCI for reducing the mortality rate and the reinfarction rate.

TIMING: The survival benefit of PCI is time-dependent, similar to thrombolytic therapy (see Figure 16.2). This is demonstrated in Figure 16.4,

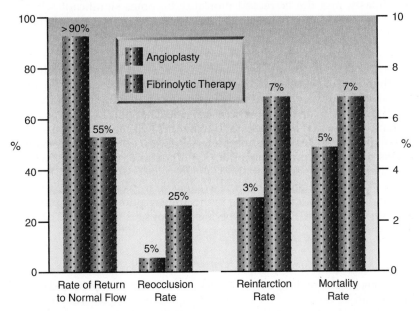

FIGURE 16.3 Comparative effects of coronary angioplasty and thrombolytic therapy on vascular events (graph on the left) and clinical outcomes (graph on the right) in patients with ST-elevation myocardial infarction. Data from references 27–29.

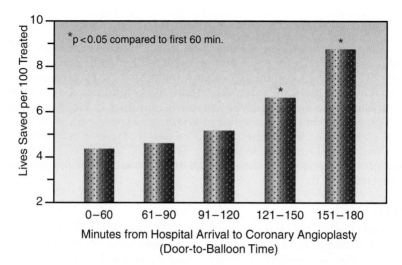

FIGURE 16.4 Mortality rate in relation to the time elapsed from hospital arrival to coronary angioplasty (door-to-balloon time). Asterisk indicates a significant difference compared to the initial time period (0–60 min). Adapted from data in Reference 30.

which shows the mortality rate (at 30 days) in relation to the time elapsed from hospital arrival to coronary angioplasty (the "door-to-balloon" time) (30). The mortality rate rises steadily with increasing delays to angioplasty, and the increased mortality becomes significant when the delay exceeds 2 hours. This is the basis for the recommendation that *PCI should be performed within 90 minutes after hospital arrival* (2–4).

INTERHOSPITAL TRANSFER: The major limitation of PCI is availability; i.e., less than 25% of hospitals in the United States can provide PCI on a timely basis. One solution for this problem is a facilitated transfer from "have-not" hospitals to hospitals that can provide emergent PCI. Clinical studies have shown that interhospital transfer for PCI can result in a survival benefit if the transfer can be completed within 1–2 hours of the patient's arrival at the "have not" hospital (31). Therefore, for patients who are candidates for reperfusion therapy, *interhospital transfer for PCI is encouraged if the total door-to-balloon time, including the transfer time, does not exceed 90 minutes* (2–4). Strict adherence to this time requirement is not inviolate because delayed PCI may still be a better option than no PCI (e.g., in patients with heart failure or hemodynamic instability).

Approach to Reperfusion Therapy in STEMI

Decisions regarding immediate reperfusion therapy in suspected cases of STEMI can be organized as a series of four questions, as shown in Table 16.4. The first two questions determine if the patient is a candidate for early reperfusion therapy, and the last two questions determine the type of reperfusion therapy that is most appropriate (i.e., PCI or thrombolytic therapy).

Other Indications for PCI

PCI is also advantageous in the following situations:

1. For patients with non-ST elevation MI (NSTEMI) who have risk factors for a poor outcome (e.g., unrelenting chest pain, heart failure, or hemodynamic instability) (4–6).

2. When thrombolytic therapy fails.

Table 16.4	Approach to Reperfusion Therapy in ST-Elevation MI

When an acute coronary syndrome is first suspected, ask yourself the following questions *immediately:*

1. Does the ECG show ST elevation (≥ 0.1 mV) in at least 2 contiguous leads, or a new left bundle branch block?

If the answer is YES, go to the next question

2. Did the chest pain begin less than 12 hours ago?

If the answer is YES, go to the next question

3. Can PCI be performed in a timely manner (here or elsewhere?)

If the answer is YES, proceed to PCI
If the answer is NO, go to the next question

4. Does the patient have any reason to withhold lytic therapy?

If the answer is NO, begin thrombolytic therapy

ADJUNCTIVE ANTITHROMBOTIC THERAPY

Antithrombotic therapy with heparin and antiplatelet agents other than aspirin have proven benefits in ACS when used with or without reperfusion therapy.

Heparin

Anticoagulation with heparin is beneficial in most patients with ACS. It is particularly advantageous after thrombolytic therapy, to counteract the prothrombotic actions of thrombin released by clot dissolution. The following is a summary of the recommendations for unfractionated heparin (UFH) and low-molecular-weight heparin (LMWH) in acute coronary syndromes. (See Chapter 6 for a description of the differences between UFH and LMWH.)

1. Short-term therapy with UFH is preferred for patients who receive reperfusion therapy with fibrinolytic agents or PCI. The recommended dosing regimens are as follows:

   a. *UFH with PCI:* Use intravenous (IV) bolus doses of 70–100 Units/kg to maintain an activated clotting time of 250–350 seconds during the procedure (3).

Reduce dose to 50–70 Units/kg if UFH is combined with glycoprotein receptor antagonists (see later) (7).

b. *UFH with Thrombolytic Therapy:* Start with an IV bolus dose of 60 Units/kg, and follow with an infusion of 12 Units/kg/hr for at least 48 hours (3). Adjust dosing to maintain an activated PTT (aPTT) at 1.5–2 times control. For a body weight > 70 kg, the maximum doses are 4,000 Units (IV bolus) and 1,000 Units hourly (3).

2. LMWH is preferred for patients who do not receive reperfusion therapy. The dosing regimen for a popular LMWH (enoxaparin) is as follows:

   a. *Enoxaparin in ACS:* 30 mg IV bolus, then 1 mg/kg by subcutaneous injection every 12 hours for the duration of hospitalization (7).

   b. *Enoxaparin in Renal Insufficiency:* When creatinine clearance < 30 mL/min, reduce the daily dose by 50% (e.g., 1 mg/kg every 24 hours) (7).

3. For patients with a history of heparin-induced thrombocytopenia (see Chapter 19), the following alternative regimens are available:

   a. For PCI: *Bivalirudin* (a direct thrombin inhibitor), 0.7 mg/kg as IV bolus, followed by an infusion of 1.75 mg/kg/hr (7). Discontinue after successful PCI.

   b. For Thrombolytic Therapy or No Reperfusion Therapy: *Fondaparinux* (factor Xa inhibitor), 2.5 mg by subcutaneous injection daily (7,8).

Thienopyridines

The thienopyridines (clopidogrel, ticlodipine, tigrecalor, prasugrel) are antiplatelet agents that irreversibly block surface receptors involved in ADP-induced platelet aggregation (32). This mechanism of action differs from that of aspirin, so these drugs can be used in addition to aspirin or as an alternative to aspirin. The thienopyridines are prodrugs that require activation in the liver, and are ineffective in patients with liver failure.

Clopidogrel

Clopidogrel (Plavix) is the most popular thienopyridine, and has a proven survival benefit when combined with aspirin in both STEMI and NSTEMI patients, with or without reperfusion therapy (1–6,32,33). Clopidogrel is also recommended as a replacement for aspirin in aspirin-allergic patients (3,5). The dosing recommendations for clopidogrel are as follows:

1. *Clopidogrel without PCI:* Start with an oral loading dose of 300 mg, given as soon as possible, and follow with an oral maintenance dose of 75 mg daily. The same dose is used when clopidogrel is added to aspirin or used as a replacement for aspirin.

2. *Clopidogrel with PCI:* Use an oral loading dose of 600 mg prior to PCI (4,6), and follow with the standard maintenance dose of 75 mg daily.

3. *Clopidogrel and Surgery:* Clopidogrel must be discontinued at least 5 days before major surgery is performed (4,6), so it is wise to avoid the drug if emergency coronary bypass surgery is anticipated.

The activation of clopidogrel in the liver is blocked by protein pump inhibitors (5,6,32). The clinical significance of this interaction is unclear, but it seems wise to avoid proton pump inhibitors for stress ulcer prophylaxis in patients receiving clopidogrel.

Glycoprotein Receptor Antagonists

When platelets are activated, specialized glycoprotein receptors on the platelet surface (named IIb and IIIa) change their configuration and begin to bind fibrinogen. This allows fibrinogen molecules to form bridges between adjacent platelets, which promotes platelet aggregation. Glycoprotein receptor antagonists (also called *IIb/IIIa inhibitors*) block fibrinogen binding to activated platelets and inhibit platelet aggregation. These drugs are the most potent antiplatelet agents available, and are sometimes referred to as the *superaspirins*.

Table 16.5	Antiplatelet Therapy with Glycoprotein Receptor Antagonists
Drug	**Dosing Regimen**
Abciximab	Dosing: Load with 0.25 mg as IV bolus, then infuse at 0.125 µg/kg/min (maximum rate is 10 µg/min) for up to 12 hr.
Eptifibatide	Dosing: Load with 180 µg/kg as IV bolus, then infuse at 2 µg/kg/min for 12–18 hr. For PCI in STEMI, repeat bolus dose in 10 min if renal function is normal. Reduce infusion rate by 50% when creatinine clearance is <50 mL/min.
Tirofiban	Dosing: Load with 25 µg/kg as IV bolus, then infuse at 0.1 µg/kg/min for 12–24 hr. Reduce infusion rate by 50% when creatinine clearance is <30 mL/min.

From the clinical practice guidelines in Reference 6.

Drugs and Dosing Regimens

The IIb/IIIa inhibitors available for clinical use include *abciximab* (ReoPro), *eptifibatide* (Integrilin), and *tirofiban* (Aggrastat). All three are given by intravenous infusion using the dosing regimens in Table 16.5. These drugs are used in high-risk patients who receive emergent PCI, and are given just before or at the start of the procedure (6,32). They are managed primarily by invasive cardiologists, and are described only briefly here.

Abciximab is (an almost unpronounceable name for) a monoclonal antibody that is the most potent, most expensive, and longest-acting IIb/IIa inhibitor. After discontinuing abciximab, bleeding times can take 12 hours to normalize (32). Eptifibatide (a synthetic peptide) and tirofiban (a tyrosine derivative) are short-acting agents that are cleared by the kidneys. After discontinuing these drugs, bleeding times return to normal in 15 minutes for eptifibatide and 4 hours for tirofiban (32). Dose adjustments are recommended for both drugs in renal insufficiency, as indicated in Table 16.5.

COMPLICATIONS

The appearance of decompensated heart failure and cardiogenic shock in the first few days after an acute MI is an ominous sign, and usually indicates a catastrophic structural defect like acute mitral regurgitation, or extensive muscle injury resulting in cardiac pump failure. Fatal outcomes are common in these conditions despite timely interventions.

Structural Defects

The following defects are usually the result of transmural (ST-elevation) infarctions.

Acute Mitral Regurgitation

Acute mitral regurgitation is the result of papillary muscle rupture, and presents with the sudden onset of pulmonary edema and the characteristic holosystolic murmur radiating to the axilla. The pulmonary artery occlusion pressure should show prominent V waves, but this can be a non-specific finding. Diagnosis is by echocardiography, and arterial vasodilators (e.g., hydralazine) are used to relieve pulmonary edema pending surgery. Mortality is 70% without surgery and 40% with surgery (34).

Rupture of Ventricular Septum

Rupture of the septum separating the two ventricles can occur anytime in the first 5 days after an acute MI, and the diagnosis can be elusive without cardiac ultrasound. There is a step-up in O_2 saturation from right atrial to pulmonary artery blood, but this is rarely measured. Initial management involves vasodilator (e.g., nitroglycerin) infusions and the intra-aortic balloon pump if needed. Mortality is 90% without surgery and 20% to 50% with surgery (3).

Rupture of Ventricular Wall

Ventricular free wall rupture occurs in up to 6% of cases of STEMI, and is more common with anterior MI, fibrinolytic or steroid therapy, and advanced age (3). The first signs of trouble are usually return of chest pains and new ST-segment abnormalities on the ECG. Accumulation of blood in the pericardium often leads to rapid deterioration and cardiovascular collapse from pericardial tamponade. Diagnosis is made by cardiac ultrasound (if time permits), and prompt pericardiocentesis combined with aggressive volume resuscitation is required for hemodynamic support. Immediate surgery is the only course of action, but fewer than half of the patients survive despite surgery (3).

Cardiac Pump Failure

About 10% of cases of ST-elevation MI (STEMI) result in enough muscle damage to produce decompensated heart failure and cardiogenic shock (35). Management involves hemodynamic support followed by coronary angioplasty or coronary bypass surgery. Unfortunately, the mortality rate in cardiogenic shock can be as high as 80% (36), but hospitals that provide timely PCI can expect 10% fewer deaths (36).

Hemodynamic Support

Hemodynamic support for acute heart failure and cardiogenic shock is described in Chapter 13. When these conditions are the result of coronary insufficiency, hemodynamic support should be designed to augment cardiac output without increasing cardiac work and myocardial oxygen consumption. Table 16.6 shows the effects of hemodynamic support measures on the determinants of myocardial O_2 consumption (preload, contractility, afterload, and heart rate) for acute heart failure and cardiogenic shock. As judged by the net effect on myocardial O_2 consumption, vasodilator therapy is the best choice for acute heart failure, and the intra-aortic balloon pump is the best choice for cardiogenic shock.

Reperfusion

Hemodynamic support is, of course, a bridge to interventions that re-establish flow in the infarct-related blood vessels. The ACC/AHA guidelines (3) recommend immediate PCI when cardiogenic shock appears within 36 hours of STEMI and when the angioplasty can be performed within 18 hours of the onset of shock. Coronary artery bypass surgery is considered if the cardiac catheterization reveals multivessel disease that is not amenable to angioplasty.

Table 16.6	Hemodynamic Support and Myocardial O_2 Consumption			
Parameter	**Heart Failure**		**Cardiogenic Shock**	
	Vasodilators	**Dobutamine**	**IABP**	**Dopamine**
Preload	↓	↓	↓	↑
Contractility	—	↑↑	—	↑↑
Afterload	↓↓	↓	↓	↑
Heart Rate	—	↑↑	—	↑↑
Net effect on myocardial VO_2	↓↓↓	↑↑	↓↓	↑↑↑↑↑↑

IABP = intra-aortic balloon pump; VO_2 = oxygen consumption

ACUTE AORTIC DISSECTION

Aortic dissection involving the ascending aorta can be mistaken as ACS, and can also be a cause of ACS. However, unlike ACS, aortic dissection is a surgical emergency that is often fatal if not managed appropriately.

Pathophysiology

Aortic dissection occurs when a tear in the aortic intima allows blood to dissect between the intimal and medial layers of the aorta, creating a false lumen. This process can be the result of atherosclerotic damage in the aorta from hypertension, or accelerated degradation of the aortic wall from a genetic disorder (e.g., Marfan's syndrome). The dissection can originate in the ascending or descending aorta, and can propagate in antegrade and retrograde directions. When a dissection involves the ascending aorta, retrograde propagation can result in coronary insufficiency, aortic insufficiency, and pericardial tamponade, while antegrade propagation can result in neurologic deficits (from involvement of the aortic arch vessels) (37).

Clinical Manifestations

The most common complaint is the abrupt onset of chest pain. The pain is often sharp, and can be substernal (ascending aortic dissection) or in the back (descending aortic dissection). Most importantly, *the chest pain can subside spontaneously for hours to days (39.40), and this can be a source of missed diagnoses*. The return of the pain after a pain-free interval is often a sign of impending aortic rupture. About 5% of patients with acute aortic dissection are devoid of pain (37).

Clinical Findings

The most common clinical findings are hypertension (50% of patients) and aortic insufficiency (50% of patients) (38,39). Unequal pulses in the upper extremities (from obstruction of the left subclavian artery in the aortic arch) are found in as few as 15% of patients (39). The chest x-ray can show mediastinal widening (60% of cases) (39), but normal chest x-rays are reported in up to 20% of cases (37). The ECG can show ischemic changes (15% of cases) or evidence of MI (5% of cases), but the ECG is normal in 30% of cases (37). Because of the limited sensitivity of clinical findings, additional imaging studies are required for the diagnosis.

Diagnostic Tests

The diagnosis of aortic dissection requires one of four imaging modalities (40): magnetic resonance imaging (MRI) (sensitivity and specificity 98%), transesophageal echocardiography (sensitivity 98%, specificity 77%), contrast-enhanced computed tomography (sensitivity 94%, specificity 87%), and aortography (sensitivity 88%, specificity 94%). As indicated *MRI is the most sensitive and specific imaging modality for the diagnosis aortic dissection*. However, the immediate availability of MRI is limited in some hospitals, and CT angiography is often the diagnostic test when aortic dissection is suspected.

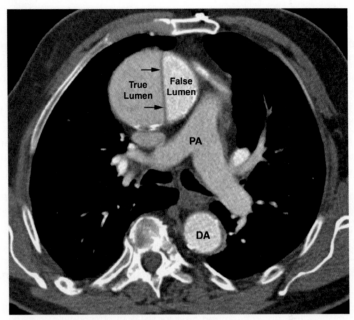

FIGURE 16.5 Contrast-enhanced CT image showing an aortic dissection involving the ascending aorta. The characteristic finding is the intimal flap that separates the true and false lumens (indicated by the small arrows). PA = main pulmonary artery, DA = descending aorta.

The CT image in Figure 16.5 shows an aortic dissection involving the ascending aorta. The small arrows point to the intimal flap that separates the dissecting blood in the wall of the aorta (false lumen) from blood in the aortic lumen (true lumen). The presence of this flap distinguishes an aortic dissection from a saccular aneurysm of the aorta.

Management

There are two essential management goals in aortic dissection: i.e., control of hypertension (to prevent aortic rupture) and prompt surgical correction.

Antihypertensive Therapy

There is one major caveat for blood pressure control in aortic dissection: *the reduction in blood pressure should not be accompanied by an increase in cardiac stroke output* because increased flow in the aorta can promote further dissection. As a result, *β-receptor antagonists are preferred* for blood pressure control in aortic dissection because of their ability to reduce the force of ventricular contraction (negative inotropic effect). The drug regimens used for blood pressure control in aortic dissection are presented in Table 16.7, and outlined below.

1. The β-blocker that is most favored is *esmolol* (Brevibloc), which has a short duration of action (9 minutes) and can be rapidly titrated to achieve the desired end-point (i.e., systolic blood pressure of 120 mm Hg and a heart rate of 60 bpm).

2. If the β-blocker does not achieve the desired effect, a vasodilator like *nitroprusside* can be added. Vasodilators should, however, never be used as monotherapy because they will increase cardiac output and increase the risk of progressive aortic dissection.

3. An alternative to dual therapy with a β-blocker and a vasodilator is the drug *labetalol*, which is a combined α-, β-receptor antagonist that can be used as monotherapy for blood pressure control in aortic dissection.

With medical management alone, the mortality in acute aortic dissection increases 1–2% per hour after the onset of symptoms (37). Surgical repair reduces the mortality rate to 10% at 24 hours and 12% at 48 hours (37).

Table 16.7	Antihypertensive Therapy in Acute Aortic Dissection	
Drug	**Dosing Regimen and Comments**	
Esmolol	Dosing:	500 μkg IV bolus, then infuse at 50 μg/kg/min. Increase rate by 25 μg/kg/min every 5 min until systolic BP 120 mm Hg or heart rate 60 bpm. Maximum dose is 200 μg/kg/min.
	Comment:	An ultra rapid-acting β-blocker, which is the preferred drug for BP control in aortic dissection.
Nitroprusside	Dosing:	Start infusion at 0.2 μg/kg/min and titrate to achieve a systolic BP of 120 mm Hg. (See Table 13.3 for further dosing recommendations.)
	Comment:	Use only in combination with β-blockers. Do not use in renal failure (risk of thiocyanate toxicity).
Labetalol	Dosing:	20 mg IV over 2 min, then give 20–40 mg IV every 10 min if needed or infuse at 1–2 mg/min to the same endpoints as esmolol. Maximum cumulative dose is 300 mg.
	Comment:	A combined α- and β-blocker that can be used as monotherapy in aortic dissection.

Dosing regimens are manufacturer's recommendations.

A FINAL WORD

Blood Clots vs. O_2 Transport

The discovery that acute myocardial infarctions are caused by blood clots that obstruct a coronary artery is at odds with the traditional teaching that global decreases in myocardial oxygen delivery (e.g., from anemia and hypoxemia) can promote ischemic injury in patients with coronary artery disease. This teaching is responsible for the current emphasis on blood transfusions and oxygen breathing to prevent myocardial ischemia in ICU patients with coronary artery disease. However, since *blood clots cause heart attacks, not anemia or hypoxemia*, these practices are unfounded.

Ever wonder why myocardial infarction is an uncommon occurrence during progressive circulatory shock and multiorgan failure (where myocardial O_2 delivery is progressively threatened)? Now you have the answer.

REFERENCES

1. Roger V, Go AS, Lloyd-Jones D, et al. Heart disease and stroke statistics—2012 update: a report from the American Heart Association. Circulation 2012; 125:e2–e220.

Clinical Practice Guidelines

2. O'Connor RE, Brady W, Brooks SC, et al. Part 10: Acute coronary syndromes. 2010 American Heart Association Guidelines for Cardiopulmonary Resuscitation and Emergency Cardiovascular Care. Circulation 2010; 122(Suppl 3):S787–S817.

3. Antman EM, Anbe DT, Armstrong PW, et al. ACC/AHA guidelines for the management of patients with ST-elevation myocardial infarction—executive summary. Circulation 2004; 110:588–636.

4. Kushner FG, Hand M, Smith SC Jr, et al. 2009 focused updates: ACC/AHA guidelines for the management of patients with ST-elevation myocardial infarction (updating the 2004 guideline and 2007 focused update) and ACC/AHA/SCAI guidelines for percutaneous coronary intervention (updating the 2005 guideline and the 2007 focused update). J Am Coll Cardiol 2009; 54:2205–2241.

5. Andersen JL, Adams CD, Antman EM. ACC/AHA 2007 guidelines for the management of patients with unstable angina/non-ST-elevation myocardial infarction: executive summary. Circulation 2007; 116:803–877.

6. Jneid H, Anderson JL, Wright RS, et al. 2012 ACCF/AHA focused update of the guideline for the management of patients with unstable angina/non-ST-elevation myocardial infarction (updating the 2007 guideline and replacing the 2011 focused update). Circulation 2012; 212:1–36.

Reviews

7. Trost JC, Lange RA. Treatment of acute coronary syndrome: Part 1: non ST-segment acute coronary syndrome. Crit Care Med 2011; 39:2346–2353.

8. Trost JC, Lange RA. Treatment of acute coronary syndrome: Part 2: ST-segment elevation myocardial infarction. Crit Care Med 2012; 40:1939–1945.

Coronary Thrombosis

9. Davies MJ, Thomas AC. Plaque fissuring: the cause of acute myocardial infarction. Br Heart J 1985; 53:363–373.

10. Van der Wal AC, Becker AE, van der Loos CM, Das PK. Site of intimal rupture or erosion of thrombosed coronary atherosclerotic plaques is characterized by an inflammatory process irrespective of the dominant plaque morphology. Circulation 1994; 89:36–44.

11. Malek AM, Alper SL, Izumo S. Hemodynamic shear stress and its role in atherosclerosis. JAMA 1999; 282:2035–2042.

Routine Measures

12. Moradkan R, Sinoway LI. Revisiting the role of oxygen therapy in cardiac patients. J Am Coll Cardiol 2010; 56:1013–1016.

13. Bulkley GB. Reactive oxygen metabolites and reperfusion injury: aberrant triggering of reticuloendothelial function. Lancet 1994; 344:934–936.

14. Burls A, Cabello JB, Emperanza JI, et al. Oxygen therapy for acute myocardial infarction. A systematic review and meta-analysis. Emerg Med J 2011; 28:917–923.

15. Eikelboom JW, Hirsh J, Spencer FA, et al. Antiplatelet drugs. Chest 2012; 141 (Suppl): e89S–e119S.

16. ISIS-2 (Second International Study of Infarct Survival) collaborative group. Randomized trial of intravenous streptokinase, oral aspirin, both, or neither among 17,187 cases of suspected acute myocardial infarction: ISIS-2. Lancet 1988; 2:349–360.

17. Roux S, Christellar S, Ludin E. Effects of aspirin on coronary reocclusion and recurrent ischemia after thrombolysis: a meta-analysis. J Am Coll Cardiol 1992; 19:671–677.

Thrombolytic Therapy

18. Gruppo Italiano per lo Studio della Streptochinasi nell'Infarto Miocardico (GISSI). Effectiveness of intravenous thrombolytic treatment in acute myocardial infarction. Lancet 1986; 1:397–401.

19. Fibrinolytic Therapy Trialists Collaborative Group. Indications for fibrinolytic therapy in suspected acute myocardial infarction: collaborative overview of early mortality and major morbidity results from all randomized trials of more than 1000 patients. Lancet 1994; 343:311–322.

20. Boden WE, Kleiger RE, Gibson RS, et al. Electrocardiographic evolution of posterior acute myocardial infarction: importance of early precordial ST-segment depression. Am J Cardiol 1987; 59:782–787.

21. GUSTO Investigators. An international randomized trial comparing four thrombolytic strategies for acute myocardial infarction. N Engl J Med 1993; 329:673–682.

22. Smalling RW, Bode C, Kalbfleisch J, et al. More rapid, complete, and stable coronary thrombolysis with bolus administration of reteplase compared with alteplase infusion in acute myocardial infarction. Circulation 1995; 91:2725–2732.

23. GUSTO-III Investigators. An international, multicenter, randomized comparison of reteplase with alteplase for acute myocardial infarction. N Engl J Med 1997; 337:1118–1123.

24. Llevadot J, Giugliano RP, Antman EM. Bolus fibrinolytic therapy in acute myocardial infarction. JAMA 2001; 286:442–449.

25. Assessment of the Safety and Efficacy of a New Thrombolytic (ASSENT-2) Investigators. Single-bolus tenecteplase compared with front-loaded alteplase in acute myocardial infarction. Lancet 1999; 354:716–722.

26. Young GP, Hoffman JR. Thrombolytic therapy. Emerg Med Clin 1995; 13:735–759.

Percutaneous Coronary Intervention

27. The GUSTO IIb Angioplasty Substudy Investigators. A clinical trial comparing primary coronary angioplasty with tissue plasminogen activator for acute myocardial infarction. New Engl J Med 1997; 336:1621–1628.

28. Keeley EC, Boura JA, Grines CL. Primary angioplasty versus intravenous thrombolytic therapy for acute myocardial infarction: a quantitative review of 23 randomized trials. Lancet 2003; 361:13–20.

29. Stone GW, Cox D, Garcia E, et al. Normal flow (TIMI-3) before mechanical reperfusion therapy is an independent determinant of survival in acute myocardial infarction. Circulation 2001; 104:636–641.

30. Cannon CP, Gibson CM, Lambrew CT, et al. Relationship of symptom onset to balloon time and door-to-balloon time with mortality in patients undergoing angioplasty for acute myocardial infarction. JAMA 2000; 283:2941–2947.

31. Andersen HR, Nielsen TT, Rasmussen K, et al. for the DANAMI-2 Investigators. A comparison of coronary angioplasty with fibrinolytic therapy in acute myocardial infarction. New Engl J Med 2003; 349:733–742.

Adjunctive Therapies

32. Patrono C, C, Coller B, Fitzgerald G, et al. Platelet-active drugs: the relationship among dose, effectiveness, and side effects. Chest 2004; 126:234S–264S.

33. COMMIT (Clopidogrel and Metoprolol in Myocardial Infarction Trial) collaborative group. Addition of clopidogrel to aspirin in 45,852 patients with acute myocardial infarction: randomized placebo-controlled trial. Lancet 2005; 366:1607–1621.

Complications

34. Thompson CR, Buller CE, Sleeper LA, et al. Cardiogenic shock due to acute severe mitral regurgitation complicating acute myocardial infarction: a report from the SHOCK trial registry. J Am Coll Cardiol 2000; 36:1104–1109.

35. Samuels LF, Darze ES. Management of acute cardiogenic shock. Cardiol Clin 2003; 21:43–49.

36. Babaev A, Frederick PD, Pasta D, et al. Trends in the management and outcomes of patients with acute myocardial infarction complicated by cardiogenic shock. JAMA 2005; 294:448–454.

Aortic Dissection

37. Tsai TT, Nienaber CA, Eagle KA. Acute aortic syndromes. Circulation 2005; 112:3802–3813.

38. Khan IA, Nair CK. Clinical, diagnostic, and management perspectives of aortic dissection. Chest 2002; 122:311–328.

39. Knaut AL, Cleveland JC. Aortic emergencies. Emerg Med Clin N Am 2003; 21:817–845.

40. Zegel HG, Chmielewski S, Freiman DB. The imaging evaluation of thoracic aortic dissection. Appl Radiol 1995; (June):15–25.

Chapter 17

CARDIAC ARREST

When we all think alike, then no one is thinking.

Walter Lippmann
(1889–1974)

In 1960, an article was published in the *Journal of the American Medical Association* that would eventually change the way we approach the dying process. The article, titled "Closed-Chest Cardiac Massage" (1), was a report of 5 cases of cardiorespiratory arrest that were successfully managed with chest compressions, defibrillation shocks, and assisted ventilation. This report marks the birth of what is known today as *cardiopulmonary resuscitation* (CPR). In the more than 50 years since its inception, CPR has become a universally mandated practice that requires certification, and is withheld only on request. All this for an intervention that doesn't work in most cases, as demonstrated in Figure 17.1 (2,3).

This chapter describes the essential elements of resuscitation for cardiac arrest, including induced hypothermia for patients who remain comatose after successful resuscitation. The material in this chapter is drawn heavily from the most recent guidelines on CPR from the American Heart Association (4,5).

BASIC LIFE SUPPORT

The essential elements of basic life support are chest compressions, establishing a patent airway in the oropharynx, and periodic lung inflations. The original mnemonic for these elements, ABC (*A*irway, *B*reathing, and *C*irculation), has been rearranged to CAB (*C*irculation, *A*irway, *B*reathing), reflecting a recent *shift in emphasis from ventilation to chest compressions in the resuscitation effort.*

The Time Factor

One of the limiting factors in the success of CPR is the narrow time window between the cessation of blood flow and irreversible cell death. This time period can be estimated using the determinants of systemic oxygenation described in Chapter 10. The volume of O_2 in circulating blood

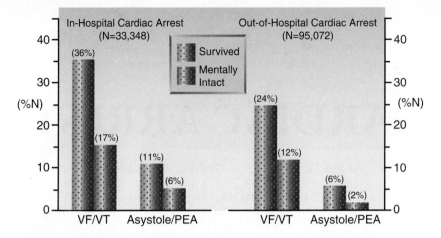

FIGURE 17.1 Rates of survival and satisfactory neurologic recovery in cardiac arrests that occur inside the hospital (graph on the left) and outside the hospital (graph on the right), grouped according to the responsible rhythm disturbance. N=number of cases included in each survey, VF=ventricular fibrillation, VT=ventricular tachycardia, PEA=pulseless electrical activity. Data from References 2 and 3.

is normally about 800 mL (see Table 10.1), which is equivalent to the total-body O_2 content (because oxygen is not stored in tissues). The whole-body O_2 consumption in adults at rest is about 250 mL/min (see Table 10.2), which will consume the total-body O_2 content of 1 liter in just 4 minutes. Therefore, *following the cessation of blood flow from a cardiac arrest, oxygen depletion and anoxic cell death can be expected after 4–5 minutes.* Therefore, CPR must be initiated within this limited time period to have any chance of success.

Chest Compressions

The most recent recommendations for chest compressions are summarized in Table 17.1 (6). The principal feature is the *emphasis on early and uninterrupted chest compressions.*

Early Chest Compressions

For the initial resuscitation, first responders should *begin with a series of 30 chest compressions, followed by 2 rescue breaths.* Chest compressions should be delivered at a rate of at least 100/min. The initial compression:ventilation ratio of 30:2 should be repeated until an advanced airway (e.g., endotracheal tube) is placed. Thereafter, lung inflations are provided at regular intervals (see later), while the chest compressions continue without interruption.

RATIONALE: The emphasis on early chest compressions is based on the observation that delays to initiating CPR have an adverse effect on survival (see later) (6). The importance of chest compressions over ventilation is demonstrated by the practice of *hands-only bystander CPR* (chest compressions only), which has the same survival benefit as standard CPR (chest compressions plus rescue breaths) in the initial resuscitation period (7). Chest compressions can produce cardiac outputs that are 25% or 30% of normal (6), but this effect diminishes rapidly with delays to initiating CPR.

Table 17.1	Recommendations for Chest Compressions
1. Chest compressions should be delivered at a rate of at least 100/min.	
2. Each chest compression should depress the mid-sternum at least 2 inches (5 cm), and the chest should be allowed to recoil completely to allow the heart to fill before the next compression.	
3. First responders should begin CPR with a series of 30 chest compressions, followed by 2 rescue breaths. This compression:ventilation ratio (30:2) is continued until an advanced airway is placed (e.g., endotracheal tube).	
4. Chest compressions should not be interrupted unless absolutely necessary (e.g., to deliver electric countershocks).	
5. When possible, those performing chest compressions should be replaced every 1–2 minutes to prevent shallow compressions from fatigue.	

From Reference 6.

Avoiding Interruptions

Avoiding unnecessary interruptions in chest compressions is also emphasized. Observational studies have shown that interruptions in chest compressions are common, and the accumulated time of these interruptions can be as much as 50% of the total resuscitation time (8). Prolonging the time without chest compressions is considered to have a negative effect on outcomes (6), although there is evidence that is contrary to this view (9).

Ventilation

Prior to endotracheal intubation, rescue breathing is provided by a face mask that is connected to a self-inflating ventilation bag (e.g., Ambu Respirator) that fills with oxygen. The bag is compressed by hand to deliver the breath, and 2 breaths are provided for every 30 chest compressions, as mentioned earlier. After an endotracheal tube is in place, *lung inflations are delivered at 6- to 8-second intervals (8 to 10 breaths/min)* using the same type of self-inflating ventilation bag that is used for the bag-mask device. The *recommended volume for each lung inflation is 6–7 mg/kg* (6), or about 500 mL in a normal sized adult.

Inflation Volumes

The volume of lung inflations is not monitored during "bagged ventilation," and large inflation volumes are considered to be common during CPR (6), resulting in troublesome hyperinflation of the lungs (10).

Adherence to the recommended inflation volumes (6–7 mL/kg) is possible if the volume capacity of the inflation bag is known. For example, if the inflation bag has a volume capacity of 1 liter, compressing the bag until it is about half full will deliver close to 500 mL for lung inflation. (The volume capacity of most adult ventilation bags is 1 to 2 liters.) An alternative method is to use one hand to compress the ventilation bag; this generates a volume of 600 to 800 mL (personal observation), and is unlikely to produce short-term hyperinflation.

Hyperventilation During CPR

Rapid lung inflation rates are common during CPR (10,11), and average rates of 30 inflations/min (3 times the recommended rate) have been reported (11). Rapid breathing is problematic because there is insufficient time for the lungs to empty, and this results in progressive hyperinflation and positive end-expiratory pressure (PEEP). This is called *dynamic hyperinflation*, and is described in more detail Chapter 27. The increased intrathoracic pressure associated with PEEP has two adverse effects. First, it reduces venous return to the heart, which limits the ability of chest compressions to augment cardiac output. Secondly, it reduces coronary perfusion pressure (10), which is an important determinant of outcome in cardiac arrest. These adverse effects provide a reason to avoid rapid rates of "bagged ventilation."

High-Quality CPR

The practices listed in Table 17.2 (which have all been described in this section) are considered essential for providing high-quality CPR (6). This table is included to provide you with a checklist for achieving the highest level of performance in CPR.

Table 17.2	The Elements of High-Quality CPR
	1. Rate of chest compressions at least 100 per minute
	2. Depth of chest compressions at least 2 inches (5 cm)
	3. Allow chest to recoil completely after each compression.
	4. Minimize interruptions in chest compressions.
	5. Avoid excessive ventilation.

From Reference 6.

ADVANCED LIFE SUPPORT

Advanced cardiovascular life support, or *ACLS*, includes a variety of interventions such as airway intubation, mechanical ventilation, defibrillation, and the administration of life-supporting drugs (12). This section will focus on defibrillation and life-supporting drugs, and will describe these interventions using a rhythm-based approach. This approach divides the management of cardiac arrest into 2 pathways: one for the management of ventricular fibrillation (VF) and pulseless ventricular tachycardia (VT), and the other for the management of pulseless electrical activity (PEA) and asystole.

VF and Pulseless VT

The outcomes in cardiac arrest are most favorable when the initial rhythm is VF or pulseless VT, as demonstrated in Figure 17.1. This is the result of prompt electrical cardioversion, as described next.

Defibrillation

Electrical cardioversion using asynchronous shocks (i.e., not timed to the QRS complex), which is called *defibrillation*, is the most effective resuscitation measure for cardiac arrest associated with VF and pulseless VT. The survival benefit from defibrillation is time-dependent; i.e., *the time elapsed from the cardiac arrest to the first electric shock is the most important factor in determining the likelihood of survival* (12–14). This is demonstrated in Figure 17.2 (14). Note that 40% of patients survived when the first shock was delivered 5 minutes after the arrest, while only 10% of patients survived if defibrillation was delayed until 20 minutes after the arrest. These results emphasize the importance of prompt defibrillation when VF or pulseless VT is first apparent in a cardiac arrest victim.

IMPULSE ENERGY: Modern defibrillators deliver current based on stored energy, and the strength of the impulses is expressed in joules (J), which is a unit of thermal energy (see Appendix 1). The appropriate strength for effective cardioversion is determined by the waveform of the energy

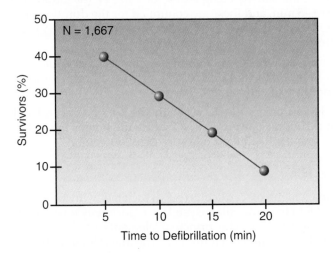

FIGURE 17.2 Survival in out-of-hospital cardiac arrests with "shockable" arrhythmias (VF/pulseless VT) in relation to the time elapsed from the onset of the cardiac arrest to the initial defibrillation attempt. N=number of cases studied. Data from Reference 14.

impulse. Biphasic waveforms (used by newer defibrillators) are effective at lower energy levels than monophasic waveforms (used by older defibrillators). *For termination of VF and pulseless VT, the effective impulse strengths are 120 to 200 J for biphasic shocks, and 360 J for monophasic shocks* (12,13). Manual defibrillators used in hospitals require the operator to select the desired energy level of the impulse, while automated external defibrillators (AEDs) use a preselected energy level.

Management Protocol

The flow diagram in Figure 17.3 is the ACLS algorithm for cardiac arrest in adults. The left half of the diagram is the management of cardiac arrest associated with VF and pulseless VT. The major features of the management are summarized below.

1. The management includes a series of 3 defibrillation attempts, if needed, and the impulse strength should be the same for each defibrillation. The recommended impulse strength is 120–200 J for biphasic waveforms, and 360 J for monophasic waveforms (12,13).

2. For each defibrillation attempt, one member of the resuscitation team charges the defibrillator and selects the impulse strength, while another member of the team provides chest compressions. The chest compressions are withheld when the defibrillation shock is delivered, and are resumed immediately thereafter. At least 2 minutes of uninterrupted chest compressions are recommended after defibrillation before the compressions are interrupted again to check the post-shock rhythm. If the rhythm is unchanged, the process is repeated twice, if necessary.

3. If a second defibrillation attempt is required, bolus injections of epinephrine are started using a dose of 1 mg IV (or intraosseous – IO) every 3–5 min, and these are continued for the duration of the resuscitation effort. A single dose of *vasopressin* (40 Units IV) can replace the first or second dose of epinephrine.

4. If a third defibrillation attempt is required, *amiodarone* is administered in an IV (or IO) dose of 300 mg, which can be followed by a second dose of 150 mg, if needed.

Failure to terminate VF or VT with the first or second defibrillation attempt carries a poor prognosis because the longer the arrhythmia persists, the less the likelihood of a successful outcome.

Asystole/PEA

The management of cardiac arrest associated with pulseless electrical activity (PEA) or ventricular asystole is notoriously unsuccessful, as indicated in Figure 17.1. The principal elements of the management are shown in the right half of Figure 17.3. The major intervention is vasopressor therapy with epinephrine using the same dosing regimen used for VF and pulseless VT. Defibrillation is not attempted unless the cardiac rhythm changes to VF or VT.

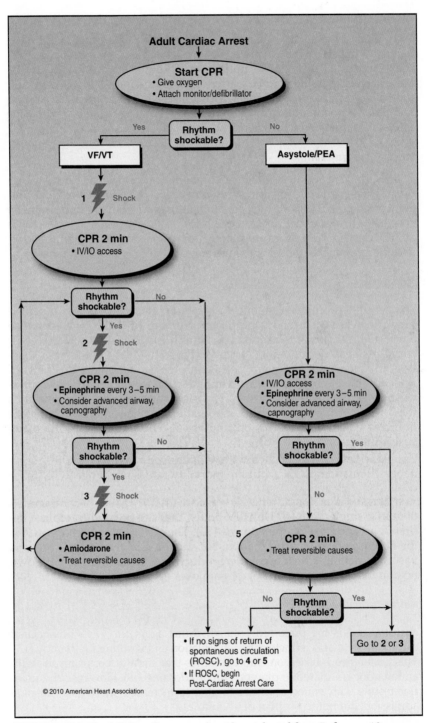

FIGURE 17.3 The ACLS cardiac arrest algorithm. Adapted from Reference 12.

Reversible Causes of PEA

PEA offers some hope because there are reversible causes, and the prominent ones are easily remembered with the letter T: i.e., Tension pneumothorax, pericardial Tamponade, pulmonary Thromboembolism, and Thrombotic occlusion of the coronary arteries. Unfortunately, there is little time for a diagnostic workup during a cardiac arrest, but pericardial tamponade and tension pneumothorax can be rapidly identified at the bedside using ultrasound imaging, which is readily available in many ICUs.

Resuscitation Drugs

The use of drugs is considered a second-line treatment in cardiac arrest because there is no documented survival benefit (12). This may not be surprising, considering that the drugs are administered at a time of cardiovascular collapse, when drug delivery to target sites is sluggish and may not occur at all. The cardiac arrest drugs are either vasopressors or antiarrhythmic agents, and the recommended dosing regimen for each drug is shown in Table 17.3.

Vasopressors

EPINEPHRINE produces systemic vasoconstriction, which is accompanied by an increase in coronary perfusion pressure (the difference between aortic and right atrial relaxation pressures during the time between chest compressions). This is demonstrated in Figure 17.4 (15). In this case, there is a 30% increase in coronary perfusion pressure following IV epinephrine, and the effect lasts at least 3 minutes (the recommended time interval between epinephrine doses). The disadvantage with epinephrine is the β-receptor-mediated cardiac stimulation, which can erase the benefit of increased coronary perfusion, and has also been implicated in postresuscitation heart failure (15).

Epinephrine use is associated with an increased rate of return to spontaneous circulation (ROSC), but the mortality rate is unchanged (12,16).

VASOPRESSIN is a non-adrenergic vasoconstrictor that is recommended only as a single dose (40 Units IV bolus) that can be used to replace the first or second dose of epinephrine (12). The advantage of vasopressin is the absence of cardiac stimulation, but vasopressin also causes coronary vasoconstriction, which is counterproductive. Clinical trials have shown no apparent advantage of vasopressin over epinephrine (17).

Antiarrhythmic Agents

AMIODARONE is the preferred antiarrhythmic agent for VF/VT-associated cardiac arrest that is refractory to defibrillation and vasopressor therapy (12). This preference is based on clinical studies that show superior results with amiodarone compared to placebo (18) or lidocaine (19). However, the superior results with amiodarone are limited to increased survival to hospital admission, but not to hospital discharge.

LIDOCAINE is the original antiarrhythmic agent used for shock-resistant

VF and pulseless VT, but it is less effective than amiodarone, and should be used only when amiodarone is not available.

MAGNESIUM is used for polymorphic VT, but only when the arrhythmia is associated with QT prolongation (torsade de pointes). The recognition and treatment of polymorphic VT are described in Chapter 15.

The Endotracheal Route

In the rare instance when intravenous or intraosseous access is not available, some ACLS drugs (i.e., epinephrine, vasopressin, and lidocaine) can be administered by injection into the upper airway through an endotracheal tube. The drug dose for endotracheal injection should be 2–2.5 times the intravenous dose (e.g., 2–2.5 mg for epinephrine) (12).

Table 17.3	Advanced Cardiac Life Support Drugs	
Drug	**Dosing Regimen and Comments**	
Vasoconstrictor Drugs		
Epinephrine	Dosing:	1 mg IV/IO every 3–5 minutes.
	Comment:	Vasopressor effect can increase coronary perfusion pressure, but cardiac stimulation is counterproductive.
Vasopressin	Dosing:	40 Units IV/IO as a single dose.
	Comment:	Can be used to replace the 1st or 2nd dose of epinephrine, to reduce cardiac stimulation. No proven advantage.
Antiarrhythmic Agents		
Amiodarone	Dosing:	300 mg IV/IO, then another 150 mg if needed.
	Comment:	Antiarrhythmic drug of choice for VF/VT that is refractory to defibrillation and vasopressors.
Lidocaine	Dosing:	1–1.5 mg/kg IV/IO, then 0.5–0.75 mg/kg every 5–10 min, as needed, to a total of 3 mg/kg. Can use a 1–4 mg/min for maintenance.
	Comment:	Alternative to amiodarone, but much less effective.
Magnesium	Dosing:	1–2 grams IV/IO over 5 minutes.
	Comment:	Used for polymorphic VT associated with prolonged QT interval (torsade de pointes).

From the ACLS guidelines in Reference 12.

RESUSCITATION MONITORING

Monitoring for the return of spontaneous circulation (ROSC) is typically limited to palpation for carotid artery pulsations, but this is discouraged as

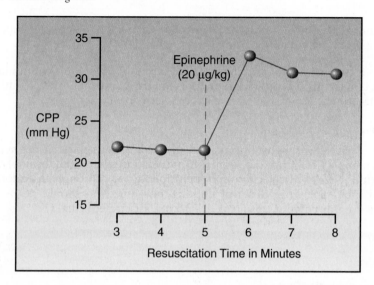

FIGURE 17.4 The effect of intravenous epinephrine on coronary perfusion pressure (CPP) during resuscitation of cardiac arrest with VF/pulseless VT. Data from Reference 15.

a sole practice (12) because the search for pulses often requires interruption of chest compressions for extended periods of time, and there are often uncertainties about the presence or absence of pulses (20a). The end-tidal PCO_2 and central venous O_2 saturation provide a more reliable evaluation of the circulation, and can be used to predict the likelihood of ROSC.

End-Tidal PCO_2

The end-tidal PCO_2 measurement is described in detail in Chapter 21. The PCO_2 in exhaled gas at the end of expiration (end-tidal PCO_2) is a measure of the balance between ventilation and perfusion in the lungs (V/Q balance). The end-tidal PCO_2 varies directly (in the same direction) with changes in cardiac output relative to ventilation, and when *alveolar ventilation is constant, changes in end-tidal PCO_2 reflect proportional changes in cardiac output* (e.g., a 30% decrease in end-tidal PCO_2 indicates a 30% decrease in the cardiac output). The end-tidal PCO_2 is normally equivalent to the arterial PCO_2 (i.e., about 40 mm Hg), but it can be lower than the arterial PCO_2 in pulmonary conditions associated with increased physiologic dead space (i.e., V/Q ratio > 1).

Predictive Value

End-tidal CO_2 monitoring provides a measure of exhaled PCO_2 for each breath, and serial measurements during CPR can be used to identify when ROSC occurs, or is unlikely to occur. The graph in Figure 17.5 shows the serial changes in end-tidal PCO_2 during 20 minutes of CPR in patients who achieved ROSC and in patients who did not achieve ROSC (20b). Note that patients who achieved ROSC showed a progressive increase in end-tidal PCO_2 during the resuscitation period, whereas patients who did not achieve ROSC showed a progressive decline in end-tidal PCO_2. The end-tidal PCO_2 that separated responders from nonresponders in this study was 15 mm Hg after 20 minutes of CPR. Other studies have shown a discriminant value of 10 mm Hg separating survivors and nonsurvivors (21,22).

The available studies indicate that a *successful outcome is unlikely if the end-tidal PCO_2 is not higher than 10–15 mm Hg after 20 minutes of CPR.* When the end-tidal PCO_2 remains above this level, continued resuscitation for as long as 1 1/2 hours has been associated with a favorable outcome (23).

Central Venous O_2 Saturation

As described in Chapter 10, the O_2 saturation of hemoglobin in central venous (superior vena cava) blood ($ScvO_2$) is a measure of the balance between systemic O_2 delivery (DO_2) and systemic O_2 uptake (VO_2). When VO_2 is constant, a decrease in DO_2 (e.g., from a low cardiac output) is accompanied by a decrease in $ScvO_2$. The normal $ScvO_2$ is about 70–80% (see Chapter 10), and there is evidence that *failure to achieve an $ScvO_2$ $\geq 30\%$ during CPR is associated with failure to achieve ROSC* (24). The value of $ScvO_2$ during CPR is limited by the need for a central venous catheter.

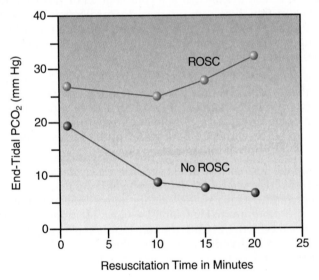

FIGURE 17.5 Serial changes in end-tidal PCO_2 in relation to return of spontaneous circulation (ROSC) during the resuscitation of cardiac arrest with VF/pulseless VT. Data points represent mean values for the patients in each group. From Reference 20b.

POST-RESUSCITATION PERIOD

The immediate goal of CPR is a return of spontaneous circulation (ROSC), but this does not ensure a satisfactory outcome. In fact, surveys of cardiac arrest victims who survive the initial resuscitation indicate that *about 70% do not survive to leave the hospital* (25). This section describes the common problems encountered in the days following ROSC, and a few treatment modalities that can alleviate some of these problems.

Post-Cardiac Arrest Syndrome

The release of blood from areas of ischemia triggers an inflammatory response that can damage vital organs. This *reperfusion injury* is responsible for the *post-cardiac arrest syndrome*, which is characterized by dysfunction in one or more major organs (most often involving the brain and heart) in the early period following successful resuscitation of cardiac arrest (25,26). The principal features of this syndrome are summarized below:

1. *Brain injury* is the most common manifestation of the post-cardiac arrest syndrome, and is *responsible for 23% to 68% of deaths following cardiac arrest* (25). Clinical manifestations include failure to awaken, myoclonus, and generalized seizures. The high prevalence of brain injury after cardiac arrest is attributed to a limited tolerance to ischemia, and a predisposition to oxidative reperfusion injury.

2. Post-arrest *cardiac dysfunction* is a combination of systolic and diastolic dysfunction that can progress to cardiogenic shock within hours after ROSC (25). The underlying problem is a type of reperfusion injury known as myocardial "stunning," which usually resolves within 72 hours (25).

3. *Systemic inflammatory response syndrome* (see Table 14.2) is almost universal after cardiac arrest, and can result in widespread inflammatory injury with multiorgan failure and circulatory shock. This condition can be described as a "whole-body reperfusion injury," and is usually apparent within 24 hours after cardiac arrest. (See Chapter 14 for a description of inflammatory shock.)

The nexus of the post-cardiac arrest syndrome is *inflammatory injury mediated by toxic oxygen metabolites* (see Figure 14.1) (27). As with other life-threatening conditions involving oxidant injury, little attention has been given to supporting antioxidant defenses as a therapeutic modality. Of possible relevance in this regard, the consumption of endogenous antioxidants is reduced by hypothermia (28), which is also the most effective treatment for post-arrest brain injury (see next).

Targeted Temperature Management

Induced hypothermia, previously known as *human refrigeration* (29), was introduced for the management of post-cardiac arrest victims in the mid-twentieth century (30), but was abandoned because of uncertain benefit and the risks of severe hypothermia (< 30°C) used at the time. About 40 years later (in 2002), two studies were published showing that comatose survivors of cardiac arrest who were treated with 12 to 24 hours of mild hypothermia (32–34°C) had more favorable neurologic outcomes and fewer deaths (31,32). The results of one of these studies (the larger one) is shown in Figure 17.6 (31). According to these results, mild hypothermia prevented one unfavorable neurologic outcome for every 6 patients treated, and prevented one death for every 7 patients treated. Since these results were published, mild induced hypothermia, now called *targeted temperature management* or TTM (33), has been adopted with enthusiasm for patients who do not awaken after ROSC. The general features of TTM are presented in Table 17.4 (26,27,30–33).

Who Benefits?

The original reports of benefit with mild hypothermia included cases of out-of-hospital cardiac arrest associated with VF/pulseless VT (31,32), and this condition was initially considered the only indication for mild hypothermia. However, because of the great promise with TTM, it is now a consideration *for any patient who does not awaken following ROSC* (26), regardless of the associated rhythm or location of the cardiac arrest. The only absolute contraindications to TTM are pre-existing hypothermia (< 34°C), major bleeding, or cryoglobulinemia. Hemodynamic instability and cardiogenic shock are not considered absolute contraindications to TTM (26).

The Method

Surface cooling has been the most popular method of TTM, but endovascular cooling is gaining favor because it creates less risk of shivering, and avoids the problem of erratic surface cooling caused by cold-induced vasoconstriction in the skin. The endovascular cooling method requires insertion of a specialized central venous catheter, but this is easily accomplished during the induction phase of cooling (see next). Both types of cooling are optimal when automated, and a number of automated systems are commercially available.

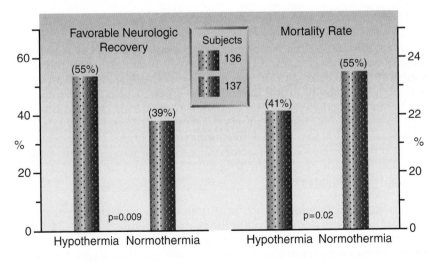

FIGURE 17.6 Clinical outcomes with mild hypothermia (32–34°C) and conventional management (normothermia) in comatose survivors of out-of-hospital cardiac arrest with VF/pulseless VT. Data from Reference 31.

Patients who receive TTM are intubated and mechanically ventilated, and have thermistor-equipped bladder catheters to monitor body temperature. Although the patients are comatose, infusions of sedative agents (e.g., midazolam, propofol, or fentanyl) are often used to alleviate anticipated shivering. The cooling process in TTM is divided into 3 phases: induction, maintenance, and rewarming.

Table 17.4	Targeted Temperature Management
Indications	Patients who do not awaken after ROSC
Contraindications	Body temp <34°C, major bleeding, cryoglobulinemia
Treatment Plan	Reduce body temp to 32–34°C, for 24 hrs. Begin as soon as possible after ROSC.
Cooling Methods	Surface cooling and endovascular cooling
Protocol	Infuse ice-cold (4°C) saline until body temp at 34°C, then maintain temp at 32–34°C for 24 hrs, and rewarm at 0.25–0.5°C/hr.
Complications	Shivering, bradycardia, hypotension, diuresis, hypokalemia, infection
Benefit	Prevents one unfavorable neurologic outcome for every 6 patients treated, and prevents one fatal outcome for every 7 patients treated.†

†Reported for out-of-hospital cardiac arrests with VF/pulseless VT (31).
From References 25, 26, 30–33. ROSC = return of spontaneous circulation.

INDUCTION: Rapid cooling is advised with ice-cold (4°C) saline or lactated Ringers fluid infused in 500 mL aliquots every 10 minutes until the body temperature falls to 34°C or the infusion volume reaches 30 mL/kg. Shivering is common during the induction phase, and is counterproductive because it increases the body temperature. Shivering can be controlled with *propofol* (0.1–0.2 mg/kg/min IV), *midazolam* (0.02–0.1 mg/kg/hr IV), or *fentanyl* (25–100 μg/hr IV), while *magnesium* (5 grams IV over 5 hours) can also be effective (25). Refractory shivering is managed with neuromuscular blockade (e.g., *cisatracurium*, 0.15–0.2 mg/kg IV bolus, then 1–2 μg/kg/min, if needed).

MAINTENANCE: Following induction, automated surface cooling or endovascular cooling systems maintain the body temperature at 32–34°C for the next 24 hours. *Bradycardia* is common during hypothermia, but usually requires no intervention. *Hypotension* can occur as a result of cold-induced diuresis and cardiac depression, and is managed with volume infusions initially, followed by a vasopressor (e.g., norepinephrine) if needed. *Hypokalemia* is common (from potassium moving into cells), and should be treated cautiously to prevent hyperkalemia during rewarming. If available, continuous EEG recording is advised during TTM because *nonconvulsive status epilepticus has been reported an about 10% of patients* (34).

REWARMING: Slow rewarming (0.25–0.5°C/hr) is recommended, and is usually managed by the automated cooling system. Watch for hyperkalemia during rewarming (when potassium moves back out of cells), especially when aggressive potassium replacement was used during hypothermia.

After rewarming, it is important to discontinue sedation as soon as possible, because residual sedation can prolong the time to awaken. The evaluation of patients who fail to awaken soon after rewarming is described later.

Fever

As expected from the beneficial effects of hypothermia, fever following a cardiac arrest is associated with unfavorable neurologic outcomes (35). Therefore, prompt antipyretic therapy is advised for patients with fever who do not receive TTM, or for rebound fever that can follow TTM. *Acetaminophen* is the standard antipyretic agent, and is given in doses of 650 mg or 1000 mg IV or via feeding tube every 6 hours, with a maximum daily dose of 4 grams. Patients with hepatic insufficiency should not receive acetaminophen.

Glycemic Control

Hyperglycemia following cardiac arrest is associated with a poor neurologic outcome (36), although there is no evidence that glycemic control after cardiac arrest improves neurologic outcome. Strict glycemic control in ICU patients is associated with frequent episodes of hypoglycemia (37), so a higher-than-normal *range of 144–180 mg/dL* for blood glucose is considered a reasonable target (26). As an adjunct to this practice, it is wise to avoid dextrose-containing intravenous solutions whenever possible.

Predicting Neurologic Recovery

In patients who do not regain consciousness after CPR or induced hypothermia, the single most important determination is the likelihood of neurologic recovery. The traditional signs that predict a poor neurologic outcome are based on observations performed before hypothermia was adopted as a treatment modality (38,39), and these signs may not apply to patients who are treated with hypothermia (40–42). The following sections describe the signs that predict a poor neurologic outcome after CPR, and whether or not these signs also apply to patients treated with hypothermia. This information is summarized in Table 17.5

Table 17.5	Predictive Signs of a Poor Outcome in Patients Who Do Not Awaken After CPR or Induced Hypothermia	
Poor Prognostic Signs	**After CPR**	**After Hypothermia**
No pupillary light reflex on day 3	✔	✔
No corneal reflexes on day 3	✔	✔
GCS motor score ≤ 2 on day 3†	✔	
Generalized status epilepticus	✔	
Myoclonic status epilepticus on day 1	✔	✔

†A motor score of ≤2 on the Glasgow Coma Score indicates no motor response or an abnormal extensor motor response (decerebrate posturing) to a painful stimulus.
From References 38–43.

Time to Awaken

Following CPR, most (80–95%) of the patients who regain consciousness are awake after 72 hours (38,40), but it can take 7 days or even longer for all the patients to awaken (38). There is a perception that hypothermia prolongs the time to awaken, but this remains unproven. In one retrospective study (40), the median time to awaken was the same (2 days) after CPR and after hypothermia, and a larger percentage of the patients who received hypothermia were awake at 72 hours (91%) compared to patients who did not receive hypothermia (79%). In general, the time to awaken can be a poor predictor of neurologic outcome in the first week following CPR, with or without hypothermia. Residual sedation may play a role in prolonging the time to awaken, particularly in patients who are treated with hypothermia (40).

Brainstem Reflexes

Absence of brainstem reflexes is highly predictive of a poor outcome in patients who remain comatose after CPR and hypothermia. When papillary light reflexes or corneal reflexes are absent 3 days after CPR or hypothermia, none of the patients have a satisfactory neurologic recovery (39,41,42).

Best Motor Response

Patients who remain comatose for 72 hours after CPR have no chance of a satisfactory neurologic recovery if they show no motor response to pain, or an abnormal extensor response (i.e., decerebrate posturing) (38,39). However, when hypothermia is used, as many as 25% of patients who show no motor response at 72 hours will have a satisfactory recovery (43). Therefore, poor motor responses at 72 hours do not predict a poor outcome in patients treated with hypothermia.

Status Epilepticus

Myoclonic status epilepticus (repetitive, irregular movements of the face, trunk, and extremities) often appears in the first 24 hours after a cardiac arrest (41), and is a poor prognostic sign for recovery in all patients, including those who receive hypothermia (39,41,42). Generalized status epilepticus (repetitive, tonic-clonic movements of the face, trunk, and extremities), including nonconvulsive status epilepticus (no seizure-like movements), is a poor prognostic sign without hypothermia, but does not always indicate a poor outcome following hypothermia (41).

Sedation and Prognosis

The prognostic evaluation following hypothermia requires further study; however, one issue that is emerging is the possible interference of unsuspected sedation in the neurologic evaluation following hypothermia. The administration of opiates and other sedating drugs is commonplace during hypothermia and rewarming (which can last for 30 hours or longer), and slowed drug metabolism from hypothermia could result in prolonged sedation after the procedure. This could prolong the time to awaken, and create misleading signs of a poor neurologic recovery. Attention to limiting the use of sedating drugs, if possible, during hypothermia and rewarming will limit the risk of errors in interpreting persistent unresponsiveness, and can avoid the embarrassing situation where a patient wakes up after you have assured the family that there is little or no chance of awakening.

A FINAL WORD

Perception

Cardiopulmonary resuscitation has always enjoyed a popularity far greater than deserved. This is evident in surveys of the general public, where 95% of respondents have unrealistic expectations about CPR (44), including the perception that more than half of cardiac arrest victims not only survive, but return to daily life with no residual effects (45). Television shows mirror this perception, where CPR is portrayed as a success in 67 to 75% of cases (46).

Reality

The reality of CPR is far removed from perception; i.e., on average, less than 10% of patients who receive CPR survive to leave the hospital (47), and when the responsible rhythm is asystole or PEA, as few as 2% of patients have a satisfactory recovery (see Table 17.1). Thus, the reality of CPR is that it doesn't produce satisfactory results in most instances, even when trained personnel are immediately available.

Why is this discrepancy between perception and reality so important? Because perception is dictating CPR practices; i.e., patients decide whether CPR is performed, not clinical practitioners.

REFERENCES

1. Kouwenhoven WB, Ing, Jude JR, Knickerbocker GG. Closed-chest cardiac massage. JAMA 1960; 173:1064–1067.

Clinical Outcomes

2. Nadkarni VM, Laarkin GL, Peberdy MA, et al, for the National Registry of Cardiopulmonary Resuscitation Investigators. First documented rhythm and clinical outcome from in-hospital cardiac arrest among children and adults. JAMA 2006; 295:50–57.

3. Yasanuga H, Horiguchi H, Tanabe S, et al. Collaborative effects of bystander-initiated cardiopulmonary resuscitation and prehospital advanced cardiac life support by physicians on survival of out-of-hospital cardiac arrest: a nationwide population-based observational study. Crit Care 2010; 14:R199–R210.

American Heart Association Guidelines

4. 2010 American Heart Association Guidelines for Cardiopulmonary Resuscitation and Emergency Cardiovascular Care Science with Treatment Recommendations. Circulation, volume 122, issue 16, supplement 2, October 16, 2010. (Available online @ http:// circ.ahajournals.org/ content/122/16_suppl_2.toc)

5. Advanced Cardiovascular Life Support Provider Manual. Dallas, TX: Amer-ican Heart Association, 2011.

Basic Life Support

6. Berg RA, Hemphill R, Abella BS, et al. Part 5: Adult basic life support: 2010 American Heart Association Guidelines for Cardiopulmonary Resuscitation and Emergency Cardiovascular Care. Circulation 2010; 122 (suppl 3):S685–S705.

7. Hupfl M, Selig H, Nagele P. Chest compression-only CPR: a meta-analysis. Lancet 2010; 376:1552–1557.

8. Wit L, Kramer-Johansen J, Mykelbust H, et al. Quality of cardiopulmonary resuscitation during out-of-hospital cardiac arrest. JAMA 2005; 293:299–304.

9. Jost D, Degrance H, Verret C, et al. DEFI 2005: a randomized controlled trial of the effect of automated external defibrillator cardiopulmonary resuscitation protocol on outcome from out-of-hospital cardiac arrest. Circulation 2010; 121:1614–1622.

10. Aufderheide TP, Lurie KG. Death by hyperventilation: A common and life-threatening problem during cardiopulmonary resuscitation. Crit Care Med 2004; 32(Suppl):S345–S351.

11. Abella BS, Alvarado JP, Mykelbust H, et al. Quality of cardiopulmonary resuscitation during in-hospital cardiac arrest. JAMA 2005; 293:305–310.

Advanced Life Support

12. Neumar RW, Otto CW, Link MS, et al. Part 8: adult advanced cardiovascular life support: 2010 American Heart Association Guidelines for Cardiopul-

monary Resuscitation and Emergency Cardiovascular Care. Circulation 2010; 122 (suppl 3):S729–S767.

13. Link MS, Atkins DL, Passman RS, et al. Part 6: electrical therapies: automated external defibrillators, defibrillation, cardioversion, and pacing: 2010 American Heart Association Guidelines for Cardiopulmonary Resuscitation and Emergency Cardiovascular Care. Circulation 2010; 122 (suppl 3):S706–S719.

14. Larsen MP, Eisenberg M, Cummins RO, Hallstrom AP. Predicting survival from out of hospital cardiac arrest: a graphic model. Ann Emerg Med 1993; 22:1652–1658.

15. Sun S, Tang W, Song F, et al. The effects of epinephrine on outcomes of mormothermic and therapeutic hypothermic cardiopulmonary resuscitation. Crit Care Med 2010; 38:2175–2180.

16. Herlitz J, Ekstrom L, Wennerblom B, et al. Adrenaline in out-of-hospital ventricular fibrillation. Does it make any difference? Resuscitation 1995; 29:195–201.

17. Aung K, Htay T. Vasopressin for cardiac arrest: a systematic review and meta-analysis. Arch Intern Med 2005; 165:17–24.

18. Kudenchuk PJ, Cobb LA, Copass MK, et al. Amiodarone for out-of-hospital cardiac arrest due to ventricular fibrillation. New Engl J Med 1999; 341:871–878.

19. Dorian P, Cass D, Schwartz B, et al. Amiodarone as compared to lidocaine for shock-resistant ventricular fibrillation. New Engl J Med 2002; 346:884–890.

Resuscitation Monitoring

20a. Ochoa FJ, Ramalle-Gomara E, Carpintero JM, et al. Competence of health professionals to check the carotid pulse. Resuscitation 1998; 37:173–175.

20b. Kolar M, Krizmaric M, Klemen P, Grmec S. Partial pressure of end-tidal carbon dioxide predicts successful cardiopulmonary resuscitation – a prospective observational study. Crit Care 2008; 12:R115. Full text available on PubMed; accessed on 10/15/2012

21. Sanders AB, Kern KB, Otto CW, et al. End-tidal carbon dioxide monitoring during cardiopulmonary resuscitation. JAMA 1989; 262:1347–1351.

22. Wayne MA, Levine RL, Miller CC. Use of end-tidal carbon dioxide to predict outcome in prehospital cardiac arrest. Ann Emerg Med 1995; 25:762–767.

23. White RD, Goodman BW, Svoboda MA. Neurologic recovery following prolonged out-of-hospital cardiac arrest with resuscitation guided by continuous capnography. Mayo Clin Proc 2011; 86:544–548.

24. Rivers EP, Martin GB, Smithline H, et al. The clinical implications of continuous central venous oxygen saturation during human CPR. Ann Emerg Med 1992; 21:1094–1101.

Post-Resuscitation Period

25. Nolan JP, Neumar RW, Adrie C, et al. Post-cardiac arrest syndrome: epidemiology, pathophysiology, and prognostication. A scientific statement from the International Liaison Committee on Resuscitation; the American Heart Association Emergency Cardiovascular Care Committee; the Council

on Cardiovascular Surgery and Anesthesia; the Council on Cardiopulmonary, Perioperative, and Critical Care; the Council on Clinical Cardiology; the Council on Stroke. Resuscitation 2008; 79:350–379.

26. Peberdy MA, Callaway CW, Neumar RW, et al. Part 9: post-cardiac arrest care. 2010 American Heart Association Guidelines for Cardiopulmonary Resuscitation and Emergency Cardiovascular Care. Circulation 2010; 122 (suppl 3):S768–S786.

27. Huet O, Dupic L, Batteux F, et al. Post-resuscitation syndrome: potential role of hydroxyl radical-induced endothelial cell damage. Crit Care Med 2011; 39:1712–1720.

28. Karibe H, Chen SF, Zarow GJ, et al. Intraischemic hypotherma suppresses consumption of endogenous antioxidants after temporary focal ischemia in rats. Brain Res 1994; 649:12–18.

29. Fay T. Observations on prlonged human refrigeration. NY State J Med 1940; 40:1351–1354.

30. Williams GR, Spencer FC. The clinical use of hypothermia after cardiac arrest. Am Surg 1959; 148:462–468.

31. The Hypothermia After Cardiac Arrest Study group. Mild therapeutic hypo-thermia to improve the neurologic outcome after cardiac arrest. N Engl J Med 2002; 346: 549–556.

32. Bernard SA, Gray TW, Buist MD, et al. Treatment of comatose survivors of out-of-hospital cardiac arrest with induced hypothermia. N Engl J Med 2002; 346:557–563.

33. Holzer M. Targeted temperature management for comatose survivors of cardiac arrest. N Engl J Med 2010; 363:1256–1264.

34. Rittenberger JC, Popescu A, Brenner RP, et al. Frequency and timing of non-convulsive status epilepticus in comatose, post-cardiac arrest subjects treated with hypothermia. Neurocrit Care 2012; 16:114–122.

35. Zeiner A, Holzer M, Sterz F, et al. Hyperthermia after cardiac arrest is associated with an unfavorable neurologic outcome. Arch Intern Med 2001; 161:2007–2012.

36. Calle PA, Buylaert WA, Vanhaute OA. Glycemia in the post-resuscitation period. The Cerebral Resuscitation Study group. Resuscitation 1989; 17 (suppl):S181–S188.

37. Marik PE, Preiser J-C. Towards understanding tight glycemic control in the ICU. A systematic review and meta-analysis. Chest 2010; 137:544–551.

38. Levy DE, Caronna JJ, Singer BH, et al. Predicting outcome from hypoxic-ischemic coma. JAMA 1985; 253:1420–1426.

39. Wijdicks EFM, Hijdra A, Young GB, et al. Practice parameter: Prediction of outcome incomatose survivors after cardiopulmonary resuscitation (an evidence-based review). Report of the Quality Standards Subcommittee of the American Academy of Neurology. Neurology 2006; 67:203–210.

40. Fugate JE, Wijdicks EFM, White RD, Rabinstein AA. Does therapeutic hypothermia affect time to awakening in cardiac arrest survivors? Neurology 2011; 77:1346–1350.

41. De Georgia M, Raad B. Prognosis of coma after cardiac arrest in the era of hypothermia. Continuum Lifelong Learning Neurol 2012; 18:515–531.

42. Fugate JE, Wijdicks EFM, Mandrekar J, et al. Predictors of neurologic outcome in hypothermia after cardiac arrest. Ann Neurol 2010; 68:907–914.

43. Rosetti AO, Oddo M, Logroscino G, et al. Prognostication after cardiac arrest and hypothermia. A prospective study. Ann Neurol 2010; 67:301–307.

A Final Word

44. Jones GK, Brewer KL, Garrison HG. Public expectations of survival following cardiopulmonary resuscitation. Acad Emerg Med 2000; 7:48–53.

45. Marco CA, Larkin GL. Cardiopulmonary resuscitation: knowledge and opinions among the U.S. general public. State of the science-fiction. Resuscitation 2008; 79:490–498.

46. Diem SJ, Lantos JD, Tulsky JA. Cardiopulmonary resuscitation on television. Miracles and misinformation. N Engl J Med 1996; 334:1578–1582.

47. Bohm K, Rosenqvist M, Herlitz J, et al. Survival is similar after standard treatment and chest compressions only in out-of-hospital bystander cardiopulmonary resuscitation. Circulation 2007; 116:2908–2912.

BLOOD COMPONENTS

The golden rule is there are no golden rules.

George Bernard Shaw

Chapter 18

ANEMIA AND RED BLOOD CELL TRANSFUSIONS

Fundamental progress requires the reinterpretation of basic ideas.

Alfred North Whitehead

(1861–1947)

Anemia is almost universal in patients who spend a few days in the ICU (1), and about 50% of ICU patients receive erythrocyte transfusions to alleviate anemia (1,2). Unfortunately, few ICUs employ guidelines to standardize transfusion therapy (2), and erythrocyte transfusions are typically guided by personal preference and tradition rather than evidence of need or benefit. The discovery in recent years that erythrocyte transfusions often create risks instead of benefits has prompted a mandate for change in this fickle and arbitrary practice.

This chapter describes the effects (physiological and clinical) of anemia and erythrocyte transfusions, and presents the indications, methods, and risks of erythrocyte transfusions in critically ill patients (3,4). Transfusion practices that lack a scientific basis or justification are highlighted to comply with Whitehead's edict in the introductory quote.

ANEMIA IN THE ICU

The variety of erythrocyte-related measurements and their reference ranges are shown in Table 18.1. The use of hematocrit and hemoglobin concentration as measures of anemia is problematic in ICU patients, as described next.

Definition of Anemia

Anemia is defined as a *decrease in the oxygen (O_2) carrying capacity of blood.* The most accurate measure of the O_2 carrying capacity of blood is the *red* *cell mass*, which is measured using chromium-tagged erythrocytes. This measurement is not readily available for clinical use, so the hematocrit and hemoglobin (Hb) concentration are used as clinical measures of O_2 carrying capacity.

Table 18.1	Reference Ranges for Red Cell Parameters in Adults	

Red Cell Count	**Mean Cellular Volume (MCV)**
Males: 4.6×10^{12}/L	Males: $80–100 \times 10^{-15}$/L
Females: 4.2×10^{12}/L	Females: same
Reticulocyte Count	**Hematocrit**
Males: $25–75 \times 10^9$/L	Males: 40–54%
Females: same	Females: 38–47%
Red Cell Mass[†]	**Hemoglobin[#]**
Males: 26 mL/kg	Males: 14–18 g/dL
Females: 24 mL/kg	Females: 12–16 g/dL

[†]Normal values are 10% lower in the elderly ($\geq$ 65 years of age).

[#]Normal values are 0.5 g/dL lower in blacks

Sources: (1) Walker RH (ed.) Technical Manual of the American Association of Blood Banks, 10th ed., VA: American Association of Blood Banks, 1990:649–650; (2) Billman RS, Finch CA. Red cell manual. 6th ed. Philadelphia, PA: Davis, 1994:46.

Influence of Plasma Volume

The problem with the hematocrit and Hb concentration as measures of O_2 carrying capacity is the influence of plasma volume on these variables. This is demonstrated in Figure 18.1, which shows the postural changes in hematocrit and plasma volume in a group of healthy adults (5). When changing from the standing to supine positions, there is a decrease in the hydrostatic pressure in the veins and capillaries in the legs (due to loss of the gravitational effect), and interstitial fluid moves into the bloodstream and increases the plasma volume (by 420 mL in this study). The hematocrit then decreases by dilution, but there is no change in the O_2 carrying capacity of blood. The postural change in hematocrit (4.1%) is equivalent to one unit of erythrocytes (packed red blood cells), so a dilutional drop in Hct similar to the one in Figure 18.1 could be misinterpreted as indicating a decrease in O_2 carrying capacity equivalent to one unit of blood.

Increased plasma volume is common in critically ill patients (see Figure 11.3 in Chapter 11), which means the hematocrit and Hb concentration will overestimate the occurrence and severity of anemia. Clinical studies have confirmed that *the Hct and Hb concentration are unreliable measures of anemia in critically ill patients* (6,7). Unfortunately, these are the measures used in all the clinical studies evaluating anemia and erythrocyte transfusions in critically ill patients.

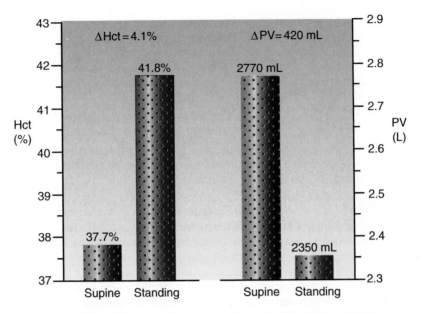

FIGURE 18.1 Postural changes in hematocrit (Hct) and plasma volume (PV) in a group of healthy adults. The numbers above the columns are mean values for each measurement. From Reference 5.

ICU-Related Anemia

Two conditions have been implicated in the anemia that appears during the ICU stay (8): systemic inflammation, and repeated phlebotomy for laboratory studies.

Anemia of Inflammation

Inflammation is responsible for the *anemia of chronic disease*, which *is now called the anemia of inflammation* (8). The hematologic effects of inflammation include inhibition of erythropoietin release from the kidneys, reduced marrow responsiveness to erythropoietin, iron sequestration in macrophages, and increased destruction of RBCs (12,13). The changes in plasma include a decrease in plasma iron, total iron binding capacity, and transferrin levels, and an increase in plasma ferritin levels.

Phlebotomy

An average of 40–70 mL of blood is withdrawn daily from each ICU patient to perform laboratory tests (9,10), which is at least 4 times more than the daily phlebotomy volume in non-ICU patients (9). The cumulative phlebotomy volume can reach 500 mL (one unit of whole blood) after one week, and this volume loss can result in an iron-deficiency anemia if allowed to continue.

The daily phlebotomy volume can be reduced by ordering fewer laboratory tests, and by reducing the volume of blood discarded for each laboratory blood draw. When blood is withdrawn through vascular catheters for laboratory testing, the initial aspirate is discarded to eliminate interference from intravenous fluid in the lumen of the catheter. The volume of discarded blood is typically about 5 mL for each laboratory blood draw, and returning this blood to the patient can reduce the daily phlebotomy volume by 50% (11).

Physiological Effects of Anemia

Anemia elicits two responses that help to preserve tissue oxygenation: (a) an increase in cardiac output, and (b) an increase in O_2 extraction from capillary blood.

Cardiac Output

The graph in Figure 9.9 (page 166) shows the increase in cardiac output that occurs in response to a progressive decrease in hematocrit. This response is explained by the influence of anemia on blood viscosity. The hematocrit is the principal determinant of blood viscosity, and decreases in hematocrit are accompanied by similar decreases in blood viscosity. The relationship between hematocrit and blood viscosity is shown in Table 9.2 (page 165). The final section of Chapter 9 contains a detailed description of blood viscosity and its influence on circulatory blood flow.

Systemic Oxygenation

The influence of progressive anemia on measures of systemic oxygenation are shown in Figure 18.2 (12). The principal findings are explained using the following relationships between O_2 uptake (VO_2), O_2 delivery (DO_2), and O_2 extraction:

$$VO_2 = DO_2 \times O_2 \text{ Extraction} \qquad (18.1)$$

1. The progressive decrease in hematocrit is associated with a steady decrease in O_2 delivery (DO_2). However, there is also an equivalent increase in O_2 extraction, and the reciprocal changes in DO_2 and O_2 extraction results in an unchanged O_2 uptake (VO_2).
2. When the hematocrit falls below 10%, the increase in O_2 extraction is no longer able to match the decrease in DO_2, and the VO_2 begins to fall. The decrease in VO_2 represents a decrease in O_2 availability in tissues, and is accompanied by lactate accumulation in the blood.
3. The maximum O_2 extraction is about 50%, and it marks the threshold for impaired tissue oxygenation. Therefore, an O_2 extraction of 50% could be used as a trigger point for transfusion of erythrocytes. This point will be revisited later in the chapter.

Lowest Tolerable Hematocrit

Animal studies have shown that, when the intravascular volume is maintained, hematocrits as low as 5 to 10% (Hb=1.5 to 3 g/dL) do not adversely affect tissue oxygenation (12–14), even in awake animals breathing room air (14). The lowest tolerable hematocrit or hemoglobin has not been determined in humans, but in one study of progressive hemodilution in healthy adults, Hb levels of 5 g/dL showed no apparent harm (15). The important message from studies of severe anemia is not the lowest tolerable hematocrit, but the realization that *severe anemia is tolerated when the intravascular volume is maintained.*

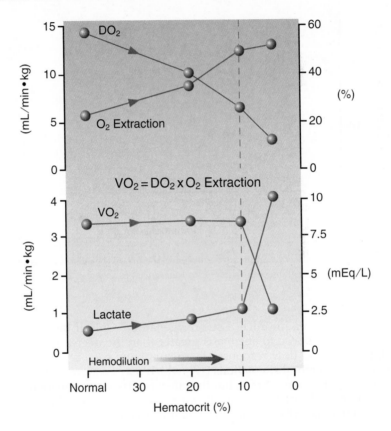

FIGURE 18.2 The influence of progressive isovolemic anemia on measures of systemic oxygenation. DO_2 = systemic O_2 delivery, VO_2 = systemic O_2 uptake. Data from Reference 12.

Paradoxical Effect

The graph in Figure 18.3 reveals an effect of anemia that few would predict; i.e., enhanced tissue oxygenation! The data in this graph is from a study that used direct measurements of the PO_2 in subcutaneous tissue to evaluate normovolemic hemodilution in isolated skin flaps (16). As indicated in the graph, progressive decreases in hematocrit were accompanied by increases in the subcutaneous PO_2 in both normal and ischemic skin regions, and this relationship continued until the hematocrit fell to 15%. Similar results in other studies has led to the use of normovolemic anemia to promote the viability of skin flaps.

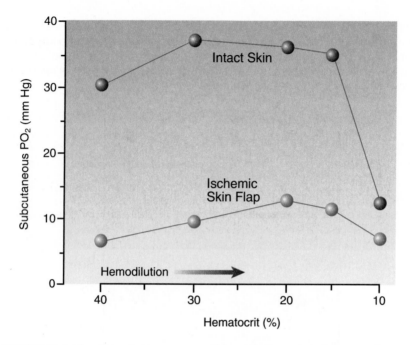

FIGURE 18.3 The effect of progressive isovolemic anemia on the subcutaneous PO_2 in normal and ischemic regions of the skin. From Reference 16.

So how can anemia improve tissue oxygenation? Only if the flow augmentation in response to anemia is greater than the decrease in hematocrit. Exaggerated flow responses to anemia have been reported in the coronary and cerebral circulations (17), which may be a protective mechanism for the heart and brain, but the effect on tissue oxygenation is not known. Regional variations in the flow response to anemia add further to the problem of selecting an appropriate transfusion trigger.

TRANSFUSION TRIGGERS

Surveys indicate that 90% of the erythrocyte transfusions in ICU patients are given to alleviate anemia (18), and are guided by the hemoglobin concentration in blood. This is a flawed practice, as described in this section.

Hemoglobin

In 1942, a hemoglobin (Hb) level < 10 g/dL was recommended as an indication for erythrocyte transfusions (19), and this was the standard transfusion trigger for the next 60 years, until clinical studies showed that adopting a lower transfusion trigger (i.e., Hb < 7 g/dL) had no adverse consequences (20,21). This lower transfusion trigger is now included in the clinical practice guidelines for RBC transfusions.

Guidelines

The most recent guidelines on erythrocyte transfusions in critically ill patients (3) contain the following statement:

1. The use of only the Hb level as a "trigger" for transfusion *should be avoided* (italics mine)

Despite this recommendation, the guidelines also contain the following inconsistent statements:

2. Consider transfusion if Hb < 7 g/dL in critically ill patients who require mechanical ventilation.
3. Consider transfusion if Hb < 7 g/dL in resuscitated critically ill trauma patients.
4. Consider transfusion if Hb < 7 g/dL in critically ill patients with stable cardiac disease.
5. RBC transfusion may be beneficial in patients with acute coronary syndromes (ACS) who are anemic (Hb < 8 g/dL).

What's Wrong

There are two fundamental problems with the Hb as a transfusion trigger.

1. The Hb concentration in blood provides absolutely no information about the adequacy of tissue oxygenation, so transfusions based on the Hb level have no relationship to tissue oxygenation.
2. Decreases in the Hb concentration can be a dilutional effect, and may not reflect decreases in the O_2 carrying capacity of blood.

Clinical practice guidelines published over the past 25 years have recommended abandoning the Hb level as a transfusion trigger and adopting more physiologic measures of tissue oxygenation, like the ones described next (3,22). However, instead of abandoning the Hb level, physicians have abandoned the recommendation!

Oxygen Extraction

As described earlier (and shown in Figure 18.2) anemia elicits a compensatory increase in O_2 extraction from capillary blood, which serves to maintain a constant rate of O_2 uptake into tissues. However, the O_2 extraction cannot increase much further than 50%, and, when the O_2 extraction is maximum at 50%, further decreases in Hb are accompanied by proportional decreases in O_2 uptake into tissues (indicating tissue dysoxia). Therefore, an O_2 extraction of 50% can be used as a transfusion trigger because it identifies the threshold for impaired tissue oxygenation. The O_2 extraction is roughly equivalent to the $(SaO_2 - ScvO_2)$, and can be monitored continuously using pulse oximetry (for the SaO_2) and a central venous oximetry catheter (PreSep Catheter, Edwards Life sciences) to monitor the central venous O_2 saturation $(ScvO_2)$. The $(SaO_2 - ScvO_2)$ is very appealing as a transfusion trigger (23) because it provides information about the adequacy of tissue oxygenation.

Central Venous O_2 Saturation

When the SaO_2 is close to 100%, the $(SaO_2 - ScvO_2)$ is equivalent to $(1 - ScvO_2)$, and the $ScvO_2$ can be used as a transfusion trigger. An $ScvO_2$ < 70% has been proposed as a transfusion trigger (24), although it seems a lower $ScvO_2$ (i.e., closer to 50%) would be more appropriate for identifying the threshold for impaired tissue oxygenation.

ERYTHROCYTE TRANSFUSIONS

Whole blood is stored only on request, and is otherwise separated into its component parts; i.e., red blood cells, platelets, plasma, and cryoprecipitate. This practice allows each unit of donated blood to serve multiple transfusion needs. The erythrocyte preparations that are available for transfusion are shown in Table 18.2.

Table 18.2	Erythrocyte Transfusion Preparations
Preparation	**Features**
Packed RBCs	1. Each unit has a volume of 350 mL and hematocrit of about 60%.
	2. Contains leukocytes and residual plasma (15–30 mL per unit).
	3. Can be stored for 42 days with appropriate additives.
Leukocyte-Poor RBCs	1. Donor RBCs are passed through specialized filters to remove most of the leukocytes. This reduces the risk of febrile reactions to RBC and platelet transfusions.
	2. Indicated for patients with a history of febrile transfusion reactions.
Washed RBCs	1. Saline washing of packed RBCs removes residual plasma, which reduces the risk of hypersensitivity reactions.
	2. Used in patients with a history of transfusion-related allergic reactions, and in patients with IgA deficiency, who are at risk for transfusion-related anaphylaxis.

From Reference 25.

Packed Red Blood Cells

The erythrocyte fraction of donated blood is placed in a preservative fluid and stored at 1 to 6°C. Newer preservative solutions contain adenine, which helps to maintain ATP levels in stored erythrocytes, and allows storage of donor erythrocytes for up to 42 days (25). Each unit of donor erythrocytes, known as *packed red blood cells* (packed RBCs), has a hematocrit of about 60% and a volume of about 350 mL. Packed RBCs also contain 30–50 mL of residual plasma, and a considerable numbers of leukocytes (1–3 billion leukocytes per unit of packed RBCs) (25).

Leukocyte Reduction

The leukocytes in packed RBCs can trigger an antibody response in the recipient after repeated transfusions, and this is responsible for febrile nonhemolytic transfusion reactions (see later). To reduce the occurrence of this reaction, donor RBCs are passed through specialized filters to remove most of the leukocytes. This is performed routinely in many blood banks, but universal leukocyte reduction has yet to be adopted in the United States. Leukocyte-reduced RBCs are recommended for patients with prior febrile nonhemolytic transfusion reactions (25).

Washed Red Blood Cells

Donor RBCs can be washed with isotonic saline to remove residual plasma. This reduces the risk of hypersensitivity reactions caused by prior sensitization to plasma proteins in donor blood. Washed RBC preparations are recommended for patients with a history of hypersensitivity reactions to blood transfusions, and for patients with immunoglobulin A deficiency, who have an increased risk of transfusion-related anaphylaxis (25). Saline washing does not effectively remove leukocytes.

Infusing Packed RBCs

The infusion of packed RBCs is described in Chapter 11 (see page 205). Rapid infusion rates are not necessary when packed RBCs are used to alleviate anemia, and this eliminates the need for infusion pumps or dilution with saline to increase infusion rates. The gravity-driven flow rate of packed RBCs through an 18-gauge peripheral catheter is 5 mL/min (see Figure 11.5 on page 206), which corresponds to 70 minutes for the transfusion of one unit (350 mL) of packed RBCs. This is well within the recommended transfusion time of 2 hrs per unit of packed RBCs for hemodynamically stable patients (26).

Blood Filters

Standard blood filters (pore size 170 to 260 microns) are required for the transfusion of all blood products (26). These filters trap blood clots and other debris, but they do not trap leukocytes, and are not effective for leukocyte reduction (25). These filters can become an impediment to flow as they collect trapped debris, and sluggish infusion rates should prompt replacement of the blood filter.

Systemic Oxygenation

In an average sized adult, one unit of packed RBCs is expected to raise the hemoglobin concentration and hematocrit by 1 g/dL and 3%, respectively (25). The effects of RBC transfusions on measures of systemic oxygenation are shown in Figure 18.4. The data in this figure is from a group of postoperative patients with severe normovolemic anemia (Hb < 7 g/dL) who were transfused with 1–2 units of packed RBCs to raise the Hb above 7 g/dL. The RBC transfusions increased the mean Hb concentration from 6.4 to 8 g/dL (25% increase), and there was a similar increase in O_2 delivery (DO_2). However, the systemic O_2 uptake (VO_2) was unchanged. The constant VO_2 in the face of an increased DO_2 indicates that O_2 extraction was reduced by the RBC transfusions, as predicted by equation 18.1. These changes in DO_2 and O_2 extraction are the reverse of the changes produced by anemia, as shown in Figure 18.2.

Tissue Oxygenation

The lack of an effect on VO_2 indicates that RBC transfusions do not enhance tissue oxygenation. This has been confirmed in several clinical studies (27–30), and prolonged storage of RBCs can actually impair tissue oxygenation after transfusion (31). These studies have prompted the following statement in the most recent clinical practice guidelines for red blood cell transfusions (3): "*RBC transfusion should not be considered an absolute method to improve tissue oxygenation in critically ill patients.*" If RBC transfusions do not provide a benefit for tissue oxygenation, then why do we give RBC transfusions? Unfortunately, there is no satisfying answer to this question.

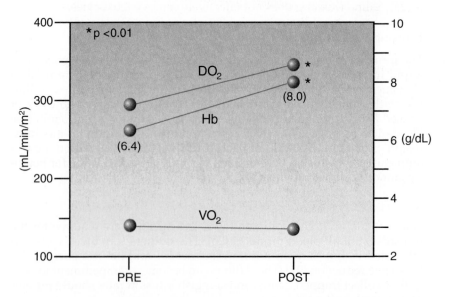

FIGURE 18.4 Effects of erythrocyte transfusions (1–2 units packed RBCs) on hemoglobin concentration (Hb), systemic oxygen delivery (DO_2), and systemic oxygen uptake (VO_2) in 11 postoperative patients with severe anemia (Hb <7 g/dL). Data points represent mean values for each parameter. Numbers in parentheses are the mean hemoglobin concentrations before and after transfusion. Data from personal observations.

The inability of RBC transfusions to enhance tissue oxygenation raises serious questions about the practice of transfusing RBCs simply to raise the blood Hb level. Adding to the concern are studies indicating that RBC transfusions are a source of morbidity and even mortality in critically ill patients (32). The risks associated with RBC transfusions are described next.

TRANSFUSION RISKS

The spectrum of adverse events associated with blood transfusions are shown in Table 18.3, along with the incidence of each event expressed in relation to the number of units transfused (33–37). (Only acute events are included.) Note that transfusion errors are much more frequent than the feared transmission of HIV or the hepatitis B virus. The following is a brief description of the principal transfusion reactions (37–41).

Table 18.3	Adverse Events Associated with RBC Transfusions (per units transfused)
Immune Reactions	**Other Risks**
Nonhemolytic fever (1 in 200)	Transmitted Infections:
Hypersensitivity Reactions:	Bacterial (1 in 500,000)
Urticaria (1 in 100)	Hepatitis B virus (1 in 220,000)
Anaphylaxis (1 in 1,000)	Hepatitis C virus (1 in 1.6 million)
Anaphylactic shock (1 in 50,000)	HIV (1 in 1.6 million)
†Acute lung injury (1 in 12,000)	Transfusion Errors:
*Nosocomial Infections (?)	Wrong person transfused (1 in 15,000)
Acute hemolytic reaction (1 in 35,000)	Incompatible transfusion (1 in 33,000)
Fatal hemolytic reaction (1 in 1 million)	

Includes only acute complications. From References 33–39.
†The leading cause of transfusion-elated deaths.
*May be the most common adverse consequence of RBC transfusions.

Acute Hemolytic Reactions

Acute hemolytic reactions are prompted by the transfusion of RBCs that are ABO-incompatible with the recipient. When this occurs, antibodies in recipient blood bind to ABO antigens on the donor RBCs , and the ensuing lysis of donor RBCs triggers a systemic inflammatory response that can be accompanied by hypotension and multiorgan failure. These reactions are usually the result of human error.

Clinical Features

The hallmark of acute hemolytic reactions is the abrupt onset of fever, dyspnea, chest pain, low back pain, and hypotension within minutes after starting the transfusion. Severe reactions are accompanied by a consumptive coagulopathy and progressive multiorgan dysfunction.

Management

1. If a hemolytic reaction is suspected, STOP the transfusion immediately and verify that the correct blood was given to the correct patient. It is imperative to stop the transfusion as soon as possible because the severity of hemolytic reactions is a function of the volume of blood transfused (33).

2. If the donor blood is correctly matched to the patient, an acute hemolytic reaction is unlikely. However, the blood bank must be notified, and they will ask for blood samples to perform a plasma-free hemoglobin determination (for evidence of intravascular hemolysis) and a direct Coomb's test (for evidence of the anti-ABO antibody).

3. If an acute hemolytic reaction is confirmed, support blood pressure and ventilation as needed. The management of severe hemolytic reactions is similar to septic shock (i.e., volume resuscitation and a vasopressor, if necessary) because inflammation is the culprit in both conditions. Most patients with hemolytic reactions should survive the condition.

Febrile Nonhemolytic Reactions

A febrile nonhemolytic transfusion reaction is defined as a temperature elevation >1°C (1.8°F) that occurs during transfusion or up to 6 hours after transfusion, and is not attributed to another cause (e.g., acute hemolytic reaction) (35). The culprit is the presence of antileukocyte antibodies in recipient blood that react with antigens on donor leukocytes. This triggers the release of endogenous pyrogens from phagocytes, which is the source of the fever. This reaction is reported in 0.5% of RBC transfusions (once per 200 transfusions), and occurs in patients who have received prior transfusions, and in multiparous women. Transfusion of leukocyte-reduced RBCs reduces, but does not eliminate, the risk of this reaction (35).

Clinical Features

The fever typically does not appear in the first hour after the start of transfusion (unlike the fever associated with acute hemolytic reactions), and it can be accompanied by rigors and chills.

Management

1. The initial approach to transfusion-related fever is the same as described for hemolytic transfusion reactions, even though the fever may not appear until after the transfusion is completed. The diagno-

sis is confirmed by excluding the presence of hemolysis with the tests described previously.

2. The blood bank will perform a Gram stain on the donor blood, and may request blood cultures on the recipient. This is usually unrewarding because microbial contamination in stored blood is rare (1 per 5,000,000 units). The organism most frequently isolated in stored RBCs is *Yersinia enterocolitica* (34).

3. More than 75% of patients with a nonhemolytic fever will not experience a similar reaction to subsequent transfusions (34). Therefore, no special precautions are needed for future transfusions. If a second febrile reaction occurs, leukocyte-reduced RBCs are advised for all subsequent transfusions.

Hypersensitivity Reactions

Hypersensitivity reactions are the result of sensitization to plasma proteins in donor blood from prior transfusions. Patients with IgA deficiency are prone to hypersensitivity transfusion reactions, and prior exposure to plasma products is not required. The most common hypersensitivity reaction is urticaria, which is reported in one of every 100 units transfused (36). More severe anaphylactic reactions (e.g., bronchospasm) are much less common, and anaphylactic shock is rare.

Clinical Features

The usual manifestation is mild urticaria that appears during the transfusion and is not accompanied by fever. The abrupt onset of dyspnea during a transfusion could represent laryngeal edema or bronchospasm, and hypotension from anaphylactic shock can be mistaken for an acute hemolytic reaction.

Management

1. Mild urticaria without fever does not require interruption of the transfusion. However, the popular practice is to stop the transfusion temporarily and administer an antihistamine for symptom relief (e.g., diphenhydramine, 25–50 mg PO, IM, or IV).

2. Severe anaphylactic reactions should be managed as described in Chapter 14. The transfusion should be stopped immediately if severe anaphylaxis is suspected.

3. Washed RBCs should be used for all future transfusions in patients with hypersensitivity reactions. However, in patients with severe anaphylactic reactions, future transfusions are risky, even with washed RBCs, and should be avoided unless absolutely necessary.

4. Patients who develop hypersensitivity reactions should be tested for an underlying IgA deficiency.

Acute Lung Injury

Transfusion-related acute lung injury (TRALI) is an inflammatory lung injury associated with RBC and platelet transfusion (38), and resembles the acute respiratory distress syndrome (ARDS), which is described in Chapter 23. Recent surveys show an incidence of 1 per 12,000 transfusions (38), and a mortality rate of 6% (37). TRALI is considered the leading cause of transfusion-related deaths (37).

Etiology

The prevailing theory is that TRALI is the result of antileukocyte antibodies in donor blood that bind to antigens on circulating neutrophils in the recipient. This triggers neutrophil activation, and the activated neutrophils become sequestered in pulmonary capillaries and migrate into the lungs to produce the inflammatory injury. The risk of TRALI is higher when donor blood contains high levels of antileukocyte antibodies, and in donor blood from females (37). The link between female blood and TRALI is not well understood.

Clinical Features

Signs of respiratory compromise (dyspnea, tachypnea, hypoxemia, etc.) can appear for up to 6 hours after the start of a transfusion, but they usu-

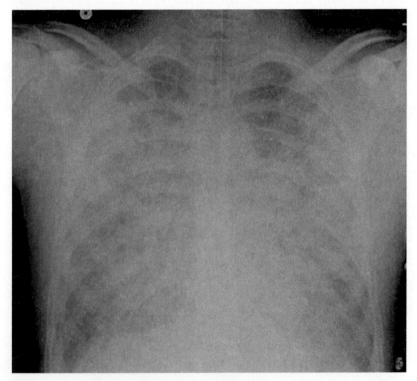

FIGURE 18.5 Portable chest film from a patient with transfusion-related acute lung injury. Note the homogeneous pattern of infiltration in the lungs, and the fine "ground-glass" appearance of the infiltrates, which are characteristics of inflammatory lung injury.

ally appear within the first hour after the transfusion begins (37). Fever is common, and the chest x-ray eventually looks like the one in Figure 18.5, with diffuse, homogeneous infiltrates in both lungs that are indistinguishable from ARDS. The diagnosis of TRALI is based on the clinical setting (i.e., ARDS that appears within 6 hours after the start of a blood transfusion). The chest x-ray can be mistaken for acute hydrostatic pulmonary edema, but this can be excluded based on the clinical setting. TRALI can be severe at the outset, and often requires mechanical ventilation, but the condition typically resolves within a week (37).

Management

1. If the transfusion is not completed, it should be stopped at the first signs of respiratory difficulty. The blood bank should be notified for all cases of TRALI. (Assays for antileukocyte antibodies are available, but are not currently used in the diagnostic evaluation of TRALI.)

2. The management of TRALI is supportive, and is very similar to the management of ARDS described in Chapter 23.

3. There are no firm recommendations regarding future transfusions in patients who develop TRALI. Some recommend using washed RBCs to remove antibodies from donor blood, but the effectiveness of this measure is not known.

Nosocomial Infections

The immunosuppressive effects of blood transfusions became evident with the discovery (in the early 1970s) that pre-transplant blood transfusions improved the survival rate of renal allografts (39). Since then, a multitude of clinical studies have shown that patients who receive blood transfusions have a higher incidence of nosocomial infections (32,39–41). The risk of infection increases with the volume of blood transfused (see Figure 18.6), and with the storage time of donor blood (42). There has been some concern that the association between blood transfusions and infection is not a causal relationship, but instead is a reflection of severity of illness (i.e., sicker patients develop more infections and they also require more blood transfusions). However, at least 22 studies have shown that blood transfusion is an independent risk factor for nosocomial infections (32).

Transfusion-related immunosuppression is poorly understood, but the emerging opinion is that *nosocomial infections are a major source of transfusion-related morbidity and mortality in critically ill patients* (32).

Clinical Outcomes

A review of 45 clinical studies evaluating RBC transfusions in critically ill patients, which included 272,596 patients, revealed the following findings (32):

1. In 42 of the 45 studies, the adverse effects of RBC transfusions outweighed any benefits.

2. Only 1 of 45 studies showed that the benefits of RBC transfusions outweighed the adverse effects.

3. Eighteen studies evaluated the relationship between RBC transfusions and survival, and 17 of the 18 studies showed that RBC transfusions were an independent risk factor for death. The likelihood of a fatal outcome was, on average, 70% higher in patients who received an RBC transfusion.

Not a very good report card, is it? These observations, combined with those showing that RBC transfusions do not improve tissue oxygenation, suggest that the current practice of transfusing RBCs to increase the Hb concentration in blood may simply be *bad medicine.*

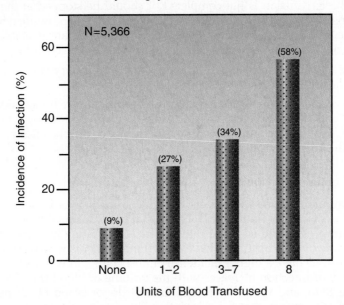

FIGURE 18.6 Results of a large multicenter study showing the relationship between the incidence of nosocomial infections and the volume of blood transfused in critically ill patients. N = number of patients in the study. From Reference 40.

A FINAL WORD

Blood Volume vs. RBCs

The practice of transfusing RBCs to raise the Hb level in blood is rooted in the belief that anemia is a threat to tissue oxygenation. However, as described earlier in the chapter, the severest anemias do not threaten tissue oxygenation as long as the intravascular volume (and hence cardiac output) is maintained. The supremacy of blood volume over RBCs in supporting tissue oxygenation is evident when you consider that hypovolemia is a recognized cause of impaired tissue oxygenation (i.e., hypovolemic shock), but anemia is not (i.e., "anemic shock" is not a clinical entity). The importance of blood volume is often overlooked, even by the American Red Cross, whose popular slogan, *blood saves lives*, deserves a more accurate update, as shown in Figure 18.7. Awareness of the attributes of blood volume would help to curb the undeserved emphasis on the transfusion of RBCs to support tissue oxygenation.

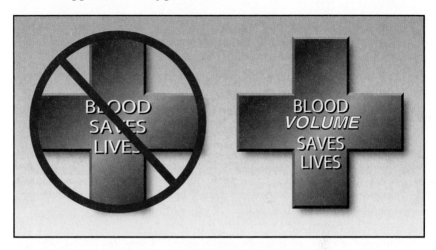

FIGURE 18.7 A popular slogan of the American Red Cross on the left, and an amended version on the right that recognizes the contribution of intravascular volume in the survival benefit of blood transfusions.

REFERENCES

King KE (ed). Blood Transfusion Therapy: A Physician's Handbook. 9th ed. Bethesda, MD: American Association of Blood Banks, 2008.

Introduction

1. Hebert PC, Tinmouth A, Corwin HL. Controversies in RBC transfusions in the critically ill. Chest 2007; 131:1583–1590.
2. Bennet-Guerrero E, Zhao Y, O'Brien SM, et al. Variation in the use of blood transfusion in coronary artery bypass graft surgery. JAMA 2010; 304:1568–1575.

Clinical Practice Guidelines

3. Napolitano LM, Kurek S, Luchette FA, et al. Clinical practice guideline: Red blood cell transfusion in adult trauma and critical care. Crit Care Med 2009; 37:3124–3157.
4. Ferraris VA, Ferraris SP, Saha SP, et al. Perioperative blood transfusion and blood conservation in cardiac surgery; the Society of Thoracic Surgeons and the Society of Cardiovascular Anesthesiologists Clinical Practice Guideline. Ann Thorac Surg 2007; 83(suppl):S27–S86.

Anemia in the ICU

5. Jacob G, Raj SR, Ketch T, et al. Postural pseudoanemia: posture-dependent change in hematocrit. Mayo Clin Proc 2005; 80:611-614.

6. Jones JG, Holland BM, Wardrop CAJ. Total circulating red cells versus hematocrit as a primary descriptor of oxygen transport by the blood. Br J Hematol 1990; 76:228-232.

7. Cordts PR, LaMorte WW, Fisher JB, et al. Poor predictive value of hematocrit and hemodynamic parameters for erythrocyte deficits after extensive elective vascular operations. Surg Gynecol Obstet 1992; 175:243-248.

8. Prakash D. Anemia in the ICU. Crit Care Clin 2012; 28:333-343.

9. Smoller BR, Kruskall MS. Phlebotomy for diagnostic laboratory tests in adults: Pattern of use and effect on transfusion requirements. N Engl J Med 1986; 314:1233-1235.

10. Corwin HL, Parsonnet KC, Gettinger A, et al. RBC transfusion in the ICU: Is there a reason? Chest 1995; 108:767-771.

11. Silver MJ, Li Y-H, Gragg LA, et al. Reduction of blood loss from diagnostic sampling in critically ill patients using a blood-conserving arterial line system. Chest 1993; 104:1711-1715.

12. Wilkerson DK, Rosen AL, Gould SA, et al. Oxygen extraction ratio: a valid indicator of myocardial metabolism in anemia. J Surg Res 1987; 42:629-634.

13. Levine E, Rosen A, Sehgal L, et al. Physiologic effects of acute anemia: implications for a reduced transfusion trigger. Transfusion 1990; 30:11-14.

14. Nielsen VG, Baird MS, Brix A, Matalon S. Extreme, progressive isovolemic hemodilution with 5% albumin, PentaLyte, or hextend does not cause hepatic ischemia or histologic injury in rabbits. Anesthesiology 1999; 90:1428-1435.

15. Weiskopf RB, Viele M, Feiner J, et al. Human cardiovascular and metabolic response to acute, severe, isovolemic anemia. JAMA 1998; 279:217-221.

16. Hansen ES, Gellett S, Kirkegard L, et al. Tissue oxygen tension in random pattern skin flaps during normovolemic hemodilution. J Surg Res 1989; 47:24-29.

17. Hebert PC, McDonald BJ, Tinmouth A. Clinical consequences of anemia and red cell transfusion in the critically ill. Crit Care Clin 2004; 20:225-235.

Transfusion Triggers

18. Corwin HL, Gettinger A, Pearl R, et al. The CRIT study: anemia and blood transfusion in the critically ill – Current clinical practice in the United States. Crit Care Med 2004; 32:39-52.

19. Adam RC, Lundy JS. Anesthesia in cases of poor risk: Some suggestions for decreasing the risk. Surg Gynecol Obstet 1942; 74:1011-1101.

20. Hebert PC, Wells G, Blajchman MA, et al. A multicenter, randomized, controlled clinical trial of transfusion requirements in critical care. N Engl J Med 1999; 340:409-417.

21. Hebert PC, Yetisir E, Martin C, et al. Is a low transfusion threshold safe in critically ill patients with cardiovascular disease. Crit Care Med 2001; 29:227-234.

22. Consensus Conference on Perioperative Red Blood Cell Transfusion. JAMA 1988; 260:2700–2702.

23. Levy PS, Chavez RP, Crystal GJ, et al. Oxygen extraction ratio: a valid indicator of transfusion need in limited coronary vascular reserve? J Trauma 1992; 32:769–774.

24. Vallet B, Robin E, Lebuffe G. Venous oxygen saturation as a physiologic transfusion trigger. Crit Care 2010; 14:213–217.

Erythrocyte Transfusions

25. King KE (ed). Blood Transfusion Therapy: A Physician's Handbook. 9th ed. Bethesda, MD: American Association of Blood Banks, 2008:1–18.

26. Ibid, pp. 91–95.

27. Conrad SA, Dietrich KA, Hebert CA, Romero MD. Effects of red cell transfusion on oxygen consumption following fluid resuscitation in septic shock. Circ Shock 1990; 31:419–429.

28. Dietrich KA, Conrad SA, Hebert CA, et al. Cardiovascular and metabolic response to red blood cell transfusion in critically ill volume-resuscitated nonsurgical patients. Crit Care Med 1990; 18:940–944.

29. Marik PE, Sibbald W. Effect of stored-blood transfusion on oxygen delivery in patients with sepsis. JAMA 1993; 269:3024–3029.

30. Fuller BM, Gajera M, Schorr C, et al. Transfusion of packed red blood cells is not associated with improved central venous oxygen saturation or organ function in patients with septic shock. J Emerg Med 2012; 43:593–598.

31. Kiraly LN, Underwood S, Differding JA, Schreiber MA. Transfusion of aged packed red blood cells results in decreased tissue oxygenation in critically ill trauma patients. J Trauma 2009; 67:29–32.

32. Marik PE, Corwin HL. Efficacy of red blood cell transfusion in the critically ill: A systematic review of the literature. Crit Care Med 2008; 36:2667–2674.

Transfusion Risks

33. Kuriyan M, Carson JL. Blood transfusion risks in the intensive care unit. Crit Care Clin 2004; 237–253.

34. Goodnough LT. Risks of blood transfusion. Crit Care Med 2003; 31:S678–S686.

35. King KE (ed). Acute transfusion reactions. In: Blood Transfusion Therapy: A Physician's Handbook 9th ed. Bethesda, MD: American Association of Blood Banks, 2008:148–173.

36. Greenberger PA. Plasma anaphylaxis and immediate-type reactions. In: Rossi EC, Simon TL, Moss GS (eds). Principles of transfusion medicine. Philadelphia: Williams & Wilkins, 1991:635–639.

37. Transfusion reactions: newer concepts on the pathophysiology, incidence, treatment, and prevention of transfusion-related acute lung injury. Crit Care Clin 2012; 28:363–372.

38. Toy P, Gajic O, Bachetti P, et al. Transfusion-related acute lung injury: incidence and risk factors. Blood 2012; 119:1757–1767.

39. Vamvakas EC, Blajchman MA. Transfusion-related immunomodulation (TRIM): an update. Blood Rev 2007; 21:327–348.

40. Agarwal N, Murphy JG, Cayten CG, Stahl WM. Blood transfusion increases the risk of infection after trauma. Arch Surg 1993; 128:171–177.

41. Taylor RW, O'Brien J, Trottier SJ, et al. Red blood cell transfusions and nosocomial infections in critically ill patients. Crit Care Med 2006; 34:2302–2308.

42. Juffermans NP, Prins DJ, Viaar AP, et al. Transfusion-related risk of secondary bacterial infections in sepsis patients: a retrospective cohort study. Shock 2011; 35:355–359.

Chapter 19

PLATELETS AND PLASMA

Hemorrhage upon a strong pulsation in wounds is bad.

Hippocrates
Aphorisms
(400 B.C.)

The last chapter was devoted to the red blood cell and its relationship with tissue oxygenation. The spotlight now shifts to the platelet and plasma components of blood, and their relationship with the tendency to bleed.

OVERVIEW OF HEMOSTASIS

The vascular endothelium is a thromboresistant surface that helps to maintain the "fluidity" of blood in three ways (1). First, endothelial cells secrete substances like nitric oxide and prostacyclin that inhibit platelet adhesiveness. Secondly, a glycoprotein on the surface of endothelial cells, known as *thrombomodulin*, serves as an endogenous anticoagulant by activating protein C (which inactivates clotting factors V and VII). Finally, the endothelium serves as a barrier that separates the blood from tissue elements that can trigger thrombosis.

Response to Injury

When the endothelium is disrupted, platelets adhere to exposed collagen in the subendothelium and begin to form a *platelet plug*. The platelets release calcium, which activates the glycoprotein receptor IIb/IIIa complex on the platelet surface. This receptor complex binds irreversibly to von Willebrand factor on the surrounding endothelial cells, which helps to anchor the platelet plug to the vessel wall. The IIb/IIIa receptor complex also binds fibrinogen, and the subsequent formation of fibrin bridges between adjacent platelets allows the platelet plug to grow and mature into a fibrin-platelet thrombus. (Drugs that inhibit the IIb/IIIa receptor complex are used in the management of acute coronary syndromes—see page 315).

Endothelial and tissue injury also promote the formation of fibrin, which is essential for the growth and stability of the developing thrombus. There are two pathways to fibrin formation (2). The major pathway is called the *Tissue Factor Pathway* (formerly called the Extrinsic Pathway), and is activated by the release of thromboplastin (tissue factor) from the subendothelium. The second pathway is the *Contact Activation Pathway* (formerly called the Intrinsic Pathway), and is activated by endogenous peptides known as kininogens, which are precursors of bradykinin. Both pathways involve the activation of specific procoagulant proteins known as clotting factors, and they both lead to the activation of prothrombin (factor II) and the subsequent conversion of fibrinogen (factor I) to fibrin monomers.

The end-product of the response to injury is the *thrombus*, which is essentially a clump of platelets embedded in a meshwork of fibrin strands and anchored to vessel wall in the area of injury.

THROMBOCYTOPENIA

Thrombocytopenia is the most common hemostatic disorder in critically ill patients, with a reported incidence as high as 60% (3,4). The traditional definition of thrombocytopenia is a platelet count below 150,000/μL, but the ability to form a hemostatic plug is retained until the platelet count falls below 100,000/μL (4), so a platelet count < 100,000/μL is more appropriate for identifying clinically significant thrombocytopenia. However, *the risk of major bleeding is not determined by the platelet count alone*, but also requires a structural lesion that is prone to bleeding. In the absence of such a lesion, platelet counts as low as 5,000/μL can be tolerated without evidence of major hemorrhage (5). The major risk with a platelet count < 10,000/μL is spontaneous intracerebral hemorrhage, which is uncommon (4).

Pseudothrombocytopenia

Pseudothrombocytopenia is a condition where antibodies to EDTA (the anticoagulant in blood collection tubes) produce clumping of platelets in vitro. The clumped platelets are misread as leukocytes by automated machines that perform cell counts, and this results in a spuriously low platelet count (4,6). This phenomenon has been reported in 2% of platelet counts performed in hospitalized patients (6), and is most often seen in patients with severe sepsis or autoimmune, neoplastic, or liver disease (4).

Suspicion of pseudothrombocytopenia is usually prompted by a platelet count that is lower than expected, or by the presence of clumped platelets on the peripheral blood smear. If suspected, blood collection tubes that use citrate or heparin as an anticoagulant should be used for subsequent platelet counts.

Critically Ill Patients

The most likely causes of thrombocytopenia in the ICU setting are listed in Table 19.1. Systemic sepsis is the most common cause of thrombocy-topenia in ICU patients (7), and is the result of increased platelet destruc-tion by macrophages (8). Other less common but more life-threatening causes of thrombocytopenia include heparin and the thrombotic micro-angiopathies; i.e., disseminated intravascular coagulation (DIC), throm-botic thrombocytopenia purpura (TTP), and the pregnancy-related HELLP syndrome.

Table 19.1	Most Likely Causes of Thrombocytopenia in ICU Patients	
Nonpharmacological	**Pharmacological**	
Cardiopulmonary Bypass	Anticonvulsants:	
	Phenytoin	
Disseminated Intravascular	Valproic Acid	
Coagulation (DIC)	Antimicrobial Agents:	
HELLP Syndrome	β-Lactams	
	Linezolid	
Hemolytic-Uremic Syndrome	TMP/SMX	
	Vancomycin	
HIV Infection	Antineoplastic Agents	
Intra-Aortic Balloon Pump	Antithrombotic Agents	
	Heparin	
Liver Disease/Hypersplenism	IIb/IIIa Inhibitors	
Massive Transfusion	Histamine H_2 Blockers	
Renal Replacement Therapy	Miscellaneous Drugs	
	Amiodarone	
Systemic Sepsis[†]	Furosemide	
Thrombotic Thrombocytopenia	Thiazides	
Purpura (TTP)	Morphine	

[†]The most common cause of thrombocytopenia in the ICU setting.
From References 3, 4, 8, 9.

Drugs like antineoplastic agents can produce thrombocytopenia by sup-pressing platelet production in the bone marrow, but the most common mechanism for drug-induced thrombocytopenia is the production of antibodies that cross-react with platelets (8). This immune-mediated thrombocytopenia is most frequently observed with heparin, and less frequently with platelet glycoprotein receptor (IIb/IIIa) antagonists and selected antibiotics (particularly linezolid, β-lactams, and vancomycin).

Heparin-Induced Thrombocytopenia

There are two types of thrombocytopenia associated with heparin. The first is a nonimmune response that results in mild thrombocytopenia (platelet counts may not fall below 100,000/μL) in the first few days after starting heparin. This reaction is reported in 10 to 30% of patients receiving heparin (10), and it resolves spontaneously without interruption of heparin, and without adverse consequences. The second type of thrombocytopenia is an immune response that typically appears 5 to 10 days after starting heparin (10,11). This reaction is much less common (incidence = 1–3%) but is much more serious; i.e., it can produce life-threatening thrombosis (not hemorrhage), and has a mortality rate as high as 30% if left unnoticed (10). The term *heparin-induced thrombocytopenia* (HIT) is reserved for the immune-mediated thrombocytopenia, and this condition is the focus of the current presentation.

Pathogenesis

Heparin is not immunogenic itself, but it binds to a protein (platelet factor 4) on platelets to form an antigenic complex that can trigger the formation of IgG antibodies. These antibodies bind to platelets and induce a strong platelet activation response to promote thrombosis. These antibodies can also bind to endothelial cells and promote the release of tissue factor from the endothelium; this promotes fibrin formation and further accelerates the thrombotic process. The reticuloendothelial system can clear antibody-coated platelets, and this helps to limit the incidence of thrombosis. Heparin-associated antibodies usually disappear within 3 months after discontinuing heparin (10).

Risk Factors

One of the most important features of HIT is the fact that it is *not a dose-dependent reaction*, and can occur as a result of heparin exposure from heparin-based flushes of intravascular catheters, or even heparin-coated pulmonary artery catheters (12). The type of heparin preparation does, however, influence the risk of HIT; i.e., *the risk of HIT is ten times greater with unfractionated heparin (UFH) than with low-molecular-weight heparin (LMWH)* (11). The risk of HIT also varies by patient population; i.e., it is highest in patients undergoing orthopedic and cardiac surgical procedures, and lowest in medical patients (10,11). The reported incidence of HIT with UFH is 1–5% following orthopedic or cardiac surgery, and 0.1–1% in medical patients (11).

Clinical Features

HIT typically appears 5 to 10 days after the first exposure to heparin, but can appear within 24 hours in patients with HIT antibodies due to heparin exposure within the past 3 months (11). Platelet counts are usually between 50,000/μL and 150,000/μL. Severe thrombocytopenia (< 20,000/mL) is uncommon in HIT (10,11). *In up to 25% of cases of HIT, the thrombosis precedes the thrombocytopenia* (11).

THROMBOSIS: Venous thrombosis is more common than arterial thrombosis. Reports indicate that 17% to 55% of patients with untreated HIT develop deep vein thrombosis in the legs and/or pulmonary embolism, whereas only 1% to 3% of patients develop arterial thromboses resulting in limb ischemia, thrombotic stroke, or acute myocardial infarction (11). Limb gangrene from thrombotic veno-occlusion has been reported in 5% to 10% of patients with HIT who are treated with a vitamin K antagonist (e.g., coumadin).

Diagnosis

About 8 different assays are currently used to detect HIT antibodies. The most popular of these is an enzyme-linked immunosorbent assay (ELISA) for antibodies to the platelet factor 4-heparin complex. A negative assays helps to exclude the diagnosis of HIT, but a positive assay does not confirm the diagnosis because HIT antibodies do not always promote thrombocytopenia or thrombosis (11). The diagnosis of HIT requires a positive antibody assay in combination with a high index of clinical suspicion.

Table 19.2	Anticoagulation with Direct Thrombin Inhibitors
Drug	**Dosing Regimen and Comments**
Argatroban	Dosing: Infuse at 2 µkg/kg/min and titrate dose to achieve aPTT = 1.5–3 × control. Max. dose is 10 µg/kg/min. In patients with liver failure, reduce initial infusion rate to 0.5 µkg/kg/min.
	Comment: Argatroban is cleared by the liver, and may be preferred in patients with renal insufficiency.
Lepirudin	Dosing: Start with IV bolus of 0.4 mg in cases of life-threatening thrombosis. Begin infusion at 0.15 mg/kg/h and titrate to achieve aPTT = 1.5–3 × control. In renal failure, reduce IV bolus to 0.2 mg/kg and adjust infusion rate as follows:

Serum Creatinine	Reduce Initial Infusion by
1.6–2 mg/dL	50%
2.1–3	70%
3.1–6	85%
>6	Avoid

	Comment: Severe anaphylactic reactions can occur with re-exposure to lepirudin, so only a single course of therapy is advised.

From References 10, 11, 14.

Acute Management

Heparin must be discontinued immediately (don't forget to discontinue heparin flushes and remove heparin-coated catheters). Therapeutic anticoagulation with one of the *direct thrombin inhibitors* shown in Table 19.2

should be started immediately, even in cases where HIT is not accompanied by thrombosis (11). The recommendation for full anticoagulation without evidence of thrombosis is based on studies showing a 10-fold higher incidence of thrombosis following the appearance of HIT when anticoagulation is delayed (13).

ARGATROBAN: Argatroban is a synthetic analogue of L-arginine that reversibly binds to the active site on thrombin. It has a rapid onset of action, and is given by continuous infusion using the dosing regimen in Table 19.2. The therapeutic goal is an activated partial thromboplastin time (aPTT) of 1.5 to 3 times control values. The drug is cleared primarily by the liver, and a dose adjustment is necessary in hepatic insufficiency. Argatroban is *recommended in patients with renal insufficiency* (11) because a dose adjustment is not necessary.

LEPIRUDIN: Lepirudin is a recombinant form of hirudin, an anticoagulant found in leech saliva (!) that binds irreversibly to thrombin. Lepirudin is also given by continuous infusion, which can be preceded by a bolus injection in cases of life-threatening thrombosis. The therapeutic goal is the same as with argatroban (aPTT = 1.5–3 × control). Lepirudin is cleared by the kidneys, and a dose adjustment is necessary when renal function is even mildly impaired (i.e., when the serum creatinine is above 1.5 mg/dL), as shown in Table 19.2 (14). Using argatroban in patients with renal impairment will avoid dosing adjustments. Finally, re-exposure to lepirudin can produce life-threatening anaphylactic reactions (11), so the treatment of HIT with lepirudin is usually a one-time affair.

DURATION OF TREATMENT: Full anticoagulation with argatroban or lepirudin is recommended until the platelet count rises above 150,000/µL (11). Thereafter, coumadin can be used for long-term anticoagulation if HIT is associated with thrombosis, but there are 2 caveats: (a) coumadin should NOT be started until the platelet count increases beyond 150,000/µL, and (b) the initial coumadin dose should not exceed 5 mg (11). These precautions are intended to reduce the *risk of limb gangrene associated with coumadin therapy* during the active phase of HIT (as mentioned earlier). The antithrombin agents should be continued until coumadin achieves full anticoagulation.

Thrombotic Microangiopathies

A *thrombotic microangiopathy* is a clinical disorder with the following features:

1. Widespread microvascular thrombosis with multiorgan dysfunction or failure.

2. A consumptive thrombocytopenia.

3. Fragmentation of erythrocytes in the clot-filled microvasculature, resulting in a *microangiopathic hemolytic anemia*.

These features are identified in the following clinical disorders:

A. Disseminated intravascular coagulation (DIC).

B. Thrombotic thrombocytopenia purpura (TTP).

C. The HELLP syndrome: hemolysis, elevated liver enzymes, and low platelets.

The comparative features of these 3 conditions are shown in Table 19.3.

Table 19.3	Comparative Features of the Thrombotic Microangiopathies		
Feature	**DIC**	**TTP**	**HELLP**
Schistocytes	Present	Present	Present
Platelets	Low	Low	Low
INR	Elevated	Normal	Normal
aPTT	Prolonged	Normal	Normal
Fibrinogen	Low	Normal	Normal
Plasma D-dimer	Elevated	Normal	Normal
Liver Enzymes	Variable	Normal	Elevated

From Reference 4.

Disseminated Intravascular Coagulation

Disseminated intravascular coagulation (DIC) is a secondary disorder that is triggered by conditions that produce widespread tissue injury such as multisystem trauma, severe sepsis and septic shock, and obstetric emergencies (amniotic fluid embolism, abruptio placentae, eclampsia, and retained fetus syndrome). The inciting event is release of *tissue factor*, which (as described earlier) activates a series of clotting factors in the bloodstream that culminates in the formation of fibrin. This leads to widespread microvascular thrombosis and secondary depletion of platelets and clotting factors, resulting in a *consumptive coagulopathy* (15).

Clinical Features

The microvascular thrombosis in DIC can lead to multiorgan failure, most often involving the lungs, kidneys, and central nervous system, while depletion of platelets and coagulation factors can promote bleeding, particularly from pre-existing lesions in the GI tract such as stress ulcers. DIC can also be accompanied by symmetrical necrosis and ecchymosis involving the limbs, a condition known as *purpura fulminans* that is usually seen with overwhelming systemic sepsis, most notably with meningococcemia (7).

HEMATOLOGIC ABNORMALITIES: In addition to thrombocytopenia, DIC is usually (but not always) associated with elevation of the INR (i.e., prolongation of the prothrombin time) and prolongation of the activated partial thromboplastin time (aPTT), both abnormalities being the result of consumption and subsequent depletion of clotting factors in blood. The enhanced thrombosis is also accompanied by enhanced fibrinolysis, which elevates the fibrin degradation products in plasma (i.e., plasma D-dimers). Finally, the microangiopathic hemolytic anemia is identified by the presence of damaged or fragmented erythrocytes in a peripheral blood smear, like the ones in Figure 19.1. The fragmented erythrocytes are known as *schistocytes*, and they are the hallmark of the thrombotic microangiopathies.

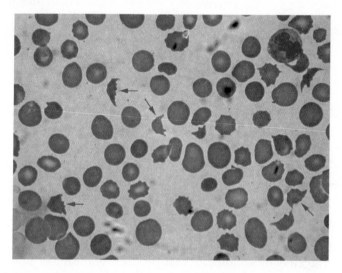

FIGURE 19.1 Peripheral blood smear from a patient with DIC. The arrows are pointing to schistocytes, which are fragmented erythrocytes. Their presence in a peripheral blood smear confirms the presence of a microangiopathic hemolytic anemia.

Management

There is no specific treatment for DIC other than supportive care. Uncontrolled bleeding often prompts consideration of replacement therapy with platelets and coagulation factors (plasma products), but this rarely helps and can be deleterious by "adding fuel" to the microvascular thrombosis. In severe cases of DIC associated with multiorgan failure, the mortality rate is 80% or higher (7,15).

Thrombotic Thrombocytopenia Purpura

Thrombotic thrombocytopenia purpura (TTP) is thrombotic microangiopathy that is caused by platelet binding to abnormal von Willebrand factor on microvascular endothelium (4). This can be a devastating condition that is fatal within 24 hours of onset. There is often no predisposing condition, although it seems to follow a nonspecific viral illness in some cases.

Clinical Features

TTP presents with a characteristic *pentad* of clinical manifestations that includes fever, altered mental status, acute renal failure, thrombocytopenia, and microangiopathic hemolytic anemia. The presence of all 5 conditions is not necessary for the diagnosis of TTP, but the diagnosis does require thrombocytopenia and evidence of a microangiopathic hemolytic anemia (e.g., schistocytes in the peripheral blood smear). TTP can be distinguished from DIC because clotting factors are not depleted in TTP, *so the INR, aPTT, and fibrinogen levels are normal in TTP.*

Management

Platelet transfusions are contraindicated in TTP because they can aggravate the underlying thrombosis. *The treatment of choice for TTP is plasma exchange* (16,17), where blood from the patient is diverted to a device that separates and discards the patient's plasma and reinfuses plasma from a healthy donor. This is continued until 1.5 times the normal plasma volume is exchanged, and this process is repeated daily for 3–7 days. Acute fulminant TTP is almost always fatal if untreated, but if plasma exchange is started early (with 48 hours of symptom onset), as many as 90% of patients can survive the illness (16,17).

HELLP Syndrome

HELLP (Hemolysis, Elevated Liver enzymes, Low Platelets) syndrome is a thrombotic microangiopathy that occurs late in pregnancy or in the early postpartum period (18). About 20% of cases are associated with severe pre-eclampsia, and there is also an association with the antiphospholipid syndrome (19). The culprit in the HELLP syndrome is unexplained activation of clotting factors and platelets leading to microvascular thrombosis. There is also an unexplained elevation in liver enzymes, principally the transaminases (18).

Clinical Features

As the name indicates, HELLP is identified by the characteristic *triad* of hemolysis, thrombocytopenia, and elevated liver enzymes. HELLP can be confused with DIC (which can occur in the same clinical settings), but the INR and aPTT are usually normal in HELLP because there is no depletion of clotting factors, and this feature should distinguish HELLP from DIC (see Table 19.3).

The HELLP syndrome is an obstetric emergency, and a detailed description of this condition is beyond the scope of this text. For more information on HELLP, some recent reviews are included in the bibliography at the end of the chapter (18,19).

PLATELET TRANSFUSIONS

Platelet Products

Platelets are obtained either by pooling the platelets from multiple donors, or by extracting platelets from a single donor using apheresis techniques.

Pooled Platelets

Platelets are separated from fresh whole blood by differential centrifugation, and the resulting platelet concentrates from 5 units of whole blood (from 5 individual donors) are pooled together prior to storage. The pooled platelet concentrate contains about 38×10^{10} platelets in 260 mL plasma, which is equivalent to a platelet count of about $130 \times 10^9/\mu L$. This is six orders of magnitude higher than the normal platelet count in blood ($150-400 \times 10^3/\mu L$). Platelets are stored at $20-24°C$, and can be stored for up to 5 days.

Apheresis Platelets

Apheresis platelets are collected from a single donor and have a platelet count and volume that is equivalent to the pooled platelets from 5 donors. The presumed benefit of single-donor platelet transfusions is a lower risk of transmitted infections and a lower incidence of platelet *alloimmunization* (i.e., developing antibodies to donor platelets). However, neither of these proposed benefits has been documented in clinical trials (20), and when leukocytes are removed from platelet products, there is no difference in the risk of platelet alloimmunization with single-donor and multiple-donor platelet transfusions (22).

Leukoreduction

Leukocytes in donor blood have been implicated in several adverse reactions, and leukocyte removal using specialized filters is now a routine practice for erythrocyte transfusions (see last chapter). Platelet concentrates are not free of leukocytes, and leukocyte reduction for platelet transfusions has the following advantages (20,22): a lower incidence of cytomegalovirus transmission (because this organism is transmitted in leukocytes), fewer febrile reactions, and a lower incidence of platelet alloimmunization. Because of these advantages, leukocyte reduction is becoming a routine practice for platelet transfusions.

Response to Transfused Platelets

In an average sized adult with no ongoing blood loss, *a platelet concentrate from one unit of whole blood should raise the circulating platelet count by 7,000 to 10,000/μL at one hour post-transfusion* (20). Since an average of 5 platelet concentrates are pooled together for each platelet transfusion, the expected (or ideal) increase in platelet count is 35,000 to 50,000/μL at one hour post-transfusion. The increment is about 40% lower after 24 hours, as shown in Figure 19.2. Note: The number of platelet concentrates that are pooled together can differ slightly (by ± 1 unit) in individual platelet transfusions, so if you want to be precise about estimating post-transfusion platelet increments (which is usually not necessary), you need to enquire about the number of units of platelets included in the transfusion pack.

Multiple Transfusions

The increment in platelet count declines with multiple transfusions. This is shown in Figure 19.2, where the platelet increment is about 25% lower after 5 platelet transfusions (23). As mentioned earlier, this phenomenon of "platelet refractoriness" is the result of antiplatelet antibodies in the recipient directed at ABO antigens on donor platelets. This effect can be mitigated by transfusing ABO-matched platelets.

Indications for Platelet Transfusions

Active Bleeding

In the presence of active bleeding other than ecchymoses or petechiae, platelet transfusions are recommended to maintain a platelet count >50,000/μL (21). For intracranial hemorrhage, higher platelet counts (>100,000/μL) should be maintained (21).

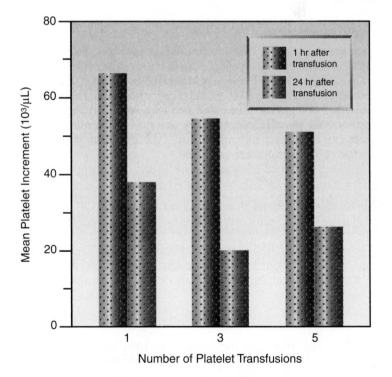

FIGURE 19.2 Post-transfusion increment in platelet counts in relation to the time elapsed after the transfusion (one hour versus 24 hours) and the number of transfusions given. Data from Reference 23.

No Active Bleeding

Despite evidence that spontaneous bleeding through an intact vascular system is uncommon with platelet counts down to 5,000/μL (20), most experts are reluctant to adopt a platelet transfusion trigger as low as 5,000/μL. In the absence of bleeding (other than ecchymoses or petechiae), prophylactic platelet transfusions are usually recommended when the platelet count reaches 10,000/μL (21).

Procedures

In the absence of associated coagulation abnormalities:

1. Platelet counts >40,000/μL are sufficient to perform laparotomy, craniotomy, tracheotomy, percutaneous liver biopsy, and bronchoscopic or endoscopic biopsy (20).

2. Platelet counts >20,000/μL are sufficient to perform lumbar punctures (20).

3. Platelet counts >10,000/μL are sufficient to perform central venous cannulation safely (24,25).

Adverse Effects

Bacterial Transmission

Bacteria are much more likely to flourish in platelet concentrates than in RBC concentrates (packed cells) because platelets are stored at room temperature (22°C), while RBCs are refrigerated at about 4°C. It is estimated that one in every 2,000 to 3,000 platelet concentrates harbors bacteria, and that one in 5,000 concentrates will produce sepsis in the recipient (16). Cultures of all platelet concentrates are now required (16) but, since platelets can be stored for only 5 days, the platelets can be transfused before the culture results are available.

Fever

Febrile nonhemolytic reactions have been reported in as many as 30% of platelet transfusions (26), which is much greater than the 0.5% rate of similar reactions reported with RBC transfusions (see Table 18.3 on page 359). Part of this difference may be related to the multiple donors used for platelet transfusions. Since antibodies to donor leukocytes are implicated in this reaction, leukoreduction of platelet products will help to alleviate this problem.

Hypersensitivity Reactions

Hypersensitivity reactions (urticaria, anaphylaxis, anaphylactic shock) are also more common with platelet transfusions that with erythrocyte transfusions (20). Since this is a reaction to proteins in donor plasma, removing the plasma from platelet concentrates will reduce the risk of hypersensitivity transfusion reactions.

Acute Lung Injury

Transfusion-related acute lung injury (TRALI) is described in Chapter 18 (see pages 361–363). This condition, which is an inflammatory lung injury similar to the acute respiratory distress syndrome (ARDS), is most often associated with erythrocyte transfusions, but has also been reported in association with platelet transfusions (27). The culprit is believed to be antileukocyte antibodies in donor blood that activate neutrophils in the recipient. TRALI usually appears within 6 hours after the start of a transfusion, and management is supportive.

PLASMA PRODUCTS

Plasma products are used as a source of coagulation factors, but surveys indicate that about 50% of plasma transfusions are inappropriate (28).

Fresh Frozen Plasma

Plasma is separated from donor blood and frozen at −18°C within 8 hours of blood collection. This *fresh frozen plasma* (FFP) has a volume of about 230 mL, and can be stored for one year. Once thawed, FFP can be stored at 1 to 6°C for up to 5 days. The principal uses of FFP include the resuscitation of massive blood loss, and the reversal of excess anticoagulation with coumadin.

Massive Blood Loss

As described in Chapter 11 (see pages 209–210), the use of FFP in massive blood loss (blood loss equivalent to one blood volume within 24 hours) has become more aggressive in recent years, mostly as a result of experiences in combat injuries. Whereas the traditional practice was to transfuse one unit of FFP for every 6 units of packed RBCs to prevent a dilutional coagulopathy, there is now evidence that severe trauma is accompanied by a coagulopathy (30), and survival rates have improved with FFP:RBC ratios of 1:2 to 1:3 during massive transfusion (31,32). This approach is called *hemostatic resuscitation*, and the goal is an INR that remains below 1.5. (Note: the international normalized ratio or INR is the ratio of the patient's prothrombin time and an international standard for the normal or control prothrombin time; i.e., INR = Patient's PT/standardized control PT.)

Warfarin-Induced Hemorrhage

The annual incidence of major bleeding during warfarin anticoagulation is 3 to 12%, and the incidence of fatal hemorrhage is 1 to 3% (33), with intracerebral hemorrhage causing most of the fatalities. The management of major or life-threatening hemorrhage related to excessive warfarin anticoagulation is shown in Table 19.4 (34,35). Since warfarin acts by inhibiting vitamin K-dependent clotting factors (i.e., factors II, VII, IX, X), vitamin K is administered to block ongoing anticoagulant activity. Clotting factors are then replenished, and this has traditionally involved the infusion of FFP at a volume of 15 mL/kg. There are two shortcomings with the use of FFP in this setting: the time to normalize the INR can be prolonged, and the volume of fluid required can aggravate the bleeding. These problems can be mitigated by using the plasma product described next.

PROTHROMBIN COMPLEX CONCENTRATE: Normalizing the INR quickly with a limited infusion volume is possible with *prothrombin complex concentrates* (PCC) using the dosing recommendations in Table 19.4. There are 3-factor and 4-factor PCC preparations (the name indicating the number of vitamin K-dependent clotting factors in the preparation), but only the 3-factor PCC is approved for clinical use. PCC is a lyophilized powder that is quickly reconstituted, thereby avoiding the time delays involved in thawing FFP. Whereas FFP can take hours to normalize the INR, PCC can accomplish this task in less than 30 minutes (34,35). The rapid response and limited volume associated with PCC make it well suited for the treatment of warfarin-induced bleeding, particularly intracerebral hemorrhage (35).

Table 19.4	Management of Warfarin-Induced Hemorrhage

1. Give 10 mg vitamin K intravenously over 10 minutes. (Do not exceed 1 mg/min to avoid hypersensitivity-like reactions.)

2. If available, give *prothrombin complex concentrate* (PCC) using the dosing recommendations shown below. Check the INR 30 min after each dose of PCC.

INR	PCC Dose
2–3.9	35–39 IU/kg
4–6	40–45 IU/kg
>6	46–50 IU/kg

3. If PCC is not available, give fresh frozen plasma, 15 mL/kg.

4. The management goal is an INR <1.5.

From References 34, 35.

Cryoprecipitate

When FFP is allowed to thaw at 4°C, a milky residue forms that is rich in cold-insoluble proteins (cryoglobulins) like fibrinogen, von Willebrand factor, and factor VIII. This cryoprecipitate can be separated from plasma and stored at –18°C for up to one year. The storage volume is 10 to 15 mL.

Cryoprecipitate was introduced in 1965 as a concentrated source of factor VIII for the management of hemophilia, but it has been replaced by recombinant factor VIII preparations. The current use of cryoprecipitate in the ICU is limited to uncontrolled uremic bleeding and selected cases of hypofibrinogenemia.

Uremic Bleeding

Platelet adhesion is impaired in renal failure (acute and chronic) as a result of abnormal platelet binding to fibrinogen and von Willebrand factor (which anchors the platelet plug to the endothelium, as mentioned previously). Bleeding times are prolonged when the serum creatinine climbs above 6 mg/dL, and dialysis corrects the bleeding time in only 30 to 50% of patients (36).

The significance of the impaired platelet adhesiveness in renal failure is unclear. However, upper GI bleeding is the second leading cause of death in acute renal failure (36), so there is reason to be concerned about this platelet function abnormality. There are two treatment options for uremic bleeding: desmopressin and cryoprecipitate.

DESMOPRESSIN: Desmopressin is a vasopressin analogue (deamino-arginine vasopressin or DDAVP) that does not have the vasoconstrictor or antidiuretic effects of vasopressin, but is capable of elevating plasma levels of von Willebrand factor and correcting the abnormal bleeding time in 75% of patients with renal failure (36,37). The recommended dose is *0.3 µg/kg IV or by subcutaneous injection, or 30 µg/kg by intranasal spray* (36,37). The effect lasts only 6 to 8 hours, and repeat dosing leads to tachyphylaxis.

Although desmopressin can correct the bleeding time in renal failure, the effect on uremic bleeding is not known. When uremic bleeding is worrisome, desmopressin can be given empirically in one or two doses (6 to 8 hours apart). If the bleeding persists, cryoprecipitate can be given (because it is rich in fibrinogen and von Willebrand factor, which are both involved in the platelet function abnormality in renal failure). The standard dose of cryoprecipitate for uremic bleeding is 10 units.

Hypofibrinogenemia

Cryoprecipitate can also be used as a source of fibrinogen in bleeding episodes associated with fibrinogen deficiency, such as variceal bleeding from liver failure. One unit of cryoprecipitate contains about 200 mg of fibrinogen, and infusion of 10 units of cryoprecipitate (2 grams of fibrinogen) should raise the serum fibrinogen level by about 70mg/dL in an average sized adult (38). The goal is a serum fibrinogen level above 100 mg/dL.

Adverse Effects

The risks associated with transfusion of plasma products are essentially the same risks associated with transfusion of erythrocytes and/or platelets. The exception is nonhemolytic febrile transfusion reactions, which are caused by donor leukocytes and thus should not occur with plasma transfusions.

Acute Hemolytic Reactions

Acute hemolytic reactions are caused by anti-A and anti-B antibodies in the transfused plasma that react with A and B antigens on recipient RBCs. Since cross-matching of plasma transfusions is not a universal practice, acute hemolytic reactions continue to be reported with plasma transfusions. The evaluation of suspected acute hemolytic transfusion reactions is described in Chapter 18 (see pages 359–360).

Transmitted Infections

Plasma transfusions carry a minimal risk of transmitting infections. The risk of hepatitis B transmission is 1 per 900,000 transfusions, the risk of hepatitis C transmission is 1 per 30 million transfusions, and the risk of HIV transmission is one per 8 million transfusions (39). The risk of bacterial transmission is reported as "rare" and CMV transmission, which occurs in transfused leukocytes, has not been reported with plasma transfusions (39).

Hypersensitivity Reactions

Hypersensitivity reactions (urticaria, anaphylaxis, anaphylactic shock), which are caused by sensitization to proteins in donor plasma, are more common with plasma transfusions than with erythrocyte or platelet transfusions. These reactions are, however, uncommon; e.g., the reported incidence of allergic reactions in the United Kingdom is approximately 1 case per 17,000 plasma transfusions (39).

Acute Lung Injury

Transfusion-related acute lung injury (TRALI) is attributed to antileukocyte antibodies in donor blood, and is a complication of erythrocyte, platelet, and plasma transfusions. The reported incidence of TRALI after platelet transfusions is 1 per 60,000 units (39), which is much less than the reported incidence following RBC transfusions (1 per 12,000 units). The clinical features of TRALI are described in Chapter 18 (see pages 361–363).

A FINAL WORD

The following points in this chapter deserve emphasis.

1. The transfusion of platelets or plasma is rarely indicated in the absence of active bleeding. In fact, in most life-threatening cases of thrombocytopenia (e.g., HIT, DIC, TTP, HELLP), the major problem is thrombosis, not hemorrhage.

2. The presence of a coagulopathy is not an absolute contraindication to inserting central venous catheters, even with platelet counts as low as 10,000/µL.

3. If heparin-induced thrombocytopenia is suspected, don't forget to remove heparin from catheter flushes, and to remove heparin-coated catheters.

4. For the management of major hemorrhage associated with warfarin anticoagulation, prothrombin complex concentrate is superior to fresh frozen plasma for correcting the coagulopathy, especially if the bleeding is intracranial.

REFERENCES

Hemostasis

1. King KE (ed). Overview of hemostasis. In: Blood transfusion therapy: A physician's handbook. 9th ed. Bethesda, MD: American Association of Blood Banks, 2008.

2. Wheeler AP, Rice TW. Coagulopathy in critically ill patients. Part 2 – Soluble clotting factors and hemostatic testing. Chest 2010; 137:185–194.

Thrombocytopenia in the ICU

3. Parker RI. Etiology and significance of thrombocytopenia in critically ill patients. Crit Care Clin 2012; 28:399–411.

4. Rice TR, Wheeler RP. Coagulopathy in critically ill patients. Part 1:Platelet disorders. Chest 2009; 136:1622–1630.

5. Slichter SJ, Harker LA. Thrombocytopenia: mechanisms and management of defects in platelet production. Clin Haematol 1978; 7:523–527.

6. Payne BA, Pierre RV. Pseudothrombocytopenia: a laboratory artifact with potentially serious consequences. Mayo Clin Proc 1984; 59:123–125.

7. DeLoughery TG. Critical care clotting catastrophes. Crit Care Clin 2005; 21:531–562.

8. Francois B, Trimoreau F, Vignon P, et al. Thrombocytopenia in the sepsis syndrome: role of hemophagocytosis and macrophage colony-stimulating hormone. Am J Med 1997; 103:114–120.

9. Priziola JL, Smythe MA, Dager WE. Drug-induced thrombocytopenia in critically ill patients. Crit Care Med 2010; 38(Suppl):S145–S154.

10. Shantsila E, Lip GYH, Chong BH. Heparin-induced thrombocytopenia: a contemporary clinical approach to diagnosis and management. Chest 2009; 135:1651–1664.

11. Linkins L-A, Dans AL, Moores LK, et al. Treatment and prevention of heparin-induced thrombocytopenia. Antithrombotic Therapy and Prevention of Thrombosis, 9th ed: American College of Chest Physicians Evidence-Based Clinical Practice Guidelines. Chest 2012; 141(Suppl):495S–530S.

12. Laster J, Silver D. Heparin-coated catheters and heparin-induced thrombocytopenia. J Vasc Surg 1988; 7:667–672.

13. Greinacher A, Eichler P, Lubenow N, et al. Heparin-induced thrombocytopenia with thromboembolic complications: a meta-analysis of 2 prospective trials to assess the value of parenteral treatment with lepirudin and its therapeutic aPTT range. Blood 2000; 96:846–851.

14. Lepirudin drug monograph. In McEvoy GK, ed. AHFS Drug Information, 2012. Bethesda, MD: American Society of Health System Pharmacists, 2012:1476–1478.

15. Senno SL, Pechet L, Bick RL. Disseminated intravascular coagulation (DIC). Pathophysiology, laboratory diagnosis, and management. J Intensive Care Med 2000; 15:144–158.

16. Rock GA, Shumack KH, Buskard NA, et al. Comparison of plasma exchange with plasma infusion in the treatment of thrombotic thrombocytopenia purpura. N Engl J Med 1991; 325:393–397.

17. Hayward CP, Sutton DMC, Carter WH Jr, et al. Treatment outcomes in patients with adult thrombotic thrombocytopenic purpura-hemolytic uremic syndrome. Arch Intern Med 1994; 154:982–987.

18. Kirkpatrick CA. The HELLP syndrome. Acta Clin Belg 2010; 65:91–97.

19. Di Prima FAF, Valenti O, Hyseni E, et al. Antiphospholipid syndrome during pregnancy: the state of the art. J Prenat Med 2011; 5:41–53.

Platelet Transfusions

20. Slichter SJ. Platelet transfusion therapy. Hematol Oncol Clin N Am 2007; 21:697–729.

21. Slichter SJ. Evidence-based platelet transfusion guidelines. Hematol 2007; 2007:172–178.

22. The Trial to Reduce Alloimmunization to Patients Study Group. Leukocyte reduction and ultraviolet B irradiation of platelets to prevent alloimmunization and refractoriness to platelet transfusions. N Engl J Med 1997; 337:1861–1869.

23. Slichter SJ, Davis K, Enright H, et al. Factors affecting post-transfusion platelet increments, platelet refractoriness, and platelet transfusion intervals in thrombocytopenic patients. Blood 2005; 105:4106–4114.

24. Doerfler ME, Kaufman B, Goldenberg AS. Central venous catheter placement in patients with disorders of hemostasis. Chest 1996; 110:185–188.

25. DeLoughery TG, Liebler JM, Simonds V, et al. Invasive line placement in critically ill patients: Do hemostatic defects matter? Transfusion 1996; 36:827–831.

26. Gelinas J-P, Stoddart LV, Snyder EL. Thrombocytopenia and critical care medicine. J Intensive Care Med 2001; 16:1–21.

27. Sayah DM. Looney MR, Toy P. Transfusion reactions. Newer concepts on the pathophysiology, incidence, treatment, and prevention of transfusion-related acute lung injury. Crit Care Clin 2012; 28:363–372.

Plasma Products

28. Lauzier F, Cook D, Griffith L, et al. Fresh frozen plasma transfusion in critically ill patients. Crit Care Med 2007; 35:1655–1659.

29. Roback JD, Caldwell S, Carson J, et al. Evidence-based practice guidelines for plasma transfusion. Transfusion 2010; 50:1227–1239.

30. Brohi K, Singh J, Heron M, Coats T. Acute traumatic coagulopathy. J Trauma 2003; 54:1127–1130.

31. Beekley AC. Damage control resuscitation: a sensible approach to the exsanguinating surgical patient. Crit Care Med 2008; 36:S267–S274.

32. Magnotti LJ, Zarzaur BL, Fischer PE, et al. Improved survival after hemostatic resuscitation: does the emperor have no clothes? J Trauma 2011; 70:97–102.

33. Landefeld CS, Goldman L. Major bleeding in outpatients treated with warfarin: incidence and prediction by factors known at the start of outpatient therapy. Ann Intern Med 1989; 87:144–152.

34. Zareh M, Davis A, Henderson S. Reversal of warfarin-induced hemorrhage in the emergency department. West J Emerg Med 2011; 12:386–392.

35. Imberti D, Barillari G, Biasioli C, et al. Emergency reversal of anticoagulation with a three-factor prothrombin complex concentrate in patients with intracerebral hemorrhage. Blood Transfus 2011; 9:148–155.

36. Salman S. Uremic bleeding: pathophysiology, diagnosis, and management. Hosp Physician 2001; 37:45–76.

37. Mannucci PM. Desmopressin (DDAVP) in the treatment of bleeding disorders. The first 20 years. Blood 1997; 90:2515–2521.

38. Callum JL, Karkouti K, Lin Y. Cryoprecipitate: the current state of knowledge. Transfus Med Rev 2009; 23:177–184.

39. MacLennan S, Williamson LM. Risks of fresh frozen plasma and platelets. J Trauma 2006; 60(Suppl):546–550.

ACUTE RESPIRATORY FAILURE

I breathe for my own necessity, for my survival.

Ayn Rand
The Fountainhead
1943

Chapter 20

HYPOXEMIA AND HYPERCAPNIA

> *Respiration is thus a process of combustion, in truth very slow,*
> *but otherwise exactly like that of charcoal.*
>
> Antoine Lavoisier

Antoine Lavoisier was an 18th-century French scientist who was the first to identify oxygen as the essential element for metabolism, and the first to discover that aerobic metabolism is essentially a combustion reaction, where oxygen reacts with an organic fuel and produces carbon dioxide as a by-product. (One of the many tragedies of the French Revolution was the senseless beheading of Antoine Lavoisier in 1794.) Providing the oxygen and removing the carbon dioxide is the responsibility of the lungs, and this chapter describes how the lungs perform this task, and how abnormalities in lung function can lead to deficits in arterial oxygenation (hypoxemia) and accumulation of carbon dioxide (hypercapnia). The last part of the chapter presents a physiological approach to the evaluation of hypoxemia and hypercapnia in individual patients.

PULMONARY GAS EXCHANGE

The efficiency of gas exchange in the lungs is determined by the balance between alveolar ventilation and pulmonary capillary blood flow (1–4). This balance is commonly expressed as the ventilation–perfusion (V/Q) ratio. The influence of V/Q ratios on pulmonary gas exchange can be described using an alveolar–capillary unit, as shown in Figure 20.1. The upper panel shows a perfect match between ventilation and perfusion (V/Q = 1). This is the reference point for defining the abnormal patterns of gas exchange.

Dead Space Ventilation

A V/Q ratio above 1.0 (Fig. 20.1, middle panel) describes the condition where ventilation is excessive relative to pulmonary capillary blood flow.

The excess ventilation, known as *dead space ventilation*, does not participate in gas exchange with the blood. Dead space ventilation includes *anatomic dead space*, which is the gas in the large conducting airways that does not come in contact with capillary blood (about half of the anatomic dead space is in the pharynx), and *physiologic dead space*, which is alveolar gas that does not equilibrate fully with capillary blood. In normal subjects, dead space ventilation (V_D) accounts for 20% to 30% of the total ventilation (V_T); i.e., $V_D/V_T = 0.2$ to 0.3 (1,3).

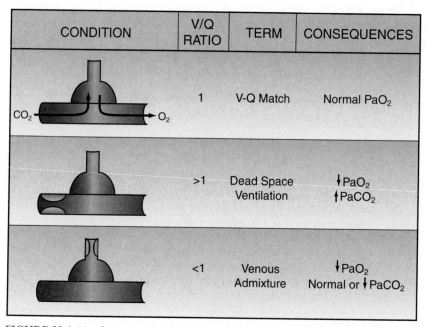

CONDITION	V/Q RATIO	TERM	CONSEQUENCES
CO_2 ⟶ O_2	1	V-Q Match	Normal PaO_2
	>1	Dead Space Ventilation	↓PaO_2 ↑$PaCO_2$
	<1	Venous Admixture	↓PaO_2 Normal or ↓$PaCO_2$

FIGURE 20.1 Ventilation–perfusion (V/Q) relationships and associated blood gas abnormalities.

Pathophysiology

Dead space ventilation increases in the following situations:

1. When the alveolar–capillary interface is destroyed; e.g., emphysema
2. When blood flow is reduced; i.e., low cardiac output
3. When alveoli are overdistended; e.g., during positive-pressure ventilation

ARTERIAL BLOOD GASES: An increase in V_D/V_T above 0.3 results in both hypoxemia (decreased arterial PO_2) and hypercapnia (increased arterial PCO_2), which is analogous to what would happen if you held your breath. The hypercapnia usually appears when the V_D/V_T is above 0.5 (5).

Intrapulmonary Shunt

A V/Q ratio below 1.0 (Fig. 20.1, lower panel) occurs when pulmonary capillary blood flow is excessive relative to ventilation. The excess blood flow, known as *intrapulmonary shunt*, does not participate in pulmonary gas exchange. There are two types of intrapulmonary shunt. *True shunt* indicates the total absence of gas exchange between capillary blood and alveolar gas (V/Q = 0), and is equivalent to an anatomic shunt between the right and left sides of the heart. *Venous admixture* represents the capillary flow that does not equilibrate completely with alveolar gas (0 < V/Q < 1). As the venous admixture increases, the V/Q ratio decreases until it becomes a true shunt (V/Q = 0).

The fraction of the cardiac output that represents intrapulmonary shunt is known as the *shunt fraction*. In normal subjects, intrapulmonary shunt flow (Qs) represents less than 10% of the total cardiac output (Qt), so the shunt fraction (Qs/Qt) is less than 10% (1,2,4).

Pathophysiology

Intrapulmonary shunt fraction is increased in the following situations:

1. When the small airways are occluded; e.g., asthma

2. When the alveoli are filled with fluid; e.g., pulmonary edema, pneumonia

3. When the alveoli collapse; e.g., atelectasis

4. When capillary flow is excessive; e.g., in nonembolized regions of the lung in pulmonary embolism

ARTERIAL BLOOD GASES: The influence of shunt fraction on arterial O_2 and CO_2 tensions (PaO_2, $PaCO_2$, respectively) is shown in Figure 20.2. The PaO_2 falls progressively as shunt fraction increases, but the $PaCO_2$ remains constant until the shunt fraction exceeds 50% (4). The $PaCO_2$ is often below normal in patients with increased intrapulmonary shunt as a result of hyperventilation triggered by the disease process or by the accompanying hypoxemia.

Inhaled Oxygen

The shunt fraction also determines the influence of inhaled oxygen on the arterial PO_2. This is shown in Figure 20.3 (4). As intrapulmonary shunt increases from 10 to 50%, an increase in fractional concentration of inspired oxygen (FiO_2) produces less of an increment in the arterial PO_2. When the shunt fraction exceeds 50%, the arterial PO_2 is independent of changes in FiO_2, and the condition behaves like a true (anatomic) shunt. This means that, *in conditions associated with a high shunt fraction* (e.g., acute respiratory distress syndrome), *the FiO_2 can often be lowered to non-toxic levels (FiO_2 below 60%) without further compromising arterial oxygenation*. This can be a valuable maneuver for preventing pulmonary oxygen toxicity.

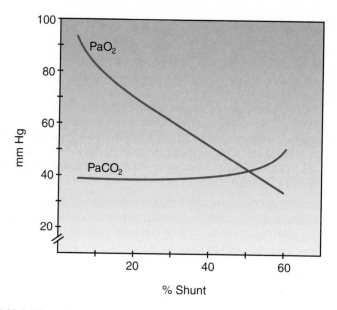

FIGURE 20.2 The influence of shunt fraction on arterial PO$_2$ (PaO$_2$) and arterial PCO$_2$ (PaCO$_2$). From Reference 4.

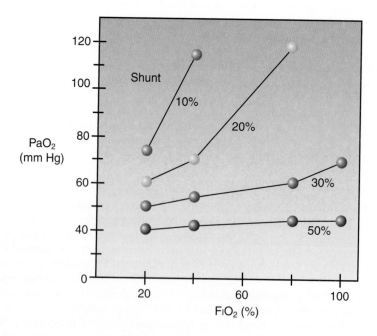

FIGURE 20.3 The influence of shunt fraction on the relationship between the inspired oxygen (FiO$_2$) and the arterial PO$_2$ (PaO$_2$). From Reference 4.

MEASURES OF GAS EXCHANGE

The calculation of dead space ventilation (V_D/V_T) is based on the difference between the PCO_2 in exhaled gas and end-capillary (arterial) blood. In the normal lung, the capillary blood equilibrates fully with alveolar gas, and the exhaled PCO_2 ($PECO_2$) is equivalent to the arterial PCO_2 ($PaCO_2$). As dead space ventilation (V_D/V_T) increases, the $PECO_2$ decreases relative to the $PaCO_2$. The Bohr equation shown below (derived by Christian Bohr, father of Neils Bohr, one of the founders of quantum mechanics) is based on this principle.

$$V_D / V_T = \frac{PaCO_2 - PECO_2}{PaCO_2} \tag{20.1}$$

Thus, when the $PECO_2$ decreases relative to the $PaCO_2$, the calculated V_D/V_T rises. The $PECO_2$ is measured in a random sample of expired gas (mean exhaled PCO_2), and is not measured at the end of expiration (end-tidal PCO_2).

Intrapulmonary Shunt Fraction

The intrapulmonary shunt fraction (Qs/Qt) is derived by the relationship between the O_2 content in arterial blood (CaO_2), mixed venous blood (CvO_2), and pulmonary capillary blood (CcO_2).

$$Qs/\, Qt = \frac{CcO_2 - CaO_2}{CcO_2 - CvO_2} \tag{20.2}$$

The problem with this formula is the inability to measure the pulmonary capillary O_2 content (CcO_2) directly. As a result, pure oxygen breathing (to produce 100% oxyhemoglobin saturation in pulmonary capillary blood) is recommended for the shunt calculation. However in this situation, Qs/Qt measures only true shunt.

The A-a PO_2 Gradient

The PO_2 difference between alveolar gas and arterial blood ($PAO_2 - PaO_2$) is an indirect measure of ventilation–perfusion abnormalities (5–7). The $PAO_2 - PaO_2$ (A-a PO_2) gradient is determined with the alveolar gas equation shown below.

$$PAO_2 = PIO_2 - (PaCO_2 / RQ) \tag{20.3}$$

This equation defines the relationship between the PO_2 in alveolar gas (PAO_2), the PO_2 in inhaled gas (PIO_2), the PCO_2 in arterial blood ($PaCO2$), and the respiratory quotient (RQ). The RQ defines the relative rates of exchange of O_2 and CO_2 across the alveolar–capillary interface: i.e., RQ = VCO_2/VO_2. The PIO_2 is determined using the fractional concentration of inspired oxygen (FIO_2), the barometric pressure (P_B), and the partial pressure of water vapor (P_{H_2O}) in humidified gas:

$$PIO_2 = FIO_2 (P_B - P_{H_2O}) \tag{20.4}$$

If equations 20.3 and 20.4 are combined (for the alveolar PO_2), the A–a PO_2 gradient can be calculated as follows:

$$\text{A-a } PO_2 = [FiO2 (P_B - P_{H_2O}) - (PaCO_2/RQ)] - PaO_2 \tag{20.5}$$

In a healthy subject breathing room air at sea level, $FiO_2 = 0.21$, $P_B = 760$ mm Hg, $P_{H_2O} = 47$ mm Hg, $PaO_2 = 90$ mm Hg, $PaCO_2 = 40$ mm Hg, and $RQ = 0.8$:

$$\text{A-a } PO_2 = [0.21 (760 - 47) - (40/0.8)] - 90 = 10 \text{ mm Hg} \tag{20.6}$$

This represents an idealized rather than normal A-a PO_2 gradient, because the A-a PO_2 gradient varies with age and with the concentration of inspired oxygen.

Influence of Age

As shown in Table 20.1, *the normal A-a PO_2 gradient rises steadily with advancing age* (6). Assuming that most adult patients in an ICU are 40 years of age or older, the normal A-a PO_2 gradient in an adult ICU patient can be as high as 25 mm Hg when the patient is breathing room air. However, few ICU patients breathe room air, and the A-a PO_2 gradient is increased further when oxygen is added to inhaled gas (see next).

Table 20.1	Normal Arterial Blood Gases		
Age (Years)	PaO_2 (mm Hg)	$PaCO_2$ (mm Hg)	A-a PO_2 (mm Hg)
20	84–95	33–47	4–17
30	81–92	34–47	7–21
40	78–90	34–47	10–24
50	75–87	34–47	14–27
60	72–84	34–47	17–31
70	70–81	34–47	21–34
80	67–79	34–47	25–38

All values pertain to room air breathing at sea level.
From the Intermountain Thoracic Society Manual of Uniform Laboratory Procedures. Salt Lake City, 1984:44–45.

Influence of Inspired Oxygen

The influence of inspired oxygen on the A-a PO_2 gradient is shown in Figure 20.4 (7). The A-a PO_2 gradient increases from 15 to 60 mm Hg as the FiO_2 increases from 21% (room air) to 100%. According to this relationship, *the normal A-a PO_2 gradient increases 5 to 7 mm Hg for every 10% increase in FiO_2*. This effect is presumably caused by the loss of regional hypoxic vasoconstriction in the lungs. Hypoxic vasoconstriction in poorly ventilated lung regions diverts blood to more adequately ventilated regions, and this helps to preserve the normal V/Q balance. Loss of regional hypoxic vasoconstriction during supplemental O_2 breathing maintains blood flow in poorly ventilated lung regions, and this increases intrapulmonary shunt fraction and increases the A-a PO_2 gradient.

The FIO_2 is difficult to estimate accurately when supplemental O_2 is delivered via nasal prongs or "open" face masks (see Chapter 22), and this limits the accuracy of the A-a PO_2 gradient in these situations.

Positive-Pressure Ventilation

Positive-pressure mechanical ventilation elevates the pressure in the airways above the ambient barometric pressure. Therefore, when determining the A-a PO_2 gradient in a ventilator-dependent patient, the mean airway pressure should be added to the barometric pressure (8). In the example presented in equation 20.6, a mean airway pressure of 30 cm H_2O would increase the A-a PO_2 gradient from 10 to 16 mm Hg (a 60% increase). Thus, neglecting the contribution of positive airway pressure during mechanical ventilation will underestimate the degree of abnormal gas exchange.

The a/A PO_2 Ratio

Unlike the A-a PO_2 gradient, the a/A PO_2 ratio is relatively unaffected by the FIO_2. This is demonstrated in Figure 20.4. The independence of the a/A PO_2 ratio in relation to the FIO_2 is explained by the equation below.

$$a/A\ PO_2 = 1 - (A\text{-}a\ PO_2)/P_AO_2 \qquad (20.7)$$

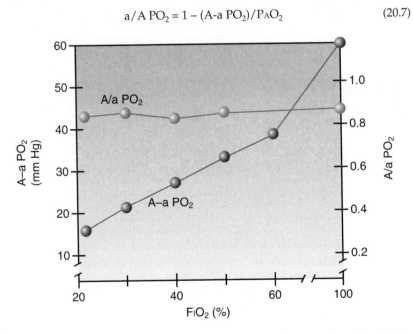

FIGURE 20.4 The influence of FIO_2 on the alveolar-arterial PO_2 gradient (A-a PO_2) and the arterial-alveolar PO_2 ratio (a/A PO_2) in normal subjects. From Reference 7.

Because the alveolar PO_2 is in both the numerator and denominator of the equation, the influence of FIO_2 on the PAO_2 is eliminated. Thus, *the a/A PO_2 ratio is a mathematical manipulation that eliminates the influence of FIO_2 on the A-a PO_2 gradient.* The normal a/A PO_2 ratio is 0.74 to 0.77 when breathing room air, and 0.80 to 0.82 when breathing 100% oxygen (7).

The PaO_2/FIO_2 Ratio

The PaO_2/FIO_2 ratio is used as an indirect estimate of shunt fraction. The following correlations have been reported (9).

PaO_2/FIO_2	Qs/Qt
<200	>20%
>200	<20%

The major limitation of the PaO_2/FIO_2 ratio is the inability to estimate the FIO_2 accurately when supplemental O_2 is delivered through nasal prongs or "open" face masks (see Chapter 22). (This limitation has also been described for the A-a PO_2 gradient.)

Blood Gas Variability

The arterial PO_2 and PCO_2 can vary spontaneously without a change in the clinical condition of the patient. This is demonstrated in Table 20.2, which shows the spontaneous variation in arterial PO_2 and PCO_2 over a one-hour period in a group of clinically stable trauma victims (10). Note that the *arterial PO_2 varied by as much as 36 mm Hg*, while the *arterial PCO_2 varied by as much as 12 mm Hg.* This variability has also been observed in patients in a medical ICU (11). Because of this degree of spontaneous variation, *routine monitoring of arterial blood gases can be misleading.*

Table 20.2	Spontaneous Blood-Gas Variability	
Variation	**PaO₂**	**PaCO₂**
Mean	13 mm Hg	2.5 mm Hg
95th Percentile	±18 mm Hg	±4 mm Hg
Range	2–37 mm Hg	0–12 mm Hg

Represents variations over a 1-hour period in 26 ventilator-dependent trauma victims who were clinically stable.

From Reference 10.

HYPOXEMIA

Hypoxemia can be defined as an arterial PO_2 below what is expected for a patient's age, as defined in Table 20.1. However, hypoxemia usually doesn't raise red flags until the arterial PO_2 falls below 60 mm Hg (or the arterial O_2 saturation falls below 90%). The causes of hypoxemia can be separated into 3 categories based on the physiological process involved (12,13).

Each group of disorders can be distinguished by the A-a PO_2 gradient and/or the mixed venous PO_2, as shown in Table 20.3.

Table 20.3	Sources of Hypoxemia	
Source	**A-a PO_2**	**PvO_2**
Hypoventilation	Normal	Normal
V/Q mismatch	Increased	Normal
DO_2/VO_2 imbalance	Increased	Decreased

Hypoventilation

Alveolar hypoventilation causes both hypoxemia and hypercapnia, similar to breath-holding. There is no V/Q imbalance in the lungs, so the A-a PO_2 gradient is not elevated. The common causes of alveolar hypoventilation are listed in Table 20.4. Most cases of hypoventilation in the ICU are the result of drug-induced respiratory depression or neuromuscular weakness. Obesity-related hypoventilation (Pickwickian syndrome) is also a consideration, as this condition is present in up to one-third of morbidly obese patients (body mass index > 35 kg/m²) (14).

Table 20.4	Alveolar Hypoventilation in the ICU
Brainstem Respiratory Depression	
1. Drugs (e.g., opiates)	
2. Obesity-hypoventilation syndrome	
Peripheral Neuropathy	
1. Critical illness polyneuropathy	
2. Guillain-Barré syndrome	
Muscle Weakness	
1. Critical illness myopathy	
2. Hypophosphatemia	
3. Myasthenia gravis	

Respiratory Muscle Weakness

Most cases of respiratory muscle weakness in the ICU are the result of an idiopathic polyneuropathy and myopathy that is specific to ICU patients, particularly those with sepsis, prolonged mechanical ventilation, and prolonged neuromuscular paralysis (15). The standard method of evaluating respiratory muscle strength is to measure the *maximum inspiratory pressure* (PI_{max}), which is the maximum pressure recorded during a maximum inspiratory effort against a closed valve. The normal PI_{max} varies with age and gender, but most healthy adults can generate a negative PI_{max} of at least 80 cm H_2O (16). A PI_{max} that does not exceed -25 cm H_2O is considered evidence of respiratory muscle failure (17). (See Chapter 45 for more information on neuromuscular weakness syndromes in the ICU.)

V/Q Mismatch

Most cases of hypoxemia are the result of a V/Q mismatch in the lungs. Virtually any lung disease can be included in this category, but the common ones encountered in the ICU are pneumonia, inflammatory lung injury (acute respiratory distress syndrome), obstructive lung disease, hydrostatic pulmonary edema, and pulmonary embolism. The A-a PO_2 gradient is almost always elevated in these conditions, but the elevation can be minimal in patients with severe airways obstruction (which behaves like hypoventilation).

DO_2/VO_2 Imbalance

As explained in Chapter 10, a decrease in systemic O_2 delivery (DO_2) is usually accompanied by an increase in O_2 extraction from capillary blood, and this serves to maintain a constant rate of O_2 uptake (VO_2) into the tissues. The increased O_2 extraction from capillary blood results in a decrease in the PO_2 of venous blood, and this can have an deleterious effect on arterial oxygenation, as explained below.

Mixed Venous PO$_2$

The O_2 in arterial blood represents the sum of the O_2 in mixed venous (pulmonary artery) blood and the O_2 added from alveolar gas. When gas exchange is normal, the PO_2 in alveolar gas is the major determinant of the arterial PO_2. However, when gas exchange is impaired, the contribution of the alveolar PO_2 declines and the contribution of the mixed venous PO_2 rises (18). The greater the impairment in gas exchange, the greater the contribution of the mixed venous PO_2 to the arterial PO_2. (If there is no gas exchange in the lungs, the mixed venous PO_2 would be the sole determinant of the arterial PO_2.)

The diagram in Figure 20.5 demonstrates the influence of mixed venous PO_2 on the arterial PO_2 when gas exchange is impaired. The curves in the graph represent the transition from mixed venous PO_2 to arterial PO_2 as blood flows through the lungs. The slope of each curve reflects the efficiency of gas exchange in the lungs. Note that the curve representing the V/Q abnormality results in a lower arterial PO_2 because the slope is decreased (indicating impaired oxygen exchange in the lungs). If this curve begins at a lower mixed venous PO_2, as indicated, the curve shifts downward, resulting in a further decrease in arterial PO_2. This illustrates how a decrease in mixed venous PO_2 can aggravate the hypoxemia caused by a V/Q abnormality. It also indicates that, in the presence of a V/Q abnormality, the mixed venous PO_2 is an important consideration in the evaluation of hypoxemia.

The relationship between O_2 delivery (DO_2), O_2 uptake (VO_2), and the mixed venous PO_2 (PvO_2) can be stated as follows:

$$PvO_2 = k \times (DO_2/VO_2) \qquad (20.8)$$

(k is a proportionality constant.) Thus, any condition that reduces DO_2 (e.g., low cardiac output, anemia) or increases VO_2 (e.g., hypermetabolism) can decrease the PvO_2 and aggravate the hypoxemia caused by abnormal gas exchange in the lungs.

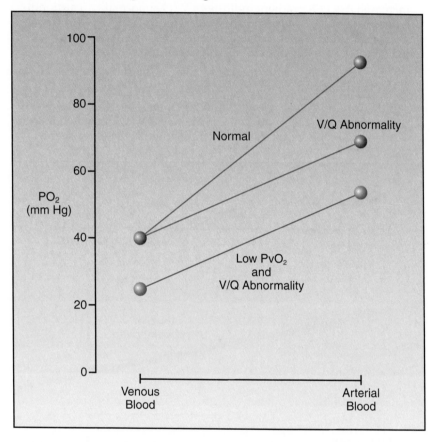

FIGURE 20.5 The influence of a V/Q abnormality on the transition from venous to arterial PO_2, and the added effect of a low mixed venous PO_2 (PvO_2).

Diagnostic Evaluation

The evaluation of hypoxemia can proceed according to the flow diagram in Figure 20.6. This approach uses three measures: A-a PO_2 gradient, mixed venous PO_2, and maximum inspiratory pressure. The PO_2 in superior vena cava blood (central venous PO_2) can be used as the mixed venous PO_2 when there is no indwelling pulmonary artery catheter.

The first step in the approach involves a determination of the A-a PO_2 gradient. After correcting for age and FiO_2, the A-a PO_2 gradient can be interpreted as follows:

1. Normal A-a PO_2 gradient indicates hypoventilation rather than a cardiopulmonary disorder. In this situation, the most likely problems are drug-induced respiratory depression and neuromuscular weakness. The latter condition can be uncovered by measuring the maximum inspiratory pressure (PI_{max}), which is described earlier.

2. Increased A-a PO_2 gradient indicates a V/Q abnormality (cardiopulmonary disorder) and a possible superimposed DO_2/VO_2 imbalance (e.g., a decrease in cardiac output). The mixed venous (or central venous) PO_2 will help to identify a DO_2/VO_2 imbalance.

   a. If the venous PO_2 is 40 mm Hg or higher, the problem is solely a V/Q mismatch in the lungs.

   b. If the venous PO_2 is below 40 mm Hg, there is a DO_2/VO_2 imbalance adding to the hypoxemia created by a V/Q mismatch in the lungs. The source of this imbalance is either a decreased DO_2

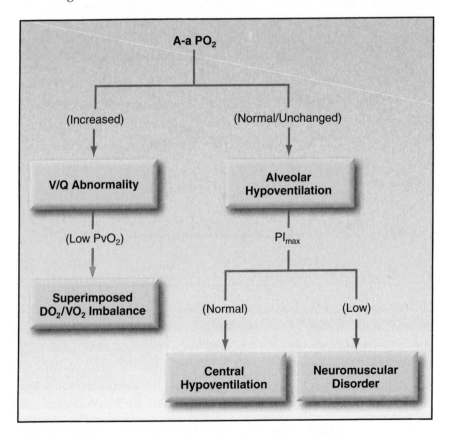

FIGURE 20.6 Flow diagram for the evaluation of hypoxemia.

(from anemia or a low cardiac output) or an increased VO_2 (from hypermetabolism).

Spurious Hypoxemia

Spurious hypoxemia is a rarely reported phenomenon that is character-ized by hypoxemia in an arterial blood sample without corresponding hypoxemia in circulating blood (as measured by pulse oximetry) (19). This phenomenon seems to occur only in patients with hematologic malignancies who have marked leukocytosis (WBC > 100,000) or throm-bocytosis (platelet count > 1,000,000). The reduced PO_2 in the blood sam-ple has been attributed to O_2 consumption by activated leukocytes in the sample, a phenomenon that has been called *leukocyte larceny* (20). This does not explain why marked thrombocytosis can also produce spurious hypoxemia because platelets are not oxygen-guzzlers like activated leukocytes. Regardless of the mechanism, there is no accepted method of preventing spurious hypoxemia (rapid cooling of blood samples has had inconsistent results), so you should be aware of the phenomenon and the value of pulse oximetry for validating in vitro PO_2 measurements (pulse oximetry is described in the next chapter).

HYPERCAPNIA

Hypercapnia is defined as an arterial PCO_2 ($PaCO_2$) above 46 mm Hg that does not represent compensation for a metabolic alkalosis (21). The causes of hypercapnia can be identified by considering the determinants of $PaCO_2$ in the following relationship, where VCO_2 is the rate of CO_2 production in the body, V_A is the rate of alveolar ventilation, and k is a proportionality constant (1).

$$PaCO_2 = k \times (VCO_2/V_A) \tag{20.9}$$

Alveolar ventilation is the portion of the total ventilation (V_E) that is not dead space ventilation (V_D/V_T); that is, $V_A = V_E (1 - V_D/V_T)$. Therefore, equation 20.9 can be restated as follows:

$$PaCO_2 = k \times [VCO_2/V_E (1 - V_D/V_T)] \tag{20.10}$$

This equation identifies three major sources of hypercapnia: (a) increased CO_2 production (VCO_2), (b) hypoventilation ($1/V_E$), and (c) increased dead space ventilation (V_D/V_T).

Hypoventilation

Hypoventilation was discussed briefly in the last section on hypoxemia, and Table 20.4 shows the common causes of hypoventilation. Because hypoxemia is so common in ICU patients, hypercapnia may be the first sign of hypoventilation from neuromuscular weakness or drug-induced respiratory depression. This is also the case in obesity-hypoventilation syndrome, where hypercapnia while awake is often the first evidence of hypoventilation. On the other hand, *hypercapnia is a relatively late sign in neuromuscular disorders,* and does not appear until the maximum inspiratory pressure or PI_{max} (described earlier) is below 50% of normal (17).

V/Q Abnormality

As mentioned earlier, hypercapnia is not a feature of increased intrapulmonary shunt until late in the process (which is why hypercapnia is not a feature of pulmonary edema or other infiltrative lung processes until they are far advanced). Hypercapnia is more a feature of increased dead space ventilation (such as occurs in advanced emphysema, where there is destruction of the alveolar-capillary interface), and *the $PaCO_2$ usually begins to rise when dead space ventilation accounts for more than 50% of total ventilation ($V_D/V_T > 0.5$).*

Increased CO_2 Production

An increase in CO_2 production is usually related to oxidative metabolism, but non-metabolic CO_2 production is possible when extracellular acids generate hydrogen ions that combine with bicarbonate ions and generate CO_2. Whatever the source, increased CO_2 production is normally accompanied by an increase in minute ventilation, which eliminates the excess CO_2 and maintains a constant arterial PCO_2. Therefore, excess CO_2 production does not normally cause hypercapnia. However, when CO_2 excretion is impaired, an increase in CO_2 production can lead to an increase in $PaCO_2$. Thus, *increased CO_2 production is an important factor in promoting hypercapnia only when the ability to eliminate CO_2 is impaired.*

Overfeeding

Overfeeding, or the provision of calories in excess of daily needs, is a recognized cause of hypercapnia in patients with severe lung disease and acute respiratory failure (22). Nutrition-associated hypercapnia occurs predominantly in ventilator-dependent patients, and can delay weaning from mechanical ventilation. Overfeeding with carbohydrates is particularly problematic because the oxidative metabolism of carbohydrates generates more carbon dioxide than the other nutrient substrates (lipids and proteins). This is described in more detail in Chapter 47.

Diagnostic Evaluation

The bedside evaluation of hypercapnia is shown in Figure 20.7. The evaluation of hypercapnia, like hypoxemia, begins with the A-a PO_2 gradient (23). A normal or unchanged A-a PO_2 gradient indicates that the problem is alveolar hypoventilation (the same as described for the evaluation of hypoxemia). An increased A-a PO_2 gradient indicates a V/Q abnormality (an increase in dead space ventilation) that may or may not be accompanied by an increase in CO_2 production.

Measuring CO_2 Production

The rate of CO_2 production (VCO_2) can be measured at the bedside with

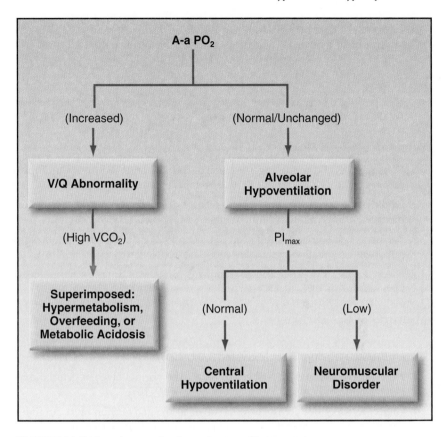

FIGURE 20.7 Flow diagram for the evaluation of hypercapnia.

specialized metabolic carts that are normally used to perform nutritional assessments. These carts are equipped with infrared devices that can measure the CO_2 in expired gas (much like the end-tidal CO_2 monitors described in Chapter 21), and can determine the volume of CO_2 excreted per minute. In steady-state conditions, the rate of CO_2 excretion is equivalent to the VCO_2. The *normal VCO_2 is 90 to 130 L/minute/m², which is roughly 80% of the VO_2.* As mentioned earlier, an increased VCO_2 is evidence for one of the following conditions: generalized hypermetabolism, overfeeding (excess calories), or metabolic acidoses.

A FINAL WORD

It is important to remember that *the arterial PO_2 is not a useful measure for determining the amount of oxygen in the blood* (this requires the hemoglobin concentration in blood and the percent saturation of hemoglobin with oxygen, as shown in Equation 10.6 in Chapter 10). Instead, the PaO_2 (along with the $PaCO_2$) is used to evaluate gas exchange in the lungs, and can be useful in identifying the source of the problem with gas exchange.

406 Acute Respiratory Failure

An approach to O_2 and CO_2 balance that is superior in many ways to the measurement of arterial blood gases is described in the next chapter.

REFERENCES

Bell SM. Lavoisier in the Year One. New York: W.H. Norton & Co., 2005.

Pulmonary Gas Exchange

1. Dantzger DR. Pulmonary gas exchange. In: Dantzger DR, ed. Cardiopulmonary critical care. 2nd ed. Philadelphia: WB Saunders, 1991; 25–43.

2. Lanken PN. Ventilation-perfusion relationships. In: Grippi MA, ed. Pulmonary Pathophysiology. Philadelphia: JB Lippincott, 1995; 195–210.

3. Buohuys A. Respiratory dead space. In: Fenn WO, Rahn H, eds. Handbook of physiology: respiration. Bethesda: American Physiological Society, 1964; 699–714.

4. D'Alonzo GE, Dantzger DR. Mechanisms of abnormal gas exchange. Med Clin North Am 1983; 67:557–571.

Measures of Gas Exchange

5. Gammon RB, Jefferson LS. Interpretation of arterial oxygen tension. UpToDate Web Site, 2006. (Accessed 3/11/2006)

6. Harris EA, Kenyon AM, Nisbet HD, et al. The normal alveolar-arterial oxygen tension gradient in man. Clin Sci 1974; 46:89–104.

7. Gilbert R, Kreighley JF. The arterial/alveolar oxygen tension ratio. An index of gas exchange applicable to varying inspired oxygen concentrations. Am Rev Resp Dis 1974; 109:142–145.

8. Carroll GC. Misapplication of the alveolar gas equation. N Engl J Med 1985; 312:586.

9. Covelli HD, Nessan VJ, Tuttle WK. Oxygen derived variables in acute respiratory failure. Crit Care Med 1983; 11:646–649.

10. Hess D, Agarwal NN. Variability of blood gases, pulse oximeter saturation, and end-tidal carbon dioxide pressure in stable, mechanically ventilated trauma patients. J Clin Monit 1992; 8:111–115.

11. Sasse SA, Chen P, Mahutte CK. Variability of arterial blood gas values over time in stable medical ICU patients. Chest 1994; 106:187–193.

Hypoxemia

12. Duarte A, Bidani A. Evaluating hypoxemia in the critically ill. J Crit Illness 2005; 20:91–93.

13. White AC. The evaluation and management of hypoxemia in the chronic critically ill patient. Clin Chest Med 2001; 22:123–134.

14. Nowbar S, Burkhart KM, Gonzalez R, et al. Obesity-associated hypoventilation in hospitalized patients: prevalence, effects, and outcome. Am J Med 2004; 116:1–7.

15. Rich MM, Raps EC, Bird SJ. Distinction between acute myopathy syndrome and critical illness polyneuropathy. Mayo Clin Proc 1995; 70:198–199.

16. Bruschi C, Cerveri I, Zoia MC, et al. Reference values for maximum respiratory mouth pressures: A population-based study. Am Rev Respir Dis 1992; 146:790–793.

17. Baydur A. Respiratory muscle strength and control of ventilation in patients with neuromuscular disease. Chest 1991; 99:330–338.

18. Rossaint R, Hahn S-M, Pappert D, et al. Influence of mixed venous PO_2 and inspired oxygen fraction on intrapulmonary shunt in patients with severe ARDS. J Appl Physiol. 1995; 78:1531–1536.

19. Lele A, Mirski MA, Stevens RD. Spurious hypoxemia. Crit Care Med 2005; 33:1854–1856.

20. Fox MJ, Brody JS, Weintraub LR. Leukocyte larceny: A cause of spurious hypoxemia. Am J Med 1979; 67:742–746.

Hypercapnia

21. Weinberger SE, Schwartzstein RM, Weiss JW. Hypercapnia. N Engl J Med 1989; 321:1223–1230.

22. Talpers SS, Romberger DJ, Bunce SB, Pingleton SK. Nutritionally associated increased carbon dioxide production. Chest 1992; 102:551–555.

23. Gray BA, Blalock JM. Interpretation of the alveolar-arterial oxygen difference in patients with hypercapnia. Am Rev Respir Dis 1991; 143:4–8.

Chapter 21

OXIMETRY AND CAPNOMETRY

The killing vice of the young doctor is intellectual laziness.

Sir William Osler
*On the Educational Value
of the Medical Society,* in
Aequanimitas, 1904

The introduction of optical techniques for the continuous and noninvasive measurement of oxyhemoglobin saturation in blood (oximetry) and carbon dioxide in exhaled gas (capnometry) has provided the most useful advances in critical care monitoring in the last 30 years. Oximetry has had an enormous impact on patient care throughout the hospital, and the arterial O_2 saturation has been called the *fifth vital sign* (1,2), while infrared capnometry has emerged as an indispensable component of cardiopulmonary resuscitation (see pp. 334–335).

Despite the prominent role of oximetry and capnography in critical care management, surveys have shown that 97% of house staff and ICU nurses have little or no understanding of these techniques or the parameters that are monitored (3). The material in this chapter should help to correct this situation.

OXIMETRY

All atoms and molecules absorb specific wavelengths of light, and this property is the basis for the technique known as *spectrophotometry*, where light waves of specific wavelengths are transmitted through a medium to determine the molecular composition of the medium. The absorption of specific wavelengths of light as they pass through a medium is proportional to the concentration of the substance that absorbs the light waves, and the length of the path that the waves travel (as defined by the Lambert-Beer Law). The application of this principle to the detection of hemoglobin in its different forms is known as *oximetry*.

Light Absorption by Hemoglobin

Hemoglobin (like all proteins) changes its structural configuration when it participates in a chemical reaction, and each of the configurations has a distinct pattern of light absorption. The patterns of light absorption for the different forms of hemoglobin are shown in Figure 21.1 (4). Four different forms of hemoglobin are represented in the figure: oxygenated hemoglobin (HbO_2), deoxygenated hemoglobin (Hb), methemoglobin (metHb), and carboxyhemoglobin (COHb). In the red region of the light spectrum (represented by the wavelength of 660 nm), oxygenated hemoglobin (HbO), does not absorb light as well as deoxygenated hemoglobin (Hb), which is why oxygenated blood is more intensely red than deoxygenated blood. The opposite is true in the infrared region of the spectrum (represented by the wavelength of 940 nm), where HbO_2 absorbs light more effectively than Hb. Based on these absorption patterns, two wavelengths of light (660 nm and 940 nm) can be used to identify oxygenated and deoxygenated hemoglobin.

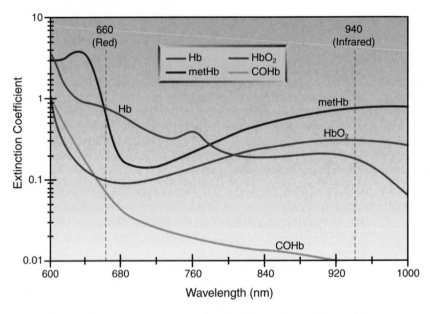

FIGURE 21.1 The absorption spectrum for the different forms of hemoglobin: oxygenated hemoglobin (*HbO₂*), deoxygenated hemoglobin (*Hb*), carboxyhemoglobin (*COHb*), and methemoglobin (*metHb*) The vertical lines represent the two wavelengths of light (660 nm and 940 nm) used by pulse oximeters. Adapted from Reference 4.

Early Oximetry

Oximetry was introduced in the 1940s to detect hypoxemia in fighter pilots. Early oximetry, which measured the transmission of red and infrared light waves through the earlobe, had two major shortcomings: (a) the transmission of light was influenced by factors other than hemoglobin (e.g., skin pigments, and the thickness of the earlobe), and (b) it was not possible to differentiate between hemoglobin in arteries and veins. As a result of these problems, oximetry failed to gain acceptance as a monitoring tool, but this situation changed in the 1970s with the introduction of *pulsatile* oximetry.

Pulse Oximetry

When a light beam passes through a pulsating artery, the phasic changes in arterial blood volume create pulsatile variations in the intensity of the transmitted light beam. Therefore, restricting the analysis of light transmission to pulsatile light waves will focus the analysis on arterial blood, and will eliminate errors due to light absorption by non-pulsatile elements (e.g., hemoglobin in veins). This is the basic principle of *pulse oximetry* (4,5), which employs an alternating-current (AC) amplifier to process pulsatile light transmission from arteries while rejecting non-pulsatile light transmission through veins, connective tissue, and skin.

The basic features of pulse oximetry are illustrated in Figure 21.2. The upper panel shows a standard pulse oximeter probe that is placed on a finger. (These probes are usually placed on the index or middle finger, but can be placed on any digit, including the great toe.) One side of the probe contains two light-emitting diodes that emit monochromatic light at wavelengths of 660 nm and 940 nm. These light waves pass through the finger and are sensed by a photodetector on the opposite side of the probe. The transmitted light waves are then passed through an AC amplifier that amplifies the pulsatile light waves and blocks the non-pulsatile waves. The intensity of light transmission at 660 nm and 940 nm is a reflection of the deoxygenated hemoglobin (Hb) and oxygenated hemoglobin (HbO_2) concentrations in arterial blood, respectively. The pulse oximeter converts "light density" to "chemical density" (concentration) for Hb and HbO_2 using proprietary algorithms. The ratio of HbO_2 to total hemoglobin ($HbO_2 + Hb$) is then used to define the fraction of hemoglobin that is saturated with oxygen. The resulting "pulse oximeter saturation" (SpO_2) is expressed as a percentage;

$$SpO_2 = \frac{HbO_2}{HbO_2 + Hb} \times 100 \qquad (21.1)$$

The lower panel of Figure 21.2 shows the pulsatile output of the pulse oximeter, which is strikingly similar to an arterial pressure waveform.

Reliability

At clinically acceptable levels of arterial oxyhemoglobin saturation ($SaO_2 > 70\%$), the O_2 saturation recorded by pulse oximeters (SpO_2) differs by less than 3% from the actual SaO_2 (6,7). In addition to accuracy, the SpO_2 shows little tendency for spontaneous variations, as indicated in Table 21.1 (8).

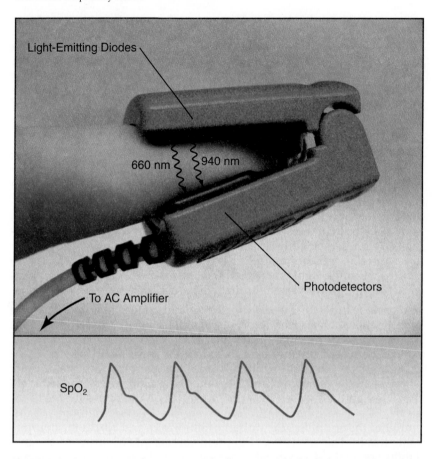

FIGURE 21.2 Fingertip pulse oximetry. The fingertip probe has light-emitting diodes (LEDs) on one side that emit light in the red (660 nm) and infrared (940 nm) spectrum, and a photodetector on the opposite side that processes light waves of alternating intensity (using an AC amplifier). The lower panel shows the pulsatile oximetry signal (SpO_2) that is displayed on the bedside monitor.

Table 21.1	Variability in Oximetry and Capnometry Recordings		
Study Parameters	**SpO_2***	**SvO_2****	**$P_{ET}CO_2$***
Time period	60 min	120 min	60 min
Mean variation	1%	6%	2 mm Hg
Range of variation	0–5%	1–19%	0–7 mm Hg

Clinically stable patients. 95% of measurements obtained during mechanical ventilation.
*From Reference 8.
**From Reference 23.

Dyshemoglobinemias

Standard pulse oximeters do not detect carboxyhemoglobin (COHb) or methemoglobin (metHb) in blood. Normally, these hemoglobin variants account for less than 5% of the total hemoglobin pool in blood (7,9). When metHb or COHb levels are abnormally elevated, the arterial O_2 saturation (SaO_2) decreases because HbO_2 is a lower fraction of the total hemoglobin pool. However, the SpO_2 from pulse oximetry is not influenced by COHb or metHb levels (10,11). Therefore, *in cases of methemoglobinemia and carbon monoxide poisoning, the SpO_2 overestimates the true SaO_2, and is not a reliable marker of arterial O_2 desaturation.*

Hospital laboratories have large oximeters that use 8 wavelengths of light to measure all the hemoglobin variants in blood. Therefore, when abnormal elevations of metHb or COHb are suspected, an arterial blood sample should be sent to the hospital laboratory for a complete oximetry assessment. Newer blood gas analyzers are also equipped with 8 wavelengths of light, and can measure the levels of metHb and COHb in blood. (Carbon monoxide poisoning and methemoglobinemia are described in Chapter 55.)

Note: A pulse oximeter is now available that uses multiple wavelengths of light to detect all forms of hemoglobin (Rainbow Pulse CO-oximeter, Masimo Corp, Irvine, CA) (12). These devices are used by firefighters and emergency first responders for rapid, on-site detection of carbon monoxide exposure, and are not meant for routine SpO_2 monitoring in a hospital setting.

Hypotension

Although pulse oximetry is based on the presence of pulsatile blood flow, SpO_2 is an accurate reflection of SaO_2 at blood pressures as low as 30 mm Hg (13). Damped pulsations also do not affect the accuracy of fingertip SpO_2 recordings distal to a cannulated radial artery (14). When fingertip SpO_2 recordings are unreliable as a result of hypotension or peripheral vasoconstriction, the forehead is an alternate site for SpO_2 monitoring (see later).

Anemia

In the absence of hypoxemia, pulse oximetry is accurate down to hemoglobin levels as low as 2 to 3 g/dL (15). At hemoglobin levels between 2.5 and 9 g/dL, SpO_2 is within 1% of the SaO_2 (15).

Pigments

The influence of skin and fingernail color on the accuracy of SpO_2 measurements has been severely curtailed by the introduction of pulse oximetry. Dark skin can produce a up to a 10% discrepancy between SpO_2 and SaO_2, but this occurs at O_2 saturations between 70% and 80% (16), which are much lower than allowed in ICU patients. Dark fingernail polish produces a very small (2%) discrepancy between SpO_2 and SaO_2 (17), but the clinical significance of this effect is in doubt.

Forehead Pulse Oximetry

The forehead is an appealing site for pulse oximetry because the arterial circulation in the forehead (which originates from the internal carotid artery) is less prone to vasoconstriction than the digital arteries in the fingers (18). Clinical studies have shown that pulse oximetry in the forehead can provide suitable SpO_2 measurements when fingertip SpO_2 recordings are compromised by hypotension or peripheral vasoconstriction (19). The basic features of forehead pulse oximetry are shown in Figure 21.3. Forehead SpO_2 sensors are placed just above the eyebrows, where vascular density is greatest. The forehead sensors have light-emitting diodes and photodetectors positioned next to each other, and they record the light intensity reflected back from the underlying arteries to derive the SpO_2. This method of *reflectance oximetry* differs from the method of *transmission oximetry* used by the fingertip SpO_2 sensors.

Venous Pulsations

The major limitation of forehead pulse oximetry is the risk of spuriously low SpO_2 readings when there is localized venous congestion (e.g., from positive-pressure mechanical ventilation). This effect is attributed to enhanced venous pulsations, which are misread as arterial pulsations, resulting in SpO_2 readings that include reflections from HbO_2 and Hb in venous blood. This effect can be minimized with an elastic headband, as shown in Figure 21.3, which helps to dispel venous blood from the forehead (20). These headbands are often provided with the forehead SpO_2 sensors.

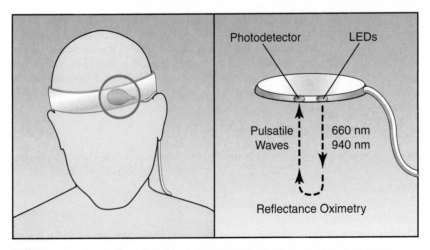

FIGURE 21.3 Forehead pulse oximetry. The forehead probe (circled in red) is placed just above the eyebrows, and an elastic headband is used to reduce venous pulsations. The probe has light-emitting diodes (LEDs) and photodetectors placed next to each other, and the intensity of pulsatile light waves that are reflected back from the underlying arteries is used to determine the SpO_2.

Using Pulse Oximetry

In theory, pulse oximetry is indicated in any situation where arterial oxygenation is a concern. In reality, pulse oximetry is considered a requirement for patient safety in certain areas of the hospital (e.g., ICUs and operating suites), and pulse oximetry is mandatory for all patients in these areas. Therefore, the important issue concerning the use of pulse oximetry in the ICU is not when to use it, but how to use it. The following information is relevant in this regard.

SpO_2 and Arterial O_2 Content

As a surrogate measure of the O_2 saturation of hemoglobin in arterial blood (SaO_2), the SpO_2 is one of the determinants of the O_2 concentration in arterial blood (CaO_2), as described in the following equation.

$$CaO_2 = 1.34 \times [Hb] \times SaO_2 \ (mL/dL) \qquad (21.2)$$

(1.34 is the oxygen binding capacity of hemoglobin in mL/g, and [Hb] is the hemoglobin concentration in blood in g/dL.) In an idealized situation where [Hb] = 15 g/dL and SpO_2 = 0.98, the CaO_2 is 19.7 mL/dL (or 197 mL/L). A 10% decrease in SpO_2 (from 0.98 to 0.88), which is considered a clinically relevant change, results in a 10% decrease in CaO_2 (from 19.7 to 17.7 mL/dL). Based on this information, the following statements about the SpO_2 are valid:

1. Since the SaO_2 is not the sole determinant of the arterial O_2 content, monitoring the SpO_2 provides only partial information about arterial oxygenation.

2. Changes in SpO_2 that are considered clinically relevant are associated with only minor changes in the O_2 content of arterial blood.

Lowest Tolerable SpO_2

A standard practice in the management of respiratory failure is to maintain the SpO_2 above a certain level by adjusting the O_2 concentration in inspired gas. However, opinions vary about the lowest tolerable SpO_2. In one survey of 25 ICU directors, the lowest acceptable SpO_2 varied from 85% to 95% (21). Studies in ventilator-dependent patients have shown that the threshold for hypoxemia (PaO_2 = 60 mm Hg) occurs at SpO_2 levels of 92% to 95% (21). However, it is important to emphasize that *the lowest SpO_2 needed to support aerobic metabolism has never been identified*, so the choice of a minimally acceptable SpO_2 is largely empirical.

Venous Oximetry

Specialized oximetry catheters are available that can monitor the O_2 saturation of hemoglobin in the superior vena cava or pulmonary artery, and the operation of these catheters is illustrated in Figure 21.4. Oximetry catheters contain fiberoptic bundles that transmit two wavelengths of light (red and infrared) from an external light source to the tip of the catheter. Another channel of the catheter is connected to a photodetector

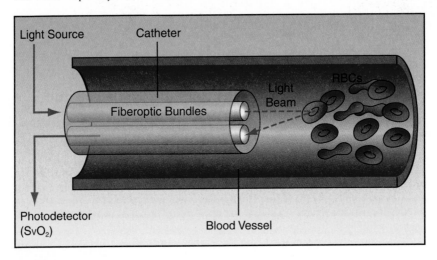

FIGURE 21.4 Venous oximetry using a specialized catheter that records the venous O_2 saturation (SvO_2) using reflectance oximetry.

that records the intensity of light that is reflected back from the hemoglobin in circulating erythrocytes. This technique (reflectance ox-imetry) is similar to the one used in forehead pulse oximetry. Oximetry catheters process and display the venous O_2 saturation every 5 seconds.

Venous O_2 Saturation

The O_2 saturation in mixed venous (pulmonary artery) blood and central venous (superior vena cava) blood (SvO_2 and $ScvO_2$, respectively) are described in Chapter 10 (see pp. 183–184). Both measurements are influenced by the balance between systemic O_2 delivery (DO_2) and O_2 consumption (VO_2), as described below:

$$SvO_2 \text{ or } ScvO_2 = 1 - VO_2/DO_2 \tag{21.3}$$

(For the derivation of this equation, see Equations 10.17 and 10.18 on page 183.) A decrease in venous O_2 saturation below the normal range ($SvO_2 < 65\%$ or $ScvO_2 < 70\%$) identifies a condition where O_2 delivery is low relative to O_2 consumption. This condition can be the result of a decrease in DO_2 (from low cardiac output, anemia, or arterial O_2 desaturation) or an increase in VO_2 (from hypermetabolism).

Mixed Venous O_2 Saturation

Measurements of SvO_2 with pulmonary artery oximetry catheters are typically within 1–2% of in vitro measurements (22). The spontaneous variations in SvO_2 can be considerable, as demonstrated in Table 21.1 (23). As a general rule, *a greater than 5% change in SvO_2 that persists for longer than 10 minutes is considered a significant change* (24).

Central Venous O_2 Saturation

Measurements of $ScvO_2$ with central venous oximetry catheters (PreSep

Catheter, Edwards Life Sciences) are slightly lower than the SvO_2, and this difference is magnified in the presence of circulatory shock (25). Single measurements of $ScvO_2$ can differ from SvO_2 by as much as 10%, but the difference is reduced (to within 5%) when multiple measurements are obtained (26).

Dual Oximetry

The predictive value of SvO_2 or $ScvO_2$ can be increased by adding the SpO_2 from pulse oximetry. The difference (SpO_2-SvO_2) or (SpO_2-ScvO_2) is roughly equivalent to the O_2 extraction from capillary blood (27). Therefore, using the equation for the O_2 extraction ratio (see Equation 10.12 on page 181), the following relationships can be defined (using SvO_2 instead of $ScvO_2$):

$$SpO_2 - SvO_2 = (VO_2/DO_2) \times 100 \qquad (21.4)$$

An increase in (SpO_2-SvO_2) above the normal range (above 30%) can be the result of an increasing VO_2 (hypermetabolism), or a decreasing DO_2 (from progressive anemia or a declining cardiac output). An (SpO_2-SvO_2) that reaches 50% can also be used as a marker of tissue hypoxia, as shown in Figure 10.5 (see page 182).

CAPNOMETRY

Capnometry is the measurement of CO_2 in exhaled gas using colorimetric techniques or infrared spectrophotometry.

Colorimetric Capnometry

The colorimetric detection of CO_2 in exhaled gas is a quick and simple method of determining if an endotracheal tube has been placed in the lungs (28). This is a standard of care following placement of an endotracheal tube because *auscultation for breath sounds is an unreliable method of determining if an endotracheal tube is in the esophagus or trachea* (29).

A popular device for the colorimetric detection of CO_2 in exhaled gas is shown in Figure 21.5. The central area of the device contains filter paper that is impregnated with a pH-sensitive indicator that changes color as a function of pH. When exhaled gas passes over the filter paper, the CO_2 in the gas is hydrated by a liquid film on the filter paper, and the resulting pH is detected by a color change. The outer perimeter of the device contains color-coded sections indicating the concentrations of exhaled CO_2 associated with each color change.

Predictive Value

The accuracy of this colorimetric device for predicting the success of endotracheal intubation is shown in Table 21.2 (28). A color change from purple to tan or yellow almost always indicates successful intubation of the trachea. The absence of a color change from purple indicates that the endotracheal tube is not in the trachea, except during a cardiac arrest, when successful intubation of the trachea does not always produce a

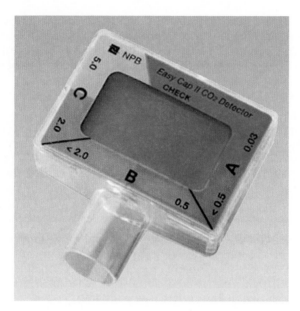

FIGURE 21.5 A disposable device (Nellcor Easy Cap II CO_2 Detector) for the colorimetric detection of CO_2 in exhaled gas. See text for explanation.

color change from purple. This latter observation is explained by the fact that exhaled CO_2 decreases when cardiac output is reduced, and the absence of a functional cardiac output during a cardiac arrest will result in very low levels of exhaled CO_2. Therefore, *the lack of a color change from purple on the colorimetric CO_2 detector is not evidence of failure to intubate the lungs during a cardiac arrest.*

Table 21.2	Performance of Colorimetric CO_2 Detector[†]	
	Color on CO_2 Detector	
Patient Group	**Purple** **(CO_2 <0.5%)**	**Tan or Yellow** **(CO_2 ≥0.5%)**
No cardiac arrest (n=83)	Tube in esophagus in 100% of cases	Tube in trachea in 99% of cases
Cardiac arrest (n=144)	Tube in trachea in 77% of cases and tube in esophagus in 23% of cases	Tube in trachea in 100% of cases

†From Reference 28.

Infrared Capnography

Carbon dioxide absorbs light in the infrared spectrum, which is the basis for the use of infrared light absorption to measure the PCO_2 in exhaled gas (30). This provides a more quantitative measure of exhaled CO_2 than the colorimetric method. Figure 21.6 shows an infrared CO_2 probe that has an airway attachment (which is placed in series with the expiratory tubing during mechanical ventilation) and a fitted transducer. When in place, the probe emits a continuous infrared light beam that travels through the exhaled gas. The photodetector has a rapid response, and can measure changes in PCO_2 during a single exhalation. This is recorded as an expiratory *capnogram* like the one in Figure 21.6.

The Capnogram

The shape of the normal capnogram has been described as "the outline of a snake that has swallowed an elephant" (31). The PCO_2 at the onset of expiration is negligible because the gas in the upper airways is first to leave the lungs. As exhalation proceeds, gas from the alveoli begins to contribute to the exhaled gas, and the PCO_2 begins to rise steadily. The rate of rise eventually declines, and the exhaled PCO_2 reaches a plateau. When gas exchange is normal, the PCO_2 at the end of expiration (called the *end-tidal PCO_2*) is equivalent to the PCO_2 in end-capillary (arterial) blood.

End-Tidal vs. Arterial PCO_2

When pulmonary gas exchange is normal, the end-tidal PCO_2 is only 2 to 3 mm Hg lower than the arterial PCO_2 (30). However, when gas exchange in the lungs is impaired, and specifically when there is increased dead space ventilation, the end-tidal PCO_2 decreases relative to the arterial PCO_2. In this situation, the $PaCO_2 - P_{ET}CO_2$ difference is greater than 3 mm Hg. The conditions associated with an increased $PaCO_2 - P_{ET}CO_2$ difference are listed in Table 21.3.

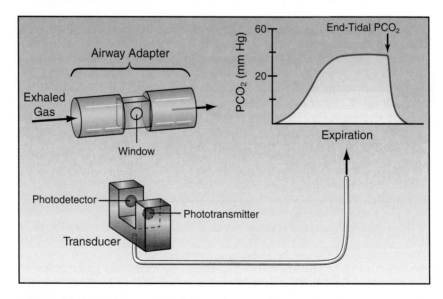

FIGURE 21.6 Infrared capnography. The airway adapter and fitted transducer allow for a steady beam of infrared light to pass through exhaled gas. The photodetector records the PCO_2 continuously during each exhalation, which is displayed in the expired capnogram.

Table 21.3	Conditions Associated with an Increased $PaCO_2$–$P_{ET}CO_2$ Gradient
Gas Exchange Abnormality	**Conditions**
Increased Anatomic Dead Space	• Open ventilator circuit • Shallow breathing
Increased Physiologic Dead Space	• Obstructive lung disease • Excessive lung inflation • Low cardiac output • Pulmonary embolism

The end-tidal PCO_2 can be higher than arterial PCO_2 in the following situations (32): (a) when CO_2 production is high (from hypermetabolism or a metabolic acidosis) and there is a low inflation volume or a high cardiac output, or (b) when the concentration of inhaled O_2 is very high (the O_2 displaces CO_2 from Hb).

Nonintubated Patients

End-tidal PCO_2 can be monitored in nonintubated patients using a modified nasal cannula. These are commercially available (Salter divided nasal cannula, DRE Medical, Louisville, KY), or a nasal cannula can be modified as shown in Figure 21.7 (33). The tubing between the two nasal prongs must be occluded (either with a cotton ball inserted through one of the nasal prongs or with a small screw clamp). This allows one nasal prong to be used for oxygen inhalation, while the other nasal prong is used to transmit exhaled gas. A 14-gauge intravascular catheter (2 inches long) is inserted into the exhalation side of the nasal cannula to transmit gas to a CO_2 detector. A sidestream CO_2 detector (i.e., one that applies suction to draw gas from the tubing) is best suited for this application. If one of these is not available, a mainstream infrared CO_2 detector (such as the one shown in Fig. 20.5) can be used with a suction pump to draw gas samples from the cannula (at 150 mL/minute). The respiratory therapy department can help with this modification.

Clinical Applications

The following are some useful applications of end-tidal CO_2 monitoring.

Arterial PCO_2

The end-tidal PCO_2 can be used as a noninvasive method of monitoring the arterial PCO_2. The arterial PCO_2 should be measured simultaneously with the end-tidal PCO_2 to establish the baseline $PaCO_2$–$P_{ET}CO_2$ gradient. This gradient should remain the same as long as no other process intervenes to disturb pulmonary gas exchange. Changing ventilator settings will influence the $PaCO_2$–$P_{ET}CO_2$ gradient (34), so the arterial

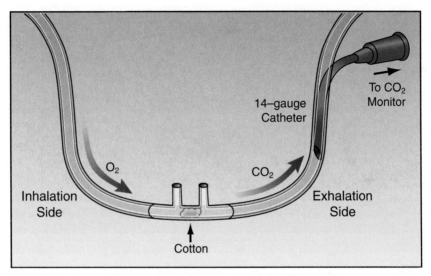

FIGURE 21.7 A modified nasal cannula to monitor end-tidal PCO_2 during spontaneous breathing.

PCO_2 should be measured after each change in ventilator settings to determine the new relationship between arterial and end-tidal PCO_2.

Cardiac Output

The most promising application of end-tidal PCO_2 monitoring is the noninvasive detection of changes in cardiac output. There is a close correlation between changes in end-tidal PCO_2 and changes in cardiac output, as demonstrated in Figure 21.8 (35). This can be useful for detecting acute changes in cardiac output (e.g., in response to volume loading), and is proving *very useful for monitoring changes in cardiac output during cardiopulmonary resuscitation* (see pages 334–335).

Nosocomial Complications

A sudden decrease in end-tidal PCO_2 with an increase in the $PaCO_2$–$PetCO_2$ gradient can be an early warning sign for any of the following conditions:

1. Overdistension of alveoli from high tidal volumes or PEEP.

2. Migration of an endotracheal tube into a mainstem bronchus (36).

3. Acute pulmonary embolism (37).

4. Acute pulmonary edema.

5. Pneumonia.

Ventilator Weaning

During weaning from mechanical ventilation, end-tidal PCO_2 monitoring can serve several purposes (38). In uneventful weaning (e.g., following surgery), it serves as a noninvasive measure of $PaCO_2$. In difficult or

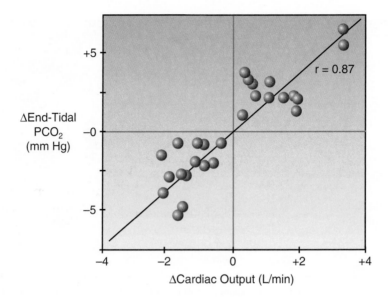

FIGURE 21.8 Relationship between changes in end-tidal PCO_2 and changes in cardiac output in a group of postoperative patients. r = correlation coefficient. Data from Reference 35.

complicated weaning, it can help determine the success or failure of the wean attempt. For example, a progressive rise in end-tidal PCO_2 can be a sign of an increase in the work of breathing (a sign of wean failure), while a decrease in end-tidal PCO_2 can be a sign of respiratory muscle weakness with shallow breathing (another sign of failure to wean).

A FINAL WORD

Filling the Void

The fall from grace of the pulmonary artery catheter has created a void in the ability to monitor the cardiac output, but the techniques described in this chapter can help to fill this void. Both dual oximetry (i.e., combining pulse oximetry and central venous oximetry) and end-tidal PCO_2 monitoring can be useful for evaluating the adequacy of cardiac output, and for detecting changes in cardiac output (e.g., in response to volume loading). End-tidal PCO_2 monitoring has the advantage of being totally noninvasive, while dual oximetry has the advantage of monitoring the balance between systemic O_2 delivery (DO_2) and O_2 uptake (VO_2). Of course, nothing can replace the pulmonary artery catheter (at least at the present time) for monitoring cardiac output and systemic oxygenation.

REFERENCES

Introduction

1. Neff TA. Routine oximetry. A fifth vital sign? Chest 1988; 94:227.
2. Mower WR, Myers G, Nicklin EL, et. al. Pulse oximetry as a fifth vital sign in emergency geriatric assessment. Acad Emerg Med 1998; 5:858–869.
3. Stoneham MD, Saville GM, Wilson IH. Knowledge about pulse oximetry among medical and nursing staff. Lancet 1994; 344:1339–1342.

Oximetry

4. Barker SJ, Tremper KK. Pulse oximetry: applications and limitations. Internat Anesthesiol Clin 1987; 25:155–175.
5. Ortega R, Hansen CJ, Elterman K, Woo A. Videos in clinical medicine: pulse oximetry. N Engl J Med 2011; 364:e33.
6. Wahr JA, Tremper KK. Noninvasive oxygen monitoring techniques. Crit Care Clin 1995; 11:199–217.
7. Severinghaus JW, Kelleher JF. Recent developments in pulse oximetry. Anesthesiology 1992; 76:1018–1038.
8. Hess D, Agarwal NN. Variability of blood gases, pulse oximeter saturation, and end-tidal carbon dioxide pressure in stable, mechanically ventilated trauma patients. J Clin Monit 1992; 8:111–115.
9. Soubani AO. Noninvasive monitoring of oxygen and carbon dioxide. Am J Emerg Med 2001; 19:141-146.
10. Hampson NB, Piantidosi CA, Thom SR, Weaver LK. Practice recommendations in the diagnosis, management, and prevention of carbon monoxide poisoning. Am J Respir Crit Care Med 2012; 186:1095–1101.
11. Barker SJ, Kemper KK, Hyatt J. Effects of methemoglobinemia on pulse oximetry and mixed venous oximetry. Anesthesiology 1989; 70:112–117.
12. Barker SJ, Badal JJ. The measurement of dyshemoglobins and total hemoglobin by pulse oximetry. Curr Opin Anesthesiol 2008; 21:805–810.
13. Severinghaus JW, Spellman MJ. Pulse oximeter failure thresholds in hypotension and vasoconstriction. Anesthesiology 1990; 73:532–537.
14. Morris RW, Nairn M, Beaudoin M. Does the radial arterial line degrade the performance of a pulse oximeter? Anesth Intensive Care 1990; 18:107–109.
15. Jay GD, Hughes L, Renzi FP. Pulse oximetry is accurate in acute anemia from hemorrhage. Ann Emerg Med 1994; 24:32–35.
16. Feiner JR, Severinghaus JW, Bickler PE. Dark skin decreases the accuracy of pulse oximeters at low oxygen saturation: the effects of oximeter probe type and gender. Anesth Analg 2007; 105(Suppl):S18–S23.
17. Chan ED. What is the effect of fingernail polish on pulse oximetry? Chest 2003; 123:2163–2164.

18. Branson RD, Manheimer PD. Forehead oximetry in critically ill patients: the case for a new monitoring site. Respir Care Clin N Amer 2004; 10:359–367.

19. Palve H. Reflection and transmission pulse oximetry during compromised peripheral perfusion. J Clin Monit 1992; 8:12–15.

20. Agashe GS, Coakely J, Mannheimer PD. Forehead pulse oximetry. Headband use helps alleviate false low recordings likely related to venous pulsation artifact. Anesthesiology 2006; 105:1111–1116.

21. Jubran A, Tobin M. Reliability of pulse oximetry in titrating supplemental oxygen therapy in ventilator-dependent patients. Chest 1990; 97:1420–1435.

22. Armaganidis A, Dhinaut JF, Billard JL, et al. Accuracy assessment for three fiberoptic pulmonary artery catheters for SvO_2 monitoring. Intensive Care Med 1994; 20:484–488.

23. Noll ML, Fountain RL, Duncan CA, et al. Fluctuation in mixed venous oxygen saturation in critically ill medical patients: a pilot study. Am J Crit Care 1992; 3:102–106.

24. Krafft P, Steltzer H, Heismay M, et al. Mixed venous oxygen saturation in critically ill septic shock patients. Chest 1993; 103:900–906.

25. Rivers EP, Ander DS, Powell D. Central venous oxygen saturation monitoring in the critically ill patient. Curr Opin Crit Care 2001; 7:204–211.

26. Dueck MH, Kilmek M, Appenrodt S, et al. Trends but not individual values of central venous oxygen saturation agree with mixed venous oxygen saturation during varying hemodynamic conditions. Anesthesiology 2005; 103:249–257.

27. Bongard FS, Leighton TA. Continuous dual oximetry in surgical critical care. Ann Surg 1992; 216:60–68.

Colorimetric Capnometry

28. Ornato JP, Shipley JB, Racht EM, et al. Multicenter study of a portable, hand-size, colorimetric end-tidal carbon dioxide detection device. Ann Emerg Med 1992; 21:518–523.

29. Mizutani AR, Ozake G, Benumoff JL, et al. Auscultation cannot distinguish esophageal from tracheal passage of tube. J Clin Monit 1991; 7:232–236.

Infrared Capnography

30. Stock MC. Capnography for adults. Crit Care Clin 1995; 11:219–232. .

31. Gravenstein JS, Paulus DA, Hayes TJ. Capnography in clinical practice. Boston ButterworthHeinemann, 1989; 11.

32. Moorthy SS, Losasso AM, Wilcox J. End-tidal PCO2 greater than $PaCO_2$. Crit Care Med 1984; 12:534–535.

33. Roy J, McNulty SE, Torjman MC. An improved nasal prong apparatus for end-tidal carbon dioxide monitoring in awake, sedated patients. J Clin Monit 1991; 7:249–252.

34. Hoffman RA, Kreiger PB, Kramer MR, et al. End-tidal carbon dioxide in critically ill patients during changes in mechanical ventilation. Am Rev Respir Dis 1989; 140:1265–1268.

35. Shibutani K, Shirasaki S, Braatz T, et al. Changes in cardiac output affect PETCO2, CO2 transport, and O_2 uptake during unsteady state in humans. J Clin Monit 1992; 8:175–176.

36. Gandhi SK, Munshi CA, Bardeen-Henschel A. Capnography for detection of endobronchial migration of an endotracheal tube. J Clin Monit 1991; 7:35–38.

37. Rodger MA, Gwynne J, Rasuli P. Steady-state end-tidal alveolar dead space fraction and D-dimer. Bedside tests to exclude pulmonary embolism. Chest 2001; 120:115–119.

38. Healey CJ, Fedullo AJ, Swinburne AJ, Wahl GW. Comparison of noninvasive measurements of carbon dioxide tension during weaning from mechanical ventilation. Crit Care Med 1987; 15:764–767.

Chapter 22

OXYGEN THERAPY

Carbon structures life. Oxygen ignites it.

Eric Roston
The Carbon Age
2008

One of the rare sights in any ICU is a patient who is NOT receiving supplemental oxygen to breathe. Oxygen is used liberally in ICU patients, and oxygen therapy is guided by measures (i.e., the arterial PO_2 and O_2 saturation) that have no proven relationship with tissue oxygenation. As emphasized in this chapter, the excessive use of oxygen without evidence of impaired tissue oxygenation is problematic because it promotes the formation of toxic oxygen metabolites, which are capable of lethal cell injury.

This chapter begins with some insights on the design of the human body in relation to oxygen and oxygen therapy. This is followed by a description of the different oxygen delivery systems. The final section is devoted to the dark side of oxygen; i.e., the propensity for oxygen to damage aerobic organisms.

INSIGHTS

The Paucity of Oxygen in Tissues

Despite our dependence on oxygen for metabolic energy production, aerobic metabolism is carried out in an oxygen-restricted environment. Oxygen does not readily dissolve in water, which is why we need hemoglobin to transport oxygen, and this limits the volume of dissolved oxygen in the tissues of the body. The estimated volume of oxygen in the interstitial fluid and cells of the human body is shown in Table 22.1. According to these estimates, there is only about 13 mL of O_2 in all the tissues of the human body!

Table 22.1	The Paucity of Dissolved Oxygen in Tissues	
	Interstitial Fluid	**Intracellular Fluid**
PO$_2$	35 mm Hg	5 mm Hg
O$_2$ Content†	0.45 mL/L	0.15 mL/L
Fluid Volume$^\xi$	16 L	23 L
Volume of O$_2$	9.6 mL	3.5 mL

†Dissolved O$_2$ content = $\alpha \times$ PO$_2$ where α (solubility coefficient) = 0.03 mL/L/mm Hg for O$_2$ in water at 37°C.

$^\xi$Volume estimates are based on total body water (TBW) of 42 liters, an intracellular volume that is 55% of TBW, and an interstitial volume that is 38% of TBW.

The estimates in Table 22.1 are based on the determinants of dissolved O$_2$ in the equation shown below.

$$\text{Dissolved O}_2 \text{ (mL/L)} = 0.03 \times \text{PO}_2 \tag{22.1}$$

where 0.03 is the solubility coefficient of O$_2$ in water (expressed as mL O$_2$ per liter of body water per mm Hg of PO$_2$) at a body temperature of 37°C. Experimental studies show that the intracellular PO$_2$ is about 5 mm Hg (1) and interstitial PO$_2$ is about 15 mm Hg (2). Using these PO$_2$ values in equation 22.1, the concentration of dissolved O$_2$ will be $0.03 \times 5 = 0.15$ mL/L inside cells and $0.03 \times 15 = 0.45$ mL/L in the interstitial fluid. An average sized adult has an intracellular volume of about 23 liters and an interstitial fluid volume of about 16 liters, so the total volume of dissolved O$_2$ will be $0.15 \times 23 = 3.5$ mL in cells and $0.45 \times 16 = 9.6$ mL in the interstitial fluid.

Man as a Microaerophilic Organism

Humans are described as obligate aerobic organisms; i.e., organisms that require oxygen to survive. However, according to the estimates in Table 22.1, humans are more accurately described as microaerophilic organisms; i.e., organisms that require only low concentrations of oxygen to survive.

Implications

The oxygen-restricted environment in tissues can be viewed as a safeguard against the damaging effects of oxygen metabolites (described later in the chapter). This safeguard will be threatened or lost if oxygen therapy exposes the tissues to more O$_2$ than is needed to sustain aerobic metabolism. The remaining observations in this section are relevant to this issue.

Tolerance to Hypoxemia

Oxygen therapy is used to prevent hypoxemia (i.e., an arterial PO$_2$ < 60 mm Hg or an arterial O$_2$ saturation < 90%) (3). However, there is no evidence that hypoxemia impairs tissue oxygenation, regardless of severity (4–6). The data points in Figure 22.1 show the blood lactate levels in patients with severe hypoxemia (i.e., arterial $PO_2 < 40$ mm Hg) from an acute exacerbation of chronic obstructive lung disease (4). Note that the blood lactate levels fail to rise above 2 mmol/L (the threshold for hyperlactatemia) despite arterial PO_2 levels as low as 22 mm Hg. This provides evidence that severe hypoxemia did not impair aerobic metabolism in these patients. Similar observations have been reported in patients with acute respiratory distress syndrome (5), indicating that tolerance to severe hypoxemia is not an adaptation that develops over time. (*Note:* Tolerance to hypoxemia is the reason that "hypoxemic shock" is not a clinical entity.)

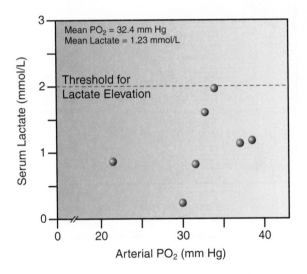

FIGURE 22.1 The relationship between arterial PO_2 and blood lactate levels in seven patients with severe hypoxemia (arterial $PO_2 < 40$ mm Hg) from acute exacerbation of chronic obstructive lung disease. All lactate levels are within the normal range (≤ 2 mmol/L), suggesting that severe hypoxemia did not impair tissue oxygenation in these patients. Data from Reference 4.

O_2 Therapy and Aerobic Metabolism

Since hypoxemia does not impair aerobic metabolism, then oxygen therapy (which is aimed at relieving hypoxemia) should not be necessary for preserving aerobic metabolism. This is supported by observations like those in Figure 22.2. The graphs in this figure show the effects of breathing 24% and 28% oxygen on the arterial PO_2 (PaO_2) and systemic oxygen consumption (VO_2) in patients with acute exacerbation of chronic obstructive lung disease. There is a significant increase in the PaO_2 with each increment in inhaled O_2, but the VO_2 remains unchanged. Similar results have been reported in other clinical studies (8,9), and since the VO_2 represents the rate of aerobic metabolism, these studies indicate that *oxygen therapy does not promote aerobic metabolism.*

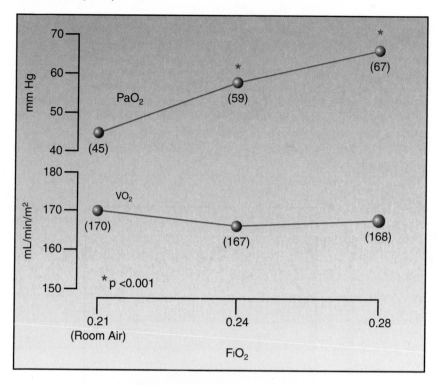

FIGURE 22.2 Acute effects of oxygen therapy on the arterial PO_2 (PaO_2) and systemic oxygen consumption (VO_2) in ICU patients with acute exacerbation of chronic obstructive lung disease. Numbers in parentheses are the mean values for each measurement. FIO_2 = fraction of O_2 in inhaled gas. Data from Reference 7.

Pure oxygen breathing (a condition known as *normobaric hyperoxia*) is accompanied by a 10% to 20% decrease in VO_2 (10,11), indicating that *hyperoxia can inhibit aerobic metabolism*(!). This effect has been attributed to oxygen-induced changes in microvascular flow (described next), and it is blocked by the antioxidant N-acetylcysteine (12), indicating that toxic oxygen metabolites are involved.

Oxygen and the Microcirculation

Oxygen therapy produces systemic vasoconstriction (not pulmonary vasoconstriction) that is most pronounced in the small arterioles that control capillary blood flow (12–14). At high concentrations of inhaled O_2, the arteriolar constriction can be accompanied by a decrease in functional capillary density (15), and this could result in a decrease in O_2 availability in the capillaries. This has been implicated in the reduction of VO_2 that occurs during normobaric hyperoxia (described above), and it may also be a mechanism for protecting the tissues from oxygen-induced injury (oxidant injury) during periods of hyperoxia.

Summary and Implications

The information just presented indicates that aerobic metabolism is normally conducted in an oxygen-restricted environment, and this condition persists in the face of severe hypoxemia. Furthermore, attempts to provide more oxygen are met with resistance, as arteriolar vasoconstriction reduces the capillary surface area available for oxygen entry into tissues. Thus, the tissues are normally oxygen-restricted, and it seems they want to remain that way. This is understandable in light of the propensity for oxygen to produce lethal cell damage, as described in the last section of the chapter.

If the scenario just presented is accurate, then oxygen therapy, which does not promote aerobic metabolism, is merely creating an added risk of oxygen-induced (oxidant) damage in the vital organs. The observation that arterial hyperoxia following cardiac arrest is associated with an increased mortality rate (16) is consistent with the notion that oxygen therapy can be dangerous. Considering the prominent role played by oxidant injury in the damaging effects of inflammation (which is a leading cause of morbidity and mortality in the ICU), the current liberal use of oxygen in critically ill patients deserves scrutiny.

OXYGEN DELIVERY SYSTEMS

Oxygen delivery systems are classified as low-flow systems, reservoir systems, and high-flow systems (17). Low-flow systems use standard nasal prongs, while reservoir systems use standard face masks and face masks with reservoir bags, and high-flow systems use air-entrainment masks or heated, humidified O_2 delivered through nasal prongs. Each system is characterized by the following features: (a) the manner in which the fractional concentration of inspired oxygen (FiO_2) is determined, (b) the achievable FiO_2 range, (c) the variability of the FiO_2, and (d) the type of patient that is most appropriate for the system. The features of different oxygen delivery systems are summarized in Table 22.2

Table 22.2	Oxygen Delivery Systems			
System or Device	Oxygen Flow Rates	Reservoir Volume	FiO_2 Range	FiO_2 Variability
Low-Flow Nasal O_2	1–6 L/min	—	24–40%	Variable
Standard Face Mask	5–10 L/min	100–200 mL	35–50%	Variable
Partial Rebreather Mask	>10 L/min	600–1000 mL	40–70%	Variable
Nonrebreather Mask	>10 L/min	600–1000 mL	60–80%	Variable
Air-Entrainment Mask	>60 L/min	100–200 mL	24–50%	Constant
High-Flow Nasal O_2	≤40 L/min	—	21–100%	Variable

Low-Flow Nasal O_2

The standard device for low-flow O_2 therapy is the nasal cannula or nasal prongs, which deliver oxygen into the nasopharynx at flow rates of 1 to 6 L/min. (The normal inspiratory flow rate during quiet breathing is about 15 L/min (0.25 L/sec), so low-flow nasal O_2 represents only a fraction of the inspiratory flow generated by the patient.) A large fraction of the inspired volume is drawn from room air, which means that low-flow nasal O_2 does not achieve high concentrations of inhaled oxygen. The FIO_2 range during quiet breathing is 24% O_2 (at 1 L/min) up to 40% O_2 (at 6 L/min), as shown in Table 22.2.

In patients with acute respiratory failure, peak inspiratory flow rates can increase to 30–120 L/min (18). In this situation, low-flow nasal O_2 provides an even smaller fraction of the inspiratory flow needs of the patient. For this reason, low-flow nasal O_2 is often not adequate for O_2 therapy in patients with high ventilatory demands.

Advantages and Disadvantages

The major advantages of nasal prongs are simplicity of use and patient acceptance, including the ability for patients to eat and converse. The major disadvantage is the inability to achieve high concentrations of inhaled O_2, particularly in patients with increased ventilatory demands.

Standard Face Masks

Face masks are considered a reservoir system because the mask encloses a volume of 100 to 200 mL. Standard face masks deliver oxygen at flow rates between 5 and 10 L/min; a minimum flow rate of 5 L/min is needed to clear exhaled gas from the mask. Exhalation ports on the side of the face mask also allow room air to be inhaled. This system can achieve a maximum FIO_2 of about 60% during quiet breathing.

Advantages and Disadvantages

Standard face masks can provide a slightly higher maximum FIO_2 than low-flow nasal prongs, but like nasal prongs, the FIO_2 varies with the ventilatory demands of the patient. Face masks are more confining than nasal prongs, and they do not permit oral feeding.

Masks with Reservoir Bags

The addition of a reservoir bag to a standard face mask increases the capacity of the oxygen reservoir by 600 to 1000 mL (depending on the size of the bag). If the reservoir bag is kept inflated, the patient will draw primarily from the gas in the bag. There are two types of reservoir bag devices: partial rebreathers and nonrebreathers.

Partial Rebreather

The device shown in Figure 22.3 is a *partial rebreather*. This device allows the gas exhaled in the initial phase of expiration to return to the reservoir bag. As exhalation proceeds, the expiratory flow rate declines, and when the expiratory flow rate falls below the oxygen flow rate, exhaled gas can no longer return to the reservoir bag. The initial part of expiration contains gas from the upper airways (anatomic dead space), so the gas that is rebreathed is rich in oxygen and largely devoid of CO_2. The patient can inhale room air through the exhalation ports on the mask, but the gas in the reservoir bag is under positive pressure, and inhalation will draw primarily from the gas in the bag. Partial rebreather devices can achieve a maximum FiO_2 of about 70%.

Nonrebreather

The device shown in Figure 22.4 is a *nonrebreather system*. The expiratory ports on the mask are covered with flaps that allow exhaled gas to escape but prevent inhalation of room air gas. There is also a one-way valve between the reservoir bag and the mask that allows inhalation of gas

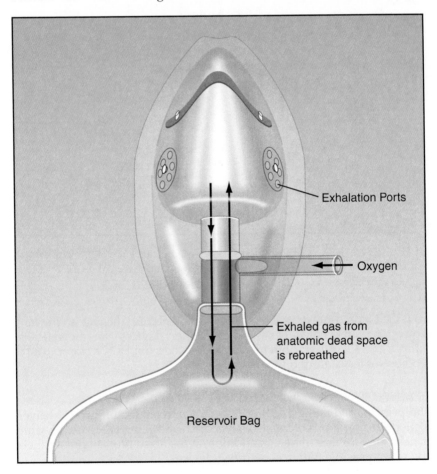

FIGURE 22.3 Partial rebreather system. The initial 100 to 150 mL of exhaled gas (anatomic dead space) is returned to the reservoir bag for rebreathing. Exhaled gas stops entering the reservoir bag when the expiratory flow rate falls below the oxygen flow rate.

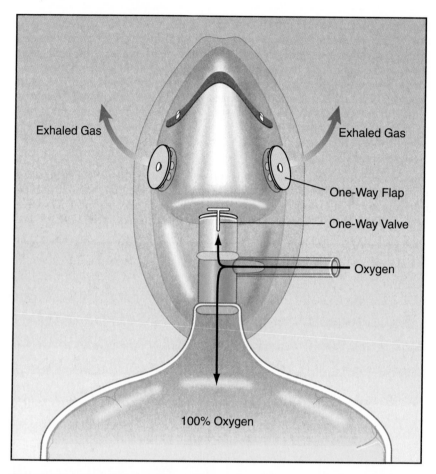

FIGURE 22.4 Nonrebreather system. Flaps on the exhalation ports of the mask prevent inhalation of room air, and a one-way valve between the mask and reservoir bag prevents exhaled gas from entering the bag for rebreathing.

from the bag but prevents exhaled gas from entering the bag (to prevent rebreathing of exhaled gas). Nonrebreather devices can theoretically achieve an FIO_2 of 100%, but in reality the maximum FIO_2 is closer to 80% (because of leaks around the mask).

Advantages and Disadvantages

The principal advantage of the reservoir bags is the ability to deliver higher concentrations of inhaled oxygen. The disadvantages are the same as described for face masks. In addition, aerosolized bronchodilator therapy is not possible with reservoir bag devices.

Air Entrainment Device

Air entrainment devices are high-flow systems that deliver a constant FIO_2.

The operation of an air-entrainment device is shown in Figure 22.5 (19). The end of the oxygen inlet port is narrowed, and this creates a high-velocity stream of gas (analogous to the nozzle on a garden hose). This creates a shearing force known as *viscous drag* that pulls room air into the device through air-entrainment ports. The greater the flow of O_2 into the mask, the greater the volume of air that is entrained, and this keeps the FiO_2 constant. The final flow created by the device is in excess of 60 L/min, which exceeds the inspiratory flow rate in most cases of respiratory distress. The FiO_2 can be varied by varying the size of the air entrainment port on the device. The FiO_2 range of these devices is 24 to 50%.

Note: The mechanism of air entrainment in these devices is known as *jet mixing* (19). However, air entrainment was originally attributed to the Venturi effect (i.e., where the pressure of a fluid decreases when the fluid flows through a constricted section of a tube), and as a result, masks that used these devices were called *Venturi masks* or *Venti-masks*.

Advantages and Disadvantages

The major advantage of air-entrainment devices is the ability to deliver a constant FiO_2. This is desirable in patients with chronic CO_2 retention, where an inadvertent increase in FiO_2 can lead to further increases in arterial PCO_2. The major disadvantage of these devices is inability to deliver high concentrations of inhaled O_2.

High-Flow Nasal O_2

The newest technique of O_2 delivery (in adults) is high-flow nasal O_2 using heated and humidified gas. Using oxygen that is heated to body temperature and supersaturated with water (to a relative humidity of

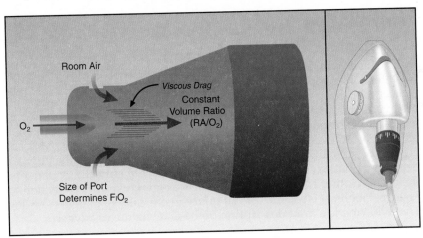

FIGURE 22.5 Function of an air-entrainment device. A narrowing at the oxygen inlet creates a high-velocity stream of gas that creates viscous drag, which pulls in room air (RA). This "jet mixing" keeps the concentration of inhaled oxygen constant, regardless of changes in the flow rate of oxygen. See text for further explanation.

99%), O_2 flow rates up to 40–60 L/min can be delivered through wide nasal prongs without discomfort and mucosal injury. A commercially available product for high-flow nasal O_2 (Vapotherm, Stevensville, MD) allows adjustments for flow rate (1–40 L/min), FIO_2 (21–100%), and temperature (usually at 37°C).

Clinical Experience

The initial experience with high-flow nasal O_2 has been very encouraging. Preliminary studies have shown that, in patients who require a high FIO_2 using mask devices, switching to humidified, high-flow nasal O_2 was associated with a significant improvement in measures of respiratory distress (e.g., reduced respiratory rate, less dyspnea), along with a decrease in the PaO_2/FIO_2 ratio (indicating improved gas exchange) (20,21). The beneficial effect on gas exchange may be explained by the observation that high-flow nasal O_2 creates positive pressure in the nasopharynx (22), which could act like positive end-expiratory pressure (PEEP) to prevent the collapse of alveoli at the end-of expiration (PEEP is described in Chapter 26). The most exciting observation regarding high-flow nasal O_2 comes from a study where the improvements resulting from high-flow nasal O_2 made it possible to avoid intubation and mechanical ventilation in 75% of the patients studied (21).

Advantages and Disadvantages

The balance sheet for high-flow nasal O_2 shows all advantages and no disadvantages (so far). The advantages include improved oxygenation and gas exchange, and a possible role in avoiding intubation and mechanical ventilation in patients with refractory hypoxemia. You will certainly hear more about this promising method of O_2 therapy in the near future.

THE TOXIC NATURE OF OXYGEN

Ever wonder why food is stored in vacuum-sealed containers, or why we wrap food in cellophane to keep it fresh? These measures are designed to protect food from exposure to oxygen, which oxidizes and disrupts all organic molecules (including the carbohydrates, proteins, and lipids in food), and is responsible for the decomposition of food. The metabolites of oxygen are even more damaging than the parent molecule, and are capable of inflicting lethal cell injury (23). In fact, contrary to the popular perception that oxygen protects cells from injury in critically ill patients, the accumulating evidence indicates that oxygen (via the production to toxic metabolites) is a *source* of cell injury in critically ill patients (23–26). The following is a brief description of the toxic nature of oxygen.

Oxygen Metabolism

The metabolism of oxygen takes place at the end of the electron transport chain in mitochondria (within the cytochrome oxidase complex), where the electrons that accumulate as a result of ATP production are cleared by the chemical reduction of oxygen to water. The reaction sequence for this process is shown in Figure 22.6. Oxygen has two unpaired electrons in its outer orbitals with the same directional spin. According to Pauli's Exclusion Principle (from the Austrian physicist Wolfgang Pauli), no two electrons can occupy the same orbital if they have the same directional spin. This means it is not possible to add an electron pair to oxygen and reduce it to water as a one-step process because one orbital would have two electrons with the same directional spin, which is a quantum impossibility. Because of this spin restriction, oxygen is metabolized in a series of single-electron reduction reactions, and this produces some highly reactive intermediates.

The intermediates in oxygen metabolism include the superoxide radical, hydrogen peroxide, and the hydroxyl radical. The behavior of these

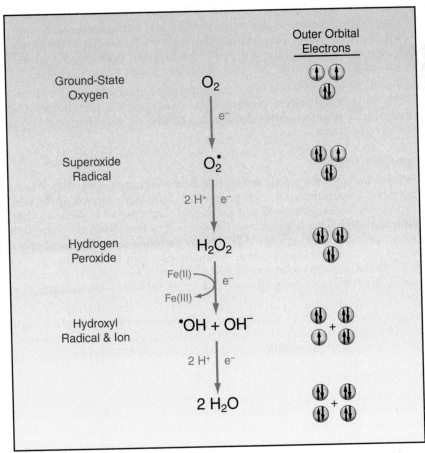

FIGURE 22.6 The metabolism of molecular oxygen to water involves a series of four single-electron reduction reactions. Orbital diagrams on the right side of the figure show the directional spin of electrons in the outer orbitals of each reactant. Free radical metabolites are indicated by a superscripted dot. See text for explanation.

metabolites is summarized in the following statements (23):

1. All the intermediates in O_2 metabolism are oxidizing agents or *oxidants* that are capable of disrupting and damaging vital cell components such as membrane lipids, cytoplasmic proteins, and nuclear DNA.

2. The superoxide and hydroxyl radicals are free radicals (i.e., they have an unpaired electron in their outer orbitals), and free radicals tend to be highly reactive. (Oxygen is also a free radical, but it is only sluggishly reactive because of the spin restriction just described.)

3. The hydroxyl radical is the most reactive molecule known in biochemistry, and enters into a reaction within three molecular diameters of its point of origin (23)! It is the most destructive O_2 metabolite, and is a major source of oxygen-induced cell injury.

4. Free iron in its reduced form (Fe^{++}) catalyses the formation of the hydroxyl radical, and thus free iron can act as a pro-oxidant (see later).

5. Hydrogen peroxide is not a free radical, and is the least reactive of the O_2 metabolites. This low reactivity allows hydrogen peroxide to move freely throughout the body, creating the potential for widespread oxidant injury.

Normally, at least 95% of oxygen is completely reduced to water, and only 3–5% of O_2 metabolism generates the damaging O_2 metabolites (27). Depletion of selected antioxidants like glutathione will change this proportion (see later).

Neutrophil Activation

Oxygen metabolites play a major role in the inflammatory response, as described in Chapter 14 (see pages 263–266). The activation of neutrophils involves a marked (up to 50-fold) increase in cellular O_2 consumption (26). This is known as the *respiratory burst*, and its purpose is not to generate high-energy ATP, but to produce toxic O_2 metabolites, which are stored in cytoplasmic granules. Oxygen metabolism in neutrophils also generates *hypochlorite* (see Figure 14.1 on page 265), which is highly microbicidal (and is the active ingredient in household bleach).

When neutrophils arrive at the sight of infection, they degranulate and release the stored O_2 metabolites to damage and destroy the invading microbes. Unfortunately, the O_2 metabolites can also damage the tissues of the host if adequate antioxidant protection is not available (25,26).

Chain Reactions

The damage produced by O_2 metabolites is magnified because of the *tendency for free radicals to create chain reactions* (28). When a free radical reacts with a non-radical, the non-radical loses an electron and is transformed into a free radical, which can then remove an electron from another nonradical to produce another free radical, and so on. This creates a self-sustaining reaction that continues after the inciting event is eliminated. A fire is a familiar example of a chain reaction involving free radicals. Chain reactions would also explain the progression of inflammatory multiorgan failure in severe sepsis and septic shock after the infection has been eradicated.

Antioxidant Protection

Oxidative (oxygen-related) injury is kept in check by a vast array of endogenous *antioxidants* (i.e., atoms or molecules that prevent or block the actions of oxidizing agents.) The following is a brief description of the major antioxidants and their possible role in critical illness.

Superoxide Dismutase

Superoxide dismutase (SOD in Figure 22.7) is an enzyme that facilitates the conversion of superoxide radicals to hydrogen peroxide. Although SOD is considered essential for aerobic life (27), its role in critical illness is unclear, and it can act as a pro-oxidant as well as an antioxidant (27,29). The pro-oxidant effect may be the result of hydrogen peroxide production.

Glutathione

Glutathione is a sulfur-containing tripeptide that is considered *the major*

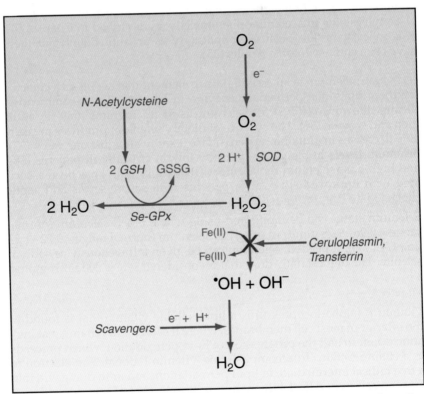

FIGURE 22.7 Actions of endogenous and exogenous antioxidants (highlighted in red). SOD = superoxide dismutase, Se-GPx = selenium-glutathione peroxidase complex, GSH = reduced glutathione, GSSG = oxidized glutathione (a dipeptide connected by a disulfide bridge). See text for explanation.

intracellular antioxidant in the human body (29,30). In its reduced form, glutathione (GSH in Figure 22.7) donates electrons to reduce hydrogen peroxide to water in a reaction that is catalyzed by a selenium-dependent enzyme, *glutathione peroxidase* (Se-GPx in Figure 22.7):

$$H_2O_2 + 2\ GSH \rightarrow 2\ H_2O + GSSG \tag{22.2}$$

Glutathione is present in high concentrations is most mammalian cells (0.5–10 mM/L), and is synthesized de novo within cells. It can be exported extracellularly, but plasma levels are three orders of magnitude lower than intracellular levels (31). However, glutathione levels in lung lavage fluid are 140-fold higher than plasma (32), suggesting that glutathione plays an important role in protecting the lung from oxidant injury. There is evidence that intracellular glutathione is depleted in critically ill patients (33).

N-ACETYLCYSTEINE: Glutathione does not move readily into cells, and exogenous glutathione administration has little effect on intracellular levels (34). However, the popular mucolytic agent *N-acetylcysteine* is a glutathione analogue that can cross cell membranes and serve as a glutathione surrogate (which is the mechanism for the beneficial effects of N-acetylcysteine in acetaminophen toxicity, as described in Chapter 54). N-acetylcysteine has been used sparingly as an antioxidant, but there have been some favorable results (35).

SELENIUM: Selenium is an essential trace element that serves as a cofactor for the glutathione peroxidase enzyme in humans. The recommended dietary allowance (RDA) for selenium is 55 micrograms daily in adult men and women (36). The absence of dietary selenium produces measurable decreases in glutathione peroxidase activity after just one week (37). Selenium levels in blood are typically low in critically ill patients (38), and high-dose selenium replacement (1000 µg IV daily) has been associated with improved survival in patients with severe sepsis and septic shock (38).

Selenium status can be monitored using whole blood selenium (normal range = 0.96–1.78 µmol/L) or serum selenium (normal range = 0.72–1.33 µmol/L) (33). If needed, selenium can be given intravenously as sodium selenite. The highest daily dose that is considered safe is 200 micrograms.

Vitamin E

Vitamin E (alpha-tocopherol) is a lipid-soluble vitamin that is found in the interior of most cell membranes, where it serves as a "chain breaking" antioxidant to halt the progression of lipid peroxidation, which proceeds as a chain reaction. To accomplish this, vitamin E donates an electron to a free radical intermediate in lipid peroxidation, and in so doing, vitamin E becomes a free radical, but an innocuous one. (*Note:* Lipid peroxidation is the oxidation of polyunsaturated fatty acids and is known as *rancidity* when it occurs in food products.)

Vitamin E depletion has been reported in patients with acute respiratory distress syndrome (39), and there is evidence that high-dose vitamin E has beneficial effects in trauma victims (see later). The normal concentration of vitamin E in plasma is 1 mg/dL, and a level below 0.5 mg/dL is evidence of deficiency (40).

Vitamin C

Vitamin C (ascorbic acid) is a water-soluble antioxidant that operates primarily in the extracellular space. The importance of vitamin C as an antioxidant is unclear, but it is a powerful reducing agent that can serve as a scavenger (i.e., donate electrons) for the superoxide and hydroxyl radicals (30). High-dose vitamin C has shown some promise in reducing pulmonary complications in trauma patients (see later).

Caeruloplasmin and Transferrin

Ceruloplasmin and transferrin account for most of the antioxidant activity in plasma (41). The antioxidant activity of both proteins is related to their actions in limiting free iron in the reduced form, Fe (II), which will limit the production of the hydroxyl radical. Caeruloplasmin oxidizes iron from the Fe (II) to the Fe (III) state, and transferrin binds iron in the oxidized or Fe (III) state. The role of free iron as a pro-oxidant (42) may explain why most of the iron in the body is bound to proteins or sequestered (e.g., in the bone marrow).

Oxidant Stress

The risk of oxidant injury is determined by the balance between oxidant and antioxidant activities. When oxidant activity exceeds the neutralizing capacity of the antioxidants, the excess or unopposed oxidation can promote tissue injury. This condition of *unopposed biological oxidation is known as oxidant stress.* Unfortunately, there is no clinical measure of oxidant stress, so the presence of this condition must be inferred.

Pulmonary Oxygen Toxicity

Pulmonary oxygen toxicity is described as an inflammatory lung injury (similar to the acute respiratory distress syndrome described in the next chapter) that occurs in patients who have inhaled gas with an $FiO_2 > 60\%$ for longer than 48 hours. This description, however, does not take into account the information that follows.

Species Differences

The tendency to develop pulmonary oxygen toxicity varies in different species. For example, laboratory rats will die of respiratory failure after 5 to 7 days of breathing 100% O_2, while sea turtles can breathe pure O_2 indefinitely without harm (43). This species-specific effect is important because experimental studies of pulmonary oxygen toxicity have been conducted almost solely in laboratory rats. There is limited information about the tendency of humans to develop pulmonary oxygen toxicity.

HUMAN STUDIES: In healthy volunteers, inhalation of 100% O_2 for 6 to 12 hours results in a tracheobronchitis and a decrease in vital capacity attributed to absorption atelectasis (44). Prolonged exposure to 100% O_2 has been reported in only 6 humans: 5 with irreversible coma who received 100% O_2 for 3 to 4 days (45), and one healthy volunteer who inhaled pure O_2 for 4.5 days (46). In all these cases, the subjects developed a pulmonary condition that was consistent with inflammatory lung injury.

What FiO_2 Is Toxic?

Based on the observation of a decreased vital capacity when the FiO_2 exceeds 60% (44), the threshold FiO_2 for pulmonary O_2 toxicity was set at 60%. However, adopting a single threshold FiO_2 for all patients neglects the contribution of endogenous antioxidants to the risk of oxygen toxicity. If the antioxidant stores in the lungs are depleted, oxygen toxicity can be expected at FiO_2 levels below 60%. Since antioxidant depletion seems to be common in ICU patients (33,38,39), it is reasonable to assume that *any FiO_2 above 21% (room air) can represent a toxic exposure to oxygen in critically ill patients.* Therefore, the best practice is to reduce the FiO_2 to the lowest tolerable level; e.g., the lowest FiO_2 needed to maintain an arterial O_2 saturation $\geq 90\%$.

Promoting Antioxidant Protection

There is no clinical measure of pulmonary O_2 toxicity. However, considering the evidence of antioxidant depletion in critically ill patients (33,38,39), antioxidant supplementation is a reasonable consideration for reducing the risk of pulmonary oxygen toxicity. Evidence of benefit from such an approach is provided by a study in trauma patients (47), which showed that a high-dose antioxidant cocktail of vitamin C (1000 mg every 8 hrs), vitamin E (1000 units every 8 hrs), and selenium (200 μg daily) for 7 days was associated with a significant decline in cases of respiratory failure and ventilator dependence (47).

Antioxidant supplementation could be guided by available measures of antioxidant protection (e.g., serum levels of selenium), or it could be used routinely in patients considered at risk for pulmonary O_2 toxicity.

A FINAL WORD

Why Is Oxygen a Vasoconstrictor?

For those who like teleological explanations for biological design, the observation that oxygen is an arteriolar vasoconstrictor merits some attention. As shown in the first section of the chapter, aerobic metabolism is normally conducted in an oxygen—restricted environment; i.e., most of the O_2 in the body is attached to hemoglobin, while very little is present in tissues because O_2 does not readily dissolve in water. Furthermore, attempts to enhance tissue oxygenation with O_2 therapy are thwarted because of oxygen's actions as an arteriolar vasoconstrictor, which reduces functional capillary flow. Thus, the body resists attempts to increase tissue oxygenation, and the likely purpose of this design is to limit the risk of oxygen-induced tissue injury. In summary, it seems *the human body is designed to maintain an oxygen-restricted environment in the tissues to limit the risk of oxygen-induced cell injury.* If this is the case, then the liberal use of oxygen therapy in critically ill patients deserves re-evaluation.

REFERENCES

Books

Lane N. Oxygen: The Molecule that Made the World. New York: Oxford University Press, 2002.

Halliwell B, Gutteridge JMC. Free Radicals in Biology and Medicine. 4th ed, New York: Oxford University Press, 2007.

Banerjee R (ed). Redox Biochemistry. Hoboken, NJ: Wiley & Sons, 2008.

Insights

1. Whalen WJ, Riley J. A microelectrode for measurement of intracellular PO_2. J Appl Physiol 1967; 23:798–801.

2. Sair M, Etherington PJ, Winlove CP, Evans TW. Tissue oxygenation and perfusion in patients with systemic sepsis. Crit Care Med 2001; 29:1343–1349.

3. American Association for Respiratory Care. Clinical practice guideline: oxygen therapy for adults in the acute care facility. Respir Care 2002; 47:717–720.

4. Eldridge FE. Blood lactate and pyruvate in pulmonary insufficiency. N Engl J Med 1966; 274:878–883.

5. Lundt T, Koller M, Kofstad J. Severe hypoxemia without evidence of tissue hypoxia in the adult respiratory distress syndrome. Crit Care Med 1984; 12:75–76.

6. Abdelsalam M. Permissive hypoxemia. Is it time to change our approach? Chest 2006; 129:210–211.

7. Lejeune P, Mols P, Naeije R, et al. Acute hemodynamic effects of controlled oxygen therapy in decompensated chronic obstructive pulmonary disease. Crit Care Med 1984; 12:1032–1035.

8. Corriveau ML, Rosen BJ, Dolan GF. Oxygen transport and oxygen consumption during supplemental oxygen administration in patients with chronic obstructive pulmonary disease. Am J Med 1989; 87:633–636.

9. Esteban A, Cerde E, De La Cal MA, Lorente JA. Hemodynamic effects of oxygen therapy in patients with acute exacerbations of chronic obstructive pulmonary disease. Chest 1993; 104:471–475.

10. Reinhart K, Bloos F, Konig F, et al. Reversible decrease of oxygen consumption by hyperoxia. Chest 1991; 99:690-694.

11. Lauscher P, Lauscher S, Kertscho H, et al. Hyperoxia reversibly alters oxygen

consumption and metabolism. Scientific World Journal, volume 2012, article ID 410321, 2012. (An open access article, accessed at www.PubMed.com on 12/24/2012.)

12. Packer M, Lee WH, Medina N, Yushak M. Systemic vasoconstrictor effects of oxygen administration in obliterative pulmonary vascular disorders. Am J Cardiol 1986; 57:853–858.

13. Bongard O, Bounameaux H, Fagrell B. Effects of oxygen on skin microcirculation in patients with peripheral arterial occlusive disease. Circulation 1992; 86:878–886.

14. Duling BR. Microvascular responses to alterations in oxygen tension. Circ Res 1972; 31:481-489.

15. Tsai AG, Cabrales P, Winslow RM, Intaglietta M. Microvascular oxygen distribution in awake hamster window chamber model during hyperoxia. Am J Physiol 2003; 285:H1537–H1545.

16. Kilgannon JH, Jones AE, Shapiro NI, et al. Association between arterial hyperoxia following resuscitation from cardiac arrest and in-hospital mortality. JAMA 2010; 303:2165–2171.

Oxygen Delivery Systems

17. Heuer AJ, Scanlan CL. Medical gas therapy. In Wilkins RL, Stoller JK, Kacmarek RM, eds. Egan's Fundamentals of Respiratory Care, 9th ed, St. Louis: Mosby Elsevier, 2009.

18. L'Her E, Deye N, Lellouche F, et al. Physiologic effects of noninvasive ventilation during acute lung injury. Am J Respir Crit Care Med 2005; 172:1112-1118.

19. Scacci R. Air entrainment masks: jet mixing is how they work. The Bernoulli and Venturi principles is how they don't. Respir Care 1979; 24:928–931.

20. Roca O, Riera J, Torres F, Masclans JR. High-flow oxygen therapy in acute respiratory failure. Respir Care 2010; 55:408–413.

21. Sztrymf B, Messika J, Bertrand F, et al. Beneficial effects of humidified high flow nasal oxygen in critical care patients: a prospective pilot study. Intensive Care Med 2011; 37:1780–1786.

22. Parke R, MacGuinness S, Eccleston M. Nasal high-flow therapy delivers low-level positive airway pressure. Br J Anesth 2009; 103:886–890.

The Toxic Nature of Oxygen

23. Halliwell B, Gutteridge JMC. Oxygen is a toxic gas – an introduction to oxygen toxicity and reactive oxygen species. In Free Radicals in Biology and Medicine. 4th ed. New York: Oxford University Press, 2007:1–28.

24. Alonso de Vega JM, Diaz J, Serrano E, Carbonell LF. Oxidative stress in critically ill patients with systemic inflammatory response syndrome. Crit Care Med 2002; 1782–1788.

25. Fink M. Role of reactive oxygen and nitrogen species in acute respiratory distress syndrome. Curr Opin Crit Care 2002; 8:6–11.

26. Anderson BO, Brown JM, Harken A. Mechanisms of neutrophil-mediated tissue injury. J Surg Res 1991; 51:170–179.

27. Michiels C, Raes M, Toussant O, Remacle J. Importance of Se-Glutathione, peroxidase, catalase, and CU/ZN-SOD for cell survival against oxidative stress Free Rad Biol Med 1994; 17:235–248.

28. Halliwell B, Gutteridge JMC. The chemistry of free radicals and related 'reactive species'. In: Free Radicals in Biology and Medicine. 4th ed. New York: Oxford University Press, 2007:30–79.

29. Halliwell B, Gutteridge JMC. Antioxidant defenses: endogenous and diet derived. In: Free Radicals in Biology and Medicine, 4th ed. New York: Oxford University Press, 2007:79–185.

30. Suttorp N, Toepfer W, Roka L. Antioxidant defense mechanisms of endothelial cells:glutathione redox cycle versus catalase. Am J Physiol 1986; 251:C671–C680.

31. Cantin AM, Begin R. Glutathione and inflammatory disorders of the lung. Lung 1991; 169:123–138.

32. Cantin AM, North SI, Hubbard RC, Crystal RG. Normal alveolar epithelial lining fluid contains high levels of glutathione. J Appl Physiol 1987; 63:152–157.

33. Hammarqvist F, Luo JL, Cotgreave IA, et al. Skeletal muscle glutathione is depleted in critically ill patients. Crit Care Med 1997; 25:78–84.

34. Robinson M, Ahn MS, Rounds JD, et al. Parenteral glutathione monoester enhances tissue antioxidant stores. J Parent Ent Nutrit 1992; 16:413–418.

35. Suter PM, Domenighetti G, Schaller MD, et al. N-acetylcysteine enhances recovery from acute lung injury in man: a randomized, double-blind, placebo-controlled clinical study. Chest 1994; 105:190–194.

36. Institute of Medicine, Food and Nutrition Board. Dietary reference intakes: vitamin C, vitamin E, selenium, and carotenoids. Washington, DC: National Academy Press, 2000.

37. Sando K, Hoki M, Nezu R, et al. Platelet glutathione peroxidase activity in long-term total parenteral nutrition with and without selenium supplementation. J Parent Ent Nutrit 1992; 16:54–58.

38. Angstwurm MWA, Engelmann L, Zimmerman T, et al. Selenium in Intensive Care (SIC): results of a prospective randomized, placebo-controlled, multiple-center study in patients with severe systemic inflammatory response syndrome, sepsis, and septic shock. Crit Care Med 2007; 35:118–126.

39. Pincemail J, Bertrand Y, Hanique G, et al. Evaluation of vitamin E deficiency in patients with adult respiratory distress syndrome. Ann NY Acad Sci 1989; 570:498–500.

40. Meydani M. Vitamin E. Lancet 1995; 345:170–176.

41. Halliwell B, Gutteridge JMC. Role of free radicals and catalytic metal ions in human disease. Methods Enzymol 1990; 186:1–85.

42. Herbert V, Shaw S, Jayatilleke E, Stopler-Kasdan T. Most free-radical injury is iron-related: it is promoted by iron, hemin, haloferritin and vitamin C, and inhibited by desferrioxamine and apoferritin. Stem Cells 1994; 12:289–303.

Pulmonary Oxygen Toxicity

43. Fanburg BL. Oxygen toxicity: why can't a human be more like a turtle? Intensive Care Med 1988; 3:134–136.

44. Lodato RF. Oxygen toxicity. Crit Care Clin 1990; 6:749–765.

45. Barber RE, Hamilton WK. Oxygen toxicity in man. N Engl J Med 1970; 283:1478–1483.

46. Winter PM, Smith G. The toxicity of oxygen. Anesthesiology 1972; 37:210–212.

47. Dossett GAM, Fleming SB, Abumrad NN, Cotton BA. High-dose antioxidant administration is associated with a reduction in post-injury complications in critically ill trauma patients. Injury 2011; 42:78–82.

Chapter 23

ACUTE RESPIRATORY DISTRESS SYNDROME

Physicians think they do a lot for a patient when they give his disease a name.

Immanuel Kant

The condition described in this chapter has had several names over the years, including shock lung, Da Nang lung (from the Vietnam war), stiff-lung syndrome, leaky capillary pulmonary edema, noncardiogenic pulmonary edema, acute lung injury, adult respiratory distress syndrome, and most recently, *acute respiratory distress syndrome, or ARDS*. None of these names provides any useful information about this disease entity, which is a diffuse inflammatory injury of the lungs, and one of the leading causes of acute respiratory failure in modern times (1).

PATHOGENESIS

The first clinical report of ARDS appeared in 1967 (2), and included 12 patients with refractory hypoxemia and diffuse infiltrates on chest x-ray. Seven patients died, and autopsy findings revealed dense infiltration of the lungs with an inflammatory exudate. There was no evidence of infection, which indicated that ARDS is an acute inflammatory lung injury.

Inflammatory Injury

The lung consolidation in ARDS is believed to originate with the activation of circulating neutrophils (3). This leads to neutrophil sequestration in the pulmonary microcirculation, where the neutrophils attach to the vascular endothelium and move between endothelial cells (by *diapedesis*) and into the lung parenchyma. The neutrophils then degranulate to release the contents of their cytoplasmic granules (i.e., proteolytic enzymes and toxic oxygen metabolites). Subsequent damage of the capillary walls then leads to exudation of protein-rich fluid, erythrocytes, and platelets into the lungs. The cellular and proteinaceous exudation eventually fills and obliterates the distal airspaces, as shown in Figure 23.1.

The inflammatory exudate contains fibrin, and progressive inflammation results in fibrin accumulation, which can lead to structural remodeling and pulmonary fibrosis (similar to the process that occurs in wound healing). The source of fibrin is a procoagulant state triggered by release of tissue factor from the lungs (4).

Predisposing Conditions

ARDS is not a primary disorder, but is a consequence of a variety of infectious and noninfectious conditions. The common conditions that predispose to ARDS are listed in Table 23.1. The most frequent offenders are pneumonia and the "sepsis syndromes" (i.e., septicemia, severe sepsis,

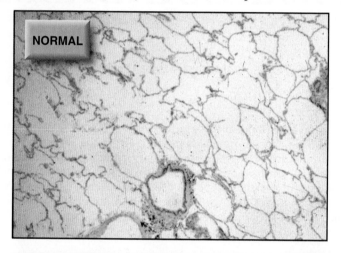

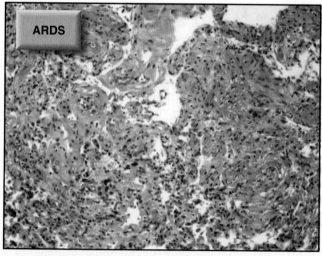

FIGURE 23.1 Microscopic images of a normal lung and a lung in the advanced stages of ARDS, which shows a dense infiltration of leukocytes and proteinaceous material that fills and obliterates the normal architecture of the lungs.

and septic shock) (1,5). One feature shared by many of these conditions is the ability to trigger a *systemic inflammatory response*, which involves neutrophil activation, the principal inciting event in ARDS.

Table 23.1	Common Sources of ARDS	
Infection-Related	**Noninfectious**	
Pneumonia	Gastric Aspiration	
	Blood Transfusions	
Septicemia		
	Multisystem Trauma	
Severe Sepsis	Pancreatitis	
Septic Shock	Drug Overdose	

Other sources of ARDS include burns, cardiopulmonary bypass, pulmonary contusion, fat embolism syndrome, inhalation injury, and pulmonary oxygen toxicity.

CLINICAL FEATURES

The clinical features of ARDS are listed in Table 23.2. The principal features include an acute onset, severe hypoxemia, and bilateral pulmonary infiltrates without evidence of left heart failure or volume overload. The earliest signs of ARDS are the sudden appearance of hypoxemia and signs of respiratory distress (e.g., dyspnea, tachypnea). The chest x-ray can be unrevealing in the first few hours after symptom onset, but bilateral pulmonary infiltrates begin to appear within 24 hours. Progressive hypoxemia requiring mechanical ventilation often occurs in the first 48 hours of the illness.

Table 23.2	Clinical Features of ARDS
1. Acute onset	
2. Bilateral infiltrates on frontal chest x-ray	
3. $PaO_2/FIO_2 \leq 300$ mm Hg[†]	
4. No evidence of left heart failure or fluid overload	
5. The presence of a predisposing condition	

[†]From Reference 7. This differs from earlier definitions of ARDS, which required a $PaO_2/FIO_2 \leq 200$ mm Hg for the diagnosis of ARDS (6). See text for further explanation.

Diagnostic Problems

Despite over 40 years of clinical experience with ARDS, there is still some uncertainty about the defining features of this condition. In 1994, a consensus conference of experts published a set of diagnostic criteria for ARDS and a clinical entity known as *acute lung injury* (ALI) (6). These criteria included: (a) PaO_2/FIO_2 ≤ 200 mm Hg for ARDS, (b) PaO_2/FIO_2 ≤ 300 mm Hg for ALI, and (c) a pulmonary artery wedge pressure (PAWP) ≤ 18 mm Hg (to rule out left heart failure). In 2012, a European task force published a set of revised criteria for the diagnosis of ARDS (7) that included the following changes: (a) ALI was eliminated as a clinical entity, and the PaO_2/FIO_2 for ARDS was set at ≤ 300 mm Hg, (b) a requirement was added that the PaO_2/FIO_2 determination should be conducted at a positive end-expiratory pressure (PEEP) of 5 cm H_2O, and (c) the wedge pressure measurement was eliminated (because of the diminished use of pulmonary artery catheters). These revised criteria are known as the *Berlin Criteria,* and they are combined with the original diagnostic criteria for ARDS in Table 23.2. Not included is the requirement for a standard level of PEEP during the $PaO_2/FIO2$ determination because PEEP requires mechanical ventilation, and the diagnosis of ARDS can occur during spontaneous breathing.

Lack of Specificity

Many of the diagnostic criteria for ARDS are non-specific, and are shared by other common causes of acute respiratory failure. This creates a tendency for misdiagnosis, which is demonstrated in Table 23.3 (8). The information in this table is from an autopsy study of patients who died with a premortem diagnosis of ARDS, and the postmortem diagnoses are listed in the table along with the prevalence of each diagnosis. Only half of the patients with the premortem diagnosis of ARDS had evidence of ARDS on postmortem examination, and the conditions most commonly mistaken for ARDS were pneumonia and hydrostatic pulmonary edema. The likelihood of identifying ARDS was 50% in this study, which is no better than the likelihood of heads or tails with a coin flip!

Table 23.3	Postmortem Diagnosis in Patients with a Premortem Diagnosis of ARDS
Postmortem Diagnosis	**% of Autopsies**
Inflammatory Injury (ARDS)	50%
Acute Pneumonia	25%
Pulmonary Congestion	11%
Invasive Aspergillosis	6%
Pulmonary Embolism	3%
Other Diagnoses	5%

From Reference 8.

Radiographic Appearance

One source of error in the diagnosis of ARDS is the appearance of the chest x-ray. The classic radiographic appearance of ARDS is shown in Figure 23.2. The infiltrate has a finely granular or *ground-glass appearance*, and is evenly distributed in all lung fields, with no evidence of a pleural effusion. Unfortunately, these characteristic features are not always present. This is demonstrated by the chest x-ray in Figure 23.3. In this case, the infiltration shows a hilar prominence and is confined to the lower lung fields, with obliteration of the left hemidiaphragm suggesting a possible pleural effusion. These features could be mistaken for cardiogenic pulmonary edema. Because of such variability in the radiographic appearance of ARDS, *it is not possible to identify ARDS reliably using the chest x-ray alone* (9).

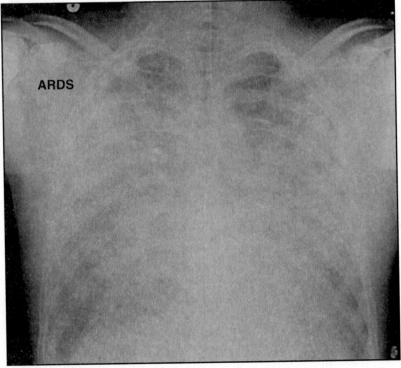

FIGURE 23.2 Portable chest x-ray showing the classic radiographic appearance of ARDS. The infiltrate has a finely granular or "ground glass" appearance, and is evenly distributed throughout both lungs, with a relative sparing of the lung bases. There is no evidence of a pleural effusion.

Pitfalls of the Wedge Pressure

When the chest-x-ray shows overlapping features of ARDS and cardiogenic pulmonary edema, like the one in Figure 23.3, the pulmonary

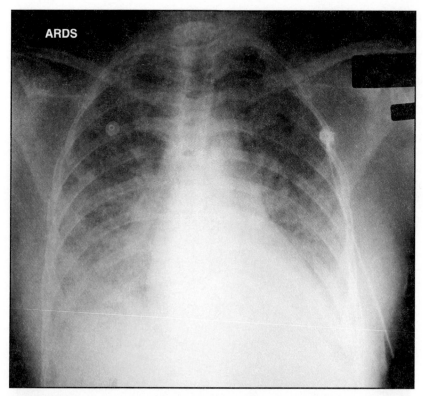

FIGURE 23.3 Portable chest x-ray of ARDS in a patient with urosepsis and Gram-negative septicemia. The infiltrates appear to emanate from the hilar areas and are confined to the lower lung fields. There is also obliteration of the left hemidiaphragm suggesting the presence of a pleural effusion. These radiographic features could be mistaken for hydrostatic pulmonary edema.

artery wedge pressure (PAWP) has been used to distinguish between these two conditions (i.e., a PAWP ≤ 18 mm Hg is considered evidence of ARDS) (6). This is problematic because *the wedge pressure is not a measure of capillary hydrostatic pressure,* as explained in Chapter 8 (see pages 140-141). The PAWP is measured in the absence of blood flow, when the static column of blood between the catheter tip and left atrium results in an equalization of pressures between the wedge pressure and left atrial pressure. However, when flow resumes, the pressure in the pulmonary capillaries must be higher than the left atrial pressure to provide a pressure gradient for flow in the pulmonary veins. Therefore, *the left atrial (wedge) pressure is lower than the capillary hydrostatic pressure, and this will lead to an overdiagnosis of ARDS.*

Bronchoalveolar Lavage

Although rarely used, bronchoalveolar lavage is a reliable method for distinguishing ARDS from cardiogenic pulmonary edema (10). This procedure is performed at the bedside using a flexible fiberoptic broncho-scope that is advanced into one of the involved lung segments. Once in place, the lung segment is lavaged with isotonic saline, and the lavage fluid is analyzed for the presence of neutrophils and protein.

1. In normal subjects, neutrophils make up less than 5% of the cells recovered in lung lavage fluid, whereas in patients with ARDS, as many as 80% of the recovered cells are neutrophils (10). A low neu-trophil count in lung lavage fluid can be used to exclude the diagno-sis of ARDS, while a high neutrophil count is evidence of ARDS.

2. Because inflammatory exudates are rich in proteinaceous material, lung lavage fluid that is rich in protein is used as evidence of ARDS. When the protein concentration in lung lavage fluid is expressed as a fraction of the protein concentration in plasma, the following cri-teria can be applied (11):

Hydrostatic Edema: Lavage fluid [protein] / plasma [protein] < 0.5

ARDS: Lavage fluid [protein] / plasma [protein] > 0.7

VENTILATOR MANAGEMENT IN ARDS

One of the most important discoveries in critical care medicine in the last quarter-century is the role of mechanical ventilation as a *source* of lung injury, particularly in patients with ARDS. This has led to a management strategy known as *lung protective ventilation* (12), which is described here.

Conventional Mechanical Ventilation

Since the introduction of positive-pressure mechanical ventilation, the use of large inflation volumes (tidal volumes) has been a standard prac-tice to reduce the tendency for atelectasis during mechanical ventilation. The conventional tidal volumes are 12 to 15 mL/kg (13), which are twice the size of tidal volumes achieved during quiet breathing (6 to 7 mL/kg). In patients with ARDS, these large inflation volumes are delivered into lungs that have only a fraction of the normal functional lung volume, as described next.

Functional Volume in ARDS

Although portable chest x-rays show an apparent homogeneous pattern of lung infiltration in ARDS, CT images reveal that the lung infiltration in ARDS is confined to dependent lung regions (13). This is shown in the CT images in Figure 23.4. Note the dense consolidation in the posterior lung regions (which are the dependent lung regions in the supine posi-tion), and the normal or uninvolved lung is restricted to the anterior half of the thorax. The uninvolved areas represent the functional portion of the lungs, and the portion that receives the inflation volumes. Therefore, the high inflation volumes used during conventional mechanical ventila-tion are being delivered to a markedly reduced volume of available lung, and this results in overdistension and rupture of the distal airspaces (15).

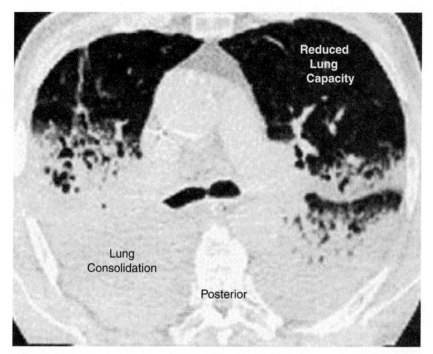

FIGURE 23.4 Computed tomographic image of lung slices in the region of the hilum from a patient with ARDS. The lung consolidation is confined to the posterior lung regions, which are the dependent regions in the supine position. The uninvolved lung in the anterior one-third of the thorax represents the functional portion of the lung. CT image is from Reference 14, and is digitally retouched.

Ventilator-Induced Lung Injury

Excessive inflation of the distal airspaces produce stress fractures in the alveolar capillary interface, and this leads to infiltration of the lung parenchyma and distal airspaces with an inflammatory exudate. This condition is known as *ventilator-induced lung injury* (VILI), and is strikingly similar to ARDS (15). The lung injury is volume-related rather than pressure-related (16), and is called *volutrauma*. (Pressure-related lung injury is called *barotrauma*, and is associated with the escape of air from the lungs.)

BIOTRAUMA: During conventional, high-volume mechanical ventilation, proinflammatory cytokines can appear in the lungs and systemic circulation, even though there is no structural damage in the lungs (17). This proinflammatory condition is known as biotrauma, and it can lead to neutrophil activation and inflammatory infiltration in the lungs (16). The systemic inflammatory response associated with biotrauma can promote inflammatory injury in other organs, which means that *mechanical ventilation can be as source of inflammatory-mediated multiorgan failure* (18)!

ATELECTRAUMA: The decrease in lung distensibility in ARDS can result in the collapse of small airways at the end of expiration. When this occurs, mechanical ventilation can be associated with cyclic opening and closing of small airways, and this process can be a source of lung injury (19). This type of lung injury is called *atelectrauma* (16), and it may be the result high-velocity shear forces created by the opening of collapsed airways, which can damage the airway epithelium.

Lung Protective Ventilation

Lung protective ventilation employs low tidal volumes (6 mL/kg) to limit the risk of volutrauma and biotrauma, and uses positive end-expiratory pressure (PEEP) to limit the risk of atelectrauma. A protocol for lung protective ventilation that has a proven survival benefit in ARDS (20) is shown in Table 23.4. This protocol was developed by the ARDS Clinical Network (a network created by governmental health agencies to evaluate potential therapies for ARDS), and is available at www.ardsnet.org. The tidal volume in this protocol is 6 mL/kg, based on *predicted body weight*, which is the body weight associated with normal lung volumes. Note that one of the stated goals is an end-inspiratory "plateau" pressure (Ppl) ≤30 cm H_2O. This pressure is described in detail in Chapter 25.

Table 23.4	Protocol for Lung Protective Ventilation in ARDS

I. 1st Stage	1. Calculate patient's **predicted** body weight (PBW)†.
	  Males: PBW = 50 + [2.3 × (height in inches − 60)]
	  Females: PBW = 45.5 + [2.3 × (height in inches − 60)]
	2. Set initial tidal volume (V_T) at 8 mL/kg PBW.
	3. Add positive end-expiratory pressure (PEEP) of 5 cm H_2O.
	4. Select the lowest FIO_2 that achieves an SpO_2 of 88–95%.
	5. Reduce V_T by 1 mL/kg every 2 hours until V_T = 6 mL/kg.

II. 2nd Stage	1. When V_T = 6 mL/kg, measure plateau pressure (Ppl). 2. If Ppl > 30 cm H_2O, decrease V_T in 1 mL/kg increments until Ppl < 30 cm H_2O or V_T = 4 mL/kg.
III. 3rd Stage	1. Monitor arterial blood gases for respiratory acidosis. 2. If pH = 7.15–7.30, increase respiratory rate (RR) until pH > 7.30 or RR = 35 bpm. 3. If pH < 7.15, increase RR to 35 bpm. If pH is still < 7.15, increase V_T in 1 mL/kg increments until pH > 7.15.
IV. Optimal Goals	V_T = 6 mL/kg, Ppl ≤ 30 cm H_2O, SpO_2 = 88–95%, pH = 7.30–7.45

Adapted from the protocol developed by the ARDS Network, available at www.ardsnet.org.
†Predicted body weight is the weight associated with normal lung volumes.

Positive End-Expiratory Pressure

(For a detailed description of this pressure, see Chapter 26.) Lung protective ventilation employs a positive end-expiratory pressure (PEEP) of at least 5 cm H_2O to prevent the collapse of small airways at the end of expiration. The goal is to prevent the cyclic opening and closing of small airways and reduce the risk of atelectrauma. Higher PEEP levels (e.g., 15 cm H_2O) have been associated with a shorter duration of mechanical ventilation and a borderline increase in survival in ARDS, but only when the PaO_2/FiO_2 ratio is ≤ 200 mm Hg (21). However, PEEP levels above 10 cm H_2O are not typically used unless there is a problem maintaining arterial oxygenation (see next).

In situations where a toxic level of inhaled oxygen ($FiO_2 > 50\%$) is needed to maintain the target SpO_2 of 88–95%, PEEP levels above 5 cm H_2O can be used to improve arterial oxygenation and reduce the FiO_2 to safer levels. However, it is important to emphasize that increases in PEEP can reduce the cardiac output, and if the goal of increasing PEEP is to maintain the same SpO_2 at a lower FiO_2, the reduced cardiac output will reduce the systemic O_2 delivery.

Permissive Hypercapnia

One of the consequences of low tidal volume ventilation is a decrease in CO_2 elimination in the lungs, which can result in hypercapnia and respiratory acidosis. Because of the benefits of low volume ventilation, hypercapnia is allowed to persist as long as there is no evidence of harm. This practice is known as *permissive hypercapnia* (22). The limits of tolerance to hypercapnia and respiratory acidosis are unclear, but data from clinical trials of permissive hypercapnia show that arterial PCO_2 levels of 60–70 mm Hg and arterial pH levels of 7.2–7.25 are safe for most patients (23). The target pH is 7.30–7.45 in the protocol for lung protective ventilation in Table 23.4.

Impact on Survival

Lung protective ventilation is one of the few measures that has been shown to improve survival in ARDS. The largest and most successful trial of lung protective ventilation was conducted by the ARDS Network (20), and enrolled over 800 ventilator-dependent patients with ARDS who were randomly assigned to receive tidal volumes of 6 mL/kg or 12 mL/kg (using predicted body weight). Ventilation with the lower tidal volume (6 mL/kg), and an end-inspiratory plateau pressure (Ppl) ≤ 30 cm H_2O, was associated with a shorter duration of mechanical ventilation and a 9% absolute reduction in mortality rate (40% to 31%, P = 0.007).

A total of 5 clinical trials have compared tidal volumes of 6 mL/kg and 12 mL/kg during mechanical ventilation in patients with ARDS. In two of the trials, low tidal volumes were associated with fewer deaths, while in three of the trials, there was no survival benefit associated with low tidal volumes (24). Despite the lack of a consistent survival benefit, lung protective ventilation using tidal volumes of 6 mL/kg has become a standard practice in patients with ARDS. A recent multicenter survey of lung protective ventilation in ARDS showed an in-hospital mortality rate of

48% (5), which is no better than mortality rates reported before the introduction of lung protective ventilation. An observation that is relevant in this context is that mortality rates for ARDS tend to be lower in controlled clinical trials than in clinical practice surveys (25).

(*Note:* A possible explanation for the lack of a consistent survival benefit with low tidal volumes is presented in Chapter 25.)

Summary

There is convincing evidence that mechanical ventilation can damage the lungs in ARDS as a result of overdistension of functional alveoli (volutrauma) and collapse of small airways (atelectrauma). Lung protective ventilation is designed to mitigate the mechanical forces that create ventilator-induced lung injury, and it has been adopted as a standard method of mechanical ventilation in ARDS.

NONVENTILATORY MANAGEMENT

The treatment of ARDS begins by treating the inciting condition (e.g., septicemia), if possible. Therapies directed at the ARDS have been marked by failure more than success. The failed therapies in ARDS include surfactant (in adults), inhaled nitric oxide, pentoxyphylline, ibuprofen, prostaglandin E1, and antifungal agents (to inhibit thromboxane) (26). Clinical benefits have been reported with fluid management that avoids fluid accumulation in the lungs, and with high-dose corticosteroids in severe or unresolving ARDS. The management described in this section is limited to the measures that have documented benefits.

Fluid Management

The lung consolidation in ARDS is an inflammatory exudate, and should not be influenced by fluid balance (for the same reason that diuresis will not clear an infiltrate caused by pneumonia). However, avoiding a positive fluid balance will prevent unwanted fluid accumulation in the lungs, which could aggravate the respiratory insufficiency in ARDS. Clinical studies have shown that avoiding a positive fluid balance in patients with ARDS can reduce the time on mechanical ventilation (27), and can even reduce mortality (28).

However, it is also important to avoid fluid deficits and maintain intravascular volume because the positive intrathoracic pressures during mechanical ventilation will magnify the tendency for the cardiac output to decrease in response to deficits in intravascular volume.

Corticosteroid Therapy

There is a long history of clinical trials evaluating steroid therapy in ARDS, and the aggregated results of these studies show *no consistent survival benefit associated with steroid therapy* (29). However, there is evidence of other benefits provided by steroid therapy in ARDS, and these include a reduction in markers of inflammation (both pulmonary and systemic inflammation), improved gas exchange, shorter duration of mechanical ventilation, and shorter length of stay in the ICU (29). *Steroid therapy is currently recommended only in cases of early severe ARDS and unresolving ARDS* (28).

Early Severe ARDS

In early severe ARDS, defined as a $PaO_2/FiO_2 < 200$ mm Hg with PEEP of 10 cm H_2O, the following steroid regimen in recommended (29):

> *Methylprednisolone:* Start with an IV loading dose of 1 mg/kg (ideal body weight) over 30 minutes, then infuse at 1 mg/kg/day for 14 days, then gradually taper the dose over the next 14 days and discontinue therapy. Five days after the patient is able to ingest oral medications, the dose can be given orally (as prednisone or prednisolone) as a single daily dose.

Unresolving ARDS

ARDS has a fibrinoproliferative phase that begins 7–14 days after the onset of illness (30), and eventually results in irreversible pulmonary fibrosis. High-dose steroid therapy started in the developing phase of fibrinoproliferation can help to halt the progression to pulmonary fibrosis. In cases where ARDS does not begin to resolve after 7 days, high-dose steroid therapy is recommended, but should begin no later than 14 days after the onset of illness. The following steroid regimen is recommended (29):

> *Methylprednisolone:* Start with an IV loading dose of 2 mg/kg (ideal body weight) over 30 minutes, then infuse at 2 mg/kg/day for 14 days, and 1 mg/kg/day for the next 7 days. After this, gradually taper the dose and discontinue therapy at 2 weeks after extubation. Five days after the patient is able to ingest oral medications, the dose can be given orally (as prednisone or prednisolone) as a single daily dose.

The risks of high-dose steroid therapy include worsening glycemic control and prolonged neuromuscular weakness when combined with neuromuscular blocking agents. There is no evidence of an increased risk of nosocomial infections with the steroid regimens described here (28).

Therapeutic Misdirection?

Although the therapeutic focus for ARDS has been the lungs, *the principal cause of death in ARDS is multiorgan failure, not respiratory failure* (5,31). As many as 70% of deaths in ARDS are the result of multiorgan failure (31), and the mortality rate is directly related to the number of organs that fail. The relationship between mortality rate and extrapulmonary organ failure is shown in Figure 23.5. This relationship indicates that mortality is a function of a progressive systemic condition, which most likely represents progressive systemic inflammation. The similarities between Figure 23.5 and Figure 14.2 (see page 267) supports the notion of a relationship between progressive systemic inflammation and mortality in ARDS. If this is the case, then limiting the therapeutic focus to the lungs in ARDS is a prescription for failure.

REFRACTORY HYPOXEMIA

A minority (10 to 15%) of patients with ARDS develop severe hypoxemia that is refractory to oxygen therapy and mechanical ventilation (32). This condition is an immediate threat to life, and the following "rescue therapies" can produce an immediate improvement in arterial oxygenation. Unfortunately, these rescue measures often provide little or no survival benefit.

High Frequency Oscillatory Ventilation

High frequency oscillatory ventilation (HFOV) delivers small tidal volumes (1–2 mL/kg) using rapid pressure oscillations (300 cycles/min). The small tidal volumes limit the risk of volutrauma, and the rapid pressure oscillations create a mean airway pressure that prevents small airway collapse and limits the risk of atelectrauma. When used in patients with severe ARDS, HFOV can improve arterial oxygenation, but there is no documented survival benefit (33). HFOV requires a specialized ventilator (Sensormedics 3100B, Viasys Healthcare, Yorba Linda, CA), and may not be available in all hospitals. This mode of ventilation is described in more detail in Chapter 27.

Inhaled Nitric Oxide

Inhaled nitric oxide (5–10 ppm) is a selective pulmonary vasodilator that can improve arterial oxygenation in ARDS by increasing flow to areas of

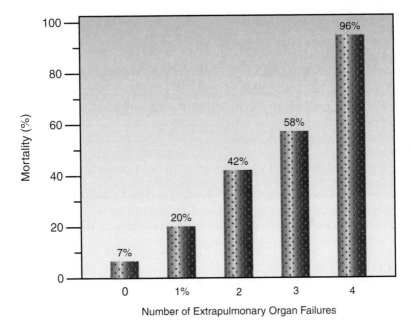

FIGURE 23.5 The relationship between extrapulmonary organ failure and mortality in ARDS. Data from the electronic supplementary material for Reference 5.

high dead space ventilation (34). However, the increase in arterial oxygenation is temporary (1–4 days), and there is no associated survival benefit (35). Adverse effects of inhaled nitric oxide include methemoglobinemia (usually mild) and renal dysfunction (35). An added risk is the potential for nitric oxide to form peroxinitrite, a potent toxin capable of oxidant cell injury.

Prone Position

Switching from the supine to prone position can improve pulmonary gas exchange by diverting blood away from poorly aerated lung regions in the posterior thorax and increasing blood flow in aerated lung regions in the anterior thorax (see Figure 23.4). Prone positioning has had little impact on mortality in ARDS, but a recent study combining lung protective ventilation with prone positioning showed a lower than expected mortality rate in patients with severe ARDS (PaO_2/FIO_2 <100 mm Hg) (36). Prone positioning is labor intensive and creates problems with nursing care (e.g., airway care and skin care), but it may be the only measure available for refractory hypoxemia in hospitals with limited resources.

ECMO

Extracorporeal membrane oxygenation (ECMO) has had variable success in patients with refractory hypoxemia, and is a consideration only in medical centers with established ECMO programs, and only when other rescue therapies have failed (37).

A FINAL WORD

The Evils of Inflammation

One of the important messages in this book is the prominent role of inflammation as a source of organ damage and multiorgan failure in critically ill patients, and the lack of an effective treatment for this destructive force. This message appears in Chapter 14, which describes inflammatory shock and multiorgan failure, and it appears again in this chapter. Although a survival benefit has been documented with lung protective ventilation in ARDS, this is not a treatment for ARDS, but rather is a lessening of the damage produced by mechanical ventilation. Until a remedy is available for the destructive effects of inflammation, conditions like ARDS will continue to be a major source of morbidity and mortality in the ICU.

REFERENCES

Review

1. Matthay MA, Ware LB, Zimmerman GA. The acute respiratory distress syndrome. J Clin Invest 2012; 122:2731–2740.

Pathogenesis

2. Ashbaugh DG, Bigelow DB, Petty TL, Levine BE. Acute respiratory distress in adults. Lancet 1967; 2:319–323.

3. Abraham E. Neutrophils and acute lung injury. Crit Care Med 2003; 31(Suppl): S195–S199.

4. Idell S. Coagulation, fibrinolysis, and fibrin deposition in acute lung injury. Crit Care Med 2003; 31(Suppl):S213–S220.

5. Villar J, Blanco J, Anon JM, et al. The ALIEN study: incidence and outcome of acute respiratory distress syndrome in the era of lung protective ventilation. Intensive Care Med 2011; 37:1932–1941.

Clinical Features

6. Bernard GR, Artigas A, Brigham KL, et al. The American–European Consensus Conference on ARDS: definitions, mechanisms, relevant outcomes, and clinical trial coordination. Am Rev Respir Crit Care Med 1994; 149:818–824.

7. The ARDS Definition Task Force. Acute respiratory distress syndrome. The Berlin definition. JAMA 2012; 307:2526–2533.

8. de Hemptinne Q, Remmelink M, Brimioulle S, et al. ARDS: A clinicopathological confrontation. Chest 2009; 135:944–949.

9. Rubenfeld GD, Caldwell E, Granton J, et al. Interobserver variability in applying a radiographic definition for ARDS. Chest 1999; 116:1347–1353.

10. Idell S, Cohen AB. Bronchoalveolar lavage in patients with the adult respiratory distress syndrome. Clin Chest Med 1985; 6:459–471.

11. Sprung CL, Long WM, Marcial EH, et al. Distribution of proteins in pulmonary edema. The value of fractional concentrations. Am Rev Respir Dis 1987; 136:957–963.

Ventilator Management in ARDS

12. Brower RG, Rubenfeld GD. Lung-protective ventilation strategies in acute lung injury. Crit Care Med 2003; 31(Suppl):S312–S316.

13. Pontoppidan H, Geffen B, Lowenstein E. Acute respiratory failure in the adult. N Engl J Med 1972; 287:799–806.

14. Rouby J-J, Puybasset L, Nieszkowska A, Lu Q. Acute respiratory distress syndrome: Lessons from computed tomography of the whole lung. Crit Care Med 2003; 31(Suppl):S285–S295.

15. Dreyfuss D, Saumon G. Ventilator-induced lung injury. Am J Respir Crit Care Med 1998; 157:294–323.

16. Gattinoni L, Protti A, Caironi P, Carlesso E. Ventilator-induced lung injury: the anatomical and physiological framework. Crit Care Med 2010; 38(Suppl):S539–S548.

17. Ranieri VM, Suter PM Tortorella C, et al. Effect of mechanical ventilation on inflammatory mediators in patients with acute respiratory distress syndrome: A randomized controlled trial. JAMA 1999; 282:54–61.

18. Ranieri VM, Giunta F, Suter P, Slutsky AS. Mechanical ventilation as a mediator of multisystem organ failure in acute respiratory distress syndrome. JAMA 2000; 284:43–44.

19. Muscedere JG, Mullen JBM, Gan K, et al. Tidal ventilation at low airway pressures can augment lung injury. Am J Respir Crit Care Med 1994; 149:1327–1334.

20. The Acute Respiratory Distress Syndrome Network. Ventilation with lower tidal volumes as compared with traditional tidal volumes for acute lung injury and the acute respiratory distress syndrome. New Engl J Med 2000; 342:1301–1308.

21. Briel M, Meade M, Mercat A, et al. Higher vs. lower positive end-expiratory pressure in patients with acute lung injury and acute respiratory distress syndrome. JAMA 2010; 303:865–873.

22. Bidani A, Tzouanakis AE, Cardenas VJ, Zwischenberger JB. Permissive hypercapnia in acute respiratory failure. JAMA 1994; 272:957–962.

23. Hickling KG, Walsh J, Henderson S, et al. Low mortality rate in adult respiratory distress syndrome using low-volume, pressure-limited ventilation with permissive hypercapnia: A prospective study. Crit Care Med 1994; 22:1568–1578.

24. Fan E, Needham DM, Stewart TE. Ventilator management of acute lung injury and acute respiratory distress syndrome. JAMA 2005; 294:2889–2896.

25. Phua J, Badia JR, Adhikari NKJ, et al. Has mortality from acute respiratory distress syndrome decreased over time? Am J Respir Crit Care Med 2009; 179:220–227.

Nonventilatory Management

26. Calfee CS, Matthay MA. Nonventilatory treatment for acute lung injury and ARDS. Chest 2007; 131:913–920.

27. The Acute Respiratory Distress Syndrome Network. Comparison of two fluid management strategies in acute lung injury. N Engl J Med 2006; 354:2564–2575.

28. Murphy CV, Schramm GE, Doherty JA, et al. The importance of fluid management in acute lung injury secondary to septic shock. Chest 2009; 136:102–109.

29. Marik PE, Meduri GU, Rocco PRM, Annane D. Glucocorticoid treatment in acute lung injury and acute respiratory distress syndrome. Crit Care Clin 2011; 27:589–607.

30. Meduri GU, Chinn A. Fibrinoproliferation in late adult respiratory distress syndrome. Chest 1994; 105(Suppl):127S–129S.

31. Estenssoro E, Dubin A, Laffaire E, et al. Incidence, clinical course, and outcome in 217 patients with acute respiratory distress syndrome. Crit Care Med 2002; 30:2450–2456.

Refractory Hypoxemia

32. Pipeling MR, Fan E. Therapies for refractory hypoxemia in acute respiratory distress syndrome. JAMA 2010; 304:2521–2527.

33. Stawicki SP, Goyal M, Sarani B. High-frequency oscillatory ventilation (HFOV) and airway pressure release ventilation (APRV): A practical guide. J Intensive Care Med 2009; 24:215–229.

34. Griffiths MJ, Evans TW. Inhaled nitric oxide therapy in adults. N Engl J Med 2005; 353:2683–2695.

35. Adhikari NK, Burns KE, Friedrich JO, et al. Effect of nitric oxide on oxygenation and mortality in acute lung injury: systematic review and meta-analysis. British Med J 2007; 334(7597):779–787.

36. Charron C, Bouferrache K, Caille V, et al. Routine prone positioning in patients with severe ARDS: feasibility and impact on prognosis. Intensive Care Med 2011; 37:785–790.

37. Raoof S, Goulet K, Esan A, et al. Severe hypoxemic respiratory failure: Part 2 – Nonventilatory strategies. Chest 2010; 137:1437–1448.

Chapter 24

ASTHMA AND COPD IN THE ICU

Asthmatic distress calls for procedures which stimulate the
sympathetic and dilate the bronchi.

Lawrason Brown, MD
The Practical Medicine Series
1931.

This chapter describes the management of severe exacerbations of asthma and chronic obstructive pulmonary disease (COPD), and includes strategies for ventilatory assistance in these conditions. The non-ventilator management of these conditions has experienced little change in recent years. In fact, Dr. Brown's comment in the introductory quote, which appeared 80 years ago, is remarkably similar to the current emphasis on adrenergic bronchodilators in the management of "asthmatic distress."

BASICS

Measures of Airway Obstruction

The management of obstructive airways disease is guided by the severity of obstruction in the airways (1,2). During acute exacerbations, *the clinical examination is often unreliable for determining the severity of airway obstruction* (3,4). As a result, more objective measures of airway obstruction like the ones described here have been recommended for guiding the management of obstructive airways diseases like asthma and COPD (1,2).

Forced Expiratory Measurements

For spontaneously breathing patients, the recommended measures of airway obstruction are the forced expiratory volume in 1 second (FEV_1), and the peak expiratory flow rate (PEFR) (1). Hand-held devices that are easy to operate are available for both measurements. The FEV_1 and PEFR vary with age, gender, and height (5), and measurements are typically expressed as "% predicted" (observed result/predicted result × 100), with the predicted values derived from standard reference equations. (The PEFR is also expressed in relation to the highest flow achieved by each patient; i.e., the "personal best" PEFR.) The correlations between the % predicted values of FEV_1 and PEFR and the severity of airway obstruction are shown below (1).

FEV_1 or PEFR	Severity of Obstruction
≥ 70%	Mild
40–69%	Moderate
< 40%	Severe

Both measurements are volume-dependent and effort-dependent, so maximum patient effort is required for reliable recordings. The FEV_1 is the preferred measurement because it is less variable and more likely to detect obstruction in the smaller airways (1,5). Comparison of both measurements in the acute care setting have shown that the PEFR underestimates the severity of airway obstruction (4).

SEVERE EXACERBATIONS: The measurement of FEV_1 and PEFR requires a maximum inspiratory effort (to total lung capacity) followed by a maximum expiratory effort (to residual lung volume), and three consecutive measurements are recommended for optimal results. Patients with severe exacerbations of asthma and COPD are often unable to perform these maneuvers because of respiratory distress, and thus the FEV_1 and PEFR have a limited role in the management of severe exacerbations of asthma and COPD (which includes most cases admitted to the ICU).

Intrinsic PEEP

For patients with asthma and COPD who require mechanical ventilation, the severity of airflow obstruction can be evaluated by monitoring a pressure known as *intrinsic PEEP*. This pressure is described in the final section of the chapter.

Aerosol Drug Therapy

Drug aerosols play a major role in the management of obstructive airways diseases. There are two basic designs for aerosol generators in clinical medicine: the *jet nebulizer* and the *metered-dose inhaler*. The operation of these devices is illustrated in Figure 24.1

Jet Nebulizer

The pneumatic or jet nebulizer uses the same principle as the air-entrainment device in Figure 22.5 (see page 435). A high-pressure gas source (e.g., 50 psi from a wall outlet) is passed through a narrow opening in the nebulizer, creating a high-velocity (jet) stream of gas that is passed over the opening of a narrow tube submerged in a drug solution. The gas jet draws the drug solution up the tube (by creating viscous drag) and then pulverizes the solution to create an aerosol spray that is inhaled by the patient. Standard jet nebulizers have a reservoir volume of 3–6 mL, and

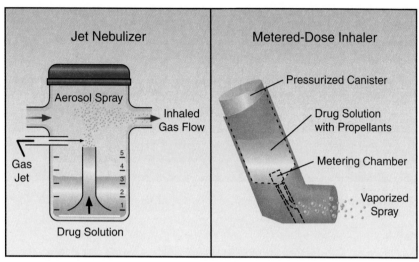

FIGURE 24.1 Devices used for aerosol drug therapy. See text for explanation.

can completely aerosolize the reservoir volume in less than 10 minutes (6). A larger version (with a reservoir volume >200 mL) is available for continuous aerosol therapy (see later).

LUNG DEPOSITION: Although small-volume nebulizers can completely aerosolize a drug solution, only a fraction of the drug aerosol reaches the lungs. This is demonstrated in Table 24.1, which shows the distribution of aerosolized albuterol with different aerosol generator systems (7). When the nebulizer is used, most of the aerosol impacts on the delivery apparatus or is exhaled, and only 12% of the intended dose reaches the lungs. Inefficient drug delivery is a characteristic feature of aerosol drug therapy, and is not specific for the jet nebulizer.

Metered-Dose Inhaler

A metered-dose inhaler (MDI) operates like a canister of hair spray. The MDI has a pressurized canister that contains a drug solution with a boiling point below room temperature. When the canister is squeezed between the thumb and fingers, a valve opens that releases a fixed volume of the drug solution. The liquid immediately vaporizes when it emerges from the canister, and a liquid propellant in the solution creates a high-velocity spray.

LUNG DEPOSITION: The spray emerging from an MDI can have a velocity in excess of 30 meters per second (over 60 miles per hour) (8), and when this high-velocity spray is delivered directly into the mouth, most of the spray impacts on the posterior wall of the oropharynx and is not inhaled. This *inertial impaction* is reduced by using a spacer device or holding chamber to reduce the velocity of aerosol delivery. The influence of a holding chamber on drug delivery is shown in Table 24.1. When the MDI is used alone, 80% of the drug aerosol is deposited in the oropharynx, but when a holding chamber is used with the MDI, drug deposition in the mouth is almost completely eliminated, and the drug dose reaching the lungs is doubled. Results like this are the reason that *holding chambers are recommended for all bronchodilator treatments with MDIs* (6).

Table 24.1	Distribution of Inhaled Albuterol by Delivery System		
Site of Deposition	Nebulizer (2.5 mg)	MDI (180 µg)	MDI + HC (180 µg)
Exhaled	20%	1%	1%
Apparatus	66%	10%	78%
Oropharynx	2%	80%	1%
Lungs	12%	9%	20%

From Reference 7. MDI = metered dose inhaler; HC = holding chamber. The MDI dose of 180 µg represents 2 puffs.

Nebulizer vs. Metered-Dose Inhaler

One of the notable features of aerosol drug therapy is the *equivalent bronchodilator responses produced by nebulizers and MDIs* despite a large difference in drug dosage. This is demonstrated in Figure 24.2, which compares the bronchodilator response to albuterol delivered by nebulizer and MDI (with a holding chamber) in patients with acute exacerbation of asthma (9). There is no difference in the response in each of the 3 treatments. Using the distribution patterns in Table 24.1, the dose of albuterol deposited in the lungs in Figure 24.2 would be 12% of 2.5 mg or 250 µg for the nebulizer and 20% of 360 µg or 72 µg for the MDI with holding chamber. Thus, there is a 3.5-fold difference in drug dose in the airways, yet the bronchodilator responses are equivalent.

Mechanical Ventilation

Equivalent responses like those in Figure 24.2 have also been observed in ventilator-dependent patients (10,11). Drug deposition in the lungs is reduced further during mechanical ventilation (11) due to condensation on the endotracheal tube and ventilator tubing. However, the impact of this loss on bronchodilator responses is not clear (12). The response to MDIs is optimal when a holding chamber is used (11): the chamber is connected to the inspiratory limb of the ventilator tubing, and 5–8 puffs from the MDI are delivered into the chamber for inhalation during the ensuing lung inflations. Regardless of the aerosol device used, drug delivery into the airways can be enhanced by decreasing the inspiratory flow rate and increasing the duration of inspiration (13).

Summary

One thing is clear about aerosol therapy; i.e., it is an inefficient method of drug administration, regardless of the type of aerosol generator that is

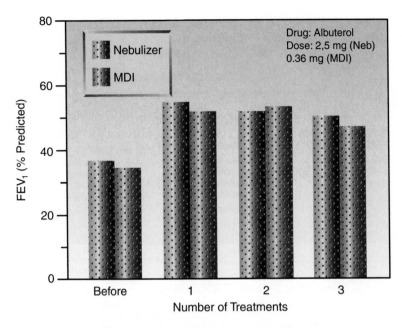

FIGURE 24.2 Equivalent responses to a bronchodilator (albuterol) given by nebulizer or metered-dose inhaler (MDI) with a holding chamber in patients with acute exacerbation of asthma. Treatments were given every 30 minutes using the doses indicated in the upper right portion of the graph (the MDI dose of 0.36 mg represents 4 puffs). FEV_1 = forced expiratory volume in one second. Data from Reference 9.

used. Yet, despite this inefficiency, drug aerosols are favored for administering bronchodilators in acute exacerbations of asthma and COPD, as described next.

ACUTE EXACERBATION OF ASTHMA

The flow diagram in Figure 24.3 summarizes the early management of adults with acute exacerbation of asthma (1). This protocol is based on objective measures of airway obstruction (i.e., FEV_1 and peak expiratory flow rate), but clinical measures of disease severity (e.g., respiratory rate, use of accessory muscles) are also suitable (14,15). The recommended drugs and dosing regimens for acute asthma are summarized in Table 24.2.

β_2-Receptor Agonists

The favored bronchodilators are drugs that stimulate β-adrenergic receptors in bronchial smooth muscle (β_2 subtype). Aerosol delivery of these *β_2-agonists* is preferred because it is more effective than oral (16) or intravenous (17) drug therapy, and has fewer side effects. Short-acting β_2-agonists are preferred for the acute management of asthma because they can be given in rapid succession with less risk of drug accumulation (1).

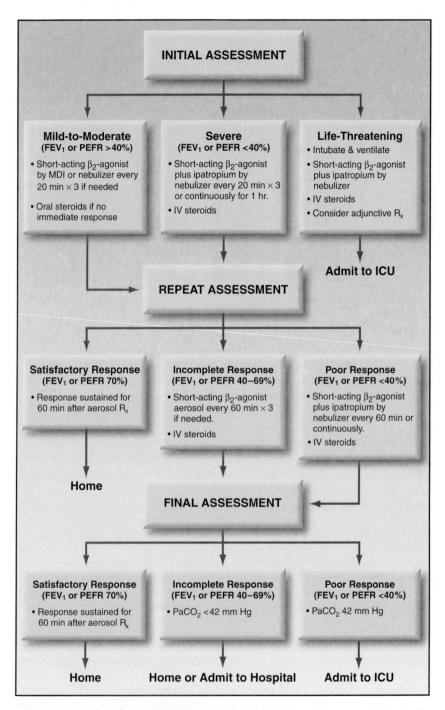

FIGURE 24.3 Flow diagram showing the early management of acute exacerbations of asthma, as recommended by the National Asthma Education Program (1). FEV_1 = forced expiratory volume in one second, PEFR = peak expiratory flow rate.

Table 24.2	Drug Regimens for Acute Exacerbations of Asthma	
Drug Preparations	**Dosing Regimen and Comments**	
Albuterol Nebulizer Solution	Dosing:	2.5–5 mg every 20 min, for 3 doses, then 2.5–10 mg every 1–4 hrs as needed, or 10–15 mg/hr by continuous infusion.
	Comment:	Nebulized drug preferred for severe exacerbations. Continuous R_x may be more effective than intermittent R_x.
MDI (90 μg/puff)	Dosing:	4–8 puffs every 20 min up to 4 hrs, then every 1–4 hrs as needed.
	Comment:	MDI with holding chamber is as effective as nebulized drug.
Levalbuterol Nebulizer Solution	Dosing:	1.25–2.5 mg every 20 min. for 3 doses, then 1.25–5 mg every 1–4 hrs as needed.
	Comment:	As effective as albuterol at half the dose, but has no proven clinical superiority over albuterol.
MDI (45 μg/puff)	Dosing:	4–8 puffs every 20 min up to 4 hrs, then every 1–4 hrs as needed.
	Comment:	MDI with holding chamber is as effective as nebulized drug.
Ipatropium Nebulizer Solution	Dosing:	0.5 mg every 20 min. for 3 doses, then use as needed.
	Comment:	Used only in combination with short-acting β_2-agonists for severe exacerbations of asthma. NOT recommended after the first few hours of therapy.
MDI (18 μg/puff)	Dosing:	8 puffs every 20 min, as needed for up to 3 hrs.
	Comment:	Nebulized drug preferred for severe exacerbations.
Corticosteroids	Dosing:	40–80 mg of prednisone (PO) or methyl-prednisone (IV) daily in 1 or 2 divided doses for 7–10 days.
	Comment:	Oral therapy as effective as intravenous therapy.

From Reference 1.

Albuterol is the most widely used short-acting β_2-agonist for the acute management of asthma (1,14,15). Aerosolized albuterol has a rapid onset of action (less than 5 minutes), and a bronchodilator effect that lasts 2–5 hours (18). *Levalbuterol* is the R-enantiomer of albuterol (a more active form of the drug) that is equally effective at half the dose. However, clinical studies have not shown an advantage with levalbuterol over albuterol (1,14).

Aerosol Regimens

The following regimens of aerosolized albuterol are recommended for acute exacerbations of asthma (1,14,15):

1. The initial treatment involves up to three 20-minute treatments using 2.5 to 5 mg albuterol by nebulizer or 4–8 puffs (90 mg albuterol per puff) by MDI with a holding chamber. Nebulizer delivery is preferred for patients with severe airflow obstruction (1), even though there is no evidence that nebulizers produce better bronchodilator responses than MDIs in acute asthma (19).

2. If further therapy is needed, albuterol can be given hourly for up to 3 hours, or can be given by continuous nebulization using doses of 5–15 mg/hr. Continuous aerosol therapy is popular, and may be more effective than intermittent aerosol therapy in patients with severe airflow obstruction (20).

3. For patients who are admitted to the hospital, albuterol (2.5–5 mg by nebulizer or 4–8 puffs by MDI) is given every 4–6 hours for the duration of the hospital stay.

Parenteral Therapy

For the rare asthmatic patient who does not tolerate bronchodilator aerosols (usually because of excessive coughing) parenteral therapy can be given using subcutaneous *epinephrine* (0.3 to 0.5 mg every 20 minutes for 3 doses) or subcutaneous *terbutaline* (0.25 mg every 20 minutes for 3 doses) (1). However, it is important to emphasize that parenteral β-agonist therapy is not more effective than aerosol therapy, and is more likely to produce unwanted side effects (21).

Side Effects

High-dose aerosol therapy with β_2-agonists can produce a number of side effects, including tachycardia, tremors, hyperglycemia, and a decrease in serum potassium, magnesium, and phosphate levels (22,23). Cardiac ischemia has been reported, but is rare (22). The decrease in serum potassium is the result of a β-receptor-mediated shift of potassium into cells. This effect is notable because large doses of inhaled β_2-agonists (e.g., 20 mg albuterol) have been used for the acute management of hyperkalemia (24). (*Note:* This is not a favored treatment for hyperkalemia because of the side effects of high-dose β_2-agonists.)

Anticholinergic Agents

Anticholinergic agents offer only marginal benefits in acute asthma, and their use is restricted to combination therapy with short-acting β_2-agonists for severe exacerbations, and only for the first 3–4 hours of management (1,25). The only anticholinergic agent approved for use in the United States is *ipatropium bromide*, a derivative of atropine that blocks muscarinic receptors in the airways. The dose in acute asthma is 0.5 mg (which can be mixed with albuterol in the nebulizer) every 20 minutes for 3 doses, then as needed, or 8 puffs (18 µg per puff) by MDI every 20 min as needed for up to 3 hours (1). Systemic absorption is minimal, and there is little risk of anticholinergic side effects (e.g., tachycardia, dry mouth, blurred vision, urinary retention). Ipatropium has no proven benefit beyond the first few hours of management, and it *should be discontinued in patients who are admitted for continued asthma management* (1).

Corticosteroids

Corticosteroids are considered a staple in the management of both acute and chronic asthma. In acute asthma, the bulk of evidence shows that corticosteroids accelerate the rate of resolution and reduce the risk of relapses (26), although not all studies show a benefit from corticosteroids (27,28). The following features of steroid therapy deserve mention:

1. There is no difference in efficacy between oral and intravenous steroids (26,29).

2. The beneficial effects of steroids are often not apparent until 12 hours after therapy is started (29), so steroid therapy will not influence the clinical course of asthma in the emergency department.

3. There is no apparent dose-response curve for steroids (29), and no evidence that doses above 100 mg of prednisone daily (or equivalent doses of other steroids) provide added benefit in acute asthma (26).

4. A 10-day course of steroids can be stopped abruptly without a tapering dose (26,30).

Regimen in Acute Asthma

The National Asthma Education Program includes the following recommendations for corticosteroid therapy in acute exacerbations of asthma (1).

1. Steroids are recommended for all patients who do not show a satisfactory response after one or two bronchodilator treatments.

2. Oral steroids are recommended for patients who can tolerate oral medications.

3. The recommended dose is 40–80 mg daily of *prednisone* (for oral therapy) or *methylprednisolone* (for intravenous therapy) in one or two divided doses, which is continued until there is evidence of satisfactory resolution.

4. If the duration of therapy is less than 10 days, there is no need for a steroid taper.

5. Inhaled corticosteroids can be started at any time during treatment of an acute exacerbation of asthma, and are continued after systemic steroids are discontinued to reduce the risk of relapses.

Mechanism of Action?

Acute asthma is considered more of an inflammatory condition than a bronchospastic condition, and the beneficial effects of steroids are attributed to their anti-inflammatory actions. However, as shown in Table 24.3, dexamethasone is the most potent anti-inflammatory corticosteroid, yet it is not recommended for the treatment of asthma. This is either an oversight, or it raises questions about the mechanism of action of steroids in asthma.

Table 24.3	Comparison of Therapeutic Corticosteroids		
Corticosteroid	Equivalent Dose (mg)	Relative Anti-inflammatory Activity	Relative Na$^+$ Retention
Hydrocortisone	20	1	20
Prednisone	5	3.5	1
Methylprednisone	4	6	0.5
Dexamethasone	0.75	30–40	0

From Zeiss CR. Intense pharmacotherapy. Chest 1992; 101(Suppl):407S.

Steroid Myopathy

An acute myopathy has been reported in ventilator-dependent asthmatic patients treated with high-dose steroids and neuromuscular blocking agents (31). Unlike the traditional steroid myopathy, which is characterized by proximal muscle weakness, this condition involves both proximal and distal muscles, and is often associated with rhabdomyolysis. The muscle weakness can be prolonged (although it usually resolves) and can hamper weaning from mechanical ventilation. Because of the risk of this myopathy, it seems wise to avoid neuromuscular paralysis whenever possible in steroid-treated ventilator-dependent asthmatic patients.

Additional Considerations

The following are some additional considerations for the management of acute asthma:

1. Asthma exacerbations are often triggered by viral infections, and empiric antibiotic therapy is not advised the absence of a treatable infection (1).

2. Intravenous *magnesium* (2 grams over 20 min) has mild bronchodilator effects (possibly as a result of calcium channel blockade), and can be used as an adjunctive measure for severe exacerbations of asthma (1). However, magnesium administration has no impact on the clinical course of acute asthma (32).

3. An arterial blood gas is advised for patients who do not show a satisfactory response to bronchodilators in the emergency department. A normal PCO_2 in acute asthma indicates severe airflow obstruction, and warrants admission to the ICU.

4. Intubation and mechanical ventilation can be problematic in acute exacerbations of asthma; this aspect of management is described in the final section of the chapter.

ACUTE EXACERBATION OF COPD

Chronic obstructive pulmonary disease (COPD) is the fourth leading cause of death in the United States (33) and, despite a marked reduction in the prevalence of cigarette smoking in adults, hospital admissions for acute exacerbations of COPD increased by 60% over a recent 10-year period (34). About half of these admissions require care in an ICU (35).

An acute exacerbation of COPD is defined as "a change in the patient's baseline dyspnea, cough, or sputum production that is beyond the normal day-to-day variation" (2). Most of these exacerbations are the result of infection (usually confined to the airways), but as *many one of every four or five cases may be the result of an acute pulmonary embolism* (36). In about one-third of patients, a precipitating event is never identified (2).

Bronchodilator Therapy

Although a distinguishing feature of COPD is lack of responsiveness to bronchodilators (in contrast to asthma), *bronchodilator therapy is used routinely in patients with COPD* (2). The same bronchodilator drugs used in acute exacerbations of asthma are also recommended for acute exacerbations of COPD, but the dosing regimens differ, as shown in Table 24.4. Ipatropium is used as combination therapy when the response to short-acting β_2-agonists is less than satisfactory, although at least three clinical studies do not support this practice (37).

Corticosteroids

A short course (7–10 days) of corticosteroid therapy is associated with fewer treatment failures and a shorter duration of mechanical ventilation in acute exacerbations of COPD (38,39). However, *at least 10 patients must be treated with corticosteroids to produce one favorable response* (38), so the impact of steroid therapy is limited. The recommended steroid regimen for acute exacerbations of COPD is shown in Table 24.4 (2). Note that the dose range is slightly lower than the dose range for treating acute asthma. *Intravenous steroids offer no advantage over oral steroids* in acute exacerbations of COPD (40), similar to the observations in acute asthma (26,29).

Antibiotics

Airways infections (viral and bacterial) are responsible for at least 50% of acute exacerbations of COPD (2), but many are nontreatable viral infections, and this limits the benefit of antimicrobial therapy.

Indications

Antibiotic therapy is not determined by sputum cultures in acute exacerbations of COPD because the same organisms are often isolated during clinically stable periods and during acute exacerbations (41). Instead, the clinical severity of disease is used to determine the need for antibiotic therapy. Clinical studies have shown that antibiotic therapy is most likely to improve clinical outcomes when exacerbations of COPD are severe

Table 24.4	Drug Regimens for Acute Exacerbations of COPD
Drugs	**Dosing Regimen and Comments**
Albuterol	Dosing: 2.5–5 mg by nebulizer or 2–8 puffs (90 µg/puff) by MDI every 4–6 hrs.
	Comment: First-line broncho-dilator that is equally effective (or ineffective) when given by nebulizer or MDI with holding chamber.
Levalbuterol	Dosing: 1.25–2.5 mg by nebulizer or 2–8 puffs (45 µg/puff) by MDI every 4–6 hrs.
	Comment: More potent form of albuterol that has no proven clinical superiority over albuterol.
Ipatropium	Dosing: 0.5 mg by nebulizer or 2–8 puffs (18 µg/puff) by MDI every 4–6 hrs..
	Comment: Used as combination therapy when response to short-acting β_2-agonists is less than satisfactory.
Corticosteroids	Dosing: 30–40 mg of prednisone (PO) or methyl-prednisone (IV) daily in 1 or 2 divided doses for 7–10 days.
	Comment: Oral therapy is equivalent to intravenous therapy.

From Reference 2.

enough to require hospitalization (34,42), and particularly when mechanical ventilation is required (2,43). This means that *all ICU patients with acute exacerbations of COPD are candidates for antibiotic therapy.*

Antibiotic Regimens

The pathogens most often isolated from the lower respiratory tract in acute exacerbations of COPD are *Hemophilus influenzae* and *Streptococcus pneumoniae* (2,41). *Pseudomonas aeruginosa* is also a prominent isolate in advanced cases of COPD and in ventilator-dependent patients (44). Antibiotics with activity against all these pathogens are advised for ICU patients with acute exacerbations of COPD. These antibiotics include *levofloxacin, pipericillin-tazobactam*, and *imipenem* or *meropenem*. Duration of antibiotic therapy is typically 5-7 days.

Oxygen Therapy

In cases of severe COPD with chronic hypercapnia, high concentrations of inhaled O_2 can promote further increases in arterial PCO_2. This was originally attributed to loss of hypoxic ventilatory drive (45), but more recent studies have shown that the oxygen-induced rise in arterial PCO_2 is not accompanied by a decrease in ventilatory drive (46). Oxygen unloading of CO_2 from hemoglobin may play a role in this phenomenon. Regardless of the mechanism involved, it is important to avoid high concentrations of inhaled O_2 in patients with chronic CO_2 retention.

The best practice for oxygen therapy in patients with chronic CO_2 retention is to keep the FiO_2 (fractional concentration of inhaled O_2) as low as possible, and use air-entrainment devices to maintain a constant FiO_2. (These devices are described on pages 434–435). If a high FiO_2 is needed to maintain adequate arterial oxygenation, then you should monitor the patient's mental status closely (for signs of CO_2 narcosis), and check the arterial PCO_2 and pH periodically. Undesirable increases in arterial PCO_2 in this situation is an indication for ventilatory assistance (noninvasive ventilation or conventional mechanical ventilation).

MECHANICAL VENTILATION

Over 50% of patients admitted to the ICU because of asthma or COPD are placed on mechanical ventilation (47,48), and the following are some of the major considerations related to positive pressure ventilation in these patients.

Dynamic Hyperinflation

During spontaneous breathing in normal subjects, inhaled gas is completely exhaled before the end of expiration. In this situation, there is no expiratory airflow at the end of expiration, so the pressure in the distal airspaces is equivalent to atmospheric (zero reference) pressure. This is illustrated in the lower pressure-volume loop in Figure 24.4. In patients with airways obstruction from asthma or COPD, exhalation is prolonged, and when the airways obstruction is severe, exhalation is not completed before the next inhalation. This results in hyperinflation, called *dynamic hyperinflation,* and the trapped gas in the distal airspaces creates a positive end-expiratory pressure (PEEP), which is called *intrinsic PEEP* or *auto-PEEP* (49). This is illustrated by the upper hysteresis loop in Figure 24.4. Note that, in the presence of hyperinflation and intrinsic PEEP, breathing occurs on a flatter portion of the pressure-volume curve, which means that the respiratory muscles must generate a higher transpulmonary pressure to draw the normal volume of air into the lungs. This creates an increased work of breathing in patients with severe airflow obstruction.

Positive Pressure Ventilation

The shift in the pressure volume curves for breathing caused by dynamic hyperinflation means that positive-pressure mechanical ventilation will create positive intrathoracic pressures that are higher than normal in patients with dynamic hyperinflation. Furthermore, mechanical ventilation can add to the hyperinflation (e.g., by delivering high inflation volumes) (50). Dynamc hyperinflation can have two adverse consequences: (a) overdistention of alveoli, which can lead to ventilator-induced lung-injury, and (b) an increase in intrathoracic pressure, which can impede venous return to the heart. The following measures can help to reduce the risk of these adverse consequences.

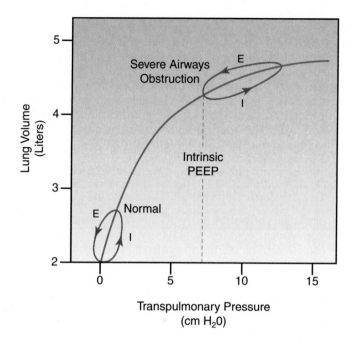

FIGURE 24.4 Pressure-volume curves showing the effects of severe airways obstruction on lung volumes and transpulmonary pressures. The hysteresis loops show the pressure and volume changes during inspiration (I) and expiration (E) for a single breath. See text for further explanation.

Monitoring

Dynamic hyperinflation can be detected by monitoring the flow waveforms displayed by mechanical ventilators. This is illustrated in Figure 24.5. The normal flow waveforms in the upper panel show that the expiratory flow ceases before the next lung inflation, while the flow waveforms in the lower panel show that expiratory flow is continuing when the next lung inflation is delivered. *The presence of expiratory flow at the end of expiration is evidence of dynamic hyperinflation.*

INTRINSIC PEEP: When there is evidence of dynamic hyperinflation on the flow waveforms, the severity of the problem can be evaluated by monitoring the level of intrinsic PEEP. (The measurement of intrinsic PEEP is described in Chapters 25 and 27). The intrinsic PEEP level provides a measure of the severity of airways obstruction in patients with asthma and COPD who require mechanical ventilation.

Ventilator Strategies

The following measures are designed to limit dynamic hyperinflation:

1. Ventilate with low tidal volumes (6 mL/kg) using the *lung protective ventilation* protocol in Table 23.4 (see page 455).

2. Maximize the time for expiration by: (a) preventing rapid respiratory rates (with sedation, if possible, or neuromuscular paralysis, if necessary) and (b) maintaining inspiratory:expiratory ratio of 1:2 or higher.

Noninvasive Ventilation

Positive pressure ventilation can be delivered with tight-fitting face masks instead of endotracheal tubes. This type of *noninvasive mechanical ventilation* avoids the adverse effects of endotracheal intubation (e.g., patient discomfort, increased risk of nosocomial pneumonia), but is not appropriate for all patients. Patients are not candidates for noninvasive ventilation if they are unresponsive, have facial trauma, have severe circulatory compromise, have impending cardiac or respiratory arrest, or have copious respiratory secretions and are unable to clear secretions effectively.

Noninvasive ventilation has been *used most successfully in acute exacerbations of COPD associated with progressive hypercapnia* (51). There is far less experience in acute asthma, but the few available studies show that noninvasive ventilation can hasten the resolution of the acute episode and reduce the number of patients who require intubation (52).

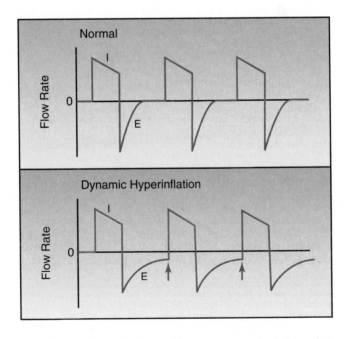

FIGURE 24.5 Flow waveforms during positive pressure mechanical ventilation. The waveforms in the lower panel show continuing expiratory flow at the end of expiration (indicated by the arrows), which indicates the presence of dynamic hyperinflation. I = inspiration, E = expiration.

Start Early

Noninvasive ventilation is a consideration in patients with acute exacerbation of asthma or COPD who do not respond adequately to initial medical management, and it *is most likely to be successful when instituted early, before progression to life-threatening CO_2 retention and impending respiratory arrest.* This is particularly important in patients with severe asthma, who do not develop hypercapnia until late in the progression to life-threatening ventilatory failure (52).

(*Note:* Noninvasive ventilation is presented in detail in Chapter 27.)

A FINAL WORD

Keeping It Simple

The management of patients admitted to the ICU because of severe exacerbations of asthma or COPD can be summarized in the following two statements:

1. Give bronchodilators and corticosteroids to all patients, plus antibiotics for patients with severe COPD.

2. If the condition progresses despite the above measures, use noninvasive ventilation if possible, or conventional mechanical ventilation if necessary.

That's about it.

REFERENCES

Clinical Practice Guidelines

1. National Asthma Education and Prevention Program Expert Panel Report 3: Guidelines for the diagnosis and management of asthma. Full Report 2007. NIH Publication No. 07–4051; August, 2007. (Available at www.nhlbi.nih.gov/guidelines/asthma)

2. Rabe KF, Hurd S, Anzueto A, et al. Global strategy for the diagnosis, management, and prevention of chronic obstructive pulmonary disease. The GOLD executive summary. Am J Respir Crit Care Med 2007; 176:532–555.

Measures of Airway Obstruction

3. Shim CS, Williams MH. Evaluation of the severity of asthma: patients versus physicians. Am J Med 1980; 68:11–13.

4. Langhan ML, Spiro DM. Portable spirometry during acute exacerbations of asthma in children. J Asthma 2009; 46:122–125.

5. Pellegrino R, Viegl G, Brusasco V, et al. Interpretive strategies for lung function tests. Eur Respir J 2005; 26:948–968.

Aerosol Drug Therapy

6. Fink J. Aerosol drug therapy. In Wilkins RL, Stoller JK, Kacmarek RM, eds. Egan's Fundamentals of Respiratory Care. St. Louis, MO: Mosby, Inc. 2009; 801–839.

7. Fink JB. Metered-dose inhalers, dry powder inhalers, and transitions. Respir Care 2000; 45:623–635.

8. Clarke SW, Newman SP. Differences between pressurized aerosol and stable dust particles. Chest 1981; 80(Suppl):907–908.

9. Idris AH, McDermott MF, Raucci JC, et al. Emergency department treatment of severe asthma. Metered-dose inhaler plus holding chamber is equivalent in effectiveness to nebulizer. Chest 1993; 103:665–672.

10. Dhand R, Tobin MJ. Pulmonary perspective: Inhaled bronchodilator therapy in mechanically ventilated patients. Am J Respir Crit Care Med 1997; 156:3–10.

11. AARC Clinical Practice Guideline. Selection of device, administration of bronchodilator, and evaluation of response to therapy in mechanically ventilated patients. Respir Care 1999; 44:105–113.

12. Smalldone GC. Aerosolized bronchodilators in the intensive care unit. Much ado about nothing? Am Rev Respir Crit Care Med 1999; 159:1029–1030.

13. Mantous CA, Hall JB. Update on using therapeutic aerosols in mechanically ventilated patients. J Crit Illness 1996; 11:457–468.

Acute Exacerbations of Asthma

14. Lazarus SC. Emergency treatment of asthma. N Engl J Med 2010; 363:755–764.

15. Mannam P, Seigel MD. Management of life-threatening asthma in adults. J Intensive Care Med 2010; 25:3–15.

16. Shim C, Williams MH. Bronchial response to oral versus aerosol metaproterenol in asthma. Ann Intern Med 1980; 93:428–431.

17. Salmeron S, Brochard L. Mal H, et al. Nebulized versus intravenous albuterol in hypercapnic acute asthma. Am J Respir Crit Care Med 1994; 149:1466–1470.

18. Dutta EJ, Li JTC. β-agonists. Med Clin N Am 2002; 86:991–1008.

19. Dhuper S, Chandra A, Ahmed A, et al. Efficacy and cost comparisons of bronchodilator administration between metered dose inhalers with disposable spacers and nebulizers for acute asthma treatment. J Emerg Med 2011; 40:247–255.

20. Peters SG. Continuous bronchodilator therapy. Chest 2007; 131:286–289.

21. Travers AH, Rowe BH, Barker S, et al. The effectiveness of IV beta-agonists in treating patients with acute asthma in the emergency department: A meta-analysis. Chest 2002; 122:1200–1207.

22. Truwit JD. Toxic effect of bronchodilators. Crit Care Clin 1991; 7:639–657.

23. Bodenhamer J, Bergstrom R, Brown D, et al. Frequently nebulized beta-agonists for asthma: effects on serum electrolytes. Ann Emerg Med 1992; 21:1337–1342.

24. Allon M, Dunlay R, Copkney C. Nebulized albuterol for acute hyperkalemia in patients on hemodialysis. Ann Intern Med 1989; 110:426–429.

25. Rodrigo G, Rodrigo C. The role of anticholinergics in acute asthma treatment. An evidence-based evaluation. Chest 2002; 121:1977–1987.

26. Krishnan JA, Davis SQ, Naureckas ET, et al. An umbrella review: corticosteroid therapy for adults with acute asthma. Am J Med 2009; 122:977–991.

27. Stein LM, Cole RP. Early administration of corticosteroids in emergency room treatment of asthma. Ann Intern Med 1990; 112:822–827.

28. Morrell F, Orriols R, de Gracia J, et al. Controlled trial of intravenous corticosteroids in severe acute asthma. Thorax 1992; 47:588–591.

29. Rodrigo G, Rodrigo C. Corticosteroids in the emergency department therapy of acute adult asthma. An evidence-based evaluation. Chest 1999; 116:285–295.

30. Cydulka RK, Emerman CL. A pilot study of steroid therapy after emergency department treatment of acute asthma: Is a taper needed? J Emerg Med 1998; 16:15–19.

31. Griffin D, Fairman N, Coursin D, et al. Acute myopathy during treatment of status asthmaticus with corticosteroids and steroidal muscle relaxants. Chest 1992; 102:510–514.

32. Rowe BH, Bretzlaff JA, Bourdon C, et al. Intravenous magnesium for treatment of acute asthma in the emergency department: a systematic review of the literature. Ann Emerg Med 2000; 36:181–190.

Acute Exacerbations of COPD

33. National Center for Health Statistics. Health, United States, 2011: with Special Feature on Socioeconomic Status and Health. Hyattville, MD, 2012.

34. Quon BS, Gan WQ, Sin DD. Contemporary management of acute exacerbations of COPD. Chest 2008; 133:756–766.

35. Stoller JK. Acute exacerbations of chronic obstructive pulmonary disease. N Engl J Med 2002; 346:988–994.

36. Rizkallah J, Man P, Sin DD. Prevalence of pulmonary embolism in acute exacerbations of COPD. Chest 2009; 135:786–793.

37. McCrory DC, Brown C, Gelfand SE, Bach PB. Management of acute exacerbations of COPD. A summary and appraisal of published evidence. Chest 2001; 119:1190–1209.

38. Walters JAE, Gibson PG, Wood-Baker R, et al. Systemic corticosteroids for acute exacerbations of chronic obstructive pulmonary disease. Cochrane Database of Systematic Reviews, 2009; 1:CD001288.

39. Immaculada A, de la Cal MA, Esteban A, et al. Efficacy of corticosteroid therapy in patients with an acute exacerbation of chronic obstructive pulmonary disease receiving ventilatory support. Arch Intern Med 2011; 171:1939–1946.

40. Lindenauer PK, Pekow PS, Lahiti MC, et. al. Association of corticosteroid dose and route of administration with risk of treatment failure in acute exacerbation of chronic obstructive pulmonary disease. JAMA 2010; 303: 2359–2367.

41. Monso E, Ruiz J, Rosell J, et al. Bacterial infection in chronic obstructive pulmonary disease. Am J Respir Crit Care Med 1995; 152:1316–1320.

42. Rothberg MR, Pekow PS, Lahti M, et al. Antibiotic therapy and treatment failure in patients hospitalized for acute exacerbations of chronic obstructive pulmonary disease. JAMA 2010; 303:2035–2042.

43. Nouira S, Marghli S, Belghith M, et al. Once daily ofloxacin in chronic obstructive pulmonary disease exacerbation requiring mechanical ventilation: a randomized, placebo-controlled trial. Lancet 2001; 358:2020–2025.

44. Murphy TF. *Pseudomonas aeruginosa* in adults with chronic obstructive pulmonary disease. Curr Opin Pulm Med 2009; 15:138–142.

45. Campbell EJM. The J. Burns Amberson Lecture. The management of acute respiratory failure in chronic bronchitis and emphysema. Am Rev Respir Crit Care Med 1967; 96:626–639.

46. Aubier M, Murciano D, Fournier M, et al. Central respiratory drive in acute respiratory failure or patients with chronic obstructive pulmonary disease. Am Rev Respir Crit Care Med 1980; 122:191–199.

Mechanical Ventilation

47. Peters JI, Stupka JE, Singh H, et al. Status asthmaticus in the medical intensive care unit: a 30-year experience. Respir Med 2012; 106:344–348.

48. Soo Hoo GW, Hakimian N, Santiago SM. Hypercapnic respiratory failure in COPD patients" response to therapy. Chest 2000; 117:169–177.

49. Blanch L, Bernabe F, Lucangelo U. Measurement of air trapping, intrinsic positive end-expiratory pressure, and dynamic hyperinflation in mechanically ventilated patients. Respir Care 2005; 50:110–123.

50. Pepe P, Marini JJ. Occult positive end-expiratory pressure in mechanically ventilated patients with airflow obstruction. The auto-PEEP effect. Am Rev Respir Dis 1982; 126:166–170.

51. Boldrini R, Fasano L, Nava S. Noninvasive mechanical ventilation. Curr Opin Crit Care 2012; 18:48–53.

52. Scala R. Noninvasive ventilation in severe acute asthma? Still far from the truth. Respir Care 2010; 55:630–637.

MECHANICAL VENTILATION

All who drink of this remedy will recover . . . except those in whom it does not help, who will die. Therefore, it is obvious that it fails only in incurable diseases.

Galen

Chapter 25

POSITIVE PRESSURE VENTILATION

"... an opening must be attempted in the trunk of the trachea, into which a tube of reed or cane should be put; you will then blow into this, so that the lung may rise again ... and the heart becomes strong ... "

Andreas Vesalius
1555

Vesalius is credited with the first description of positive pressure ventilation, but it took 400 years to apply his concept to patient care. The occasion was the polio epidemic of 1955, when the demand for assisted ventilation outgrew the supply of negative-pressure tank ventilators (known as *iron lungs*). In Denmark, all medical schools shut down and medical students worked in 8-hour shifts as human ventilators, manually inflating the lungs of afflicted patients. In Boston, the nearby Emerson Company made available a prototype positive-pressure lung inflation device, which was put to use at the Massachusetts General Hospital, and became an instant success. Thus began the era of positive pressure mechanical ventilation (and the era of intensive care medicine).

BASICS

The fundamental operation of positive pressure ventilation is to create a pressure that moves a volume of gas into the lungs. There are two general methods of positive pressure ventilation, which are summarized below and illustrated in Figure 25.1.

1. *Volume-controlled ventilation,* where the inflation volume (tidal volume) is preselected, and the ventilator automatically adjusts the inflation pressure to deliver the desired volume. The rate of lung inflation can be constant (as in Figure 25.1) or decelerating.

2. *Pressure-controlled ventilation,* where the inflation pressure is preselected, and the duration of inflation is adjusted (by the operator) to deliver the desired tidal volume. The rate of lung inflation is high at

the onset of lung inflation (to achieve the desired inflation pressure), then rapidly decelerates (to maintain a constant inflation pressure).

The uses, advantages, and disadvantages of these modes of ventilation are described in the next chapter. This section will describe the measurements that are used to evaluate the mechanical properties of the lungs and chest wall (i.e., airflow resistance and distensibility) with each method of ventilation.

During positive pressure ventilation, pressures in the thorax are monitored at the level of the endotracheal tube or ventilator. These *proximal airway pressures* can differ from pressures at the level of the alveoli (as described next).

End-Inspiratory Pressures

The proximal airway pressure at the end of a lung inflation has different interpretations for volume-cycled and pressure-cycled ventilation.

Volume-Controlled Ventilation

During volume-controlled ventilation, the pressure in the airways rises steadily until the preselected volume is delivered. The airway pressure (Paw) at the end of each lung inflation, the *peak airway pressure* (Ppeak),

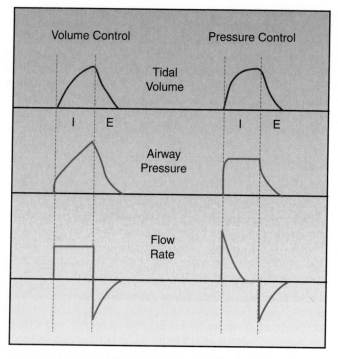

FIGURE 25.1 Waveforms for inflation (tidal) volume, airway pressure, and flow rate for volume-controlled and pressure-controlled ventilation. See text for explanation.

is the pressure needed to overcome both resistive and elastic forces in the lungs and chest wall (Pres and Pel, respectively).

$$Ppeak = Pres + Pel \qquad (25.1)$$

Pres is a function of the resistance to flow in the airways (R), and the inspiratory flow rate [Pres = R × $\dot{V}$ (insp)], while Pel is a function of the elastic recoil force of the lungs and chest wall, and the lung volume (Pel = elastance × V). The resistive component of the peak airway pressure can be eliminated by eliminating airflow. This is accomplished by occluding the expiratory circuit at the very end of lung inflation, to prevent the patient from exhaling. During this "inflation- hold" maneuver (which typically lasts for one second), the pressure in the airways decreases initially and then remains constant until the occlusion is released and the patient is allowed to exhale. This is illustrated in Figure 25.2. The steady occlusion pressure, which is called the *plateau pressure*, is the peak pressure in the alveoli (Palv) at the end of inspiration.

$$Pplateau = Palv \text{ (peak)} \qquad (25.2)$$

The difference between the plateau pressure and the level of positive end-expiratory pressure (PEEP) is the pressure needed to overcome the elastic recoil forces of the lungs and chest wall (Pel).

$$Pplateau - PEEP = Pel \qquad (25.3)$$

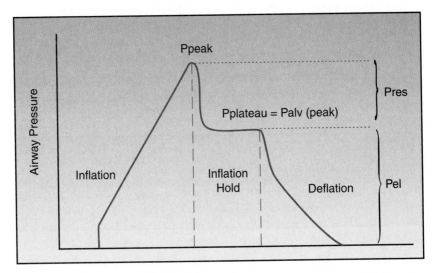

FIGURE 25.2 Airway pressure profile for a constant-flow, volume-controlled lung inflation with a brief end-inspiratory occlusion (inflation-hold). Ppeak is the peak airway pressure, Pplateau is the end-inspiratory occlusion pressure, Palv (peak) is the peak alveolar pressure at end-inspiration, Pres is the pressure attributed to airway resistance, and Pel is the pressure attributed to the elastic recoil force of the lungs and chest wall. See text for explanation.

The difference between the peak and plateau pressures represents the pressure needed to overcome the resistance to airflow at any given inspiratory flow rate.

$$Ppeak - Pplateau = Pres \qquad (25.4)$$

Pressure-Controlled Ventilation

During pressure-controlled ventilation, there should be no airflow at the end of inspiration, and the end-inspiratory airway pressure (Paw) will be equivalent to the peak alveolar pressure at the end of inspiration.

$$Paw\ (end\text{-}insp) = Palv\ (peak) \qquad (25.5)$$

The change in pressure attributed to the elastic forces of the lungs and chest wall is the pressure difference between the end-inspiratory Paw and PEEP:

$$Paw\ (end\text{-}insp) - PEEP = Pel \qquad (25.6)$$

(*Note:* These relationships are valid only when there is no airflow at the end of inspiration. Inspiratory flow may not return to zero at end-inspiration in patients who are breathing rapidly; in this situation, the end-inspiratory airway pressure will be higher than alveolar pressure.)

Since inspiratory flow is not constant during pressure-controlled ventilation, it is not possible to evaluate airway resistance during lung inflation. Resistance to expiratory flow (described later) can be used to evaluate airways resistance during pressure-controlled ventilation.

End-Expiratory Pressure

The end-expiratory pressure is the *minimum pressure in the alveoli* (not airways) during a ventilatory cycle. The different forms of end-expiratory pressure are illustrated in Figure 25.3.

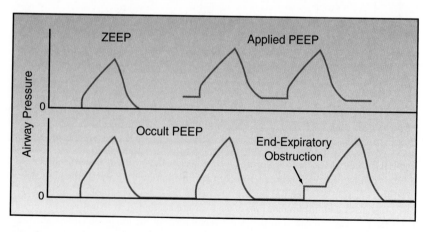

FIGURE 25.3 End-expiratory airway pressures. See text for explanation.

ZEEP

During appropriate ventilation in the normal lung, there is no airflow at the end of expiration, and the pressure in the alveoli is equivalent to atmospheric pressure. Since atmospheric pressure is a zero reference point for breathing, this condition is called *zero end-expiratory pressure*, or ZEEP.

Applied PEEP

Positive end-expiratory pressure (PEEP) can be added through the ventilatory circuit (via a pressure-sensitive valve in the expiratory limb of the circuit) so that exhalation will cease when the airway pressure falls to the preselected PEEP level. Applied PEEP is used routinely during mechanical ventilation to prevent the collapse of distal airspaces at the end of expiration, and to open collapsed alveoli (recruitment). This is described in the next chapter.

Occult PEEP

When there is continued airflow at the end of expiration, the lungs do not completely empty, and the alveolar pressure remains positive even though the proximal airway pressure falls to atmospheric (zero) pressure. This pressure is sometimes called *intrinsic PEEP* or *auto-PEEP*, but *occult PEEP* seems more appropriate because the PEEP *is not apparent in proximal airway pressure recordings* (2). Occult PEEP can be the result of dynamic hyperinflation in patients with asthma and COPD, as described in Chapter 24 (see pages 477–480), or it can be the result of ventilator settings that predispose to end-expiratory airflow (e.g., high inflation volumes, decreased time for exhalation).

Occult PEEP can be detected on the flow tracing by noting the presence of airflow at the end of expiration, as illustrated in Figure 24.5 (see page 479). If occult PEEP is present, it can be quantified by occluding the expiratory circuit at the end of expiration. During an end-expiratory occlusion, alveolar pressure will equilibrate with proximal airway pressure, and the occult PEEP becomes apparent as a abrupt increase in airway pressure, as shown in Figure 25.3. Occult PEEP is described in more detail in Chapter 28.

Mean Airway Pressure

The mean airway pressure is the average pressure in the airway during the ventilatory cycle, and is influenced by several variables, including the peak airway pressure, the contour of the pressure waveform, the PEEP level, the respiratory rate, and the inflation time relative to the total time of the ventilatory cycle (T_I/T_{tot}). The mean airway pressure that is displayed by ventilators is obtained by integrating the area under the airway pressure waveform.

The mean airway pressure is linked to the hemodynamic effects of positive pressure ventilation. (The intrapleural pressure is the important influence on cardiac function, but this pressure is measured with an intraesophageal balloon, and is not monitored routinely.) Typical values for mean airway pressure during positive pressure ventilation are 5–10 cm H_2O for normal lungs, 10–20 cm H_2O for airflow obstruction, and 20–30 cm H_2O for noncompliant (stiff) lungs (3).

Thoracic Compliance

Compliance (Δvolume/Δpressure) is the reciprocal of elastance, and is the traditional term used to express the elastic properties of structures with chambers (like the heart and lungs). Compliance expresses *distensibility*, or the tendency of a chamber to increase in volume when exposed to a given distending pressure. The compliance that is measured during mechanical ventilation is the *thoracic compliance*, and includes both the lungs and the chest wall.

Volume-Controlled Ventilation

During volume-controlled ventilation, the static compliance of the thorax (Cstat) is expressed as the preselected tidal volume (V_T) divided by the difference between the plateau pressure and the total PEEP level (applied plus occult PEEP):

$$Cstat = V_T \, / \, [Pplateau - PEEP(tot)] \qquad (25.7)$$

This is a "static" compliance because the pressures involved are measured in the absence of airflow. In patients with normal lungs, Cstat is 50–80 mL/cm H_2O (4), and in patients with infiltrative lung diseases (e.g., pulmonary edema or acute respiratory distress syndrome), Cstat is typically < 25 mL/cm H_2O (1).

Pressure-Controlled Ventilation

Compliance measurements are difficult during pressure-controlled ventilation because: (a) there must be no inspiratory flow at the end of inspiration (which is not always the case), and (b) the tidal volume varies with changes in airway resistance and thoracic compliance during pressure-controlled ventilation. Under ideal conditions (i.e., no airflow at end-inspiration and stable lung mechanics) Cstat is equivalent to the exhaled tidal volume (exhaled V_T) divided by the difference between the end-inspiratory airway pressure (Paw) and the total PEEP level:

$$Cstat = Exhaled \; V_T \, / [Paw(end\text{-}insp) - PEEP(tot)] \qquad (25.8)$$

Sources of Error

1. During passive ventilation, the chest wall can account for 35% of the total thoracic compliance (5,6), and this contribution increases when the chest wall muscles contract. Therefore, to avoid interference from respiratory muscle contraction, *static compliance measurements should be performed only in patients who are not actively breathing.*

2. Thoracic compliance is volume-dependent; i.e., it decreases as lung volume increases. Absolute lung volumes cannot be measured dur-

ing mechanical ventilation. However, *serial measurements of Cstat should be performed at the same tidal volume(s)*.

3. The *tidal volume* used for the compliance measurement *should be adjusted for the compliance of the ventilator tubing*, which is typically 3 mL/cm H_2O (1). For example, if the preselected tidal volume during volume-controlled ventilation is 500 mL and the peak airway pressure is 40 cm H_2O, then $3 \times 40 = 120$ mL of the delivered volume will be lost to expansion of the ventilator tubing, and the actual tidal volume reaching the patient will be $500 - 120 = 380$ mL. When using exhaled tidal volumes, the peak alveolar pressure at end-inspiration should be used for the volume adjustments.

Airway Resistance

Airway resistance can be measured during inspiration or expiration, although expiratory airway resistance provides more information about flow resistance in small airways.

Inspiratory Resistance

The resistance to airflow during inspiration can only be determined if the inspiratory flow rate is constant (e.g., during volume-controlled ventilation). In this case, the inspiratory resistance (Rinsp) is the pressure gradient needed to overcome the resistive forces in the lungs and chest wall (Ppeak – Pplateau) divided by the inspiratory flow rate [$\dot{V}$ (insp)]:

$$Rinsp = (Ppeak - Pplateau) / \dot{V} \text{ (insp)} \qquad (25.9)$$

An example of the Rinsp calculation for a patient with normal lungs is as follows: Ppeak = 15 cm H_2O, Pplateau = 10 cm H_2O, $\dot{V}$ (insp) = 60 L/min (1 L/sec), so Rinsp = $(15 - 10)/1 = 5$ cm H_2O/L/sec. The minimal flow resistance in large-bore endotracheal tubes is 3 to 7 cm H_2O/L/sec (6), so most of the inspiratory resistance in patients with normal lungs represents the resistance to flow in the endotracheal tube. The contribution of nonpulmonary resistive elements like endotracheal tubes is one of the shortcomings of the airway resistance determinations.

Expiratory Resistance

The resistance to expiratory airflow is more likely to detect the tendency for small airways to collapse during mechanical ventilation. The expiratory resistance (Rexp) can be measured using the driving pressure for expiratory airflow (the peak alveolar pressure at the end of inspiration minus the total PEEP level), and the peak expiratory flow rate (PEFR); i.e.,

$$Rexp = [Palv \text{ (peak)} - PEEP \text{ (tot)}] / PEFR \qquad (25.10)$$

Rexp is usually higher than Rinsp, which reflects the tendency of the airways to narrow as lung volume decreases during expiration. However, like the Rinsp, the Rexp is significantly influenced by nonpulmonary resistive elements (e.g., endotracheal tube and exhalation valves).

LUNG INJURY

Normal breathing is accomplished by pulling air into the lungs, and as much as 5 liters of air can be drawn in during a single breath (from residual volume to total lung capacity) without noticeable injury to the lungs. On the other hand, positive pressure ventilation *pushes* air into the lungs, and this push creates abnormal stresses and strains that can damage the architecture of the lungs, particularly diseased lungs, with single-breath volumes of less than one-half liter (7,8). An example of the structural damage produced by mechanical ventilation is shown in Figure 25.4 (9).

There are several types of *ventilator-induced lung injury* (VILI), as described in this section. Since VILI has been studied primarily in patients with acute respiratory distress syndrome (ARDS), a brief description of VILI is also included in the chapter describing ARDS (see pages 454–455).

Volutrauma

In the early days of positive pressure ventilation, large tidal volumes were adopted to prevent atelectasis (10). Tidal volumes of 10 to 15 mL/kg (ideal body weight) became standard during mechanical ventilation, compared to normal tidal volumes of 5 to 7 mL/kg during spontaneous breathing. From the outset, it was clear that mechanical ventilation could rupture alveoli and produce air leaks (barotrauma), but in the 1970s, a study was published showing that high inflation pressures could produce diffuse pulmonary infiltration that resembles pulmonary edema (11). This was followed by a landmark study in the 1980s showing that high inflation volumes, rather than high inflation pressures, were responsible for the lung injury produced by mechanical ventilation (12). The results of this study are shown in Figure 25.5. Note that marked increases in extravascular lung water occurred only when inflation volumes were high, regardless of the inflation pressure. As a result of this study, the term *volutrauma* was adopted to describe the underlying mechanism for the pulmonary infiltration produced by mechanical ventilation.

The lung injury in VILI is not watery pulmonary edema, but is the result of overdistension of alveoli and disruption of the alveolar-capillary interface, leading to *inflammatory infiltration of the lungs* and a clinical condition *that resembles ARDS* (13).

Infiltrative Lung Diseases

The effects of high inflation volumes are more marked in infiltrative lung diseases like pneumonia and ARDS because the inflation volumes are distributed preferentially to regions of normal lung function. In this situation, the high inflation volumes are being delivered to lungs with a decrease in functional lung volume (see Figure 23.4 on page 454), and this predisposes to volutrauma from overdistension of alveoli in normal lung regions.

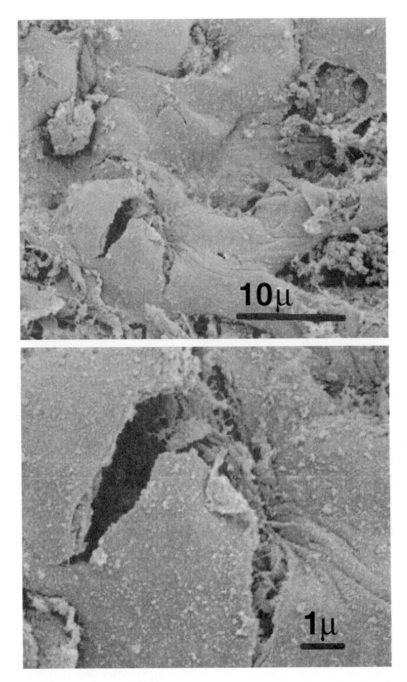

FIGURE 25.4 Electron micrographs showing a tear at the alveolar-capillary interface attributed to alveolar overdistension during mechanical ventilation. Post mortem specimen from a patient with ARDS. Scales shown in lower right corner of each image. Images from Reference 7, and digitally retouched.

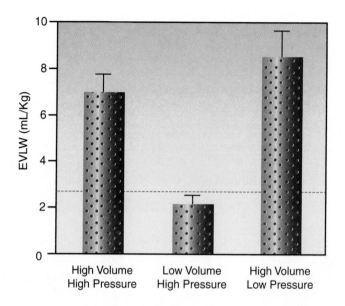

FIGURE 25.5 Effects of high pressures and high volumes on extravascular lung water (EVLW) during positive pressure ventilation. Height of the bars represents mean values, and hatched bars represent standard deviations of the mean. Dotted line represents the upper 95% limit of EVLW measurements obtained during ventilation at normal pressures and volumes. Data from Reference 12.

Low-Volume Ventilation

Concern for the risk of lung injury during conventional, high-volume ventilation prompted clinical studies evaluating lower tidal volumes during mechanical ventilation, mostly in patients with ARDS. The largest study to date included over 800 patients with ARDS (14), and compared ventilation with tidal volumes of 6 mL/kg and 12 mL/kg using *predicted body weight* (which is the weight at which lung volumes are normal). Ventilation with low tidal volumes was associated with a shorter duration of mechanical ventilation and 9% (absolute) reduction in mortality. As a result of this study (and other corroborating studies), a low-volume ventilation protocol known as *lung protective ventilation* is now recommended for all patients with ARDS. This protocol is presented later in the section.

Atelectrauma

During mechanical ventilation, small airways tend to collapse by the end of expiration, particularly in pulmonary conditions associated with reduced lung compliance (e.g., pulmonary edema, ARDS). Repetitive opening and closing of small airways during positive pressure ventilation can damage the airway epithelium, possibly by generating excessive shear forces (15). This type of lung injury is called *atelectrauma* (8), and it can be mitigated by the use of positive end-expiratory pressure (PEEP), which provides a pressurized "stent" to keep the small airways open during expiration.

Biotrauma

The most intriguing form of VILI is the ability of positive pressure ventilation to promote proinflammatory cytokine release from the lungs at inflation volumes that do not produce structural damage in the lungs (16). This is called *biotrauma*, and it can trigger the systemic inflammatory response syndrome, and can lead to inflammatory injury in the lung as well as other organs. This means that *mechanical ventilation can be a source of inflammatory-mediated multiorgan failure* (17), like that seen in severe sepsis and septic shock. This is not good.

Barotrauma

Positive pressure ventilation can also produce air leaks from a rupture in the airways and distal airspaces. The air that escapes can enter the pleural space *(pneumothorax)*, or it can move along the bronchovascular bundles into the mediastinum *(pneumomediastinum)* and up into the subcutaneous tissues *(subcutaneous emphysema)*, or it can track down the mediastinum and enter the peritoneal cavity *(pneumoperitoneum)*. This form of VILI is called *barotrauma*, even though the source of injury can be high alveolar volume (i.e., volutrauma).

Lung Protective Ventilation

The protocol shown in Table 25.1 is known as *lung protective ventilation,* and it is designed to limit the risk of all forms of VILI. The important elements of this protocol are as follows:

1. Ventilation begins with a tidal volume of 8 mL/kg, based on predicted body weight (not actual or ideal body weight), and this is gradually reduced to 6 mL/kg.

2. The plateau pressure is not allowed to rise above 30 cm H_2O. (Since the plateau pressure is equivalent to the peak alveolar pressure, a plateau pressure above 30 cm H_2O is a reflection of excessive alveolar volume.)

3. A minimum PEEP level of 5 cm H_2O is used to prevent small airways from collapsing at end-expiration (to prevent atelectrauma).

4. A rise in arterial PCO_2 is allowed during low-volume ventilation as long as the arterial pH does not fall below 7.30. This strategy is known as *permissive hypercapnia* (18).

Lung protective ventilation is now recommended for all patients with ARDS who require mechanical ventilation. The full protocol is available on the ARDS Clinical Network website (www.ardsnet.org).

Table 25.1	Protocol for Lung Protective Ventilation in ARDS

I. Tidal Volume Goal: V_T = 6 mL/kg (predicted body weight)

    1. Calculate patient's predicted body weight (PBW):
        Males: PBW = 50   + [2.3 × (height in inches − 60]
        Females: PBW = 45.5 + [2.3 × (height in inches − 60]

    2. Use volume-controlled ventilation and set initial tidal volume (V_T) to 8 mL/kg (PBW).

    3. Set respiratory rate (RR) to match baseline minute ventilation, but not >35 bpm.

    4. Set positive end-expiratory pressure (PEEP) at 5 cm H_2O.

    5. Reduce V_T by 1 mL/kg every 1 to 2 hours until V_T = 6 mL/kg (PBW)

    6. Adjust PEEP and FiO_2 to maintain SpO_2 of 88–95%.

II. Plateau Pressure Goal: Ppl ≤30 cm H_2O:

    1. If Ppl >30 cm H_2O and V_T at 6 mL/kg, decrease V_T in 1 mL/kg increments until Ppl falls to ≤30 cm H_2O or V_T reaches a minimum of 4 mL/kg.

III. pH Goal: pH = 7.30–7.45

    1. If pH = 7.15–7.30, increase RR until pH >7.30, $PaCO_2$ <25 mm Hg, or RR = 35 bpm.

    2. If pH <7.15, increase RR to 35 bpm. If pH remains <7.15, increase in V_T in 1 mL/kg increments until pH >7.15 (Ppl target may be exceeded).

    3. If pH >7.45, decrease RR, if possible.

Adapted from the protocol developed by the ARDS Clinical Network, available at www.ardsnet.org.

THE PLATEAU PRESSURE: As mentioned in Chapter 23, clinical studies have not shown a consistent survival benefit with lung protective ventilation in ARDS, and this discrepancy appears to be related to the plateau pressure; i.e., a survival benefit with low-volume, lung protective ventilation is demonstrated only when the plateau pressure is above 30 cm H_2O during conventional, high-volume (10–15 mL/kg) ventilation (19). Therefore, *a plateau pressure ≤30 cm H_2O seems more important than a low tidal volume for protecting the lungs from ventilator-induced injury.*

A STANDARD PRACTICE?: Although lung protective ventilation is recommended only for patients with ARDS, there are reports that VILI can occur during conventional ventilation in patients who do not have ARDS (20), and that lung protective ventilation is associated with improved outcomes in non-ARDS patients (21). These observations, combined with the strong physiological basis for lung protective ventilation, should lead to the adoption of lung protective ventilation for all patients who require mechanical ventilation.

CARDIAC PERFORMANCE

The influence of positive pressure ventilation on cardiac performance is complex, and involves the preload and afterload forces for the right and left sides of the heart (22). These forces are described in Chapter 9.

Preload

Positive pressure ventilation can reduce ventricular filling (preload) in several ways, and these are indicated in Figure 25.6. First and foremost, *positive intrathoracic pressure decreases the pressure gradient for venous inflow into the thorax* (although positive-pressure ventilation also increases intra-abdominal pressure, which tends to maintain the pressure gradient for venous inflow into the thorax). Second, positive pressure on the outer surface of the heart decreases the transmural pressure during diastole, and this will reduce ventricular filling. Finally, positive pressure ventilation increases pulmonary vascular resistance, and this can impede right ventricular stroke output and hence impede left ventricular filling. In this situation, the right ventricle can dilate and push the interventricular septum toward the left ventricle, and this reduces left ventricular chamber size and further reduces left ventricular filling. This phenomenon, known as *ventricular interdependence,* is one of the mechanisms whereby right heart failure can impair the performance of the left side of the heart (see Fig. 13.4 on page 247).

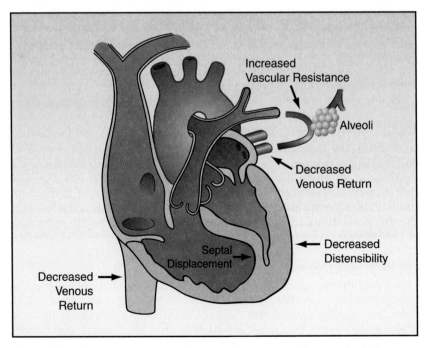

FIGURE 25.6 The mechanisms for a decrease in ventricular filling (preload) during positive pressure ventilation.

Afterload

Left ventricular afterload is a function of the peak transmural wall pressure during systole (see Figure 9.7 on page 161), which is the pressure that ventricular contraction must overcome to eject the stroke volume. Positive intrapleural pressure decreases this transmural pressure, and thereby decreases left ventricular afterload. (Conceptually, positive intrapleural pressure acts like a hand that squeezes the ventricles during systole.) Therefore, *positive pressure ventilation reduces ventricular afterload*, and this effect can augment cardiac output in certain situations (see next).

Cardiac Output

The overall effect of positive pressure ventilation on cardiac output is determined by the balance between the decrease in ventricular preload (which reduces cardiac output) and the decrease in ventricular afterload (which increases cardiac output) during positive pressure ventilation. This balance is determined by cardiac function, intravascular volume, and intrathoracic pressure.

Cardiac Function

The curves in Figure 25.7 show the superimposed influence of preload and afterload on cardiac output in the normal and failing heart. The normal heart operates on the steep portion of the preload curve and the flat portion of the afterload curve. In this situation, a decrease in preload has a greater influence on cardiac output than a decrease in afterload (as indicated by the arrows), so cardiac output is expected to decrease during positive pressure ventilation. However, as mentioned earlier, positive pressure ventilation also increases intra-abdominal pressure (by pushing the diaphragm down into the abdomen), and this serves to maintain the venous inflow into the thorax. As a result, the decrease in venous return (preload) can be minimal during positive pressure ventilation, and the cardiac output can decrease slightly, show no change, or even increase slightly (from the afterload reducing effect).

In contrast, the failing heart operates on the flat portion of the preload curve and the steep portion of the afterload curve. In this situation, the decrease in afterload during positive pressure ventilation has a greater influence on cardiac output than the decrease in preload, and cardiac output will increase during positive pressure ventilation. This is the basis for the use of positive pressure breathing as a "ventricular assist" maneuver in patients with advanced heart failure (23,24).

Low Intravascular Volume

When the intravascular volume is reduced, the preload-reducing effect of positive pressure ventilation predominates in both the normal and failing heart, and cardiac output will decline (22). This is particularly the case when intrathoracic pressures are high during mechanical ventilation. Maintaining a normal or adequate intravascular volume is essential during positive pressure ventilation to avoid significant deficits in cardiac output.

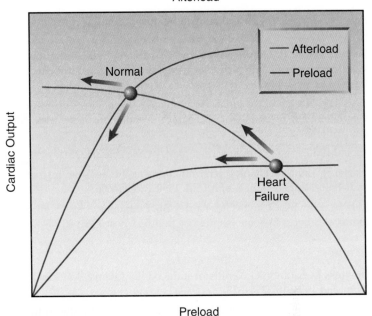

FIGURE 25.7 Superimposed curves for the relationship between preload, afterload, and cardiac output in the normal and failing heart. Arrows indicate the effects of positive pressure ventilation.

A FINAL WORD

Less Is Best

For the first 30 years after its introduction, positive pressure ventilation was dominated by large inflation volumes and high pressures, but this has changed since the discovery that pushing air into the lungs creates stresses and strains that damage the lungs, and can lead to damage in other organs as well. The emphasis now is on limiting inflation volumes and preventing overdistension of alveoli. This "less is best" strategy is currently advised only for patients with ARDS, but it seems likely that it will (and should) be adopted for all patients who require positive pressure ventilation.

REFERENCES

Books

Papadakos PJ, Lachmann B, eds. Mechanical ventilation: clinical applications and pathophysiology. Philadelphia: Saunders, Elsevier, 2008.

Basics

1. Bekos V, Marini JJ. Monitoring the mechanically ventilated patient. Crit Care Clin 2007; 23:575–611.

2. Pepe P, Marini JJ. Occult positive end-expiratory pressure in mechanically ventilated patients with airflow obstruction. The auto-PEEP effect. Am Rev Respir Dis 1982; 126:166–170.

3. Hess DR, Kacmarek RM. Basic pulmonary mechanics during mechanical ventilation. In: Essentials of Mechanical Ventilation. New York, McGraw-Hill, 1996:171–176.

4. Tobin MJ. Respiratory monitoring. JAMA 1990; 264:244–251.

5. Marini JJ. Lung mechanics determinations at the bedside: instrumentation and clinical application. Respir Care 1990; 35:669–696.

6. Katz JA, Zinn SE, Ozanne GM, Fairley BB. Pulmonary, chest wall, and lung–thorax elastances in acute respiratory failure. Chest 1981; 80:304–311.

Lung Injury

7. Dreyfuss D, Saumon G. Ventilator-induced lung injury. Am Rev Respir Crit Care Med 1998; 157:294–323.

8. Gattinoni L, Protti A, Caironi P, Carlesso E. Ventilator-induced lung injury: the anatomical and physiological framework. Crit Care Med 2010; 38(Suppl):S539–S548.

9. Hotchkiss JR, Simonson DA, Marek DJ, et al. Pulmonary microvascular fracture in a patient with acute respiratory distress syndrome. Crit Care Med 2002; 30:2368–2370.

10. Bendixen HH, Egbert LD, Hedley-White J, et al. Respiratory care. St. Louis: Mosby, 1965; 137–153.

11. Webb HH, Tierney DE. Experimental pulmonary edema due to intermittent positive pressure ventilation with high inflation pressures: protection by positive end-expiratory pressure. Am Rev Respir Dis 1974; 110:556–565.

12. Dreyfuss D, Soler P, Basset G, et al. High inflation pressure pulmonary edema: Respective effects of high airway pressure, high tidal volume, and positive end-expiratory pressure. Am Rev Respir Dis 1988; 137:1159–1164.

13. Timby J, Reed C, Zeilander S, Glauser F. "Mechanical" causes of pulmonary edema. Chest 1990; 98:973–979.

14. The Acute Respiratory Distress Syndrome Network. Ventilation with lower tidal volumes as compared with traditional tidal volumes for acute lung injury and the acute respiratory distress syndrome. N Engl J Med 2000; 342(18):1301–1308.

15. Muscedere JG, Mullen JBM, Gan K, Slutsky AS. Tidal ventilation at low airway pressures can augment lung injury. Am J Respir Crit Care Med 1994; 149:1327–1334.

16. Ranieri VM, Suter PM Tortorella C, et al. Effect of mechanical ventilation on inflammatory mediators in patients with acute respiratory distress syndrome: A randomized controlled trial. JAMA 1999; 282:54–61.

17. Ranieri VM, Giunta F, Suter P, Slutsky AS. Mechanical ventilation as a mediator of multisystem organ failure in acute respiratory distress syndrome. JAMA 2000; 284:43–44.

18. O'Croinin D, Ni Chonghaile M, Higgins B, Laffey JG. Bench-to-Bedside review: Permissive hypercapnia. Crit Care 2005; 9(1):51–59.

19. Petrucci N, Iacovelli W. Ventilation with lower tidal volumes versus traditional tidal volumes for acute lung injury and acute respiratory distress syndrome. Cochrane Database Syst Rev 2004; (2):CD003844.

20. Gajic O, Dara SI, Mendez JL, et al. Ventilator-associated lung injury in patients without acute lung injury at the onset of mechanical ventilation. Crit Care Med 2004; 32:1817–1824.

21. Serpa Neto A, Cardoso SO, Manetta JA, et al. Association between the use of lung-protective ventilation with lower tidal volumes and clinical outcomes among patients without acute respiratory distress syndrome: a meta-analysis. JAMA 2012; 308:1651–1659.

Cardiac Performance

22. Singh I, Pinsky MR. Heart-lung interactions. In Papadakos PJ, Lachmann B, eds. Mechanical ventilation: clinical applications and pathophysiology. Philadelphia: Saunders Elsevier, 2008:173–184.

23. Yan AT, Bradley TD, Liu PP. The role of continuous positive airway pressure in the treatment of congestive heart failure. Chest 2001; 120:1675–1685.

24. Boehmer JP, Popjes E. Cardiac failure: Mechanical support strategies. Crit Care Med 2006; 34(Suppl):S268–S277.

Chapter 26

CONVENTIONAL MODES OF VENTILATION

Development in most fields of medicine appears to occur according to sound scientific principles. However, exceptions can be found, and the development of mechanical ventilatory support is one of them.

J. Räsänen, MD

A recently published textbook on respiratory care equipment lists 174 specific methods of positive pressure ventilation (1), yet in the 50-plus years since positive pressure ventilation was introduced, only one method has improved clinical outcomes (2), and only because it reduces the lung damage produced by positive intrathoracic pressures. What this means is that positive pressure ventilation is much more complicated than it needs to be (3).

This chapter describes six basic methods of positive pressure ventilation (volume control, pressure control, assist-control, pressure support, intermittent mandatory ventilation, and positive end-expiratory pressure). Although this is far less than the bloated number of available methods, these six methods should be all that is needed to provide effective ventilatory support in a majority of patients.

THE VENTILATOR BREATH

As introduced in the last chapter, there are two basic methods of positive-pressure lung inflation: (a) *volume control,* where the inflation volume is constant, and (b) *pressure control,* where the inflation pressure is constant (1). The changes in pressure and flow that occur with each type of ventilator breath are shown in Figure 26.1.

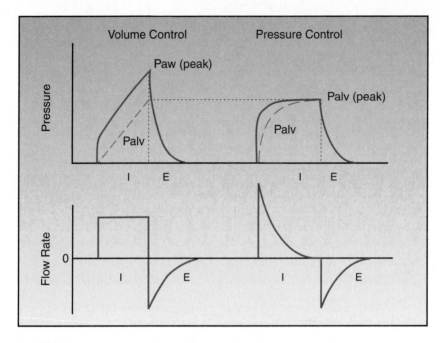

FIGURE 26.1 Pressure and flow changes during a single ventilator breath using volume control and pressure control methods of lung inflation at equivalent inflation (tidal) volumes. Changes in airway pressure (Paw) are indicated by the solid lines, and changes in alveolar pressure (Palv) are indicated by the dashed lines. I = inspiration, E = expiration.

Volume Control

With volume control ventilation (VCV), the inflation (tidal) volume is preselected, and the lungs are inflated at a constant flow rate until the desired volume is delivered. Because there is airflow at the end of inspiration, the peak pressure in the proximal airways (peak Paw) is greater than the peak pressure in the alveoli (peak Palv); and the difference (peak Paw − peak Palv) is the pressure dissipated by the resistance to flow in the airways. The peak alveolar pressure is a reflection of the alveolar volume at the end of lung inflation.

Advantages

CONSTANT TIDAL VOLUME: The major advantage of VCV is the ability to deliver a constant tidal volume despite changes in the mechanical properties of the lungs. When airways resistance increases or lung compliance decreases, the ventilator generates a higher pressure to deliver the preselected volume. This maintains the desired minute ventilation in the face of abrupt or undetected changes in airway resistance or lung compliance.

Disadvantages

AIRWAY PRESSURE: At any given tidal volume, the airway pressures at the end of inspiration are higher during VCV than during pressure control ventilation (PCV), as shown in Figure 26.1, and this is mistakenly perceived as an increased risk of ventilator-induced lung injury. However, the risk of ventilator-induced lung injury is related to the peak *alveolar* pressure (2,4), and this pressure is the same during VCV and PCV (at equivalent tidal volumes). Therefore, *the higher peak airway pressures during volume-controlled ventilation do not increase the risk of alveolar overdistension and ventilator-induced lung injury.*

INSPIRATORY FLOW: There are disadvantages related to the constant inspiratory flow rate during VCV. First, the duration of inspiration is relatively short, and this can lead to uneven alveolar filling. In addition, the maximum inspiratory flow is limited when flow is constant, and the inspiratory flow rate can be inadequate in patients with high flow demands, resulting in patient distress. A decelerating flow pattern is available for VCV, and it has been shown to improve patient comfort VCV (5).

Pressure Control

With pressure control ventilation (PCV), the desired inflation pressure is preselected, and a decelerating inspiratory flow rate provides high flows at the onset of the lung inflation, to attain the desired inflation pressure quickly. The inspiratory time is adjusted to allow enough time for the inspiratory flow rate to fall to zero at the end of inspiration. Since there is no airflow at the end of the inspiration, the end-inspiratory airway pressure is equivalent to the peak alveolar pressure (see Figure 26.1).

Advantages

ALVEOLAR PRESSURE: The major benefit of PCV is the ability to control the peak alveolar pressure, which is the pressure most closely related to the risk of alveolar overdistension and ventilator-induced lung injury. Clinical studies indicate that *the risk of ventilator-induced lung injury is negligible if the peak alveolar pressure is ≤ 30 cm H_2O* (2,4). (*Note:* Maintaining a peak alveolar pressure ≤ 30 cm H_2O is also possible during VCV by monitoring the end-inspiratory occlusion pressure or "plateau pressure," which is described on pages 489–490.)

PATIENT COMFORT: PCV is more likely to promote patient comfort than VCV (6), and this has been attributed to the high initial flow rates and the longer duration of inspiration with PCV.

Disadvantages

ALVEOLAR VOLUME: The major disadvantage of PCV is the decrease in alveolar volume that occurs when there is an increase in airway resistance or a decrease in lung compliance. This is a particular concern in acute respiratory failure, where steady-state conditions of airway resistance and lung compliance are unlikely.

Pressure-Regulated, Volume Control

Pressure-regulated, volume control ventilation (PRVC) is a hybrid mode of ventilation that provides a constant tidal volume (like volume control) but limits the end-inspiratory airway pressures (like pressure control). PRVC operates like an intelligent form of volume control; i.e., the ventilator monitors lung compliance, and uses these measurements to select the lowest airway pressure needed to deliver the desired tidal volume. Hybrid modes like PRVC are gaining in popularity, although there is no documented clinical advantage with PRVC when compared to more conventional modes of ventilation.

ASSIST-CONTROL VENTILATION

Assist-control ventilation (ACV) allows the patient to initiate a ventilator breath (assisted or patient-triggered ventilation), but if this is not possible, ventilator breaths are delivered at a preselected rate (controlled or time-triggered ventilation). The ventilator breaths during ACV can be volume-controlled or pressure-controlled.

Triggers

ACV involves two types of ventilator breaths, which are illustrated in the upper panel of Figure 26.2. The pressure waveform on the left is preceded by a negative pressure deflection, which represents a spontaneous inspiratory effort by the patient. This is a *patient-triggered* ventilator breath. The pressure waveform on the right is not preceded by a negative pressure deflection, indicating the absence of a spontaneous inspiratory effort. In this case, there is no interaction between the patient and the ventilator, and the ventilator breaths are delivered at a preselected rate. This is a *time-triggered* ventilator breath.

Patient-Related Triggers

There are two types of signals used for patient-triggered breaths: negative pressure and inspiratory flow rate.

NEGATIVE PRESSURE: Patients can trigger a ventilator breath by generating a negative airway pressure of 2 to 3 cm H_2O, which opens a pressure-sensitive valve in the ventilator. This is double the negative airway pressure generated during quiet breathing (7), which may explain why one-third of inspiratory efforts fail to trigger a ventilator breath when negative pressure is the trigger signal (8).

FLOW RATE: Flow triggering involves little or no change in pressure and volume, and thus involves less mechanical work than pressure triggering (9). For this reason, flow has replaced pressure as the standard trigger mechanism. The flow rate that is required to trigger a ventilator breath differs for each brand of ventilator, but rates of 1–10L/min are usually required. Auto-triggering from system leaks (which create flow changes)

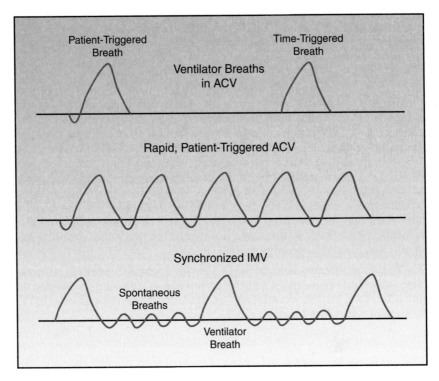

FIGURE 26.2 Airway pressure patterns in assist-control ventilation (ACV) and synchronized intermittent mandatory ventilation (SIMV). See text for further explanation.

is the major problem associated with flow triggering.

The Respiratory Cycle

A general rule of thumb during mechanical ventilation is to allow at least twice the amount of time for expiration as allowed for inspiration. This is equivalent to an inspiration:expiration time ratio (I:E ratio) of at least 1:2. The goal is to allow enough time for complete exhalation to prevent dynamic hyperinflation and intrinsic or occult PEEP (see page 491). If the duration of exhalation is too short, the I:E ratio can be increased by: (a) increasing the inspiratory flow rate, (b) reducing the tidal volume, or (c) decreasing the inspiratory time (for pressure control).

Rapid Breathing

When each breath is a patient-triggered ventilator breath, rapid breathing like that shown in Figure 26.2 can severely curtail the time for exhalation and increase the risk of incomplete alveolar emptying and intrinsic PEEP. When rapid breathing is the result of a condition other than discomfort or anxiety, attempts to reduce the respiratory rate with sedation or inspiratory flow adjustments are often unsuccessful. In this situation, the appropriate mode of ventilation is described next.

INTERMITTENT MANDATORY VENTILATION

The Method

Difficulties with rapid breathing during ACV in neonates with respiratory distress syndrome, who typically have respiratory rates above 40 breaths/minute, led to the introduction of *intermittent mandatory ventilation* (IMV). IMV is designed to allow spontaneous breathing between ventilator breaths. (Spontaneous breathing is the condition where the patient initiates and terminates each lung inflation.) This is accomplished by placing a spontaneous breathing circuit in parallel with the ventilator circuit with a unidirectional valve that opens the spontaneous breathing circuit when a ventilator breath is not being delivered. The ventilatory pattern for IMV is illustrated in the lower panel of Figure 26.2. Note that the ventilator breath is delivered in synchrony with the spontaneous breath; this is called *synchronized IMV* (SIMV).

The ventilator breaths during SIMV can be volume-controlled or pressure-controlled. The rate of ventilator breaths is adjusted as needed to match the total minute ventilation (spontaneous plus assisted breaths) to the patient's baseline level.

Adverse Effects

The principal adverse effects of IMV are: (a) an increased work of breathing, and (b) a decrease in cardiac output, primarily in patients with left ventricular dysfunction. Both effects are the result of the spontaneous breathing period.

Work of Breathing

The heightened work of breathing during the spontaneous breathing period in IMV is attributed to resistance in the ventilator circuit, which can have an exaggerated effect on ventilatory work when breathing is rapid (the condition that usually prompts the use of IMV). Pressure-support ventilation (described in the next section) overcomes the added resistance of the ventilator circuit, and thereby reduces the work of breathing (10). As a result, pressure-support ventilation (at 10 cm H_2O) is now used routinely during the spontaneous breathing periods in IMV.

Cardiac Output

As described at the end of the last chapter, positive pressure ventilation reduces left ventricular afterload and increases cardiac output, primarily in patients with left ventricular dysfunction (see Figure 25.7 on page 501) (11). IMV has the opposite effect and increases left ventricular afterload (during the spontaneous breathing periods), which results in *a decrease in cardiac output in patients with left ventricular dysfunction* (12).

Summary

The major indication for IMV is rapid breathing with incomplete exhalation during assist-control ventilation. The spontaneous breathing periods during IMV promote alveolar emptying and reduce the risk of air trapping and intrinsic PEEP. IMV can increase the work of breathing and impair cardiac output in patients with left ventricular dysfunction; as a result, *IMV is not advised for patients with respiratory muscle weakness or left heart failure.*

PRESSURE SUPPORT VENTILATION

Pressure support ventilation (PSV) is pressure-augmented spontaneous breathing (13). It differs from patient-triggered PCV because it allows the patient to terminate the lung inflation, whereas the ventilator terminates the lung inflation during patient-triggered PCV. Therefore, *PSV is a more interactive form of ventilation than PCV because it allows the patient to control the inspiratory time and tidal volume.*

The Pressure-Supported Breath

The changes in pressure, and flow during a lung inflation with PSV are shown in Figure 26.3. PSV uses a decelerating inspiratory flow rate, with high flow rates early in inspiration to achieve the desired pressure level. The pressure-augmented breath is terminated when the inspiratory flow rate falls to 25% of the peak level. This allows the patient to determine the duration of lung inflation and the tidal volume.

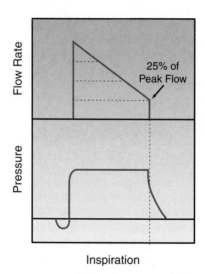

FIGURE 26.3 Changes in pressure and flow during a single lung inflation with pressure support ventilation. The lung inflation is terminated when the inspiratory flow rate falls to 25% of the peak flow rate, which allows the patient to determine the inspiratory time and tidal volume.

Clinical Uses

Low levels of PSV (5–10 cm H_2O) can be used during weaning from mechanical ventilation, to overcome the resistance to flow in the artificial airways and ventilator tubing. The goal of PSV in this setting is to reduce the work of breathing without augmenting the tidal volume (14). Higher levels of PSV (15–30 cm H_2O) can be used to augment the tidal volume; in this case, PSV is used as a form of noninvasive ventilation (which is described in the next chapter) (15).

POSITIVE END-EXPIRATORY PRESSURE

Rationale

Progressive narrowing of the airways during expiration can culminate in collapse of distal airspaces (small airways and alveoli) at the end of expiration. This normally occurs in dependent lung regions, where transpulmonary pressures are more positive (gravitational effect). The transpulmonary pressure where the distal airspaces begin to collapse, is called the *closing pressure*, and is normally about 3 cm H_2O (16). The closing pressure is higher in the presence of small airway obstruction (e.g., in COPD) and reduced lung compliance (e.g., in ARDS), and this results in more extensive airspace collapse at end-expiration. This has two adverse consequences: (a) impaired gas exchange from atelectasis, and (b) *atelectrauma* from repetetive closing and opening of the distal airspaces (17,18).

The risk of alveolar collapse at end-expiration can be eliminated by preventing the airway pressure from falling below the closing pressure at the end of expiration. This is achieved by creating a positive pressure in the airways at the end of expiration that is equivalent to the closing pressure. This *positive end-expiratory pressure* (PEEP) is created by a pressure-relief valve in the expiratory limb of the ventilator circuit that allows exhalation to proceed until the pressure falls to the preselected level, and this pressure is then maintained for the duration of expiration. Since it is not possible to identify the closing pressure in the clinical setting, a PEEP level of 5–7 cm H_2O is used to prevent alveolar collapse in all patients.

Inflation Pressures

The influence of PEEP on inflation pressures is illustrated in Figure 26.4. Note that the addition of PEEP moves the inflation pressure waveform upward, and results in a higher peak alveolar pressure and a higher mean airway pressure. The following statements are relevant in this regard.

1. The effects of PEEP are not related to the PEEP level, but are determined by the influence of PEEP on the peak alveolar pressure and the mean airway pressure.

2. The change in peak alveolar pressure determines the influence of PEEP on alveolar ventilation (and hence arterial oxygenation), and

also determines the risk of alveolar overdistension and *volutrauma (see page 494)*.

3. The change in mean airway pressure determines the influence of PEEP on cardiac output.

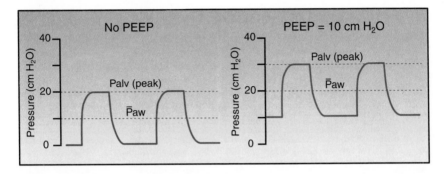

FIGURE 26.4 Airway pressure waveforms during pressure control ventilation showing the effects of positive end-expiratory pressure (PEEP) on the peak alveolar pressure (Palv) and the mean airway pressure (P̄aw).

Alveolar Recruitment

While low levels of PEEP (5–10 cm H_2O) help to prevent the collapse of distal airspaces, high levels of PEEP (20–30 cm H_2O) help to reopen distal airspaces that are persistently collapsed. This effect is demonstrated in Figure 26.5 (19). The thoracic CT image on the left shows consolidation in the posterior (dependent) regions of both lungs, and this disappears after the addition of PEEP (at 19 cm H_2O). This effect is known as *alveolar recruitment*, and it increases the available surface area in the lungs for gas exchange (19,20).

Recruitable Lung Volume

The addition of PEEP may not result in alveolar recruitment, but instead can overdistend alveoli in normal lung regions, which increases the risk of ventilator-induced lung injury. The volume of "recruitable lung" (i.e., areas of atelectasis that can be aerated) determines if PEEP will promote alveolar recruitment or alveolar overdistension; i.e., if there is a significant volume of recruitable lung, then PEEP will promote alveolar recruitment and improve pulmonary gas exchange, but if there is a negligible volume of recruitable lung, then PEEP will promote alveolar overdistension and increase the risk of ventilator-induced lung injury.

The volume of recruitable lung varies widely in individual patients (from 2% to 25% of total lung volume) (20). Although it is not possible to measure recruitable lung volume reliably, the following measures can be used to determine if PEEP is promoting alveolar recruitment (favorable response) or promoting alveolar overdistension (unfavorable response).

LUNG COMPLIANCE: When PEEP is promoting alveolar recruitment, the compliance (distensibility) of the lungs will increase, but when PEEP is overdistending alveoli in normal lung regions, lung compliance will decrease. The measurement of lung compliance during mechanical ventilation is described in Chapter 25 (see pages 492–493).

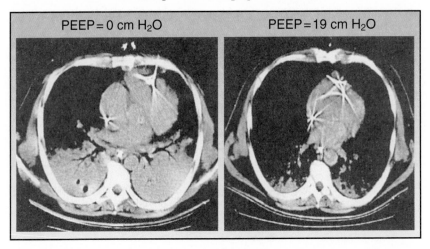

FIGURE 26.5 Thoracic CT images from a patient with ARDS showing the influence of PEEP on lung aeration (alveolar recruitment). Images from Reference 19.

PAO$_2$/FIO$_2$ RATIO: The relationship between the arterial PO$_2$ and the fractional concentration of inspired oxygen, as expressed by the PaO$_2$/FIO$_2$ ratio, is a measure of the efficiency of gas exchange in the lungs. When PEEP promotes alveolar recruitment, the PaO$_2$/FIO$_2$ ratio will increase, and when PEEP does not promote alveolar recruitment, the PaO$_2$/FIO$_2$ ratio will remain unchanged or will decrease. An example of a beneficial response in the PaO$_2$/FIO$_2$ ratio (indicating alveolar recruitment) is shown in Figure 26.6.

Systemic O$_2$ Transport

The beneficial effects of PEEP on arterial oxygenation may not be accompanied by a similar benefit in systemic oxygen transport, as described next.

Cardiac Output

The influence of positive pressure ventilation on cardiac performance is described at the end of Chapter 25 (see pages 499–501). PEEP magnifies these effects, particularly the tendency for positive pressure ventilation to decrease cardiac output. There are several mechanisms whereby PEEP can decrease cardiac output, including (a) impaired venous return, (b) decreased ventricular compliance, (c) increased right ventricular afterload, and (d) external constraint of the ventricles (21,22). These effects are more prominent in the presence of hypovolemia.

Oxygen Delivery

PEEP-induced decreases in cardiac output can erase the beneficial effects of PEEP on alveolar recruitment. This is illustrated by the following equation for systemic oxygen delivery (DO_2). (See page 178 for the derivation of this equation.)

$$DO_2 = CO \times (1.34 \times [Hb] \times SaO_2) \times 10 \ (mL/min) \tag{26.1}$$

Thus, PEEP can promote alveolar recruitment and increase arterial oxygenation (SaO_2), but systemic O_2 delivery may not improve if PEEP also decreases the cardiac output (CO). The opposing effects of PEEP on arterial oxygenation and cardiac output are demonstrated in Figure 26.6 (23).

BEST PEEP: The optimal benefit from PEEP occurs when an increase in arterial oxygenation is accompanied by an increase in systemic O_2 delivery. Therefore, the optimal or *best PEEP* for an individual patient is the level of PEEP that results in the greatest increase in systemic O_2 delivery (24). Best PEEP can be determined by measuring the systemic O_2 delivery at increasing levels of PEEP. Unfortunately, the decline in popularity of the

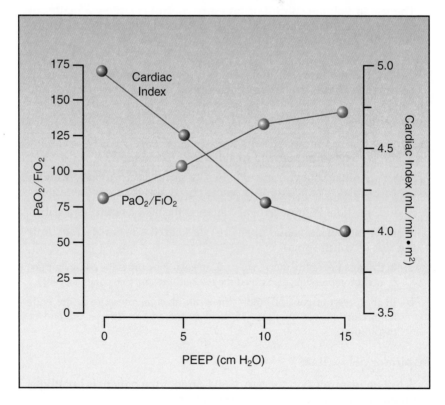

FIGURE 26.6 The opposing effects of positive end-expiratory pressure (*PEEP*) on arterial oxygenation (PaO_2/FiO_2) and cardiac index in patients with ARDS. Data from Reference 23.

pulmonary artery catheter (which provides the most reliable measurements of cardiac output) has also decreased the popularity of best PEEP determinations.

VENTILATOR SETTINGS

When mechanical ventilation is initiated, the respiratory therapist will ask you for the following parameters: (a) mode of ventilation, (b) tidal volume, (c) respiratory rate, (d) PEEP level, and (e) inspired O_2 concentration. The following is a list of suggestions for setting up mechanical ventilation.

Assist-Control Ventilation

1. Select assist-control as the initial mode of ventilation.
2. It may be necessary to switch to synchronized IMV in patients who are breathing too rapidly in the assist-control mode (see later).

Volume vs. Pressure Control

1. The use of volume control or pressure control is largely a matter of personal preference, although some patients breathe more comfortably with pressure control.
2. A suitable compromise is the pressure-regulated volume control mode of ventilation (PRVC), which allows for control of the tidal volume, but limits the airway pressures.

Tidal Volume

The following recommendations are from the *lung protective ventilation* protocol, which is summarized in Table 25.1 (see page 498).

1. Select an initial tidal volume of 8 mL/kg using *predicted* body weight. (The formulas for calculating predicted body weight are in Table 25.1.)
2. Reduce the tidal volume to 6 mL/kg over the next 2 hours, if possible.
3. Monitor the peak alveolar pressure and keep it ≤30 cm H_2O (to limit the risk of volutrauma).
   a. In the volume control mode, the peak alveolar pressure is the end-inspiratory occlusion pressure, also called the *plateau pressure* (see pages 489–491).
   b. In the pressure control mode, the peak alveolar pressure is the end-inspiratory airway pressure (as long as there is no flow at the end of inspiration).

Inspiratory Flow Rate

1. Select an inspiratory flow rate of 60 L/min if the patient is breathing quietly or has no spontaneous respirations.
2. Use higher inspiratory flow rates (e.g., ≥ 80 L/min) for patients with respiratory distress or a high minute ventilation (≥ 10 L/min).

I:E Ratio

1. The I:E ratio should be $\geq 1:2$.
2. If the I:E ratio is $< 1:2$, the options for increasing the I:E ratio include: (a) increasing the inspiratory flow rate, (b) decreasing the tidal volume, or (c) decreasing the respiratory rate, if possible.

Respiratory Rate

1. If the patient has no spontaneous respirations, set the respiratory rate to achieve your estimate of the patient's minute ventilation just prior to intubation, but do not exceed 35 breaths/minute.
2. If the patient is triggering each ventilator breath, set the machine rate just below the patient's spontaneous respiratory rate.
3. After 30 minutes, check the arterial PCO_2, and adjust the respiratory rate, if necessary, to achieve the desired PCO_2.
4. For patients who are breathing rapidly and have an acute respiratory alkalosis or evidence of occult PEEP, consider switching to synchronized IMV (SIMV) as the mode of ventilation.

PEEP

1. Set the initial PEEP to 5 cm H_2O to prevent the collapse of distal airspaces at end-expiration.
2. Further increases in PEEP may be required if either of the following conditions is present: (a) a toxic level of inhaled oxygen ($> 60\%$) is required to maintain adequate oxygenation ($SaO_2 \geq 90\%$), or (b) hypoxemia is refractory to oxygen therapy.

Occult PEEP

1. Check the flow rate at the end of expiration to detect the presence of intrinsic or occult PEEP (see Figure 24.5 on page 479).
2. If the expiratory flow rate has not returned to the zero at end-expiration (indicating the presence of occult PEEP), attempt to prolong the time for expiration by increasing the I:E ratio using the maneuvers described previously.
3. If increasing the I:E ratio is not possible or is not successful, then measure the level of occult PEEP with the end-inspiratory occlusion method, and add extrinsic PEEP at a level that is just below the occult PEEP. (The rationale for this maneuver is explained in Chapter 28.)

A FINAL WORD

Loss of Focus

Considering that the human capacity to store and process information is limited to 4 variables (25), the 174 documented modes of ventilatory assistance mentioned in the introduction represents an incomprehensible load of information. What seems to be lost in this maze of technology is the simple fact that mechanical ventilation is a temporary support measure for acute respiratory failure, and is not a treatment modality for lung disease. Therefore, if we want to improve outcomes in ventilator-dependent patients, less attention should be given to the knobs on ventilators, and more attention should be directed at the diseases that create ventilator dependency.

REFERENCES

Introduction

1. Cairo JM, Pilbean SP. Mosby's Respiratory Care Equipment. 8th ed. St. Louis: Mosby Elsevier; 2010.

2. The Acute Respiratory Distress Syndrome Network. Ventilation with lower tidal volumes as compared with traditional tidal volumes for acute lung injury and the acute respiratory distress syndrome. N Engl J Med 2000; 342(18):1301–1308.

3. Mireles-Cabodevila E, Hatipoglu U, Chatburn RL. A rational framework for selecting modes of ventilation. Respir Care 2013; 58:348–366.

The Ventilator Breath

4. Petrucci N, Iacovelli W. Ventilation with lower tidal volumes versus traditional tidal volumes for acute lung injury and acute respiratory distress syndrome. Cochrane Database Syst Rev 2004; (2):CD003844.

5. Yang SC, Yang SP. Effects of inspiratory flow waveforms on lung mechanics, gas exchange, and respiratory metabolism in COPD patients during mechanical ventilation. Chest 2002; 122:2096–2104.

6. Kallet RH, Campbell AR, Alonzo JA, et al. The effects of pressure control versus volume control on patient work of breathing in acute lung injury and acute respiratory distress syndrome. Respir Care 2000; 45:1085–1096.

Assist-Control Ventilation

7. Hess DR, Kacmarek RM. Physiologic effects of mechanical ventilation. In: Essentials of Mechanical Ventilation. New York, McGraw-Hill, 1996:1–10.

8. Leung P, Jubran A, Tobin MJ. Comparison of assisted ventilator modes on triggering, patients' effort, and dyspnea. Am J Respir Crit Care Med 1997; 155:1940–1948.

9. Laureen H, Pearl R. Flow triggering, pressure triggering, and autotriggering during mechanical ventilation. Crit Care Med 2000; 28:579–581.

Intermittent Mandatory Ventilation

10. Shelledy DC, Rau JL, Thomas-Goodfellow L. A comparison of the effects of assist-control, SIMV, and SIMV with pressure-support on ventilation, oxygen consumption, and ventilatory equivalent. Heart Lung 1995; 24:67–75.

11. Singh I, Pinsky MR. Heart-lung interactions. In Papadakos PJ, Lachmann B, eds. Mechanical ventilation: clinical applications and pathophysiology. Philadelphia: Saunders Elsevier, 2008:173–184.

12. Mathru M et al. Hemodynamic responses to changes in ventilatory patterns in patients with normal and poor left ventricular reserve. Crit Care Med 1982; 10:423–426.

Pressure-Support Ventilation

13. Hess DR. Ventilator waveforms and the physiology of pressure support ventilation. Respir Care 2005; 50:166–186.

14. Jubran A, Grant BJ, Duffner LA, et al. Effect of pressure support vs. unassisted breathing through a tracheostomy collar on weaning duration in patients requiring prolonged mechanical ventilation: a randomized trial. JAMA 2013; 309:671–677.

15. Caples SM, Gay PC. Noninvasive positive pressure ventilation in the intensive care unit: a concise review Crit Care Med 2005; 33:2651–2658.

Positive End-Expiratory Pressure

16. Hedenstierna G, Bindslev L, Santesson J. Pressure-volume and airway closure relationships in each lung of anesthetized man. Clin Physiol 1981; 1:479–493.

17. Muscedere JG, Mullen JBM, Gan K, Slutsky AS. Tidal ventilation at low airway pressures can augment lung injury. Am J Respir Crit Care Med 1994; 149:1327–1334.

18. Gattinoni L, Protti A, Caironi P, Carlesso E. Ventilator-induced lung injury: the anatomical and physiological framework. Crit Care Med 2010; 38(Suppl):S539–S548.

19. Barbas CSV. Lung recruitment maneuvers in acute respiratory distress syndrome and facilitating resolution. Crit care Med 2003; 31(Suppl):S265–S271.

20. Gattinoni L, Cairon M, Cressoni M, et al. Lung recruitment in patients with the acute respiratory distress syndrome. N Engl J Med 2006; 354:1775–1786.

21. Schmitt J-M, Viellard-Baron A, Augarde R, et al. Positive end-expiratory pressure titration in acute respiratory distress syndrome patients: Impact on right ventricular outflow impedance evaluated by pulmonary artery Doppler flow velocity measurements. Crit Care Med 2001; 29:1154–1158.

22. Takata M, Robotham JL. Ventricular external constraint by the lung and pericardium during positive end-expiratory pressure. Am Rev Respir Dis 1991; 43:872–875.

23. Gainnier M, Michelet P, Thirion X, et al. Prone position and positive end-expiratory pressure in acute respiratory distress syndrome. Crit Care Med 2003; 31:2719–2726.

24. Punt CD, Schreuder JJ, Jansen JR, et al. Tracing best PEEP by applying PEEP as a RAMP. Intensive Care Med 1998; 24:821–828.

A Final Word

25. Cowan N. The magical number 4 in short-term memory: a reconsideration of mental storage capacity. Behav Brain Sci 2001; 24:87–114.

Chapter 27

ALTERNATE MODES OF VENTILATION

The reasonable man adapts himself to the world; the unreasonable one persists in trying to adapt the world to himself. Therefore, all progress depends on the unreasonable man.

George Bernard Shaw
1903

The conventional modes of ventilation described in the last chapter are appropriate for most patients with acute respiratory failure. However, there are occasions when conventional mechanical ventilation is either unable to support gas exchange in the lungs, or is not necessary as a means of ventilatory support. This chapter describes alternate modes of ventilation that are available when conventional mechanical ventilation is either not sufficient, or not necessary, for patients with acute respiratory failure. Included are *rescue modes of ventilation* (i.e., high frequency oscillatory ventilation and airway pressure release ventilation) and *noninvasive modes of ventilation* (i.e., continuous positive airway pressure, bilevel positive airway pressure, and pressure support ventilation).

RESCUE MODES OF VENTILATION

A small percentage (10–15%) of patients with acute respiratory distress syndrome (ARDS) develop hypoxemia that is refractory to oxygen therapy and conventional mechanical ventilation (1). In this situation, the appropriate strategy for ventilatory support is defined by the concept described next.

Open Lung Concept

Alveolar collapse (atelectasis) in ARDS not only impairs alveolar ventilation, it also promotes ventilator-induced lung injury. There are two mechanisms for the lung injury produced by atelectasis. First, if the alveolar collapse is extensive, like that shown in Figure 23.4 (on page 454), the tidal volumes delivered by the ventilator will distribute in the uninvolved (normal) areas of the lungs, and this will overdistend normal alveoli and promote *volutrauma*. Secondly, if alveolar collapse occurs only at end-expiration, repetitive opening and closing of alveoli promotes *atelectrauma* by creating excessive shear forces that damage the airway epithelium. (See pages 494–497 for more information on ventilator-induced lung injury.)

The adverse consequences of alveolar collapse can be mitigated by a mode of ventilation that both prevents alveolar collapse and opens collapsed alveoli. This is the *open lung concept* of mechanical ventilation, where the goal is to: "open up the lung and keep the lung open" (2). The modes of ventilation described next are designed to achieve this goal.

High Frequency Oscillations

High frequency oscillatory ventilation (HFOV) uses high-frequency, low volume oscillations like the ones shown in Figure 27.1. These oscillations create a high mean airway pressure, which improves gas exchange in the lungs by opening collapsed alveoli (alveolar recruitment) and preventing further alveolar collapse. The small tidal volumes (typically 1–2 mL) limit the risk of alveolar overdistension and volutrauma. For optimal results, an alveolar recruitment maneuver (e.g., with high PEEP levels, as shown in Figure 26.5, page 514) is recommended just prior to switching from conventional mechanical ventilation (CMV) to HFOV (3).

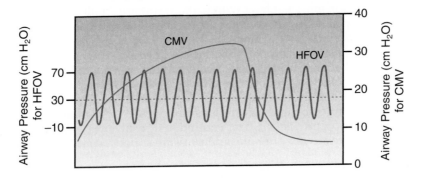

FIGURE 27.1 Airway pressure oscillations during high frequency oscillatory ventilation (HFOV), with a superimposed lung inflation during conventional mechanical ventilation (CMV). Dotted line represents mean airway pressure. From Reference 3.

Ventilator Settings

HFOV requires a specialized ventilator (Sensormedics 3100B, Viasys Healthcare, Yorba Linda, CA) that allows the following adjustments: (a) the frequency and amplitude of the oscillations, (b) the mean airway pressure, (c) the bias flow rate (similar to an inspiratory flow rate), and (d) the inspiratory time (time of the bias flow). Some recommendations for these settings are listed in Table 27.1.

OSCILLATIONS: The frequency range for the oscillations is 4–7 Hz (1 Hz is one oscillation per second or 60 oscillations/min, so a range of 4–7 Hz is 240–420 oscillations/min), and the specific frequency selected is determined by the arterial pH (which represents the CO_2 burden). The pulse amplitude (tidal volume) determines CO_2 removal, and pulse amplitude is inversely related to the frequency of oscillations; i.e., lower oscillation frequencies result in higher tidal volumes and more effective CO_2 removal. The initial pulse amplitude is set at 70–90 cm H_2O.

MEAN AIRWAY PRESSURE: The end-inspiratory alveolar pressure (e.g., the plateau pressure during volume control ventilation) should be measured just prior to switching from CMV to HFOV. This pressure is a reflection of: (a) alveolar volume, and (b) the risk of alveolar overdistension and volutrauma (see Chapter 25). The mean airway pressure is usually set 5 cm H_2O higher than the end-inspiratory alveolar pressure recorded during CMV (3), but should not exceed 30 cm H_2O (to prevent volutrauma).

Table 27.1	Suggested Initial Settings for HPOV and APRV
HPOV	**APRV**

Frequency:
    4 Hz: (pH <7.1)
    5–6 Hz: (pH 7.1–7.35)
    7 Hz: (pH >7.35)
Amplitude: 70–90 cm H_2O
Mean Paw: 5 cm H_2O >$P_{plateau}$
    on CMV to max of
    30 cm H_2O
Bias Flow: 40 L/min
Inspiratory Time: 33%
FiO_2: 100%
	Pressure:
	    High: Same as $P_{plateau}$ on CMV,
	        to max of 30 cm H_2O
	    Low: Atmospheric (zero) pressure
	Time:
	    High Pressure: 4–6 sec
	    Low Pressure: 0.6–0.8 sec
	FiO_2: 100%

From Reference 3. HFOV=high frequency oscilatory ventilation; APRV=airway pressure release ventilation; CMV=conventional mechanical ventilation; Paw=airway pressure; $P_{plateau}$=plateau pressure.

Advantages

Clinical trials comparing HFOV with CMV, primarily conducted in patients with ARDS, have shown a 16–24% increase in the PaO_2/FiO_2 ratio associated with HFOV (4). Early studies of HFOV showed no impact on mortality rate (3), but a very recent meta-analysis of all available studies shows a significant survival benefit with HFOV (4). However, HFOV has not been compared with lung protective ventilation (which also shows a survival benefit) so *it is not known if HFOV represents an advance over lung protective ventilation in patients with ARDS.*

Disadvantages

The disadvantages of HFOV are listed below (3,4):

1. A special ventilator is needed, along with trained personnel to operate the device.

2. Cardiac output is often decreased during HFOV because of the high mean airway pressures. This effect requires augmentation of the intravascular volume during HFOV.

3. Aerosolized bronchodilators are ineffective during HFOV.

Airway Pressure Release Ventilation

Airway pressure release ventilation (APRV) employs prolonged periods of spontaneous breathing at high end-expiratory pressures, which are interrupted by brief periods of pressure release to atmospheric pressure. APRV *is a variant of continuous positive airway pressure* (CPAP), which is spontaneous breathing at a positive end-expiratory pressure. The similarities between APRV and CPAP are demonstrated in Figure 27.2. The upper panel in this figure shows an airway pressure profile for CPAP; in this case, the changes in inspiratory and expiratory pressures during spontaneous breathing revolve around an end-expiratory pressure of 5 cm H_2O. The airway pressure profile for APRV (in the middle panel) shows CPAP at a much higher end-expiratory pressure (30 cm H_2O), with a brief period where the airway pressure is allowed to decrease to zero (pressure release). The high CPAP level in APRV improves arterial oxygenation by opening collapsed alveoli (alveolar recruitment) and preventing further alveolar collapse (similar to the effects of the high mean airway pressure in HFOV). The pressure release phase is designed to facilitate CO_2 removal (5).

Ventilator Settings

APRV is available in many of the modern critical care ventilators, and the variables that must be selected when initiating APRV include the high and low airway pressures, and the time spent at each pressure level. Some suggestions for the initial settings are listed in Table 27.1.

HIGH AIRWAY PRESSURE: As mentioned for HFOV, the end-inspiratory alveolar pressure (e.g., the plateau pressure during volume control ventilation) should be measured just prior to switching from CMV to APRV. (This pressure is a reflection of alveolar volume, and the risk of alveolar overdistension and volutrauma, as mentioned for HFOV). The high airway pressure should equal the end-inspiratory alveolar (plateau) pressure, but should not exceed 30 cm H_2O (to limit the risk of volutrauma).

LOW AIRWAY PRESSURE: The low pressure level is set to zero (atmospheric pressure), to maximize the driving pressure for rapid pressure release. However, the pressure never reaches the zero level because the pressure release phase is so brief, and the residual positive pressure helps to prevent alveolar collapse.

TIMING: The time spent at the high airway pressure is usually 85–90% of the total cycle time (time at high pressure plus time at low pressure). Recommended times are 4 to 6 seconds for the high pressure level and 0.6 to 0.8 seconds for the low pressure level.

Advantages

APRV can achieve nearly complete recruitment of collapsed alveoli by maintaining high airway pressures for prolonged periods of time; this not

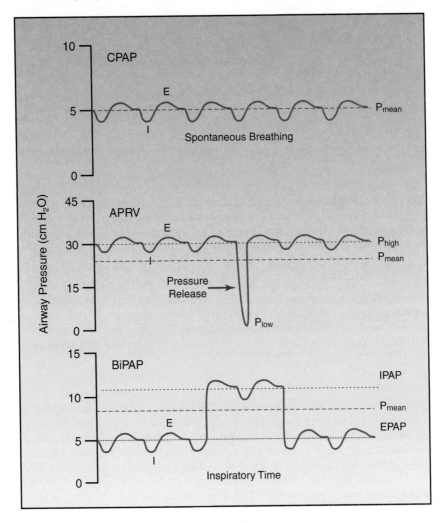

FIGURE 27.2 Related modes of pressure-regulated spontaneous ventilation. CPAP=continuous positive airway pressure, APRV=airway pressure release ventilation, BiPAP=bilevel positive airway pressure, IPAP=inspiratory positive airway pressure, EPAP=expiratory positive airway pressure, P_{mean}=mean airway pressure, I=inspiration, E=expiration. See text for explanation.

only improves arterial oxygenation, it also reduces lung compliance. As a result of the latter effect, peak airway pressures are lower during APRV than during CMV (at equivalent tidal volumes) (3). The improvement in arterial oxygenation with APRV occurs gradually over 24 hours (6).

Disadvantages

The benefits of APRV are lost if the patient has no spontaneous breathing efforts. Additional disadvantages of APRV are listed below.

1. Severe asthma and COPD are relative contraindications to APRV because of the inability to empty the lungs rapidly during the pressure release phase of APRV (3).

2. Cardiac output is often decreased during APRV because of the high mean airway pressures, but this effect is less pronounced than the cardiac depression during HFOV (3).

NONINVASIVE VENTILATION

Noninvasive ventilation (NIV) is intended for patients with acute respiratory failure who will benefit from ventilatory support, but may not need conventional mechanical ventilation (which requires endotracheal intubation). NIV is delivered via tight-fitting face masks, which obviates the need (and the complications) of endotracheal intubation. Although NIV has applications in the outpatient and inpatient setting, the following description is limited to the use of NIV in acute respiratory failure (7,8).

Modes of Ventilation

There are three modes of ventilation available for NIV: (a) continuous positive airway pressure (CPAP), (b) *bilevel positive airway pressure* (BiPAP), and (c) *pressure support ventilation* (PSV). The latter two modes of ventilation (i.e., BiPAP and PSV) are also referred to as *noninvasive positive pressure ventilation* (NPPV).

Continuous Positive Airway Pressure

Continuous positive airway pressure (CPAP) is spontaneous breathing at a positive end-expiratory pressure, as illustrated in the upper panel of Figure 27.2. CPAP is simple in design, and requires only a source of oxygen and a face mask with an expiratory valve that maintains a positive end-expiratory pressure (i.e., a CPAP mask). The principal effect of CPAP is to increase the functional residual capacity (i.e., the volume in the lungs at the end of expiration). CPAP is usually set at $5-10$ cm H_2O.

LIMITATIONS: CPAP is a limited form of ventilatory support because it does not augment the tidal volume, and this limits its use in acute respiratory failure. The principal use of CPAP in acute respiratory failure is for patients with cardiogenic pulmonary edema, and the benefits of CPAP in this condition may be the result of hemodynamic support more than ventilatory support (see later).

Bilevel Positive Airway Pressure

Bilevel positive airway pressure (BiPAP) is CPAP that alternates between two pressure levels. This is illustrated in the lower panel of Figure 27.2. BIPAP is actually a variant of airway pressure release ventilation (APRV), which is shown in the middle panel of Figure 27.2. The only difference between BiPAP and APRV is the amount of time allotted for the high pressure level and the low pressure level; i.e., with APRV, most of the time is spent at the high pressure level, and with BiPAP, most of the time is spent at the low pressure level. The high pressure level in BiPAP is called the *inspiratory positive airway pressure* (IPAP), and the low pressure level is called the *expiratory positive airway pressure* (EPAP).

BiPAP results in higher mean airway pressures than CPAP, and this helps to promote alveolar recruitment. BIPAP does not directly augment tidal volumes, but the effect of BiPAP on alveolar recruitment will increase lung compliance (lung distensibility), and this will result in larger tidal volumes at the same changes in intrathoracic pressure . Therefore, BiPAP can indirectly enhance tidal volumes.

VENTILATOR SETTINGS: BiPAP (which requires a specialized ventilator) can be started with the following initial settings: IPAP = 10 cm H_2O, EPAP = 5 cm H_2O, inspiratory time (the duration of IPAP) = 3 sec. (The IPAP is added on to the EPAP, so an IPAP of 10 cm H_2O with an EPAP of 5 cm H_2O corresponds to a peak pressure of 15 cm H_2O.) Further adjustments in pressure are determined by the resultant changes in gas exchange (i.e., PaO_2/FiO_2 ratio and $PaCO_2$), and signs of respiratory distress (e.g., respiratory rate). Peak pressures above 20 cm H_2O are not usually advised because they are poorly tolerated by patients, and also promote leaks.

Pressure Support Ventilation

Pressure support ventilation (PSV) is described in the last chapter (see pages 511–512). PSV provides patient-triggered inspirations and pressure-augmented tidal volumes. The inspiratory flow rate in PSV has a decelerating flow pattern, and the pressure-augmented tidal volume is terminated when the inspiratory flow rate decreases to 25% of the peak level (see Figure 26.3 on page 511). CPAP is usually combined with PSV to increase the functional residual capacity. The combination of tidal volume augmentation and resting lung volume augmentation makes PSV with CPAP the preferred method of noninvasive ventilation (with a few exceptions, described later).

VENTILATOR SETTINGS: PSV is usually initiated with an inflation pressure of 10 cm H_2O and a CPAP level of 5 cm H_2O. (The inflation pressure is added to the CPAP level, so an inflation pressure of 10 cm H_2O with CPAP of 5 cm H_2O results in a peak pressure of 15 cm H_2O.) As described for BiPAP, further adjustments in pressures are determined by the resultant changes in gas exchange and signs of respiratory distress, but peak pressures above 20 cm H_2O are not usually advised because they are poorly tolerated by patients, and promote leaks.

Patient Selection

Patient selection is the single most important factor in determining the success or failure of NIV (7,8). The patient selection criteria for NIV are presented as a checklist in Table 27.2.

1. The first step is to identify patients who might need ventilatory support. These patients have signs of respiratory distress (e.g., tachypnea, use of accessory muscles of respiration, abdominal paradox) plus either severe hypoxemia ($PaO_2/FIO_2 < 200$) or hypercapnia ($PaCO_2 > 45$ mm Hg).

2. The next step is to identify patients who are candidates for NIV. While some causes of acute respiratory failure are more successfully managed with NIV than others (see later), all patients should be considered candidates for NIV if all of the following conditions are present: (a) the acute respiratory failure is not an immediate threat to life, (b) there is no life-threatening circulatory disorder (e.g., circulatory shock), (c) the patient is awake or arousable and cooperative, (d) airway protective mechanisms are intact (e.g., gag and cough reflexes), (e) there is no hematemesis or recurrent vomiting, (f) there is no facial anomaly that will prevent the use of a tight-fitting face mask (e.g., recent facial trauma), and (g) there is no obstruction that will prevent effective ventilatory support through a face mask (e.g., laryngeal edema).

3. Progression of the respiratory failure can limit the success of NIV (7,8), so there should be no delays in initiating NIV for appropriate candidates.

Table 27.2	Checklist for Noninvasive Ventilation		
A. Does the patient have:		YES	NO
1. Signs of respiratory distress?		☑	☐
2. $PaO_2/FIO_2 < 200$ and/or $PaCO_2 > 45$ mm Hg?		☑	☐
B. If the answer is YES to both, answer the following questions.			
C. Does the patient have:		YES	NO
1. Respiratory failure that is an immediate threat to life?		☐	☑
2. A life-threatening circulatory disorder (e.g., shock)?		☐	☑
3. Coma, severe agitation, or uncontrolled seizures?		☐	☑
4. Inability to protect the aiways?		☐	☑
5. Hematemesis or recurrent vomiting?		☐	☑
6. Laryngeal edema, facial trauma, or recent head and neck surgery?		☐	☑
D. If the answer is NO to all of the above questions, the patient is a candidate for noninvasive ventilation.			

Efficacy

The success of NIV in avoiding endotracheal intubation varies in different clinical disorders, which can be organized according to the major blood gas abnormality associated with the respiratory failure; i.e., hypercapnia or hypoxemia.

Hypercapnic Respiratory Failure

ACUTE EXACERBATION OF COPD: The greatest benefit with NIV in acute respiratory failure is in patients with acute exacerbation of COPD and CO_2 retention (9,10). The benefits of NIV in patients with acute exacerbation of COPD are demonstrated in Figure 27.3 (9). The use of NIV is associated with a marked decline in both the rate of tracheal intubation and the mortality rate. These results are corroborated in 14 clinical studies (10); as a result, *noninvasive ventilation is considered a first-line therapy for acute exacerbations of COPD associated with hypercapnia* (7,8). The preferred mode of ventilation in this condition is PSV with CPAP.

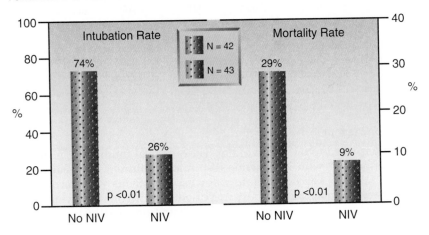

FIGURE 27.3 Impact of noninvasive ventilation (NIV) on rate of intubation and in-hospital mortality rate in patients with hypercapnic respiratory failure secondary to acute exacerbation of COPD. Patients assigned to NIV received pressure support ventilation for at least 6 hrs each day until intubation or recovery. N = number of patients in each study group. Data from Reference 9.

OBESITY HYPOVENTILATION SYNDROME: NIV reduces the severity of hypercapnia in outpatients with obesity hypoventilation syndrome (11) and, despite few studies in ICU patients, NIV is recommended as a routine measure for patients with obesity hypoventilation syndrome who are admitted with acute respiratory failure (12). Either CPAP or BiPAP can be used in this condition.

ASTHMA: NIV has not been adequately evaluated in status asthmaticus, but the available evidence shows that NIV hastens the resolution of the acute illness and decreases the length of stay in both the ICU and the hospital (13).

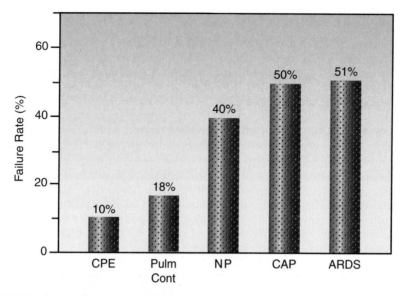

FIGURE 27.4 Failure rate of noninvasive ventilation for preventing endotracheal intubation in relation to the etiology of hypoxemic respiratory failure. CPE = cardiogenic pulmonary edema, Pulm Cont = pulmonary contusion, NP = nosocomial pneumonia, CAP = community-acquired pneumonia, ARDS = acute respiratory distress syndrome. Data from reference 14.

Hypoxemic Respiratory Failure

The failure rate of NIV for avoiding endotracheal intubation in disease states associated with hypoxemic respiratory failure is summarized in Figure 27.4 (14). The failure rate is lowest in patients with cardiogenic pulmonary edema, and highest in patients with community-acquired pneumonia and acute respiratory distress syndrome (ARDS).

CARDIOGENIC PULMONARY EDEMA: NIV is successful in reducing the need for intubation, and reducing the mortality rate, in a large majority of patients with cardiogenic pulmonary edema (15,16). Most of the experience in this condition has been with CPAP (at 10 cm H_2O), but BiPAP produces equivalent results (17). The improved outcomes may be related to improved cardiac performance because NIV can increase cardiac output in patients with systolic heart failure (17). This effect is attributed to the afterload-reducing effects of positive intrathoracic pressure (see page 500).

ARDS: NIV has had limited success in patients with ARDS. The success rate is greater with PSV plus CPAP (17) than with CPAP alone (18), and success is more likely when ARDS has an extrapulmonary source (e.g., septicemia) (14). If NIV is attempted in patients with ARDS, the preferred mode is PSV with CPAP, while CPAP alone should be avoided (8).

Monitoring

The success or failure of NIV in any individual patient should not be predetermined by the etiology of the respiratory failure, but rather by the response of the patient in the first hour after the onset of NIV. This is illustrated in Figure 27.5 for patients with hypercapnic and hypoxemic respiratory failure (14, 19). Failure to improve gas exchange significantly after one hour of NIV is evidence that NIV is failing as a support modality; at this point, the appropriate course of action is immediate endotracheal intubation. Delaying intubation only invites problems (see A FINAL WORD).

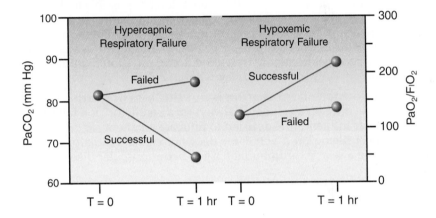

FIGURE 27.5 Responses to the first hour of noninvasive ventilation for predicting success or failure in patients with hypercapnic and hypoxemic respiratory failure. Data from References 14 and 19.

Adverse Events

Adverse events during NIV include gastric distension, pressure ulcers on the bridge of the nose from tight-fitting masks, and nosocomial pneumonia.

Gastric Insufflation

The principal concern during NIV is gastric distension from insufflated gas. However, this does not seem to be a common problem, and studies measuring upper esophageal opening pressures indicate that *pressures less than 30 cm H_2O should not cause gastric insufflation* (20). Although nasogastric tubes are commonly placed for gastric decompression during NIV, withholding nasogastric tubes is a safe practice in patients who do not develop abdominal distension during NIV (21).

Nosocomial Pneumonia

The application of positive pressure to the airways can retard mucociliary clearance and predispose to nosocomial pneumonia during NIV. In studies comparing NIV to endotracheal intubation, the incidence of nosocomial pneumonia during NIV was 8 – 10%, but this was less than half the incidence of nosocomial pneumonia during endotracheal intubation (19–22%) (22,23).

A FINAL WORD

Don't Forget to Intubate

The rising popularity of noninvasive ventilation tends to overshadow the value of endotracheal intubation. The following simple rules about endotracheal intubation deserve mention.

Rule 1: **Hesitation invites trouble.** There is a tendency to rely on noninvasive ventilation and delay intubation as long as possible in the hopes that it will be unnecessary. However, delays in intubation create unnecessary dangers for the patient because emergency intubations in patients who are *in extremis* can be troublesome as well as dangerous. As soon as intubation becomes a serious consideration, you should intubate the patient and get control of the airway without delay.

Rule 2: **Endotracheal intubation is not the 'kiss of death'.** The perception that "once on a ventilator, always on a ventilator" is a fallacy that should never influence the decision to intubate a patient for full ventilatory support. Being on a ventilator does not create ventilator dependence, having a severe cardiopulmonary or neuromuscular disease does.

REFERENCES

Rescue Modes of Ventilation

1. Pipeling MR, Fan E. Therapies for refractory hypoxemia in acute respiratory distress syndrome. JAMA 2010; 304:2521–2527.

2. Lachmann B. Open up the lung and keep the lung open. Intensive Care Med 1992; 18:319–321.

3. Stawicki SP, Goyal M, Sarini B. High-frequency oscillatory ventilation (HFOV) and airway pressure release ventilation (APRV): a practical guide. J Intens Care Med 2009; 24:215–229.

4. Sud S, Sud M, Freiedrich JO, et al. High frequency ventilation versus conventional ventilation for treatment of acute lung injury and acute respiratory distress syndrome. Cochrane Database Syst Rev 2013; Feb 28:CD004085.

5. Kallet RH. Patient-ventilator interaction during acute lung injury, and the role of spontaneous breathing: Part 2: airway pressure release ventilation. Respir Care 2011; 56:190–206.

6. Sydow M, Burchardi H, Ephraim E, et al. Long-term effects of two different ventilatory modes on oxygenation in acute lung injury. Comparison of airway pressure release ventilation and volume-controlled inverse ratio ventilation. Crit Care Med 1994; 149:1550–1556.

Noninvasive Ventilation

7. Hill NS, Brennan J, Garpestad E, Nava S. Noninvasive ventilation in acute respiratory failure. Crit Care Med 2007; 35:2402–2407.

8. Keenan SP, Sinuff T, Burns KEA, et al, as the Canadian Critical Care Trials Group /Canadian Critical Care Society Noninvasive Ventilation Guidelines Group. Clinical practice guidelines for the use of noninvasive positive-pressure ventilation and noninvasive continuous positive airway pressure in the acute care setting. Canad Med Assoc J 2011; 183:E195–E214.

9. Brochard L, Mancero J, Wysocki M, et al. Noninvasive ventilation for acute exacerbations of chronic obstructive pulmonary disease. N Engl J Med 1995; 333:817–822.

10. Ram FSF, Picot J, Lightowler J, Wedzicha JA. Non-invasive positive pressure ventilation for treatment of respiratory failure due to exacerbations of COPD. Cochrane Database Syst Rev 2009; July 8:CD004104.

11. Piper AJ, Wang D, Yee BJ, et al. Randomised trial of CPAP vs. bilevel support in the treatment of obesity hypoventilation syndrome without severe nocturnal desaturation. Thorax 2008; 63:395–401.

12. BaHamman A. Acute ventilatory failure complicating obesity hypoventilation: update on a 'critical care syndrome'. Curr Opin Pulm Med 2011 16:543–551.

13. Gupta D, Nath A, Agarwal R, Behera D. A prospective randomised controlled trial on the efficacy of noninvasive ventilation in severe acute asthma. Respir Care 2010; 55:536–543.

14. Antonelli M, Conti G, Moro ML, et al. Predictors of failure of noninvasive positive pressure ventilation in patients with acute hypoxemic respiratory failure: a multi-center study. Intensive Care Med 2001; 27:1718–1728.

15. Masip J, Roque M, Sanchez B, et al. Noninvasive ventilation in cardiogenic pulmonary edema: systematic review and meta-analysis. JAMA 2005; 294:3124–3130.

16. Vital FM, Saconato H, Ladeira MT, et al. Non-invasive positive pressure ventilation(CPAP or bilevel NPPV) for cardiogenic pulmonary edema. Cochrane Database Syst Rev 2008; July 16:CD005351.

17. Acosta B, DiBenedetto R, Rahimi A, et al. Hemodynamic effects of noninvasive bilevel positive airway pressure on patients with chronic congestive heart failure with systolic dysfunction. Chest 2000; 118:1004–1009.

18. Delclaux C, L'Her E, Alberti C, et al. Treatment of acute hypoxemic nonhypercapnic respiratory insufficiency with continuous positive airway pressure delivered by a face mask. JAMA 2000; 284:2352–2360.

19. Anton A, Guell R, Gomez J, et al. Predicting the result of noninvasive ventilation in severe acute exacerbations of patients with chronic airflow limitation. Chest 2000; 117:828–833.

20. Wenans CS. The pharyngoesophageal closure mechanism: a manometric study. Gastroenterology 1972; 63:769–777.

21. Meduri GU, Fox RC, Abou-shala N, et al. Noninvasive mechanical ventilation via face mask in patients with acute respiratory failure who refused endotracheal intubation. Crit Care Med 1994; 22:1584–1590.

22. Girou E, Schotgen F, Delclaux C, et al. Association of noninvasive ventilation with nosocomial infections and survival in critically ill patients. JAMA 200; 284:2361–2367.

23. Carlucci A, Richard J-C, Wysocki M, et al. Noninvasive versus conventional mechanical ventilation: an epidemiological study. Am J Respir Crit Care Med 2001; 163:874–880.

Chapter 28

THE VENTILATOR-DEPENDENT PATIENT

Eyes and ears are bad witnesses to men if they
have souls that understand not their language.

Heraclitus
6th Century BC

This chapter describes the practices and common concerns involved in the care of ventilator-dependent patients. The focus in this chapter is on artificial airways (endotracheal and tracheostomy tubes) and mechanical complications of positive pressure ventilation (e.g., pneumothorax). The infectious complications of mechanical ventilation (i.e., tracheobronchitis and pneumonia) are described in the next chapter.

ARTIFICIAL AIRWAYS

Positive pressure ventilation is delivered through a variety of plastic tubes that are passed into the trachea through the vocal cords (endotracheal tubes) or are inserted directly into the trachea (tracheostomy tubes). These tubes are equipped with an inflatable balloon at the distal end (called a cuff) that is used to seal the trachea and prevent inflation volumes from escaping out through the larynx.

Endotracheal Tubes

Endotracheal tubes vary in length from 25 to 35 cm, and are sized according to their internal diameter, which varies from 5 to 10 mm (e.g., a "size 7" endotracheal tube will have an internal diameter of 7 mm). For adults, *the diameter of endotracheal tubes should be at least 7 mm, and preferably 8 mm.* Smaller tubes impede the clearance of secretions, and create increased airflow resistance when weaning from the ventilator.

Proper Tube Position

Evaluation of endotracheal tube position is mandatory after intubation.

The portable chest film in Figure 28.1 shows the proper position of an endotracheal tube. When the head is in a neutral position, *the tip of the endotracheal tube should be 3 to 5 cm above the carina, or midway between the carina and vocal cords.* (If not visible, the main carina is usually over the T4-T5 interspace on a portable chest x-ray). The head is in the neutral position when the inferior border of the mandible projects over the lower cervical spine (C5-C6). Flexion or extension of the head and neck causes a 2 cm displacement of the tip of the endotracheal tube (2).

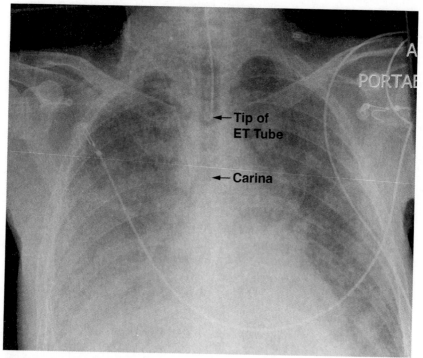

FIGURE 28.1 Portable chest x-ray showing proper position of an endotracheal tube, with the tip located midway between the thoracic inlet and the carina.

Migration of Tubes

Endotracheal tubes can migrate distally, and enter the right mainstem bronchus (which runs a straight course down from the trachea). What can happen next is shown in Figure 28.2; i.e., selective ventilation of one lung results in progressive atelectasis in the non-ventilated lung.

There are two measures that can reduce the incidence of endotracheal tube migration. First, for orotracheal intubations, don't allow the tip of endotracheal tube to advance further than 21 cm from the teeth in women and 23 cm from the teeth in men (3). Second, monitor the position of the endotracheal tube with periodic chest x-rays, and keep the tip of the tube at least 3 cm above the carina.

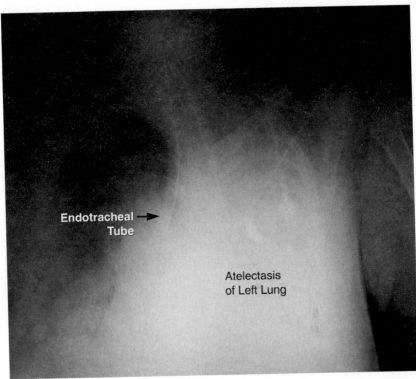

FIGURE 28.2 Portable chest x-ray showing the tip of an endotracheal tube in the right mainstem bronchus. Opacification of the left hemothorax represents atelectasis of the left lung.

Laryngeal Damage

The risk for laryngeal injury with endotracheal tubes is a major concern, and is one of the reasons for performing tracheostomies when prolonged intubation is anticipated. The spectrum of laryngeal damage includes ulceration, granulomas, vocal cord paresis, and laryngeal edema. Some type of laryngeal damage is usually evident after 72 hours of translaryngeal intubation (4), and laryngeal edema is reported in 5% of cases. Fortunately, most cases of laryngeal injury do not result in significant airways obstruction or permanent injury, and the problem resolves within weeks after extubation (5). The problem of laryngeal edema after extubation is described in Chapter 30.

Subglottic Drainage Tubes

The prominent role played by aspiration of mouth secretions in the pathogenesis of ventilator-associated pneumonia has led to the introduction of specially designed endotracheal tubes capable of draining mouth secretions that accumulate just above the inflated cuff. These tubes can reduce the incidence of ventilator-associated pneumonia (6), and they are described in more detail in the next chapter.

Tracheostomy

Tracheostomy is preferred in patients who require prolonged mechanical ventilation (> 2 weeks). There are several advantages with a tracheostomy, including greater patient comfort, easier access to the airways, and reduced risk of laryngeal injury.

Tracheostomy Timing

The optimal time for performing a tracheostomy has been debated for years. Recent studies comparing early tracheostomy (one week after intubation) with late tracheostomy (two weeks after intubation) have shown the following:

1. Early tracheostomy does not reduce the incidence of ventilator-associated pneumonia, and does not reduce the mortality rate (7,8).
2. Early tracheostomy does reduce sedative requirements and promote early mobilization (8).

Based on the pneumonia and mortality data, tracheostomy is recommended after 2 weeks of endotracheal intubation (9). If one considers patient comfort, it is not unreasonable to *consider tracheostomy after 7–10 days of intubation, if there is little chance of extubation in the following week.*

Techniques

The traditional method of performing a tracheotomy as an open surgical procedure has been replaced in popularity by *percutaneous dilatational tracheostomy*, where a guidewire is passed through a small needle puncture in the anterior wall of the trachea, and is used to advance a tracheostomy tube into the tracheal lumen (10). (This is analogous to the Seldinger technique for inserting central venous catheters, shown in Figure 1.5 on page 11.) This technique is performed at the bedside, and is associated with less blood loss and fewer local infections than surgically created tracheostomies (9,11).

The technique known as *cricothyroidotomy* is used only for emergency access to the airway. The trachea is entered through the cricothyroid membrane, just below the larynx, and there is high incidence of laryngeal injury and subglottic stenosis. Patients who survive following a cricothyroidotomy should have a regular tracheostomy (surgical or percutaneous) as soon as they are stable (12).

Complications

The morbidity and mortality associated with tracheostomy has declined in recent years. Combining surgical and percutaneous tracheostomy, the mortality rate is less than 1%, and immediate complications (i.e., bleeding and infection) occur in less than 5% of cases (11,12).

ACCIDENTAL DECANNULATION: One acute complication that deserves mention is accidental decannulation. If the tracheostomy tube is dislodged before the stoma tract is mature (which takes about one week) the tract closes quickly, and blind reinsertion of the tube can create false tracts. When a tracheostomy tube is dislodged within a few days of insertion, the patient should be reintubated before attempting to reinsert the tracheostomy tube.

TRACHEAL STENOSIS: The most feared complication of tracheostomy is tracheal stenosis, which is a late complication that appears in the first 6 months after the tracheostomy tube is removed. Most cases of tracheal stenosis occur at the site of the tracheal incision, and are the result of tracheal narrowing after the stoma closes. The incidence of tracheal stenosis ranges from zero to 15% in individual reports (12), but most cases are asymptomatic. The risk of tracheal stenosis is the same with surgical and percutaneous tracheostomies (9).

Cuff Management

Positive pressure ventilation requires a seal in the trachea that prevents gas from escaping out through the larynx. This is created by inflating the balloon (called a cuff) that surrounds the distal portion of the tracheal tube. A tracheostomy tube with an inflated cuff is shown in Figure 28.3. The cuff is attached to a pilot balloon that has a one-way valve. A syringe is attached to the pilot balloon and air is injected into the cuff until there is no audible leak around the cuff. (The pilot balloon will inflate as the cuff inflates.)

The pressure in the cuff (measured with a pressure gauge attached to the pilot balloon) should not exceed 25 mm Hg (13). This pressure limit is based on the assumption that the capillary hydrostatic pressure in the wall of the trachea is 25 mm Hg, and thus external (cuff) pressures above 25 mm Hg can compress the underlying capillaries and produce ischemic injury and tracheal necrosis. Fortunately, the elongated design of cuffs allows for greater dispersion of pressure, and also allows for a tracheal seal at relatively low pressures.

Cuff Leaks

Cuff leaks are usually detected by audible sounds during lung inflation (created by gas flowing through the vocal cords). *Cuff leaks are rarely caused by disruption of the cuff* (14), and are usually the result of nonuniform contact between the cuff and the wall of the trachea, or dysfunction of the valve on the pilot balloon.

TROUBLESHOOTING: If a cuff leak is audible, the patient should be separated from the ventilator and the lungs should be manually inflated with an anesthesia bag. If the cuff leak involves an endotracheal tube, check the position of the tube to determine if the tube is coming out of the trachea. If this is a possibility, you can deflate the cuff and advance the tube. If this is unsuccessful, the tube should be replaced (or a fiber-optic instrument can be advanced through the tube to make sure it is still in the lungs). Air should never be added to the cuff blindly because the tube may be coming out of the trachea, and cuff inflation will damage the vocal cords. If

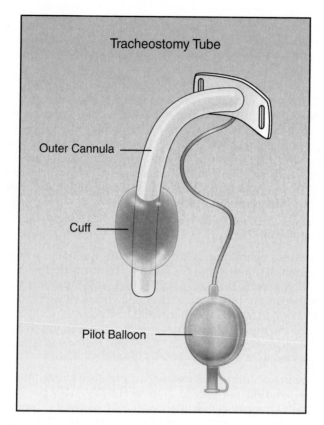

FIGURE 28.3 A tracheostomy tube with an inflated cuff.

the cuff leak involves a tracheostomy tube, air can be added to the cuff in an attempt to produce a seal. If this eliminates the leak, the cuff pressure should be measured, and should be ≤ 25 mm Hg. If the cuff pressure is above 25 mm Hg, or the leak persists despite adding volume, the tracheostomy tube should be replaced (with a larger diameter tube, if possible).

AIRWAY CARE

Suctioning

Routine suctioning to clear secretions has been a standard practice in the care of ventilator-dependent patients. However, the inner surface of artificial airways become colonized with biofilms containing pathogenic organisms (see Figure 28.4), and passing a suction catheter through the tubes can dislodge these biofilms and inoculate the lungs with pathogenic organisms (15,16). As a result, *endotracheal suctioning is no longer recommended as a routine procedure,* but should be performed only when respiratory secretions are present (17).

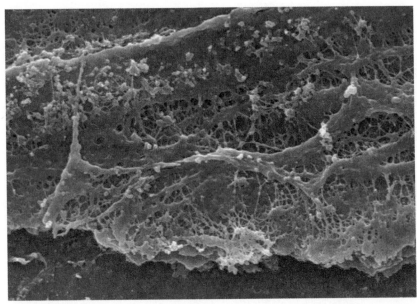

FIGURE 28.4 Electron micrograph showing a biofilm on the inner surface of an endotracheal tube. Image from Reference 16.

Saline Instillation

Saline is often instilled into the trachea to facilitate the clearing of secretions, but this practice is *no longer advised as a routine procedure* (17) for two reasons: (a) saline will not liquefy or reduce the viscosity of respiratory secretions (as described next), and (b) saline can dislodge pathogenic organisms colonizing the inner surface of tracheal tubes. One study has shown that injection of 5 mL of saline can dislodge up to 300,000 colonies of viable bacteria from the inner surface of endotracheal tubes (18).

Viscosity of Respiratory Secretions

The respiratory secretions create a blanket that covers the mucosal surface of the airways. This blanket has a hydrophilic (water soluble) layer, and a hydrophobic (water insoluble) layer. The hydrophilic layer faces inward, and keeps the mucosal surface moist. The hydrophobic layer faces outward, towards the lumen of the airways. This outer layer is composed of a meshwork of mucoprotein strands (called mucus threads) held together by disulfide bridges. This meshwork traps particles and debris in the airways, and the combination of the mucoprotein meshwork and the trapped debris is what determines the viscoelastic behavior of the respiratory secretions. Since the layer that contributes to the viscosity of respiratory secretions is not water soluble, *saline will not reduce the viscosity of respiratory secretions.* (Adding saline to thick, respiratory secretions is like pouring water over grease.)

The accumulation of viscous secretions can result in a condition like the one shown in Figure 28.5, where a tenacious "plug" is completely obstructing a major airway. In this situation, a mucolytic agent like

N-Acetylcysteine (Mucomyst) can help to disrupt the plug and relieve the obstruction. *N*-acetylcysteine (NAC) is a sulfhydryl-containing tripeptide that is better known as the antidote for acetaminophen overdose, but it is also a mucolytic agent that acts by disrupting the disulfide bridges between mucoprotein strands in sputum (19). The drug is available in a liquid preparation (10 or 20% solution) that can be given as an aerosol spray, or injected directly into the airways (Table 28.1). Aerosolized NAC should be avoided when possible because it is irritating to the airways and can provoke coughing and bronchospasm (particularly in asthmatics). Direct instillation of NAC into the tracheal tube is preferred, especially when there is an obstruction.

Table 28.1	Mucolytic Therapy with *N*-Acetylcysteine (NAC)
Aerosol Therapy:	• Use 10% NAC solution.
	• Mix 2.5 mL NAC with 2.5 mL saline and place mixture (5 mL) in a small volume ebulizer for aerosol delivery.
	• *Warning:* this can provoke bronchospasm, and is not recommended in asthmatics
Tracheal Injection:	• Use 20% NAC solution.
	• Mix 2 mL NAC with 2 mL saline and inject 2 mL aliquots into the trachea.
	• *Warning:* Excessive volumes can produce bronchorrhea.

If intratracheal injection of NAC does not relieve an obstruction, bronchoscopy should be performed (the NAC is then applied directly to the mucous plug). Following relief of the obstruction, NAC can be instilled two or three times a day for the next day or two. Daily use of NAC is not advised because the drug solution is hypertonic (even with the saline additive) and can provoke bronchorrhea.

ALVEOLAR RUPTURE

One of the manifestations of ventilator-induced lung injury is alveolar distension and volutrauma, and one of the clinical consequences of volutrauma is alveolar rupture with the escape of gas from the distal airspaces. This form of injury, which is mistakenly called *pulmonary barotrauma*, occurs in up to 25% of patients receiving mechanical ventilation (20).

Clinical Presentation

Escape of gas from the alveoli can produce a variety of clinical manifestations. The alveolar gas can dissect along tissue planes and produce *pul-*

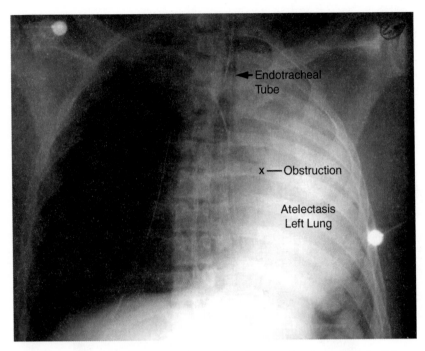

FIGURE 28.5 Portable chest x-ray of an intubated patient showing atelectasis of the left lung, which is usually caused by a mucous plug in the left mainstem bronchus.

monary interstitial emphysema, and air can move into the mediastinum and produce *pneumomediastinum.* Mediastinal gas can move into the neck to produce *subcutaneous emphysema,* or can pass below the diaphragm to produce *pneumoperitoneum.* Finally, if the rupture involves the visceral pleura, gas will collect in the pleural space and produce a *pneumothorax.* Each of these entities can occur alone or in combination (20,21).

Pneumothorax

Radiographic evidence of pneumothorax occurs in 5 to 15% of ventilator-dependent patients (20,21).

Clinical Presentation

Clinical manifestations are either absent, minimal, or nonspecific. The *most valuable clinical sign is subcutaneous emphysema* in the neck and upper thorax, which is pathognomonic of alveolar rupture. Breath sounds are unreliable in ventilator-dependent patients because sounds transmitted from the ventilator tubing can be mistaken for airway sounds.

Radiographic Detection

The radiographic detection of pleural air can be difficult in the supine position, because *pleural air does not collect at the lung apex* when patients are supine (22). Figure 28.6 illustrates this difficulty. In this case of a traumatic pneumothorax, the chest x-ray is unrevealing, but the CT scan reveals an anterior pneumothorax on the left. Pleural air will collect in the most superior region of the hemithorax and, in the supine position, this region is just anterior to both lung bases. Therefore, *basilar and subpulmonic collections of air are characteristic of pneumothorax in the supine position* (22).

REDUNDANT SKIN FOLDS: When the film cartridge used for portable chest x-rays is placed under the patient, the skin on the back can fold over on itself, and the edge of this redundant skin fold creates a radiographic shadow that can be mistaken for a pneumothorax. The radiographic

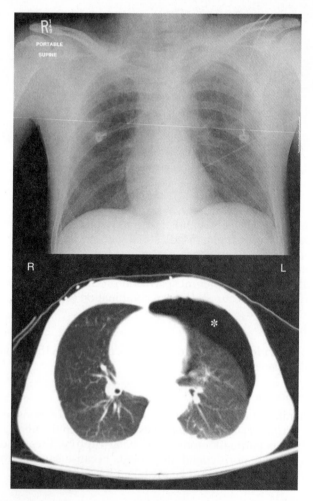

FIGURE 28.6 A portable chest x-ray and CT image of the thorax in a young male with blunt trauma to the chest. An anterior pneumothorax is evident on the CT image (indicated by the asterisk) but is not apparent on the portable chest x-ray.

appearance of a redundant skin fold is shown in Figure 28.7. Note that there is a gradual increase in radiodensity that produces a wavy line. The gradual increase in density is produced by the skin that is folded back on itself. A pneumothorax would appear as a sharp white line with dark shadows (air) on either side.

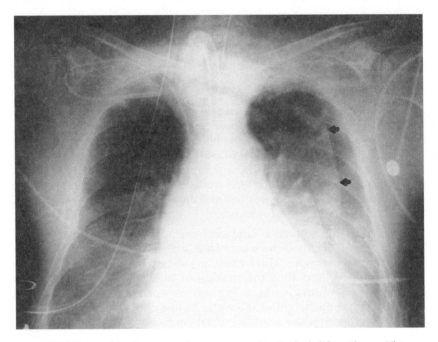

FIGURE 28.7 Portable chest x-ray showing a wavy line in the left hemithorax. This line is the edge of a redundant skin fold, and not the edge of the lung.

Pleural Evacuation

Evacuation of pleural air is accomplished by inserting a chest tube through the fourth or fifth intercostal space along the mid-axillary line. The tube should be advanced in an anterior and superior direction (because this is where pleural air collects in the supine position). The pleural space is drained of fluid and air using a three-chamber system like the one shown in Figure 28.8 (23).

Collection Bottle

The first bottle in the system collects fluid from the pleural space and allows air to pass through to the next bottle in the series. Because the inlet of this chamber is not in direct contact with the fluid, the pleural fluid that is collected does not impose a back pressure on the pleural space.

Water-Seal Bottle

The second bottle acts as a one-way valve that allows air to escape from the pleural space but prevents air from entering the pleural space. This one-way valve is created by submerging the inlet tube under water. This imposes a back-pressure on the pleural space that is equal to the depth that the tube is submerged. The positive pressure in the pleural space then prevents atmospheric air (at zero pressure) from entering the pleural space. The water thus "seals" the pleural space from the surrounding atmosphere. This water-seal pressure is usually 2 cm H_2O.

Air that is evacuated from the pleural space passes through the water in the second bottle and creates bubbles. Thus, the presence of bubbles in the water-seal chamber is evidence of a continuing bronchopleural air leak.

Suction-Control Bottle

The third bottle in the system is used to set a maximum limit on the negative suction pressure that is imposed on the pleural space. This maximum pressure is determined by the height of the water column in the air inlet tube. Negative pressure (from wall suction) draws the water down the air inlet tube, and when the negative pressure exceeds the height of the water column, air is entrained from the atmosphere. Therefore, the pressure in the bottle can never become more negative than the height of the water column in the air inlet tube.

Water is added to the suction-control chamber to achieve a water level of 20 cm. The wall suction is then activated and slowly increased until bubbles appear in the water. This bubbling indicates that atmospheric air is being entrained, and thus the maximum negative pressure has been achieved. The continuous bubbling causes water evaporation, so it is imperative that the height of the water in this chamber is checked periodically, and more water is added when necessary.

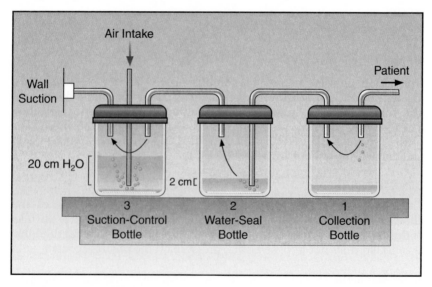

FIGURE 28.8 A standard pleural drainage system for evacuating air and fluid from the pleural space.

Why Suction?

The practice of using suction to evacuate pleural air is often unnecessary and potentially harmful. Although there is a perception that suction will help the lungs reinflate, the lungs will reinflate without the use of suction. Furthermore, creating a negative pressure in the pleural space also creates a higher transpulmonary pressure (the pressure difference between alveoli and the pleural space), and this increases the rate of the air flowing through a bronchopleural fistula. Thus *applying suction to the pleural space increases bronchopleural air leaks*, and this can prevent bronchopleural fistulas from closing. If a persistent air leak is present when suction is applied to the pleural space, the suction should be discontinued. Any air that collects in the pleural space will continue to be evacuated when the pleural pressure becomes more positive than the water-seal pressure.

INTRINSIC (OCCULT) PEEP

Intrinsic, occult PEEP (also called auto-PEEP) is described in Chapter 24 (see pages 477–479) and in Chapter 25 (see pages 490–491). The features of intrinsic PEEP are illustrated in Figure 28.9. This pressure is the result of incomplete exhalation, and can occur in patients with severe airflow obstruction, or during mechanical ventilation that is too rapid to allow complete exhalation (24). During conventional mechanical ventilation, intrinsic PEEP is probably universal in patients with severe asthma and COPD (25,26), while it is also common in patients with ARDS (27), although at low levels (<3 cm H_2O). It is important to emphasize that intrinsic PEEP is not apparent when monitoring airway pressures (hence the term "occult PEEP").

Adverse Effects

Intrinsic PEEP has several adverse effects, which are summarized below (24). As is the case with applied PEEP, many of these adverse effects are not the result of the PEEP level, but rather are due to the influence of PEEP on the end-inspiratory alveolar pressure and the mean intrathoracic pressure.

1. Intrinsic PEEP increases mean intrathoracic pressure, which impairs venous return and can decrease cardiac output.

2. The hyperinflation that produces intrinsic PEEP in patients with severe airflow obstruction can increase the work of breathing when the region of tidal breathing moves to the upper flat portion of the pressure-volume curve (see Figure 24.4 on page 478). (To appreciate this effect, take a deep breath, and then try to breathe in further.)

3. Intrinsic PEEP increases end-inspiratory alveolar pressure, which increases the risk of volutrauma and alveolar rupture.

4. When intrinsic PEEP goes undetected, the increase in end-inspiratory alveolar pressure (plateau pressure) is misinterpreted as a decrease in the compliance of the lungs and chest wall.

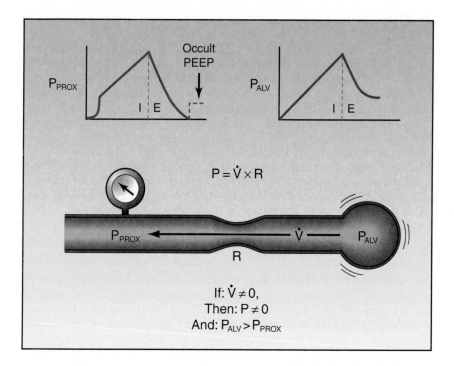

FIGURE 28.9 The features of intrinsic PEEP resulting from incomplete exhalation. The presence of airflow ($\dot{V}$) at end-expiration indicates a pressure drop from the alveolus (P_{ALV}) to the proximal airways (P_{PROX}). As shown at the top of the figure, the proximal airway pressure returns to zero at end-expiration while the alveolar pressure remains positive, hence the term *occult* PEEP. The upper left panel illustrates the end-expiratory occlusion method for measuring occult PEEP.

5. Intrinsic PEEP can be transmitted into the superior vena cava, result-ing in the mistaken impression that end-diastolic (transmural) pres-sure has increased.

Monitoring Intrinsic PEEP

Intrinsic PEEP is easy to detect but difficult to quantify. The easiest method of detection is inspecting the expiratory flow waveform for the presence of airflow at the end of expiration (see Figure 24.5 on page 479). If intrinsic PEEP is evident on the expiratory flow wave-form, the level of intrinsic PEEP can be measured with the end-expi-ratory occlusion method.

End-Expiratory Occlusion

Occlusion of the expiratory circuit at the end of expiration will "unmask" intrinsic PEEP, as shown in Figure 28.9. Accuracy requires that the occlu-sion occur at the very end of expiration, and this cannot be timed properly if patients are breathing spontaneously. Therefore, *the end-expiratory occlusion method can only be performed in the patients who are not triggering ventilator breaths.*

Management

The maneuvers used to prevent or reduce hyperinflation and intrinsic PEEP are all directed at promoting alveolar emptying during expiration. These maneuvers include reducing the tidal volume, increasing the inspiratory flow rate, reducing the inspiratory time (in pressure control ventilation), and reducing the respiratory rate, if possible. Some of these maneuvers will reduce the minute ventilation, which may not be desirable.

Applied PEEP

The addition of external PEEP can reduce hyperinflation (and intrinsic PEEP) by holding the small airways open at end-expiration. The level of applied PEEP must be enough to counterbalance the pressure causing small airways collapse (the closing pressure) but should not exceed the level of intrinsic PEEP (so that it does not impair expiratory flow) (28). To accomplish this, the level of applied PEEP should match the level of intrinsic PEEP. Since intrinsic PEEP will be difficult to quantify in spontaneously breathing patients, an alternative method in these patients is to monitor the response of the end-expiratory airflow to applied PEEP; i.e., if the applied PEEP reduces or eliminates end-expiratory flow, then it is reducing the level of intrinsic PEEP. Although the end result is still PEEP (applied PEEP instead of intrinsic PEEP), the applied PEEP will help to reduce the risk of atelectrauma from repetitive opening and closing of small airways at end-expiration.

A FINAL WORD

The patient's clinical course in the first few days of mechanical ventilation will give you a fairly accurate indication of what is coming. If the patient is not improving, proceed to a tracheostomy as soon as it can be done safely. Most of the day-to-day management of the ventilator-dependent patient involves vigilance for adverse events (e.g., pneumothorax). You will learn that, in many cases, you are not the one controlling the course of the patient's illness.

REFERENCES

Endotracheal Tubes

1. Gray AW. Endotracheal tubes. Crit Care Clin 2003; 24:379–387.

2. Goodman LR. Pulmonary support and monitoring apparatus. In: Goodman LR, Putman CE, eds. Critical care imaging. 3rd ed. Philadelphia: WB Saunders, 1992; 35–59.

3. Owen RL, Cheney FW. Endotracheal intubation: a preventable complication. Anesthesiology 1987; 67:255–257.

4. Gallagher TJ. Endotracheal intubation. Crit Care Clin 1992; 8:665–676.

5. Colice GL. Resolution of laryngeal injury following translaryngeal intubation. Am Rev Respir Dis 1992; 145:361–364.

6. Muscedere J, Rewa O, Mckechnie K, et al. Subglottic secretion drainage for the prevention of ventilator-associated pneumonia: a systematic review and meta-analysis. Crit Care Med 2011; 39:1985–1991.

Tracheostomy

7. Terragni PP, Antonelli M, Fumagalli R, et al. Early vs. late tracheotomy for prevention of pneumonia in mechanically ventilated adult ICU patients. JAMA 2010; 303:1483–1489.

8. Trouillet JL, Luyt CE, Guiguet M, et al. Early percutaneous tracheotomy versus prolonged intubation of mechanically ventilated patients after cardiac surgery: A randomized trial. Ann Intern Med 2011; 154:373–383.

9. Freeman BD, Morris PE. Tracheostomy practice in adults with acute respiratory failure. Crit Care Med 2012; 40:2890–2896.

10. Ciagla P. Technique, complications, and improvements in percutaneous dilatational tracheostomy. Chest 1999; 115:1229–1230.

11. Freeman BD, Isabella K, Lin N, Buchman TG. A meta-analysis of prospective trials comparing percutaneous and surgical tracheostomy in critically ill patients. Chest 2000; 118:1412–1418.

12. Tracheotomy: application and timing. Clin Chest Med 2003; 24:389–398.

13. Heffner JE, Hess D. Tracheostomy management in the chronically ventilated patient. Clin Chest Med 2001; 22:5; 10:561–568.

14. Kearl RA, Hooper RG. Massive airway leaks: an analysis of the role of endotracheal tubes. Crit Care Med 1993; 21:518–521.

Airway Care

15. Adair CC, Gorman SP, Feron BM, et al. Implications of endotracheal tube biofilm for ventilator-associated pneumonia. Intensive Care Med 1999; 25:1072–1076.

16. Gil-Perontin S, Ramirez P, Marti V, et al. Implications of endotracheal tube biofilm in ventilator associated pneumonia response: a state of concept. Crit Care 2012; 16:R93 (available at ccforum.com/content/16/3/R93).

17. AARC Clinical Practice Guideline. Endotracheal suctioning of mechanically ventilated patients with artificial airways 2010. Respir Care 2010; 55:758–764.

18. Hagler DA, Traver GA. Endotracheal saline and suction catheters: sources of lower airways contamination. Am J Crit Care 1994; 3:444–447.

19. Holdiness MR. Clinical pharmacokinetics of N-acetylcysteine. Clin Pharmacokinet 1991; 20:123–134.

Alveolar Rupture

20. Gammon RB, Shin MS, Buchalter SE. Pulmonary barotrauma in mechanical ventilation. Chest 1992; 102:568–572.

21. Marcy TW. Barotrauma: detection, recognition, and management. Chest 1993; 104:578–584.

22. Tocino IM, Miller MH, Fairfax WR. Distribution of pneumothorax in the supine and semirecumbent critically ill adult. Am J Radiol 1985; 144:901–905.

23. Kam AC, O'Brien M, Kam PCA. Pleural drainage systems. Anesthesia 1993; 48:154–161.

Intrinsic (Occult) PEEP

24. Marini JJ. Dynamic hyperinflation and auto-positive end expiratory pressure. Am J Respir Crit Care Med 2011; 184:756–762.

25. Blanch L, Bernabe F, Lucangelo U. Measurement of air trapping, intrinsic positive end-expiratory pressure, and dynamic hyperinflation in mechanically ventilated patients. Respir Care 2005; 50:110–123.

26. Shapiro JM. Management of respiratory failure in status asthmaticus. Am J Respir Med 2002; 1:409–416.

27. Hough CL, Kallet RH, Ranieri M, et al. Intrinsic positive end-expiratory pressure in Acute Respiratory Distress Syndrome (ARDS) Network subjects. Crit Care Med 2005; 33:527–532.

28. Tobin MJ, Lodato RF. PEEP, autoPEEP, and waterfalls. Chest 1989; 96:449–451.

Chapter 29

VENTILATOR-ASSOCIATED PNEUMONIA

Everything hinges on the matter of evidence.

Carl Sagan

The approach to pneumonias that develop during mechanical ventilation can be characterized by one word: *problematic.* The problems extend from the lack of a "gold standard" method for identifying parenchymal lung infections in ventilator-dependent patients, to the lack of standardized methods for collecting and culturing respiratory secretions and, finally, to the difficulties in eradicating multidrug-resistant organisms that are becoming prevalent in ventilator-associated pneumonias.

This chapter presents the current state of knowledge regarding ventilator-associated pneumonias, and includes recommendations from the most recent clinical practice guidelines and reviews of this topic (1–4).

GENERAL INFORMATION

The following statements include some basic information about ventilator-associated pneumonia (VAP).

1. Infections involving the lungs are the most common nosocomial infections in ICU patients, accounting for 65% of all nosocomial infections in this patient population (5). However, this prevalence is overstated because many cases of presumed ICU-acquired pneumonia are not corroborated on postmortem examination (see later).

2. Over 90% of ICU-acquired pneumonias occur during mechanical ventilation, and 50% of these ventilator-associated pneumonias (VAPs) begin in the first 4 days after intubation (2).

3. Unlike community-acquired pneumonias, where the predominant

pathogens are pneumococci, atypical organisms, and viruses, three-quarters of the isolates in VAP are Gram-negative aerobic bacilli (most frequently *Pseudomonas aeruginosa*) and *Staphylococcus aureus* (see Table 29.1).

4. The crude mortality rate associated with VAP is 5% to 65% (3). However, there is a paucity of strong evidence directly linking VAP with fatal outcomes (4,6), and several studies show no direct relationship between VAP and mortality rate (7–9). As a result, the growing consensus is that VAP is not a life-threatening illness, but it does prolong the duration of mechanical ventilation and increases the length of stay in the ICU and hospital (4).

Table 29.1	Pathogenic Isolates in Ventilator-Associated Pneumonia
Organisms	**Frequency**
Gram-Negative Bacilli	56.5%
Pseudomonas aeruginosa	18.9%
Escherichia coli	9.2%
Hemophilus spp	7.1%
Enterobacter spp	3.8%
Proteus	3.8%
Klebsiella pneumoniae	3.2%
Others	10.5%
Gram-Positive Cocci	42.1%
Staphylococcus aureus	18.9%
Streptococcus pneumoniae	13.2%
Hemophilus spp	1.4%
Others	8.6%
Fungal Isolates	1.3%

From Chastre J. et al. JAMA 2003; 290:2558.

PREVENTIVE MEASURES

Aspiration of pathogenic organisms from the oropharynx is believed to be the inciting event in most cases of VAP (10). The pathogens that most often colonize the oropharynx in ICU patients are Gram-negative aerobic bacilli (see Figure 5.5 on page 89), which explains the predominance of these pathogens in VAP. The instances of VAP that appear within 4 days of intubation are most likely caused by pathogens that have been dragged into the airways during the intubation procedure.

Oral Decontamination

The realization that VAP begins with pathogenic colonization of the oropharynx prompted the introduction of measures to decontaminate the oropharynx as a preventive measure for VAP. The methods of oral decontamination (i.e., with antiseptic agents and nonabsorbable antibiotics) are described in Chapter 5 (see pages 88–90), and the benefits of oral decontamination in reducing tracheal colonization and VAP are shown in Figure 5.6 (page 90). Oral decontamination (usually with the antiseptic agent *chlorhexidine*) is now a standard measure in all ventilator-dependent patients.

Routine Airway Care

(*Note:* This topic is described in more detail on pages 540–542 in the last chapter.) Tracheal tubes serve as a nidus for pathogenic colonization and biofilm formation, and these biofilms protect the colonized pathogens and allow them to proliferate (see Figure 28.4 on page 541). Endotracheal suctioning can disrupt the biofilms and dislodge microbes colonizing the inner surface of tracheal tubes, which introduces pathogens into the lower airways. For this reason, *endotracheal suctioning is not recommended as a routine procedure* (11), but only when necessary to clear secretions from the airways.

Clearance of Subglottic Secretions

Contrary to popular belief, *inflation of the cuff on tracheal tubes to create a seal does not prevent aspiration of mouth secretions into the lower airways.* Aspiration of saliva and liquid tube feedings has been documented in over 50% of ventilator-dependent patients with tracheostomies; in over three-fourths of the cases, this aspiration is clinically silent (12).

Concern about aspiration around inflated cuffs prompted the introduction (in 1992) of specialized endotracheal tubes equipped with a suction port just above the cuff (e.g., Mallinckrodt TaperGuard Evac Tube, Covidien, Boulder, CO). The suction port is connected to a source of continuous suction (usually not exceeding -20 cm H_2O) to clear the secretions that accumulate in the subglottic region, as illustrated in Figure 29.1.

Clinical studies have shown *a significant reduction in the incidence of VAP when subglottic secretions are cleared using specialized endotracheal tubes* (13). As a result, suction clearance of subglottic secretions is recommended as a preventive measure for VAP (3). Despite this recommendation, aspiration of subglottic secretions has yet to gain widespread acceptance.

CLINICAL FEATURES

Diagnostic Accuracy

The traditional clinical criteria for the diagnosis of VAP include: (a) fever or hypothermia, (b) leukocytosis or leukopenia, (c), an increase in volume of respiratory secretions or a change in character of the secretions, and (d) a new or progressive infiltrate on the chest x-ray (4). Unfortunately, in patients who are suspected of having VAP based on these clinical criteria, the incidence of pneumonia on postmortem exam is only 30%

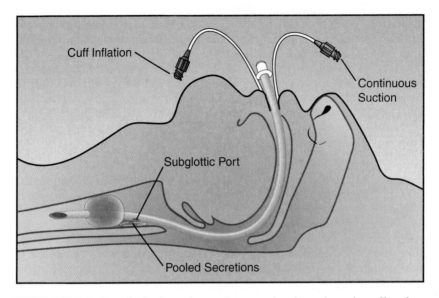

FIGURE 29.1 Endotracheal tube with a suction port placed just above the cuff to clear secretions that accumulate in the subglottic region.

to 40% (14). The diagnostic accuracy for VAP based on traditional clinical criteria is demonstrated in Table 29.2. This table shows the results of two studies that used autopsy evidence of pneumonia to evaluate the premortem diagnosis of VAP based on clinical findings (15,16). In both studies, the clinical criteria for identifying VAP were just as likely to occur in the presence or absence of pneumonia. These studies demonstrate that *the diagnosis of VAP is not possible using clinical criteria alone.*

Table 29.2	Predictive Value of Clinical Criteria in the Diagnosis of Ventilator-Associated Pneumonia	
Study	**Clinical Criteria**	**Likelihood Ratio for Pneumonia on Autopsy[†]**
Fagon et al. (15)	Radiographic infiltrate + purulent sputum + fever or leukocytosis	1.03
Timset et al. (16)	Radiographic infiltrate + 2 of the following: fever, leukocytosis, or purulent sputum.	0.96

[†]As reported in Reference 14. The likelihood ratio is the likelihood that patients with pneumonia will have the clinical findings compared to the likelihood that patients without pneumonia will have the same clinical findings. A likelihood ratio of 1 indicates that a pneumonia is just as likely to be present or absent based on the clinical findings.

Specificity of Chest Radiography

The limited diagnostic accuracy in VAP is primarily due to the nonspecific nature of pulmonary infiltrates. Pneumonia accounts for only one-third of all pulmonary infiltrates in ICU patients (17,18), which means that *conditions other than pneumonia are the most frequent cause of pulmonary infiltrates in ICU patients.* The noninfectious causes of pulmonary infiltrates in the ICU include pulmonary edema, acute respiratory distress syndrome, and atelectasis.

An example of how a decrease in lung volume can produce spurious changes in a portable chest x-ray is illustrated in Figure 29.2. Both images in this figure were obtained within minutes of each other in the same patient. The image on the left, which was taken during expiration in the supine position (a common body position in ICU patients) shows a marked reduction in lung volume accompanied by a crowding of lung markings at the base of the right lung (dotted triangle). In a patient with fever, this radiographic change could be mistaken for a basilar pneumonia.

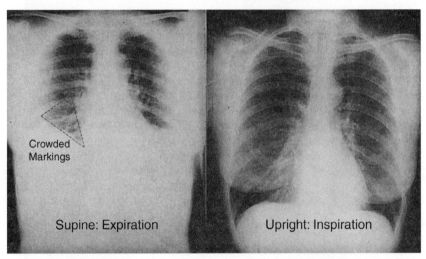

Crowded Markings

Supine: Expiration

Upright: Inspiration

FIGURE 29.2 The effect of a decrease in lung volume on the appearance of a portable chest x-ray. Both images were obtained within minutes of each other in the same patient. The dotted triangle outlines an area of crowded lung markings that could be mistaken for a basilar pneumonia in a febrile patient. Image on the left digitally enhanced.

ARDS: The most common noninfectious cause of pulmonary infiltrates in ICU patients is the acute respiratory distress syndrome (ARDS) (18). This condition, which is described in Chapter 23, is an inflammatory disorder of the lungs that produces bilateral infiltrates on chest x-ray (see Figure 23.2 on page 451). Because it is often accompanied by fever, ARDS can be difficult to distinguish from a multilobar pneumonia.

Sensitivity of Chest Radiography

The other limitation of chest radiography is a limited sensitivity for the detection of pulmonary infiltrates. This is demonstrated in Figure 29.3, where the portable chest x-ray of a patient with cough and fever shows

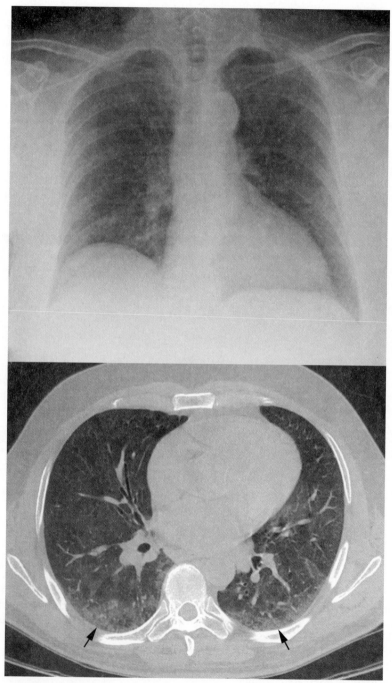

FIGURE 29.3 Demonstration of the limited sensitivity of portable chest radiography in the detection of pulmonary infiltrates. A portable chest x-ray of a patient with fever shows no apparent pulmonary infiltrates, while the CT image from the same patient reveals infiltrates in the posterior region of both lungs (indicated by the arrows).

no apparent infiltrates, while the CT image of the same patient shows a fine pattern of infiltration in the posterior region of both lungs. Since CT scans are not obtained routinely in patients with suspected pneumonia and an unrevealing chest x-ray, it is not clear how often the example in Figure 29.3 actually occurs. However, this example clearly demonstrates that *the diagnosis of pneumonia cannot be ruled out with a portable chest x-ray.*

New Clinical Criteria?

The National Healthcare Safety Network (NHSN) has recently published an algorithm for the diagnosis of VAP that does not include findings on a chest x-ray (1). This algorithm is shown in Figure 29.4. The clinical suspicion of VAP in this algorithm is triggered by a deterioration in arterial oxygenation (ventilator-associated complication) combined with a change in body temperature or leukocyte count in the blood (infection-related ventilator-associated complication). Although this algorithm has not been validated, it does recognize the limitations of chest radiography in the diagnosis of VAP.

MICROBIOLOGICAL EVALUATION

The diagnosis of VAP rests heavily on identifying a responsible pathogen, but there is little agreement on the optimal method of either collecting or culturing respiratory secretions. Blood cultures have limited value in the diagnosis of VAP because organisms isolated from blood in cases of suspected VAP are often from extrapulmonary sites of origin (14). The NHSN algorithm in Figure 29.4 relies on quantitative cultures of respiratory secretions or lung biopsies for the diagnosis of VAP, but quantitative cultures are not a standard practice in the diagnostic evaluation of suspected VAP. The following is a brief review of the methods used to collect and culture respiratory secretions in the diagnostic approach to VAP.

Tracheal Aspirate

The traditional approach to suspected VAP involves aspiration of respiratory secretions through an endotracheal or tracheostomy tube, and these specimens can be contaminated with mouth secretions that are aspirated into the upper airway. A screening method for identifying contaminated and uncontaminated specimens is described next. (This method should be performed routinely in the microbiology laboratory.)

Microscopic Analysis

The cells identified in Figure 29.5 can help to determine if secretions collected by aspiration through tracheal tubes are contaminated by mouth secretions, and if there is evidence of infection. Each type of cell can be identified and interpreted as follows.

1. The squamous epithelial cells that line the oral cavity are large and flattened with abundant cytoplasm and a small nucleus. The presence of *more than 10 squamous epithelial cells per low-power field (×100)*

I. Ventilator-Associated Condition (VAC)

After 2 days of stability or improvement on the ventilation, the patient has at least one of the following indications of worsening oxygenation:

1. Increase in daily minimum FiO_2 20% for at least 2 days.
2. Increase in daily minimum PEEP 3 cm H_2O for at least 2 days.

II. Infection-Related Ventilator-Associated Complication (IVAC)

After at least 3 days of mechanical ventilation, and within 2 days of worsening oxygenation, the patient has:

1. Body temperature 38C or <36 OR
2. WBC count 12,000/mm^3 or 4,000/mm^3.

III. Probable Ventilator-Associated Pneumonia

After at least 3 days of mechanical ventilation, and within 2 days of worsening oxygenation, the patient has one of the following:

1. Purulent secretions (25 neutrophils and 10 squamous cells per low power field) AND one of the following:
   a. Positive culture of endotracheal aspirate at 10^5 CFU/mL.[†]
   b. Positive culture of broncoalveolar lavage at 10^4 CFU/mL.[†]
   c. Positive culture of lung tissue at 10^4 CFU/mL.
   d. Positive culture of protected specimen brush at 10^4 CFU/mL.[†]

2. One of the following (with or without purulent secretions):
   a. Positive pleural fluid culture.
   b. Positive lung histopathology.
   c. Positive diagnostic test for *Legionella* spp.
   d. Positive diagnostic test on respiratory secretions for influenza virus, adenovirus, respiratory syncytial virus, rhinovirus, human metapneumovirus, or coronavirus.
   [†]Excludes the following: (a) normal respiratory flora, (b) *Candida* species or yeast not otherwise specified, (c) coagulase-negative *Staphylococcus* spp., and (d) *Enterococcus* species.

FIGURE 29.4 National Health Safety Network algorithm for the diagnosis of ventilator-associated pneumonia. From Reference 1.

indicates that the specimen is contaminated with mouth secretions, and is not an appropriate specimen for culture (1).

2. Lung macrophages are large, oval-shaped cells with a granular cyto-

plasm and a small, eccentric nucleus. The size of the nucleus in a macrophage is roughly the same size as a neutrophil. Although macrophages can inhabit the airways (20), the predominant home of the macrophage is the distal airspaces. Therefore, *the presence of macrophages, regardless of the number, is evidence that the specimen is from the lower respiratory tract.*

3. The presence of neutrophils in respiratory secretions is not evidence of infection because neutrophils can make up 20% of the cells recovered from a routine mouthwash (20). The neutrophils should be present in abundance to indicate infection. *More than 25 neutrophils per low-power field (x 100) can be used as evidence of infection (21).*

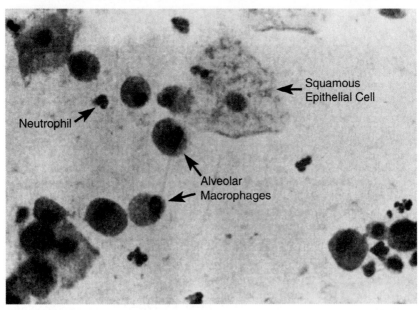

FIGURE 29.5 Microscopic appearance (magnification x400) of bronchial brushings from a ventilator-dependent patient. The paucity of squamous epithelial cells and the presence of alveolar macrophages is evidence that the specimen is from the distal airways (and thus would be an appropriate specimen for culture in a case of suspected VAP).

Qualitative Cultures

The standard practice is to perform qualitative cultures on endotracheal aspirates (where the growth of organisms is reported, but there is no assessment of growth density). These cultures have a high sensitivity (usually > 90%) but a very low specificity (15–40%) for the diagnosis of VAP (22). This means that *for qualitative cultures of tracheal aspirates, a negative culture can be used to exclude the diagnosis of VAP, but a positive culture cannot be used to confirm the presence of VAP.* The poor predictive value of positive cultures is due to contamination of tracheal aspirates with secretions from the mouth and upper airways.

Quantitative Cultures

For quantitative cultures of tracheal aspirates (where growth density on the culture plate is reported), the threshold growth for the diagnosis of VAP is 10^5 colony-forming units per mL (CFU/mL). This threshold has a sensitivity and specificity of 76% and 75%, respectively, for the diagnosis of VAP (see Table 29.3) (2,22). Comparing these results to the sensitivity and specificity of qualitative cultures (i.e., sensitivity > 90% and specificity ≤ 40%) shows that, *for cultures of tracheal aspirates, quantitative cultures are less sensitive but more specific than qualitative cultures for the diagnosis of VAP.*

Table 29.3	Quantitative Cultures for the Diagnosis of Pneumonia in Ventilator-Dependent Patients		
	TA	PSB	BAL
Diagnostic Threshhold (CFU/mL)	10^5	10^3	10^4
Sensitivity (mean)	76%	66%	73%
Specificity (mean)	75%	90%	82%
Relative Performance	Most Sensitive	Most Specific	Most Accurate

Abbreviations: TA = tracheal aspirates; PSB = protected specimen brushings; BAL = broncoalveolar lavage.

From References 2, 22, 24.

Bronchoalveolar Lavage

Bronchoalveolar lavage (BAL) is performed by wedging the bronchoscope in a distal airway and performing a lavage with sterile isotonic saline. A minimum lavage volume of 120 mL is recommended for adequate sampling of the lavaged lung segment (23), and this is achieved by performing a series of 6 lavages using 20 mL for each lavage. The same syringe is used to introduce the fluid and aspirate the lavage specimen (only 25% or less of the volume instilled will be returned via aspiration). The first lavage is usually discarded, and the remainder of the lavage fluid is pooled and sent to the microbiology lab for microscopic analysis and quantitative culture.

Quantitative Cultures

The threshold for a positive BAL culture is 10^4 CFU/mL (1). The reported sensitivity and specificity of BAL cultures are shown in Table 29.3 (2,24). BAL does not have the highest sensitivity or specificity when compared to the other diagnostic methods in Table 29.3, but when sensitivity and specificity are considered together, *BAL cultures have the highest overall accuracy for the diagnosis of pneumonia.*

Intracellular Organisms

Inspection of BAL specimens for intracellular organisms can help in guiding initial antibiotic therapy until culture results are available. *When intracellular organisms are present in more than 3% of the cells in the lavage fluid, the likelihood of pneumonia is over 90%* (25). This is not done on a routine Gram's stain, but requires special processing and staining, and will require a specific request of the microbiology lab.

BAL Without Bronchoscopy

BAL can also be performed without the aid of bronchoscopy using a sheathed catheter like the one illustrated in Figure 29.6. This catheter (COMBICATH,, KOL Bio-Medical, Chantilly, VA) is inserted through a tracheal tube and advanced "blindly" until it wedges in a distal airway. An absorbable polyethylene plug at the tip of the catheter prevents contamination while the catheter is advanced. Once wedged, an inner cannula is advanced for the BAL, which is performed with 20 mL of sterile saline. Only 1 mL of BAL aspirate is required for culture and microscopic analysis.

Nonbronchoscopic BAL (also called mini-BAL because of the lower lavage volume) is a safe procedure that can be performed by respiratory

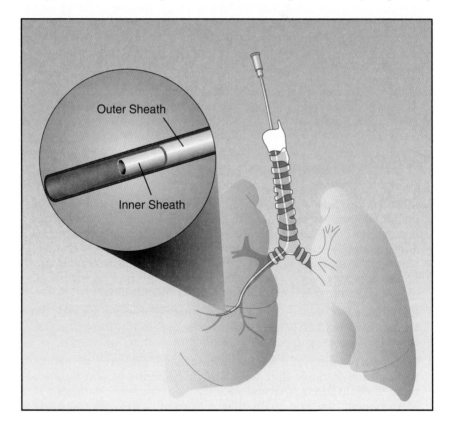

FIGURE 29.6 Protected catheter for performing bronchoalveolar lavage without the aid of bronchoscopy. See text for explanation.

therapists (26). Despite the uncertainty regarding the location of the catheter tip in relation to the region of suspected infection, the yield from quantitative cultures with mini-BAL is equivalent to the yield with bronchoscopic BAL (2,27).

Protected Specimen Brush

Aspiration of secretions through a bronchoscope produces false-positive cultures because of contamination as the bronchoscope is advanced through the tracheal tubes and upper respiratory tract (23). To eliminate this problem, a specialized brush called a *protected specimen brush* (PSB) was developed to collect uncontaminated secretions from the distal airways during bronchoscopy. The catheter design for the PSB is similar to the catheter design in Figure 29.6, and the brush is advanced from the inner cannula to collect samples from the distal airways.

Quantitative Cultures

The threshold for the diagnosis of VAP with PSB cultures is 10^3 CFU/mL (1,2), and the yield from PSB cultures is shown in Table 29.3 (2). A positive culture result has a low sensitivity (66%) but a high specificity (90%) for the diagnosis of VAP. Therefore, *a negative PSB culture does not exclude VAP, but a positive PSB culture is considered evidence of VAP.*

Which Method Is Preferred?

Despite the recommendations in clinical practice guidelines, there is little agreement about which microbiological method to use for the diagnosis of VAP, and qualitative cultures of tracheal aspirates continues to be popular. The following recommendations deserve mention.

1. The diagnostic yield from all culture methods is adversely affected by ongoing antibiotic therapy (2). Therefore, when possible, cultures should be obtained before antibiotics are started.

2. Most studies show that the mortality in VAP is not influenced by the microbiological method used to identify infection (2,28), and this observation is used to support the continued use of tracheal aspirates and qualitative cultures in the evaluation of VAP. However, there may be little mortality directly attributable to VAP, as mentioned earlier, so this observation may not be relevant to the selection of an appropriate microbiological method for the diagnosis of VAP.

3. If tracheal aspirates are used for the evaluation of suspected VAP, the specimens should be screened by microscopic examination and discarded if there is evidence of contamination with mouth secretions.

4. Quantitative cultures of tracheal aspirates are preferred to qualitative cultures because they have a higher specificity, and thus are more likely to detect VAP and identify the responsible pathogen(s). Management based on qualitative cultures of tracheal aspirates will result in the excessive use of antibiotics.

5. Non-bronchoscopic BAL provides a safe and relatively effective method of detecting VAP and identifying the responsible pathogen(s).

PARAPNEUMONIC EFFUSIONS

Pleural effusions are present in up to 50% of bacterial pneumonias (29), and these *parapneumonic effusions* typically do not require an intervention unless the conditions described next are indentified.

Indications for Thoracentesis

The typical indications for evaluation of a parapneumonic effusion include the following:

1. The effusion is large or increasing in size.
2. There is an air-fluid level in the effusion or a hydropneumothorax (indicating a bronchopleural fistula and possible empyema).
3. The patient develops severe sepsis or septic shock.
4. The patient is not responding to antimicrobial therapy.

Evaluation of the pleural fluid should focus on appropriate stains and cultures in addition to a cell count, glucose level, and pH. Tests to identify an exudate or transudate are not necessary as these will not help to identify an infection.

Indications for Drainage

The indications for immediate drainage of a parapneumonic effusion include the following:

1. Evidence of a bronchopleural air leak (i.e., hydropneumothorax).
2. Grossly purulent pleural aspirate.
3. Pleural fluid pH < 7.0
4. Pleural fluid glucose < 40 mg/dL (< 2.4 µmol/L).

Complicated parapneumonic effusions (i.e., a positive pleural fluid culture without evidence of an empyema) do not necessarily require drainage unless the patient's condition does not improve or deteriorates on antimicrobial therapy.

ANTIMICROBIAL THERAPY

Antimicrobial therapy for pneumonia accounts for half of all antibiotic use in the ICU, and 60% of this antibiotic use is for suspected pneumonias that are not confirmed by bacteriologic studies (30). The aggressive use of antibiotics in cases of suspected VAP is fueled by studies showing that the mortality rate in VAP is increased by delays in initiating appropriate antibiotic therapy (31). However, there is a paucity of strong evidence directly linking VAP with fatal outcomes (4,6), and several studies show no direct relationship between VAP and mortality rate (7–9). (See the last section of this chapter for a comment on this situation.)

Empiric Antibiotic Therapy

Empiric antimicrobial therapy for VAP should include coverage for Gram-negative aerobic bacilli and *Staphylococcus aureus* (i.e., the principal pathogens listed in Table 29.1), unless the results of a sputum Gram stain or BAL specimen indicates one prominent type of organism. Accepted regimens include *pipericillin/tazobactam or a carbepenem* (imipenem or meropenem) *or antipseudomonal cephalosporin* (ceftazidime or cefepime) plus vancomycin or linezolid (2). (See Chapter 52 for recommended dosing regimens for these antibiotics).

There is a tendency to continue empiric antibiotics despite negative culture results if patients are improving, but this is not justified unless there is some other evidence of a treatable infection (e.g., a sputum Gram stain showing a dense population of organisms) (32).

Treatment of Documented Pneumonia

Antibiotic therapy of documented VAP will be dictated by the responsible pathogen(s) and by the antibiotic susceptibilities of pathogenic organisms in your hospital (i.e., the antibiogram).

Duration of Antibiotic Therapy

The traditional duration of antibiotic therapy for VAP has been 14 to 21 days (2). However, there is evidence that 8 days of antibiotic therapy for VAP is as effective as 15 days of therapy (33), and the popular opinion now is that *one week of antibiotic therapy is adequate for most patients with VAP.*

A FINAL WORD

The paucity of evidence directly linking ventilator-associated pneumonias with a mortality rate (4,6–9) suggests one or more of the following scenarios:

1. We're really good at treating ventilator-associated pneumonias.
2. Ventilator-associated pneumonias are not life-threatening infections.
3. Ventilator-associated pneumonias are overdiagnosed, and many cases represent colonization or tracheobronchitis.

The first scenario seems unlikely, and the second scenario is the accepted choice, but it is very likely that the third scenario is the best answer, based on the results of the postmortem studies in Table 29.2.

REFERENCES

Clinical Practice Guidelines

1. Centers for Disease Control, National Healthcare Safety Network. Device-associated Module: Ventilator-Associated Event Protocol. January 2013. Available on the National Healthcare Safety Network website (www.cdc.gov/nhsn).

2. American Thoracic Society and Infectious Disease Society of America. Guidelines for the management of adults with hospital-acquired, ventilator-associated, and healthcare-associated pneumonia. Am J Respir Crit Care Med 2005; 171:388–416.

3. Muscedere J, Dodek P, Keenan S, et al. for the VAP Guidelines Committee and the Canadian Critical Care Trials Group. Comprehensive evidence-based clinical practice guidelines for ventilator-associated pneumonia: Prevention. J Crit Care 2008; 23:126–137.

General Information

4. Kollef MH. Ventilator-associated complications, including infection-related complications: The way forward. Crit Care Clin 2013; 29:33–50.

5. Vincent J-L, Rello J, Marshall J, et al. International study of the prevalence and outcomes of infection in intensive care units. JAMA 2009; 302:2323–2329.

6. Nguile-Makao M, Zahar JR, Francais A, et al. Attributable mortality of ventilator-associated pneumonia: respective impact of main characteristics at ICU admission and VAP onset using conditional logistic regression and multi-state models. Intensive Care Med 2010; 36:781–789.

7. Rello J, Quintana E, Ausina A, et al. Incidence, etiology, and outcome of nosocomial pneumonia in mechanically ventilated patients. Chest 1991; 100:439–444.

8. Papazian L, Bregeon F, Thirion X, et al. Effect of ventilator-associated pneumonia on mortality and morbidity. Am J Respir Crit Care 1996; 154:91–97.

9. Bregeon F, Cias V, Carret V, et al. Is ventilator-associated pneumonia an independent risk factor for death? Anesthesiology 2001; 94:554–560.

Preventive Measures

10. Estes RJ, Meduri GU. The pathogenesis of ventilator-associated pneumonia: I. Mechanisms of bacterial transcolonization and airway inoculation. Intensive Care Med 1995; 21:365–383.

11. AARC Clinical Practice Guideline. Endotracheal suctioning of mechanically ventilated patients with artificial airways 2010. Respir Care 2010; 55:758–764.

12. Elpern EH, Scott MG, Petro L, Ries MH. Pulmonary aspiration in mechanically ventilated patients with tracheostomies. Chest 1994; 105:563–566.

13. Muscedere J, Rewa O, Mckechnie K, et al. Subglottic secretion drainage for the prevention of ventilator-associated pneumonia: a systematic review and meta-analysis. Crit Care Med 2011; 39:1985–1991.

Clinical Features

14. Wunderink RG. Clinical criteria in the diagnosis of ventilator-associated pneumonia. Chest 2000; 117:191S–194S.

15. Fagon JY, Chastre J, Hance AJ, et al. Detection of nosocomial lung infection in ventilated patients: use of a protected specimen brush and quantitative culture techniques in 147 patients. Am Rev Respir Dis 1988; 138:110–116.

16. Timsit JF. Misset B, Goldstein FW, et al. Reappraisal of distal diagnostic testing in the diagnosis of ICU-acquired pneumonia. Chest 1995; 108:1632–1639.

17. Louthan FB, Meduri GU. Differential diagnosis of fever and pulmonary densities in mechanically ventilated patients. Semin Resp Infect 1996; 11:77–95.

18. Singh N, Falestiny MN, Rogers P, et al. Pulmonary infiltrates in the surgical ICU. Chest 1998; 114:1129–1136.

Microbiological Evaluation

19. Luna CM, Videla A, Mattera J, et al. Blood cultures have limited value in predicting severity of illness and as a diagnostic tool in ventilator-associated pneumonia. Chest 1999; 116:1075–1084.

20. Rankin JA, Marcy T, Rochester CL, et al. Human airway macrophages. Am Rev Respir Dis 1992; 145:928–933.

21. Wong LK, Barry AL, Horgan S. Comparison of six different criteria for judging the acceptability of sputum specimens. J Clin Microbiol 1982; 16:627–631.

22. Cook D, Mandell L. Endotracheal aspiration in the diagnosis of ventilator-associated pneumonia. Chest 2000; 117:195S–197S.

23. Meduri GU, Chastre J. The standardization of bronchoscopic techniques for ventilator-associated pneumonia. Chest 1992; 102:557S–564S.

24. Torres A, El-Ebiary M. Bronchoscopic BAL in the diagnosis of ventilator-associated pneumonia. Chest 2000; 117:198S–202S.

25. Veber B, Souweine B, Gachot B, et al. Comparison of direct examination of three types of bronchoscopy specimens used to diagnose nosocomial pneumonia. Crit Care Med 2000; 28:962–968.

26. Kollef MH, Bock KR, Richards RD, Hearns ML. The safety and diagnostic accuracy of minibronchoalveolar lavage in patients with suspected ventilator-associated pneumonia. Ann Intern Med 1995; 122:743–748.

27. Campbell CD, Jr. Blinded invasive diagnostic procedures in ventilator-associated pneumonia. Chest 2000; 117:207S–211S.

28. Shorr AF, Sherner JH, Jackson WL, Kollef MH. Invasive approaches to the diagnosis of ventilator-associated pneumonia: a meta-analysis. Crit Care Med 2005; 33:46–53.

29. Light RW, Meyer RD, Sahn SA, et al. Parapneumonic effusions and empyema. Clin Chest Med 1985; 6:55–62.

Antimicrobial Therapy

30. Bergmanns DCJJ, Bonten MJM, Gaillard CA, et al. Indications for antibiotic use in ICU patients: a one-year prospective surveillance. J Antimicrob Chemother 1997; 111:676–685.

31. Iregui M, Ward S, Sherman G, et al. Clinical importance of delays in the initiation of appropriate antibiotic treatment for ventilator-associated pneumonia. Chest 2002; 122:262–268.

32. Singh N, Rogers P, Atwood CW, et al. Short-course empiric antibiotic therapy for patients with pulmonary infiltrates in the intensive care unit. Am J Respir Crit Care Med 2000; 162:505–511.

33. Chastre J, Wolff M, Fagon J-Y, et al. Comparison of 8 vs. 15 days of antibiotic therapy for ventilator-associated pneumonia in adults. JAMA 2003; 290:2588–2598.

Chapter 30

DISCONTINUING MECHANICAL VENTILATION

See, and then reason and compare and control.
But see first.

Sir William Osler

Discontinuing mechanical ventilation (also known as *weaning* from mechanical ventilation) is a rapid and uneventful affair for most patients, but for one of every four or five patients, the transition from mechanical ventilation to unassisted breathing is a prolonged process that can consume almost half of the time spent on a ventilator. This chapter describes the process of removing patients from mechanical ventilation, and the difficulties that can occur in the transition to unassisted breathing (1–4).

PRELIMINARY CONCERNS

Ventilatory Support Strategies

The duration of mechanical ventilation is primarily determined by the severity of the cardiopulmonary disorder that is responsible for the ventilatory support. The measures described in this section can also contribute to shorter stays on the ventilator by facilitating the attempts to discontinue mechanical ventilation when the time arises.

Patient-Triggered Ventilation

Although the diaphragm is an involuntary muscle that contracts automatically with each lung inflation, mechanical ventilation "unloads" the diaphragm and can promote diaphragm weakness (5). This *ventilator-induced diaphragm dysfunction* is particularly prominent when contrac-

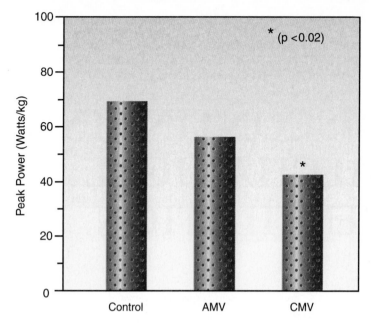

FIGURE 30.1 The power of diaphragmatic contractions (equivalent to the product of contractile force and velocity) during spontaneous breathing (control) and after 3 days of assisted (i.e., patient-triggered) mechanical ventilation (AMV) or controlled mechanical ventilation (CMV). Note that CMV (but not AMV) was associated with a significant reduction in the power output of the diaphragm. Data from Reference 5.

tions of the diaphragm are suppressed (e.g., during controlled mechanical ventilation), and is attenuated when the diaphragm is allowed to contract and initiate a ventilator breath (i.e., during patient-triggered ventilation). This is demonstrated in Figure 30.1, which shows that controlled ventilation (where diaphragmatic contractions are suppressed) is associated with a significant ($\sim 40\%$) reduction in the power output of the diaphragm, while assisted mechanical ventilation (where the diaphragm is allowed to initiate the ventilator breath) is associated with a much smaller and non-significant ($\sim 20\%$) decrement in diaphragmatic power (6).

Observations like those in Figure 30.1 indicate that allowing patients to trigger ventilator breaths (e.g., by avoiding controlled ventilation and neuromuscular paralysis) will help to preserve the strength of the diaphragm, and this should facilitate the transition from ventilatory support to spontaneous breathing. (The role of diaphragm weakness in weaning from the ventilator is described later in the chapter.)

Physical Rehabilitation

Prolonged bed rest and physical inactivity during mechanical ventilation often leads to deconditioning and generalized muscle weakness, and this is considered a contributing factor in ventilator-dependent patients who have difficulty in the transition to unassisted breathing. Supporting this contention are studies showing that early physical rehabilitation, including ambulation, is associated with a shorter duration of mechanical ventilation (7). Therefore, early and regular physical rehabilitation (including ambulation in patients who are awake and hemodynamically stable) is encouraged in selected patients to facilitate the transition to spontaneous breathing.

Sedation Practices

Several studies have shown that both deep sedation (where the patient is not arousable) and sustained use of benzodiazepines (midazolam and lorazepam) for sedation are associated with delays in discontinuing mechanical ventilation (8). As a result of these studies, the most recent guidelines on sedation in ventilator-dependent patients (8) include the following recommendations:

1. Maintain a light level of sedation, where patients are easily aroused.
2. Avoid or minimize the use of benzodiazepines for sedation. Non-benzodiazepine sedatives include propofol and dexmedetomidine, which are described in Chapter 51.

Table 30.1	Checklist for Identifying Candidates for a Trial of Spontaneous Breathing

Respiratory Criteria:
- ☑ PaO_2/FIO_2 >150–200 mm Hg with FIO_2 ≤50% and PEEP ≤8 cm H_2O.
- ☑ $PaCO_2$ normal or at baseline levels.
- ☑ Patient is able to initiate an inspiratory effort.

Cardiovascular Criteria:
- ☑ No evidence of myocardial ischemia.
- ☑ Heart rate ≤140 beats/minute.
- ☑ Blood presure adequate with minimal or no vasopressors.

Appropriate Mental Status:
- ☑ Patient is arousable, or Glasgow Coma Score ≥13.

Absence of Correctible Comorbid Conditions:
- ☑ No fever.
- ☑ No significant electrolyte abnormalities.

From References 1 and 2.

Readiness Criteria

The management of ventilator-dependent patients requires constant vigilance for signs that ventilatory support may no longer be necessary. These signs are listed in Table 30.1. Candidates for possible removal of mechanical ventilation should have adequate gas exchange in the lungs (i.e., $PaO_2/FiO_2 > 150-200$ mm Hg and a normal or baseline arterial PCO_2) while breathing non-toxic concentrations of oxygen ($FiO_2 < 50\%$) and at low levels of PEEP (< 8 cm H_2O). In addition, there should be no evidence of myocardial ischemia, severe tachycardia (> 140 beats/min), circulatory shock, or ongoing sepsis (e.g., fever).

When the criteria in Table 30.1 have been satisfied, the patient should be removed from the ventilator briefly to obtain the measurements listed in Table 30.2. These measurements (which are called "weaning parameters") are used to predict the likelihood of success or failure during a trial of spontaneous or unassisted breathing. However, as indicated by the range of likelihood ratios, each of these parameters can be a poor predictor of success or failure in individual patients. (Monitoring serial changes in these parameters during a trial of spontaneous breathing may have a greater predictive value than measurements obtained immediately after removing ventilatory support) (9). Because of the variable predictive value of the weaning parameters in Table 30.2, the emerging consensus is that *trials of spontaneous breathing can begin when the readiness criteria in Table 30.1 are satisfied.*

Table 30.2	Measurements Used to Predict a Successful Trial of Spontaneous Breathing	
Measurement[†]	**Threshold for Success**	**Range of Likelihood Ratios**[§]
Tidal Volume (V$_T$)	4 – 6 mL/kg	0.7 – 3.8
Respiratory Rate (RR)	30 – 38 bpm	1.0 – 3.8
RR/V$_T$ Ratio	60 – 105 bpm/L	0.8 – 4.7
Maximum Inspiratory Pressure (PI$_{max}$)	-15 to -30 cm H_2O	1.0 – 3.0

[†]All measurements should be obtained during the first 1–2 minutes of spontaneous breathing.

[§]The likelihood ratio is the likelihood that the measurement will predict success, divided by the likelihood that the measurement will predict failure. From Reference 2.

THE SPONTANEOUS BREATHING TRIAL

The traditional approach to discontinuing mechanical ventilation emphasized a gradual reduction in ventilatory support (over hours to days), and this created unnecessary delays in removing ventilatory support for patients who were capable of unassisted breathing. (This delayed approach is still evident in the practice of placing patients back on a ventilator at night to "rest them".) In contrast, spontaneous breathing trials (SBTs) are conducted with no ventilatory support, so that patients capable of unassisted breathing can be identified quickly. There are two methods of conducting an SBT, as described next.

Using the Ventilator Circuit

SBTs are often conducted while the patient breathes through the ventilator circuit. The advantage of this method is the ability to monitor the tidal volume (V_T) and respiratory rate (RR), since rapid, shallow breathing (indicated by an increase in the RR/V_T ratio) is a common breathing pattern in patients who fail the SBT (9). The drawback of this method is the resistance to breathing through the ventilator circuit, which can increase the work of breathing (particularly in patients who are breathing rapidly).

Pressure Support

To counteract the resistance to breathing through the ventilator circuit, low levels of pressure support (5 cm H_2O) are routinely used when SBTs are conducted through the ventilator circuit. (For a description of pressure support, see pages 511–512.) However, as demonstrated in Figure 30.2, the use of *pressure support results in only a small and insignificant decrease in the work of breathing* (10). These results suggest that the benefit of low-level pressure support is minimal, and clinically irrelevant.

Disconnecting the Ventilator

SBTs can also be conducted when the patient is disconnected from the

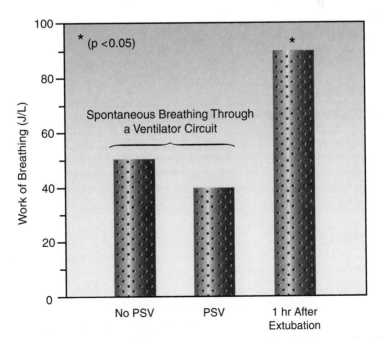

FIGURE 30.2 The work of breathing (in joules per liter) during spontaneous breathing trials conducted with and without the aid of pressure support ventilation (PSV) at 5 cm H_2O, and one hour after extubation. The asterisk indicates a significant difference at the $p = 0.05$ level. Data from Reference 10.

ventilator, using the simple circuit design illustrated in Figure 30.3. A source of O_2 (usually from a wall outlet) is delivered to the patient at a high flow rate (higher than the patient's inspiratory flow rate), and this not only facilitates the inhalation of O_2, it also carries exhaled CO_2 out to the atmosphere, to prevent CO_2 rebreathing. Because this circuit employs a T-shaped adapter, it is popularly known as a *T-piece* circuit.

The work of breathing is considered to be lower when breathing through a T-piece circuit compared to a ventilator circuit (although this is unproven). The major disadvantage of the T-piece circuit is the inability to monitor the respiratory rate and tidal volume.

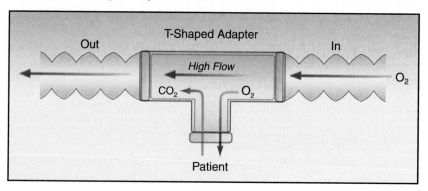

FIGURE 30.3 Simple breathing circuit for spontaneous breathing trials that are independent of the ventilator. The T-shaped adapter in the circuit is responsible for the popular term *T-piece* that is used for this circuit.

Which Method Is Preferred?

There is no clinically proven advantage with either method of SBT (3). However, the T-piece method has the following theoretical advantages: (a) it is better suited for patients with increased ventilatory demands (which is a common cause of difficulty during an SBT), and (b) it is a closer approximation of the normal conditions for breathing than breathing through a ventilator circuit with low-level pressure support as an adjunct.

Success vs. Failure

Success or failure of a trial of unassisted breathing is judged by one or more of the following parameters:

1. Signs of respiratory distress; e.g., agitation, diaphoresis, rapid breathing, and use of accessory muscles of respiration.

2. Signs of respiratory muscle weakness; e.g., paradoxical inward movement of the abdominal wall during inspiration.

3. Adequacy of gas exchange in the lungs; e.g., arterial O_2 saturation, PaO_2/FiO_2 ratio, arterial PCO_2, and gradient between end-tidal and arterial PCO_2.

4. Adequacy of systemic oxygenation; e.g., central venous O_2 saturation.

A majority of patients (~ 80%) who tolerate SBTs for 2 hours can be permanently removed from the ventilator (1,2). For patients with prolonged periods of ventilator dependence (e.g., 3 or more weeks), longer trials of spontaneous breathing may be necessary before claiming success. For patients who fail initial attempts at unassisted breathing, daily SBTs are advised to insure timely removal of ventilatory support.

Rapid Breathing

Rapid breathing during SBTs may be the result of breathlessness (dyspnea) provoked by anxiety rather than ventilatory failure (12). Monitoring the tidal volume can be useful in distinguishing anxiety from ventilatory failure; i.e., anxiety produces hyperventilation, where the respiratory rate and tidal volume are both increased, whereas ventilatory failure usually produces rapid and shallow breathing, where the respiratory rate is increased but the tidal volume is decreased. Therefore, *for the patient who develops rapid respirations during a trial of unassisted breathing, an increased tidal volume suggests anxiety as the underlying problem, while a decreased tidal volume suggests ventilatory failure.* Worsening of gas exchange may not distinguish between anxiety and ventilatory failure for the reasons described next.

Adverse Effects

Regardless of the cause, rapid breathing during SBTs can be detrimental in several ways, as summarized below.

1. In patients with asthma and COPD, rapid breathing promotes hyperinflation and intrinsic PEEP, which can: (a) decrease the cardiac output, (b) increase dead space ventilation, (c) decrease lung compliance, and (d) produce diaphragm dysfunction by flattening the diaphragm.

2. For patients with infiltrative lung disease (e.g., ARDS), rapid breathing reduces ventilation in diseased lung regions (where time constants for alveolar ventilation are prolonged), and this promotes alveolar collapse and hypoxemia.

3. For all patients with acute respiratory failure, rapid breathing can increase whole-body O_2 consumption, which places an added burden on systemic O_2 transport.

Management

If ventilatory failure is suspected as the cause of rapid breathing, the patient should be placed back on the ventilator. If anxiety is suspected as the culprit, administration of a sedative drug should be considered. Opiates may be preferred in this situation because they are particularly effective in curbing the sensation of dyspnea (13). Despite the fear of opiate use in patients with COPD, these drugs have been used safely for relief of dyspnea in patients with severe or end-stage COPD (13).

A failed trial of spontaneous breathing is usually a sign that the pathologic condition requiring ventilatory support needs further improvement. However, there are other conditions that create difficulties in discontinuing mechanical ventilation, and the principal ones are described next.

Cardiac Dysfunction

Cardiac dysfunction can develop during a trial of spontaneous breathing, and this condition has been identified in 40% of failed weaning trials (14). Potential sources of cardiac dysfunction in this situation include: (a) negative intrathoracic pressures, which increase left ventricular afterload (see pages 159–161), (b) hyperinflation and intrinsic PEEP, which impair venous return and restrict ventricular distensibility, and (c) silent myocardial ischemia (15). The adverse effects of cardiac dysfunction include pulmonary congestion, and a decrease in the contractile strength of the diaphragm (16). This latter effect is explained by the fact that the diaphragm (like the heart) maximally extracts O_2 under normal conditions, and thus is highly dependent on the cardiac output for its O_2 supply.

Monitoring

The following approaches can be used to detect cardiac dysfunction in patients who fail repeated attempts at discontinuing mechanical ventilation.

CARDIAC ULTRASOUND: Cardiac ultrasound is the most useful tool for detecting changes in systolic and diastolic function during failed trials of unassisted breathing. In fact, cardiac ultrasound is responsible for the recent discovery that diastolic dysfunction is a major determinant in the inability to wean from mechanical ventilation (17).

CENTRAL VENOUS O_2 SATURATION: A decrease in cardiac output is accompanied by a compensatory increase in peripheral O_2 extraction and a subsequent decrease in venous O_2 saturation. (See pages 183–184 for a description of the factors that influence venous O_2 saturation.) Therefore, a decrease in central venous O_2 saturation ($ScvO_2$) during a failed SBT could signal the appearance of cardiac dysfunction. The changes in mixed venous O_2 saturation (SvO_2) during successful and failed trials of spontaneous breathing are shown in Figure 30.4 (18). The SvO_2 decreased during the failed trials but not during the successful trials, suggesting that cardiac dysfunction may be responsible for the failure to sustain spontaneous breathing. The $ScvO_2$ mimics the behavior of the SvO_2, and is more easily obtained (see pages 183–184).

B-TYPE NATRIURETIC PEPTIDE: Clinical studies have shown that plasma levels of B-type natriuretic peptides are significantly increased when cardiac dysfunction develops during a trial of spontaneous breathing (14, 19). Therefore, it is possible that serial measurements of B-type natriuretic peptides can provide a simple and noninvasive method for detecting cardiac dysfunction during failed trials of spontaneous breathing. (See pages 242–243 for more information the use of B-type natriuretic peptides as biomarkers for heart failure.)

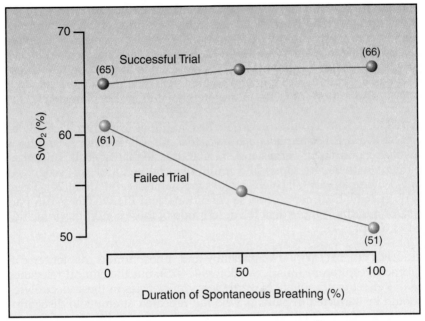

FIGURE 30.4 Mixed venous O_2 saturation (SvO_2) during successful and failed trials of spontaneous breathing. Data from Reference 17.

Management

There is surprisingly little information on methods for correcting the cardiac dysfunction that develops during spontaneous breathing trials. Patients who develop systolic dysfunction should benefit from *continuous positive airway pressure* (CPAP), which promotes cardiac output by cancelling the afterload-increasing effect of negative intrathoracic pressure (20,21). Since CPAP is delivered noninvasively, it will not prevent the removal of mechanical ventilation, including extubation.

Respiratory Muscle Weakness

Respiratory muscle weakness is always near the top of the list for potential causes of difficulty in removing ventilatory support. However, the role of respiratory muscle weakness in difficult-to-wean patients is not clear. The following are some potential sources of respiratory muscle weakness in ventilator-dependent patients.

Potential Sources

MECHANICAL VENTILATION: As mentioned earlier (and shown in Figure 30.1), mechanical ventilation is a recognized cause of diaphragm weakness (5), primarily when patients are not allowed to trigger a ventilator breath (6). However, the perception that ventilator-associated diaphragm weakness can be a source of failed SBTs is not supported by a clinical study showing that the strength of the diaphragm can actually *increase* during failed trials of spontaneous breathing (22). Furthermore, the notion that diaphragm weakness can be a source of inadequate ventilation is not supported by observations in *patients who lack functioning diaphragms* (from paralysis or injury), who *show no evidence of inadequate ventilation*, and have normal levels O_2 and CO_2 in their blood (23). These findings indicate that diaphragm weakness is not deserving of its reputation as an important factor in prolonging ventilator dependency.

CRITICAL ILLNESS NEUROMYOPATHY: The conditions known collectively as *critical illness polyneuropathy and myopathy* are inflammatory conditions involving peripheral nerves and skeletal muscle that typically appear in patients with severe sepsis and multiorgan failure, and are recognized only when patients fail to wean from mechanical ventilation (24). There is no specific treatment for these conditions, and the weakness can persist for months. A more detailed description of these conditions is included in Chapter 45.

ELECTROLYTE DEPLETION: Magnesium and phosphorous depletion can promote respiratory muscle weakness (24,25), but the clinical relevance of this effect is unproven. Nevertheless, deficiencies in these electrolytes should be corrected in patients who fail repeated attempts to discontinue mechanical ventilation.

Monitoring

Uncertainty about the role of respiratory muscle weakness in failure to remove ventilatory support is partly a reflection of the lack of reliable and readily obtained measures of respiratory muscle strength.

MAXIMUM INSPIRATORY PRESSURE: The standard clinical measure of respiratory muscle strength is the *maximum inspiratory pressure* (PI_{max}), which is the negative pressure that is generated by a maximum inspiratory effort against a closed airway (27,28). The normal values of PI_{max} vary widely, but mean values of -120 cm H_2O and -84 cm H_2O have been reported for adult men and women, respectively (28). Ventilation at rest is threatened when the PI_{max} drops to -15 to -30 cm H_2O, which are the threshold values for predicting successful trials of spontaneous breathing (see Table 30.2). Unfortunately, patients with acute respiratory failure have difficulty performing the maneuvers involved in the measurement of PI_{max}. As a result, the PI_{max} is not measured regularly in patients who require ventilatory support.

ULTRASOUND: Ultrasound has recently emerged as a potential method of assessing diaphragm strength. The ultrasound measures of diaphragm strength include the thickness of the diaphragm, and the length of excursion of the diaphragm during inspiration (29). In a preliminary study that used ultrasound assessments of diaphragm strength in patients who were weaned from mechanical ventilation, there was a significant correlation between failed SBTs and diaphragm weakness identified by ultrasound (29).

The reliability of ultrasound measurements for detecting diaphragm weakness is uncertain at the present time because the criteria for diaphragm weakness are arbitrary, and have not been validated. (This will require ultrasound measurements in large numbers of normal subjects to determine the range of normal measurements.)

Management

When respiratory muscle weakness is strongly suspected, trials of spontaneous breathing should continue, but should be terminated before patients show evidence of respiratory distress (to avoid aggravating the weakness). Strategies designed to promote muscle strength, such as patient-triggered ventilation and physical rehabilitation (described earlier), are considered particularly important in patients with documented muscle weakness.

EXTUBATION

Once there is evidence that mechanical ventilation is no longer necessary, the next step is to remove the artificial airway. This section focuses on removing endotracheal tubes, although some of the principles also apply to removing tracheostomy tubes. (The removal of tracheostomy tubes is a more gradual process, and often occurs after patients leave the ICU.)

Extubation should never be performed to reduce the work of breathing, because the work of breathing can actually *increase* after extubation, as demonstrated in Figure 30.2. (The increased work of breathing can be the result of an increased respiratory rate or breathing through a narrowed glottis, but it occurs in patients who tolerate extubation, so it is not always a cause for concern.) The considerations that must be addressed prior to extubation include: (a) the patient's ability to clear secretions from the airways, and (b) the risk of symptomatic laryngeal edema following extubation.

Airway Protective Reflexes

The ability to protect the airway from aspirated secretions is determined by the strength of the gag and cough reflexes. Cough strength can be assessed by holding a piece of paper 1–2 cm from the end of the endotracheal tube and asking the patient to cough. If wetness appears on the paper, the cough strength is considered adequate (30). Diminished strength or even absence of cough or gag reflexes will not necessarily prevent extubation, but will identify patients who need special precautions to prevent aspiration.

Laryngeal Edema

Upper airway obstruction from laryngeal edema is the major cause of failed extubations, and is reported in 5–22% of patients who have been intubated for longer than 36 hours (3,31,32). Contributing factors include difficult and prolonged intubation, endotracheal tube diameter, and self-extubation.

The Cuff-Leak Test

The cuff-leak test measures the volume of inhaled gas that escapes through the larynx when the cuff on the endotracheal tube is deflated. This test is designed to determine the risk of symptomatic upper airway obstruction from laryngeal edema after the endotracheal tube is removed. According to a recent analysis of the cuff leak test (33), the absence of an air leak indicates a high risk of upper airway obstruction following extubation, but the presence of an air leak does not indicate a low risk of upper airway obstruction following extubation, regardless of the volume of the leak.

The value of the cuff leak test has been debated for years, and the test is not universally accepted. Since the results of a cuff leak test do not alter patient management, including the decision to extubate, the clinical relevance of the test is unproven.

Pretreatment with Steroids?

Two clinical studies have shown that pretreatment with intravenous corticosteroids (methyl- prednisolone, 20–40 mg every 4–6 hrs) for 12 to 24 hours prior to extubation results in fewer cases of laryngeal edema and upper airway obstruction following extubation, and fewer reintubations (31,34). The results of one of these studies is shown in Figure 30.5. Steroid pretreatment in this study consisted of three doses of intravenous methylprednisolone (20 mg every 4 hours), with the first dose given 12 hours prior to a planned extubation. Note that this pretreatment was associated with about a 7-fold decrease in the incidence of symptomatic laryngeal edema following extubation, and a 50% drop in reintubation rate.

Although the use of corticosteroids for "anything that swells" is questionable (35), the results of the study shown in Figure 30.5 are compelling enough to consider a brief period (12 to 24 hrs) of corticosteroid therapy prior to planned extubations, particularly in patients who have a high risk of post-extubation laryngeal edema (e.g., from prior self-extubations). A single dose of methylprednisolone (40 mg IV) given one hour prior to extubation did not reduce the incidence of post-extubation laryngeal edema in one study (36), so there is no reason to administer steroids only at the time of extubation.

Postextubation Stridor

The first sign of a significant laryngeal obstruction may be *stridorous breathing* (noisy breathing), also called *stridor*. The sounds may be high-pitched and wheezy, or low-pitched and harsh, but they are always audible without a stethoscope, and they are always most apparent during inspiration. This inspiratory prominence is due to the extrathoracic location of laryngeal obstruction because negative intrathoracic pressures

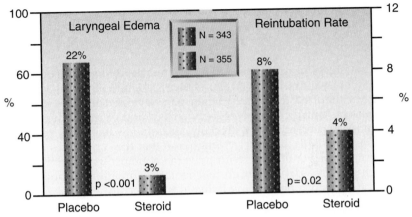

FIGURE 30.5 Results of a large, multicenter study showing the effects of pretreatment with a corticosteroid (methylprednisolone, 20 mg IV every 4 hrs for the 12 hours prior to extubation) on the incidence of post-extubation laryngeal edema and the rate of reintubation. Data from Reference 31.

generated during inspiration are transmitted to the upper airways outside the thorax, and this results in a narrowing of the extrathoracic airways during inspiration. Therefore, extrathoracic obstructions are always magnified during inspiration.

Post-extubation stridor is apparent within 30 minutes of extubation in a large majority (~80%) of cases (30), but delays in appearance of up to 2 hours can occur (personal observation). Reintubation is not always required, but close scrutiny is required because there is no proven method for reducing laryngeal edema after extubation.

Aerosolized Epinephrine

Inhalation of an epinephrine aerosol (2.5 mL of 1% epinephrine) is a popular practice for post-extubation stridor. However, while effective in children (36), this practice is unproven in adults. Aerosol therapy with a racemic mixture of epinephrine (which has equal amounts of the levo- and dextro- isomers) is also popular for post-extubation stridor, but clinical studies in children have shown no advantage with racemic epinephrine over standard (l-isomer) epinephrine (37).

Noninvasive Ventilation

Noninvasive ventilation (which is described on pages 526–531) is effective in reducing the rate of reintubation when used immediately after extubation in patients with a high risk of laryngeal edema (38), but similar success has not been demonstrated in patients who develop post-extubation respiratory failure (39). Thus, the benefit of noninvasive ventilation occurs when it is used as a preventive measure early after extubation.

A FINAL WORD

Be Vigilant

The ultimate goal of mechanical ventilation is to no longer need it, and the introductory quote by Sir William Osler is intended to emphasize that vigilance is required to identify when you have reached this goal *in a timely manner.* Vigilance involves early recognition of candidates for trials of unassisted breathing (with daily assessments using the readiness criteria in Table 30.1), and early recognition that the candidates can sustain spontaneous ventilation (with trials of spontaneous breathing). This approach will free patients from mechanical ventilation without delay, and end the misfortune of being tethered to a machine.

REFERENCES

Clinical Practice Guidelines

1. MacIntyre NR, Cook DJ, Ely EW Jr, et al. Evidence-based guidelines for weaning and discontinuing ventilatory support: a collective task force facilitated by the American College of Chest Physicians, the American Association for Respiratory Care, and the American College of Critical Care Medicine. Chest 2001; 120(Suppl):375S–395S.

Reviews

2. MacIntyre NR. Evidence-based assessments in the ventilator discontinuation process. Respir Care 2012; 57:1611–1618.

3. McConville JF, Kress JP. Weaning patients from the ventilator. New Engl J Med 2012; 367:2233–2239.

4. Thille AW, Cortes-Puch I, Esteban A. Weaning from the ventilator and extubation in ICU. Curr Opin Crit Care 2013; 19:57–64.

Preliminary Concerns

5. Petrof BJ, Jaber S, Matecki S. Ventilator-induced diaphragm dysfunction. Curr Opin Crit Care 2010; 16:19–25.

6. Sassoon CSH, Zhu E, Caiozzo VJ. Assist-control mechanical ventilation attenuates ventilator-induced diaphragm dysfunction. Am J Respir Crit Care Med 2004; 170:626–632.

7. Mendez-Tellez PA, Needham DM. Early physical rehabilitation in the ICU and ventilator liberation. Respir Care 2012; 57:1663–1669.

8. Barr J, Fraser GL, Puntillo K, et al. Clinical practice guidelines for the management of pain, agitatiom, and delirium in adult patients in the intensive care unit. Crit Care Med 2013; 41:263–306.

9. Kreiger BP, Isber J, Breitenbucher A, et al. Serial measurements of the rapid-shallow breathing index as a predictor of weaning outcome in elderly medica l patients. Chest 1997; 112:1029–1034.

Spontaneous Breathing Trials

10. Mehta S, Nelson DL, Klinger JR, et al. Prediction of post-extubation work of breathing. Crit Care Med 2000; 28:1341–1346.

11. Ely W, Baker AM, Dunagen DP, et al. Effect of duration of mechanical ventilation of identifying patients capable of breathing spontaneously. N Engl J Med 1996; 335:1864–1869.

12. Bouley GH, Froman R, Shah H. The experience of dyspnea during weaning. Heart Lung 1992; 21:471–476.

13. Raghavan N, Webb K, Amornputtisathaporn N, O'Donnell DE. Recent advances in pharmacotherapy for dyspnea in COPD. Curr Opin Pharmacol 2011; 11:204–210.

Failure of Spontaneous Breathing

14. Grasso S, Leone A, De Michele M, et al. Use of N-terminal pro-brain natriuretic peptide to detect acute cardiac dysfunction during weaning failure in difficult-to-wean patients with chronic obstructive pulmonary disease. Crit Care Med 2007; 35:96–105.

15. Srivastava S, Chatila W, Amoateng-Adjepong Y, et al. Myocardial ischemia and weaning failure in patients with coronary artery disease: an update. Crit Care Med 1999; 27:2109–2112.

16. Nishimura Y, Maeda H, Tanaka K, et al. Respiratory muscle strength and hemodynamics in heart failure. Chest 1994; 105:355–359.

17. Papanickolaou J, Makris D, Saranteas T, et al. New insights into weaning from mechanical ventilation: left ventricular diastolic dysfunction is a key player. Intensive Care Med 2011; 37:1976–1985.

18. Jubran A, Mathru M, Dries D, Tobin MJ. Continuous recordings of mixed venous oxygen saturation during weaning from mechanical ventilation and the ramifications thereof. Am Rev respir Crit Care Med 1998; 158:1763–1769.

19. Zapata L, Vera P, Roglan A, et al. B-type natriuretic peptides for prediction and diagnosis of weaning failure from cardiac origin. Intensive Care Med 2011; 37:477–485.

20. Naughton MT, Raman MK, Hara K, et al. Effect of continuous positive airway pressure on intrathoracic and left ventricular transmural pressures in patients with congestive heart failure. Circulation 1995; 91:1725–1731.

21. Bradley TD, Holloway BM, McLaughlin PR, et al. Cardiac output response to continuous positive airway pressure in congestive heart failure. Am Rev Respir Crit Care Med 1992; 145:377–382.

22. Swartz MA, Marino PL. Diaphragm strength during weaning from mechanical ventilation. Chest 1985; 88:736–739.

23. LaRoche CM, Carroll N, Moxham J, Green M. Clinical significance of severe isolated diaphragm weakness. Am Rev Respir Dis 1988; 138:862–866.

24. Hudson LD, Lee CM. Neuromuscular sequelae of critical illness. N Engl J Med 2003; 348:745–747.

25. Benotti PN, Bistrian B. Metabolic and nutritional aspects of weaning from mechanical ventilation. Crit Care Med 1989; 17:181–185.

26. Malloy DW, Dhingra S, Solren F, et al. Hypomagnesemia and respiratory muscle power. Am Rev Respir Dis 1984; 129:427–431.

27. Mier-Jedrzejowicz A, Brophy C, Moxham J, Geen M. Assessment of diaphragm weakness. Am Rev Respir Dis 1988; 137:877–883.

28. Bruschi C, Cerveri I, Zoia MC. et al. Reference values for maximum respiratory mouth pressures: A population-based study. Am Rev respir Dis 1992; 146:790–793.

29. Kim WY, Suh HJ, Hong S-S, et al. Diaphragm dysfunction assessed by ultrasonography: Influence on weaning from mechanical ventilation. Crit Care Med 2011; 39:2627–2630.

Extubation

30. Khamiees M, Raju P, DeGirolamo A, et al. Predictors of extubation outcome in patients who have successfully completed a spontaneous breathing trial. Chest 2001; 120:1262–1270.

31. François B, Bellisant E, Gissot V, et al, for the Association des Réanimateurs du Centre-Quest (ARCO). 12-h pretreatment with methylprednisolone versus placebo for prevention of postextubation laryngeal oedema: a randomized double-blind trial. Lancet 2007; 369:1083–1089.

32. Jaber S, Chanques G, Matecki S, et al. Post-extubation stridor in intensive care unit patients. Risk factors evaluation and importance of the cuff test. Intensive Care Med 2003; 29:63–74.

33. Ochoa ME, del Carmen Marín M, Frutos-Vivar F, et al. Cuff-leak test for the diagnosis of upper airway obstruction in adults: a systematic review and meta-analysis. Intensive Care Med 2009; 35:1171–1179.

34. Cheng K-C, Hou C-C, Huang H-C, et al. Intravenous injection of methylprednisolone reduces the incidence of post-extubation stridor in intensive care unit patients. Crit Care Med 2006; 34:1345–1350.

35. Shemie, S. Steroids for anything that swells: Dexamethasone and postextubation airway obstruction. Crit Care Med: 1996; 24:1613–1614.

36. Gaussorgues P, Boyer F, Piperno D, et al. Do corticosteroids prevent postintubation laryngeal edema? A prospective study of 276 adults. Crit Care Med 1988; 16:649–652.

37. Nutman J, Brooks LJ, Deakins K, et al. Racemic versus l-epinephrine aerosol in the treatment of postextubation laryngeal edema: results from a prospective, randomized, doubleblind study. Crit Care Med 1994; 22:1591–1594.

38. Nava S, Gregoretti C, Fanfulla F, et al. Noninvasive ventilation to prevent respiratory failure after extubation in high-risk patients. Crit Care Med 2005; 33:2465–2470.

39. Hess D. The role of noninvasive ventilation in the ventilator discontinuation process. Respir Care 2012; 57:1619–1625.

ACID–BASE DISORDERS

*Life is a struggle, not against sin, not against money power...
but against hydrogen ions.*

H.L. Mencken

Chapter 31

ACID-BASE ANALYSIS

Seek simplicity, and distrust it.

Alfred North Whitehead

Managing ICU patients without a working knowledge of acid-base disorders is like trying to clap your hands when you have none; i.e., it simply can't be done. This chapter presents a structured approach to the identification of acid-base disorders based on the traditional relationships between the pH, PCO_2, and bicarbonate (HCO_3) concentration in plasma. Also included is a section on the evaluation of metabolic acidosis using the anion gap and a measurement known as the "gap-gap." Alternative approaches to acid-base analysis, such as the "Stewart method," are not included here because it is unlikely, at the present time, that these methods will replace the traditional approach to acid-base analysis.

BASIC CONCEPTS

Hydrogen Ion Concentration and pH

The hydrogen ion concentration $[H^+]$ in aqueous solutions is traditionally expressed by the pH, which apparently means the *power of hydrogen*, and is a logarithmic function of the $[H^+]$; i.e.,

$$pH = \log (1/[H^+]) = - \log [H^+] \qquad (31.1)$$

The physiological range of pH and corresponding $[H^+]$ is shown in Table 31.1. The normal pH of plasma is indicated as 7.40, which corresponds to a $[H^+]$ of 40 nEq/L.

Features of the pH

The relationships in Table 31.1 illustrate 3 unfortunate features of the pH: (a) it is a dimensionless number, which has no relevance in chemical or physiological events, (b) it varies in the opposite direction to changes in [H⁺], and (c) changes in pH are not linearly related to changes in [H⁺]. Note that as the pH decreases, the changes in [H⁺] become gradually larger with each change in pH. This means that changes in pH will have different implications for acid-base balance at different points along the pH spectrum. Although it is unlikely that the pH will be abandoned, it is not a representative measure of the acid-base events in the body.

Table 31.1	pH and Hydrogen Ion Concentration		
pH	**[H⁺] (nEq/L)**	**pH**	**[H⁺] (nEq/L)**
6.9	1.26	7.4	40
7.0	100	7.5	32
7.1	80	7.6	25
7.2	64	7.7	20
7.3	50	7.8	16

Hydrogen Ions as a Trace Element

Also evident in Table 31.1 is the fact that [H⁺] is expressed as nanoequivalents per liter (nEq/L). One nanoequivalent is *one-millionth* of a milliequivalent ($1\ nEq = 1 \times 10^{-6}\ mEq$), so hydrogen ions are about a million times less dense than the principal ions in extracellular fluid (sodium and chloride), whose concentration is expressed in mEq/L. This gives hydrogen ions the status of a trace element. How can such a small quantity of an ion have all the effects attributed to acidosis and alkalosis? Other trace elements certainly have important biological effects, but it is also possible that changes in the [H⁺] are just one of several physicochemical changes that are taking place in the extracellular fluid. This would explain why the same degree of acidosis is more life-threatening in lactic acidosis than in ketoacidosis (as described in the next chapter); i.e., the acidosis is not the problem.

Classification of Acid-Base Disorders

According to traditional concepts of acid-base physiology, the [H⁺] in extracellular fluid is determined by the balance between the partial pressure of carbon dioxide (PCO_2) and the concentration of bicarbonate (HCO_3) in the fluid. This relationship is expressed as follows (1):

$$[H^+] = 24 \times (PCO_2/HCO_3) \qquad (31.2)$$

The PCO_2/HCO_3 ratio identifies the primary acid-base disorders and secondary responses, which are shown in Table 31.2.

Primary Acid-Base Disorders

According to equation 31.2, a change in either the PCO_2 or the HCO_3 will cause a change in the [H⁺] of extracellular fluid. When a change in PCO_2

is responsible for a change in [H⁺], the condition is called a *respiratory acid-base disorder*: an increase in PCO_2 is a *respiratory acidosis*, and a decrease in PCO_2 is a *respiratory alkalosis*. When a change in HCO_3 is responsible for a change in [H⁺], the condition is called a *metabolic acid-base disorder*: a decrease in HCO_3 is a *metabolic acidosis*, and an increase in HCO_3 is a *metabolic alkalosis*.

Table 31.2	Primary Acid-Base Disorders and Secondary Responses	
	$\Delta[H^+] = \Delta PCO_2 / \Delta HCO_3$	
Primary Disorder	**Primary Change**	**Secondary Response†**
Respiratory Acidosis	↑PCO_2	↑HCO_3
Respiratory Alkalosis	↓PCO_2	↓HCO_3
Metabolic Acidosis	↓HCO_3	↓PCO_2
Metabolic Alkalosis	↑HCO_3	↑PCO_2

†Secondary responses are always in the same direction as the primary change.

Secondary Responses

Secondary responses are designed to limit the change in [H⁺] produced by the primary acid-base disorder, and this is accomplished by changing the other component of the $PaCO_2/HCO_3$ ratio in the same direction. For example, if the primary problem is an increase in $PaCO_2$ (respiratory acidosis), the secondary response will involve an increase in HCO_3, and this will limit the change in [H⁺] produced by the increase in $PaCO_2$. *Secondary responses* should not be called "compensatory responses" because they *do not completely correct the change in [H⁺] produced by the primary acid-base disorder* (2). The specific features of secondary responses are described next. The equations described in the next section are included in Figure 31.1.

Responses to Metabolic Acid-Base Disorders

The response to a metabolic acid-base disorder involves a change in minute ventilation that is mediated by peripheral chemoreceptors located in the carotid body at the carotid bifurcation in the neck.

Metabolic Acidosis

The secondary response to metabolic acidosis is an increase in minute ventilation (tidal volume and respiratory rate) and a subsequent decrease in $PaCO_2$. This response appears in 30–120 minutes, and can take 12 to 24 hours to complete (2). The magnitude of the response is defined by the equation below (2).

$$\Delta PaCO_2 = 1.2 \times \Delta HCO_3 \tag{31.3}$$

Using a normal $PaCO_2$ of 40 mm Hg and a normal HCO_3 of 24 mEq/L, the above equation can be rewritten as follows:

$$\text{Expected PaCO}_2 = 40 - [1.2 \times (24 - \text{current HCO}_3)] \tag{31.4}$$

EXAMPLE: For a metabolic acidosis with a plasma HCO_3 of 14 mEq/L, the ΔHCO_3 is $24 - 14 = 10$ mEq/L, the $\Delta PaCO_2$ is $1.2 \times 10 = 12$ mm Hg, and the expected $PaCO_2$ is $40 - 12 = 28$ mm Hg. If the $PaCO_2$ is > 28 mm Hg, there is a secondary respiratory acidosis. If the $PaCO_2$ is < 28 mm Hg, there is a secondary respiratory alkalosis.

Metabolic Alkalosis

The secondary response to metabolic alkalosis is a decrease in minute ventilation and a subsequent increase in $PaCO_2$. This response is not as vigorous as the response to metabolic acidosis because the peripheral chemoreceptors are not very active under normal conditions, so they are easier to stimulate than inhibit. The magnitude of the response to metabolic alkalosis is defined by the equation below (2)

$$\Delta PaCO_2 = 0.7 \times \Delta HCO_3 \tag{31.5}$$

Using a normal $PaCO_2$ of 40 mm Hg and a normal HCO_3 of 24 mEq/L, the above equation can be rewritten as follows:

$$\text{Expected PaCO}_2 = 40 + [0.7 \times (\text{current HCO}_3 - 24)] \tag{31.6}$$

EXAMPLE: For a metabolic alkalosis with a plasma HCO_3 of 40 mEq/L, the ΔHCO_3 is $40 - 24 = 16$ mEq/L, the $\Delta PaCO_2$ is $0.7 \times 16 = 11$ mm Hg, and the expected $PaCO_2$ is $40 + 11 = 51$ mm Hg. This is only a borderline elevation in $PaCO_2$, and it demonstrates the relative weakness of the response to metabolic alkalosis.

Responses to Respiratory Acid–Base Disorders

The secondary response to changes in $PaCO_2$ occurs in the kidneys, where HCO_3 absorption in the proximal tubes is adjusted to produce the appropriate change in plasma HCO_3. This renal response is relatively slow, and can take 2 or 3 days to reach completion. Because of the delay in the secondary response, respiratory acid-base disorders are separated into acute and chronic disorders.

Acute Respiratory Disorders

Acute changes in $PaCO_2$ have a small effect on the plasma HCO_3, as indicated in the following two equations (2).

For acute respiratory acidosis:

$$\Delta HCO_3 = 0.1 \times \Delta PaCO_2 \tag{31.7}$$

For acute respiratory alkalosis:

$$\Delta HCO_3 = 0.2 \times \Delta PaCO_2 \tag{31.8}$$

EXAMPLE: For an acute increase in $PaCO_2$ to 60 mm Hg, the ΔHCO_3 is $0.1 \times 20 = 2$ mEq/L for an acute respiratory acidosis, and $0.2 \times 20 = 4$ mEq/L

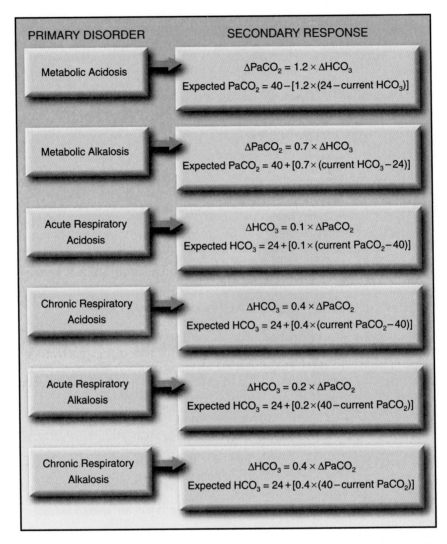

PRIMARY DISORDER	SECONDARY RESPONSE

Metabolic Acidosis

$$\Delta PaCO_2 = 1.2 \times \Delta HCO_3$$
$$\text{Expected } PaCO_2 = 40 - [1.2 \times (24 - \text{current } HCO_3)]$$

Metabolic Alkalosis

$$\Delta PaCO_2 = 0.7 \times \Delta HCO_3$$
$$\text{Expected } PaCO_2 = 40 + [0.7 \times (\text{current } HCO_3 - 24)]$$

Acute Respiratory Acidosis

$$\Delta HCO_3 = 0.1 \times \Delta PaCO_2$$
$$\text{Expected } HCO_3 = 24 + [0.1 \times (\text{current } PaCO_2 - 40)]$$

Chronic Respiratory Acidosis

$$\Delta HCO_3 = 0.4 \times \Delta PaCO_2$$
$$\text{Expected } HCO_3 = 24 + [0.4 \times (\text{current } PaCO_2 - 40)]$$

Acute Respiratory Alkalosis

$$\Delta HCO_3 = 0.2 \times \Delta PaCO_2$$
$$\text{Expected } HCO_3 = 24 + [0.2 \times (40 - \text{current } PaCO_2)]$$

Chronic Respiratory Alkalosis

$$\Delta HCO_3 = 0.4 \times \Delta PaCO_2$$
$$\text{Expected } HCO_3 = 24 + [0.4 \times (40 - \text{current } PaCO_2)]$$

FIGURE 31.1 Predictive equations for evaluating secondary responses to primary acid-base disorders. All equations are from Reference 2.

for an acute respiratory alkalosis. Neither of these changes would be recognized as significant.

Chronic Respiratory Disorders

The renal response to an increase in $PaCO_2$ is an increase in HCO_3 reabsorption in the proximal renal tubules, which raises the plasma HCO_3 concentration. The response to a decrease in $PaCO_2$ is a decrease in renal HCO_3 reabsorption, which lowers the plasma HCO_3 concentration. The magnitude of this response is similar, regardless of the directional change in $PaCO_2$, so the equation below applies to both chronic respiratory acidosis and alkalosis.

$$\Delta HCO_3 = 0.4 \times \Delta PaCO_2 \qquad (31.9)$$

Using a normal $PaCO_2$ of 40 mm Hg and a normal HCO_3 of 24 mEq/L, the above equation can be rewritten as follows:

For chronic respiratory acidosis:

$$\text{Expected } HCO_3 = 24 + [0.4 \times (\text{current } PaCO_2 - 40)] \qquad (31.10)$$

For chronic respiratory alkalosis:

$$\text{Expected } HCO_3 = 24 - [0.4 \times (40 - \text{current } PaCO_2)] \qquad (31.11)$$

EXAMPLE: For an increase in $PaCO_2$ to 60 mm Hg that persists for at least a few days, the $\Delta PaCO_2$ is $60 - 40 = 20$ mm Hg, the ΔHCO_3 is $0.4 \times 20 = 8$ mEq/L, and the expected HCO_3 is $24 + 8 = 32$ mEq/L.

STEPWISE APPROACH TO ACID-BASE ANALYSIS

The following is a structured, rule-based approach to the diagnosis of primary, secondary, and mixed acid-base disorders using the relationships between the $[H^+]$, PCO_2, and HCO_3 concentration described previously. Several examples are included as instructional aids. The reference ranges for arterial pH, PCO_2, and HCO_3 are shown below.

$$pH = 7.36 - 7.44$$
$$PCO_2 = 36 - 44 \text{ mm Hg}$$
$$HCO_3 = 22 - 26 \text{ mEq/L}$$

Stage I: Identify the Primary Acid-Base Disorder

In the first stage of the approach, the $PaCO_2$ and pH are used to identify the primary acid-base disorder.

Rule 1: If the $PaCO_2$ and/or the pH is outside the normal range, there is an acid-base disorder.

Rule 2: If the $PaCO_2$ and pH are both abnormal, compare the directional change.

   2a. If the $PaCO_2$ and pH change in the same direction, there is a primary metabolic acid-base disorder.

   2b. If the $PaCO_2$ and pH change in opposite directions, there is a primary respiratory acid-base disorder.

EXAMPLE: Consider a case where the arterial pH = 7.23 and the $PaCO_2$ = 23 mm Hg. The pH and $PaCO_2$ are both reduced (indicating a primary metabolic disorder) and the pH is low (indicating an acidosis), so the diagnosis is a primary metabolic acidosis.

Rule 3:   If only the pH or $PaCO_2$ is abnormal, the condition is a mixed metabolic and respiratory disorder (i.e., equal and opposite disorders).

   3a.   If the $PaCO_2$ is abnormal, the directional change in $PaCO_2$ identifies the type of respiratory disorder (e.g., high $PaCO_2$ indicates a respiratory acidosis), and the opposing metabolic disorder.

   3b.   If the pH is abnormal, the directional change in pH identifies the type of metabolic disorder (e.g., low pH indicates a metabolic acidosis) and the opposing respiratory disorder.

EXAMPLE: Consider a case where the arterial pH = 7.38 and the $PaCO_2$ = 55 mm Hg. Only the $PaCO_2$ is abnormal, so there is a mixed metabolic and respiratory disorder. The $PaCO_2$ is elevated, indicating a respiratory acidosis, so the metabolic disorder must be a metabolic alkalosis. Therefore, this condition is a *mixed respiratory acidosis and metabolic alkalosis.* Both disorders are equivalent in severity because the pH is normal.

Stage II: Evaluate the Secondary Responses

The second stage of the approach is for cases where a primary acid-base disorder has been identified in Stage I. (If a mixed acid-base disorder was identified in Stage I, go directly to Stage III). The goal in Stage II is to determine if there is an additional acid-base disorder.

Rule 4:   For a primary metabolic disorder, if the measured $PaCO_2$ is higher than expected, there is a secondary respiratory acidosis, and if the measured $PaCO_2$ is less than expected, there is a secondary respiratory alkalosis.

EXAMPLE: Consider a case where the $PaCO_2$ = 23 mm Hg, the pH = 7.32, and the HCO_3 = 16 mEq/L. The pH and PCO_2 change in the same direction, indicating a primary metabolic disorder, and the pH is acidemic, so the disorder is a primary metabolic acidosis. Using equations 31.3 and 31.4, the $\Delta PaCO_2$ is 1.2 × (24 − 16) = 10 mm Hg (rounded off), and the expected $PaCO_2$ is 40 − 10 = 30 mm Hg. The measured $PaCO_2$ (23 mm Hg) is lower than the expected $PaCO_2$, so there is an additional respiratory alkalosis. Therefore, this condition is a *primary metabolic acidosis with a secondary respiratory alkalosis.*

Rule 5:   For a primary respiratory disorder, a normal or near-normal HCO_3 indicates that the disorder is acute.

Rule 6:   For a primary respiratory disorder where the HCO_3 is abnormal, determine the expected HCO_3 for a chronic respiratory disorder.

   6a.   For a chronic respiratory acidosis, if the HCO_3 is lower than expected, there is an incomplete renal response, and if the HCO_3 is higher than expected, there is a secondary metabolic alkalosis.

   6b.   For a chronic respiratory alkalosis, if the HCO_3 is higher than expected, there is an incomplete renal response, and if the HCO_3 is lower than expected, there is a secondary metabolic acidosis.

EXAMPLE: Consider a case where the $PaCO_2$ = 23 mm Hg, the pH = 7.54, and the $HCO_3 = 17$ mEq/L. The $PaCO_2$ and pH change in opposite directions, indicating a primary respiratory disorder, and the pH is alkaline, so the disorder is a primary respiratory alkalosis. The HCO_3 is abnormal, indicating that this is not an acute respiratory alkalosis. Using Equations 31.9 and 31.11 for a chronic respiratory alkalosis, the ΔPCO_2 is $40 - 23 = 17$ mm Hg, the ΔHCO_3 is $0.4 \times 17 = 7$ mEq/L, and the expected HCO_3 is $24 - 7 = 17$ mEq/L. The measured HCO_3 is the same as expected for a chronic respiratory alkalosis, so this condition is a chronic respiratory alkalosis with an appropriate (completed) renal response. If the measured HCO_3 was higher than 17 mEq/L (but < 21), this condition would be a *chronic respiratory alkalosis* with an incomplete renal response, and if the measured HCO_3 was lower than 17 mEq/L, this would indicate a secondary metabolic acidosis.

Stage III: Use The "Gaps" to Evaluate a Metabolic Acidosis

The final stage of this approach is for patients with a metabolic acidosis, where the use of measurements called *gaps* can help to uncover the underlying cause of the acidosis. These are described in the next section.

THE GAPS

There are numerous potential sources of a metabolic acidosis in critically ill patients, and the measurements described in this section are designed to help in the search for the culprit.

The Anion Gap

The anion gap is a rough estimate of the relative abundance of unmeasured anions, and is used to determine if a metabolic acidosis is due to an accumulation of non-volatile acids (e.g., lactic acid) or a primary loss of bicarbonate (e.g., diarrhea) (6,7).

Determinants

To achieve electrochemical balance, the concentration of negatively charged anions must equal the concentration of positively charged cations. This electrochemical balance is expressed in the equation shown below using electrolytes that are routinely measured, including sodium (Na), chloride (CL), and bicarbonate (HCO_3), as well as the unmeasured cations (UC) and unmeasured anions (UA).

$$Na + UC = (CL + HCO_3) + UA \tag{31.12}$$

Rearranging the terms in this equation yields the following relationships:

$$Na - (CL + HCO_3) = UA - UC \tag{31.13}$$

The difference (UA − UC) is a measure of the relative abundance of unmeasured anions, and is called the *anion gap* (AG).

$$AG = Na - (CL + HCO_3) \tag{31.14}$$

REFERENCE RANGE: The original reference range for the AG was 12 ± 4 mEq/L (range = 8 to 16 mEq/L) (7). With subsequent improvements in automated systems that measure serum electrolytes, *the reference range for the AG has decreased to 7 ± 4 mEq/L* (range = 3 to 11 mEq/L) (8).

Influence of Albumin

The unmeasured anions and cations that normally contribute to the anion gap are shown in Table 31.3. Note that albumin is the principal unmeasured anion, and the principal determinant of the anion gap. Albumin is a weak (i.e., poorly dissociated) acid that contributes about 3 mEq/L to the AG for each 1 g/dL of albumin in plasma (at a normal pH) (3). A low albumin level in plasma will lower the AG, and this could mask the presence of an unmeasured anion (e.g., lactate) that is contributing to a metabolic acidosis. Since hypoalbuminemia is present in as many as 90% of ICU patients (9), the following formula for the "corrected AG" (AGc) has been proposed to include the contribution of albumin:

$$AGc = AG + 2.5 \times (4.5 - [\text{albumin in g/dL}]) \qquad (31.15)$$

(4.5 represents the normal concentration of albumin in plasma). For a patient with an AG of 10 mEq/L and a plasma albumin of 2 g/dL, the AGc is $10 + (2.5 \times 2.5) = 16$ mEq/L, which represents a 60% increase in the AG.

Table 31.3	Determinants of the Anion Gap	
Unmeasured Anions		**Unmeasured Cations**
Albumin (15 mEq/L)		Calcium (5 mEq/L)
Organic Acids (5 mEq/L)		
Phosphate (2 mEq/L)		Potassium (4.5 mEq/L)
Sulfate (1 mEq/L)		Magnesium (1.5 mEq/L)
Total UA: (23 mEq/L)		Total UC: (11 mEq/L)
Anion Gap = UA − UC = 12 mEq/L		

Using the Anion Gap

The AG can be used to identify the underlying mechanism of a metabolic acidosis, which then helps to identify the underlying clinical condition. An elevated AG occurs when there is an accumulation of fixed or nonvolatile acids (e.g., lactic acidosis), while a normal AG occurs when there is a primary loss of bicarbonate (e.g., diarrhea) (7). Table 31.4 shows the causes of metabolic acidosis grouped according to the AG.

HIGH AG: Common causes of high AG metabolic acidosis are lactic acidosis, diabetic ketoacidosis, and advanced renal failure (where there is loss of H^+ secretion in the distal tubules of the kidneys). Also included are toxic ingestions of methanol (which produces formic acid), ethylene glycol (which produces oxalic acid), and salicylates (which produce salicylic acid) (10).

Table 31.4	Classification of Metabolic Acidosis with the Anion Gap (AG)
High AG	**Normal AG**
Lactic Acidosis	Diarrhea
Ketoacidosis	Isotonic Saline Infusion
End-Stage Renal Failure	Early Renal Insufficiency
Methanol Ingestion	Renal Tubular Acidosis
Ethylene Glycol Ingestion	Acetazolamide
Salicylate Toxicity	Ureteroenterostomy

NORMAL AG: Common causes of a normal AG metabolic acidosis are diarrhea, saline infusion (see Figure 12.3), and early renal failure (where there is loss of bicarbonate reabsorption in the proximal tubules). The loss of HCO_3 is counterbalanced by a gain of chloride ions to maintain electrical charge neutrality; hence the term *hyperchloremic metabolic acidosis* is used for normal AG metabolic acidoses. (In high AG metabolic acidoses, the remaining anions from the dissociated acids balance the loss of HCO_3, so there is no associated hyperchloremia.)

RELIABILITY The AG has shown a limited ability to detect non-volatile acids, and there are several reports where the AG was normal in patients with lactic acidosis (11,12). The poor performance of the AG may be due to the confounding influence of albumin, which was not considered in early studies of the AG. A recent study shows that the albumin-corrected AG (AGc) provides a more accurate assessment of metabolic acidosis than the AG (13).

The Gap-Gap Ratio

In the presence of a high AG metabolic acidosis, it is possible to detect another metabolic acid-base disorder (a normal AG metabolic acidosis or a metabolic alkalosis) by comparing the AG excess (the difference between the measured and normal AG) to the HCO_3 deficit (the difference between the measured and normal HCO_3 in plasma). This is accomplished with the equation shown below, which includes 12 mEq/L for the normal AG and 24 mEq/L for the normal HCO_3 in plasma.

$$AG \text{ Excess}/HCO_3 \text{ Deficit} = (AG - 12)/24 - HCO_3) \qquad (31.16)$$

This ratio is sometimes called the *gap-gap ratio* because it involves two gaps (the AG excess and the HCO_3 deficit). Some applications of the gap-gap ratio are described next.

Mixed Metabolic Acidoses

In metabolic acidoses caused by non-volatile acids (high AG metabolic acidosis), the decrease in serum HCO_3 is equivalent to the increase in AG, and the gap-gap (AG Excess/HCO_3 deficit) ratio is unity or 1. However, if there is a second acidosis that has a normal AG, the decrease in HCO_3 is greater than the increase in AG, and the gap-gap ratio falls below unity (< 1). Therefore, *in the presence of a high AG metabolic acidosis, a gap-gap ratio < 1 indicates the co-existence of a normal AG (hyperchloremic) metabolic acidosis* (6,14).

DIABETIC KETOACIDOSIS: A popular question on the medicine boards is a case where the management of a patient with diabetic ketoacidosis (DKA) is associated with improvement in the blood glucose and the clinical condition of the patient, but the acidosis persists, and you are asked what to do (more insulin, more fluids, etc). The answer lies in the gap-gap ratio; i.e., DKA presents with a high AG metabolic acidosis, but the aggressive infusion of isotonic saline during the initial management creates a hyperchloremic (normal AG) metabolic acidosis, which replaces the high AG acidosis as the ketoacids are cleared. In this situation, the serum bicarbonate remains low, but the gap-gap ratio falls below 1 as the acidosis switches from a high AG to a normal AG acidosis (15). Therefore, monitoring the serum HCO_3 alone will create a false impression that the DKA is not resolving, while the gap-gap ratio provides an accurate measure of the acid-base status of the patient.

Metabolic Acidosis and Alkalosis

When alkali is added in the presence of a high AG acidosis, the decrease in serum bicarbonate is less than the increase in AG, and the gap-gap is greater than unity (> 1). Therefore, *in the presence of a high AG metabolic acidosis, a gap-gap > 1 indicates the co-existence of a metabolic alkalosis*. This is an important consideration because metabolic alkalosis is common in ICU patients (from the frequent use of nasogastric suction and diuretics).

A FINAL WORD

For more than 100 years, the evaluation of acid-base balance has been based on a single reaction sequence (which is shown below), and a single determinant of plasma pH (the PCO_2/HCO_3 ratio).

$$CO_2 + H_2O \Leftrightarrow H_2CO_3 \Leftrightarrow H^+ + HCO_3$$

This approach is appealing because of its simplicity, but as Whitehead advises in the introductory quote, the simplicity of this approach is also a reason for "distrust." The following are a few reasons to distrust the traditional view of acid-base balance.

1. The use of the PCO_2-HCO_3 relationship to identify acid-base disorders has two flaws:

   a. The PCO_2 and HCO_3 are both dependent variables, and thus it is not possible detect acid-base conditions that operate independent of these variables.

   b. Since the CO_2 in plasma is present primarily as HCO_3, it is difficult to establish an independent identity for HCO_3.

2. Bicarbonate does not act as a buffer in the physiological pH range (which is demonstrated in the next chapter). The plasma $[H^+]$ is a

function of the anionic charge equivalence of plasma proteins (which act as the buffers in plasma), and is not directly related to the plasma [HCO₃] (16).

A novel view of acid-base balance that challenges traditional concepts was introduced by Peter Stewart (a Canadian physiologist working at Brown) about 30 years ago, and I have included a textbook, and one of Stewart's original papers on the subject (17), for your interest.

REFERENCES

Books

Rose BD, Post T, Stokes J. Clinical Physiology of Acid-Base and Electrolyte Disorders. 6th ed. New York:McGraw-Hill, 2013.

Kellum JA, Elbers WG, ed. Stewart's Textbook of Acid-Base. 2nd ed. Amsterdam: AcidBase.org, 2009.

Gennari FJ, Adrogue HJ, Galla JH, Maddias N, eds. Acid-Base Disorders and Their Treatment. Boca Raton: CRC Press, 2005.

Reviews

1. Adrogue HJ, Gennari J, Gala JH, Madias NE. Assessing acid-base disorders. Kidney Int 2009; 76:1239–1247.

2. Adrogue HJ, Madias NE. Secondary responses to altered acid-base status: The rules of engagement. J Am Soc Nephrol 2010; 21:920–923.

3. Kellum JA. Disorders of acid-base balance. Crit Care Med 2007; 35:2630–2636.

4. Whittier WL, Rutecki GW. Primer on clinical acid-base problem solving. Dis Mon 2004; 50:117–162.

5. Fencl V, Leith DE. Stewart's quantitative acid-base chemistry: applications in biology and medicine. Respir Physiol 1993; 91:1–16.

6. Narins RG, Emmett M. Simple and mixed acid-base disorders: a practical approach. Medicine 1980; 59:161–187.

Selected References

7. Emmet M, Narins RG. Clinical use of the anion gap. Medicine 1977; 56:38–54.

8. Winter SD, Pearson JR, Gabow PA, et al. The fall of the serum anion gap. Arch Intern Med 1990; 150:311–313.

9. Figge J, Jabor A, Kazda A, Fencl V. Anion gap and hypoalbuminemia. Crit Care Med 1998; 26:1807–1810.

10. Judge BS. Metabolic acidosis: differentiating the causes in the poisoned patient. Med Clin N Am 2005; 89:1107–1124.

11. Iberti TS, Liebowitz AB, Papadakos PJ, et al. Low sensitivity of the anion gap as a screen to detect hyperlactatemia in critically ill patients. Crit Care Med 1990; 18:275–277.

12. Schwartz-Goldstein B, Malik AR, Sarwar A, Brandtsetter RD. Lactic acidosis associated with a normal anion gap. Heart Lung 1996; 25:79–80.

13. Mallat J, Barrailler S, Lemyze M, et al. Use of sodium chloride difference and corrected anion gap as surrogates of Stewart variables in critically ill patients. PLoS ONE 2013; 8:e56635. (Open access jounal, accessed at www.plosone.org on 4/11/2013.)

14. Haber RJ. A practical approach to acid-base disorders. West J Med 1991; 155:146–151.

15. Paulson WD. Anion gap-bicarbonate relationship in diabetic ketoacidosis. Am J Med 1986; 81:995–1000.

16. Stewart PA. Whole-body acid-base balance. In :Kellum JA, Elbers PWG, eds. Stewart's Textbook of Acid Base. 2nd ed. Amsterdam: AcidBase.org, 2009:181–197.

17. Stewart PA. Modern quantitative acid-base chemistry. Can J Physiol Pharmacol 1983; 61:1444–1461.

Chapter 32

ORGANIC ACIDOSES

It is incident to physicians, I am afraid, beyond all other men,
to mistake subsequence for consequence.

Samuel Johnson

This chapter describes the clinical conditions associated with the accumulation of organic acids; i.e., lactic acid and ketoacids (diabetic and alcoholic ketoacidosis). Also included is a presentation of the issues regarding alkali therapy for metabolic acidosis. One of the goals of this chapter is to introduce the notion that the problem with these metabolic acidoses is not the acidosis, but the metabolic derangement that produces the acidosis.

LACTIC ACIDOSIS

Lactate Metabolism

Lactate is the end-product of glucose metabolism in the cytoplasm (glycolysis), and is formed by the reduction of pyruvate in a reaction catalyzed by lactate dehydrogenase (LDH) (see Figure 32.1). About 1,500 mmoles of lactate are produced daily under aerobic conditions (1,2), and the principal sites of production are skeletal muscle (25%), skin (25%), red blood cells (20%), brain (20%), and intestine (10%). Activated neutrophils are an additional source of lactate in inflammatory conditions like acute respiratory distress syndrome (ARDS) (3,4). The concentration of lactate in plasma is usually ≤2 mmol/L, with a lactate:pyruvate ratio of 10:1 (1,2). Lactate is cleared from plasma by the liver (60%), kidneys (30%), and heart (10%).

Lactate as a Fuel

The diagram in Figure 32.1 shows the energy yield from the metabolism of glucose and lactate. Anaerobic glycolysis generates 32 kilocalories (kcal) per mole of glucose, which is only 5% of the energy yield from the oxidative metabolism of glucose (673 kcal/mole) (3). The energy deficit

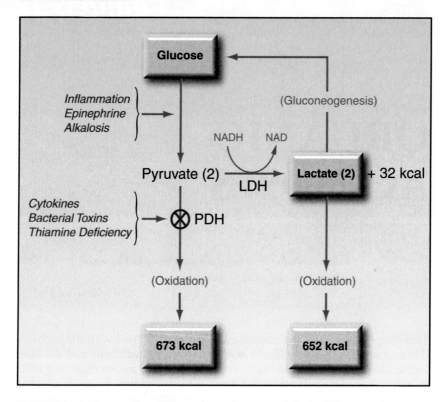

FIGURE 31.1 The energy yield from the oxidative metabolism of glucose and lactate, and the actions of selected factors that promote lactic acidosis. PDH = pyruvate dehydrogenase; LDH = lactate dehydrogenase.

from anaerobic lactate production can be corrected by the oxidative metabolism of lactate, which generates 326 kcal/mole (5), or $326 \times 2 = 652$ kcal per mole of glucose (since 1 mole of glucose produces 2 moles of lactate). In fact, lactate is classified as an organic fuel, and has a caloric density (3.62 kcal/g) equivalent to glucose (3.74 kcal/g) (5).

LACTATE SHUTTLE: Lactate is used as a fuel source during exercise (the *lactate shuttle* (6), and it is possible that lactate serves a similar function in critically ill patients (7). This is consistent with the observation that lactate uptake by the myocardium is increased in patients with septic shock (8). The possibility of a lactate shuttle in critically ill patients suggests that the enhanced production of lactate in these patients could be an adaptive response that helps to maintain energy metabolism in vital organs like the heart. This differs radically from the traditional perception of lactate as a source of fatal outcomes in critically ill patients.

Lactate as a Biomarker

The role of lactate as a biomarker is described in Chapter 10 (see pages 184–187), and is summarized in the following statements:

1. In clinical shock syndromes, the magnitude of elevation in blood lactate has a direct relationship with mortality rate, and an initial lactate level ≥ 4 mmol/L is associated with an increased mortality rate in the ensuing 72 hours (see Figure 10.6 on page 186).

2. The time required for lactate levels to return to normal (lactate clearance) has a greater prognostic value than the initial lactate level. Normalization of lactate levels within 24 hours is associated with the lowest mortality rates (see Figure 10.6 on page 186).

3. The source of elevated lactate levels in severe sepsis and septic shock is a combination of increased production of pyruvate (9) and a defect in O_2 utilization in mitochondria, called *cytopathic hypoxia* (10). The latter phenomenon may be the result of cytokine or bacterial toxin-induced inhibition of pyruvate dehydrogenase (11,12), the enzyme responsible for pyruvate entry into mitochondria (see Figure 32.1). Thus, tissue oxygenation is not impaired in severe sepsis and septic shock (see Figure 14.3 on page 269).

Lactate and Acidosis

The end-product of glycolysis is lactic acid, which acts like a strong acid (i.e., loses its H^+) in the physiological pH range, and exists as the negatively-charged lactate ion (1). *The lactate moiety released by cells is the lactate ion, not lactic acid.* So how does hyperlactatemia produce an acidosis? This cannot be explained by the traditional Brønsted-Lowry concept of acid base balance (i.e., an acid donates H^+), but can be explained using Peter Stewart's concept of the *strong ion* difference and its role in acid-base balance (13–15).

Strong Ion Difference

The strong ion difference (SID) is the difference in the summed concentrations of strong (readily dissociated) cations and anions in extracellular fluid (13,14). The strong ions in extracellular fluid are sodium (Na), chloride (CL), potassium (K), magnesium (Mg), calcium (Ca), and lactate, so the SID is determined as follows (15):

$$SID = (Na + K + Mg + Ca) - (CL + Lactate) \qquad (32.1)$$

The principle of electrical neutrality requires the following relationship between the SID and the ions that dissociate from water ($H^+ + OH^-$):

$$SID + [H^+] + [OH^-] = 0 \qquad (32.2)$$

Since OH^- has a negligible influence on $[H^+]$ in the physiological pH range, the above equation can be simplified to:

$$SID + [H^+] = 0 \text{ or } SID = - [H^+] \qquad (32.3)$$

According to this relationship, a change in SID will be accompanied by an opposite change in $[H^+]$ and, if pH is used instead of $[H^+]$, *the SID and pH will change in the same direction* (see Figure 12.4 on page 222).

Therefore, to summarize equations 32.2–32.4, an increase in the plasma lactate concentration will decrease the SID, and this will decrease the plasma pH. The SID of plasma is normally about 40 mEq/L (14).

Causes of Hyperlactatemia

Clinical Shock Syndromes

The most notable, and most feared, sources of hyperlactatemia are the *clinical shock syndromes*; i.e., hypovolemic, cardiogenic, and septic shock. Although the mechanisms for the hyperlactatemia may be different, the plasma lactate level has prognostic value in these syndromes, as mentioned previously.

Systemic Inflammatory Response Syndrome

Systemic inflammation (fever, leukocytosis, etc.) can be accompanied by mild elevations of blood lactate (2 to 5 mEq/L) with a normal lactate:pyruvate ratio and a normal plasma pH. This condition is called *stress hyperlactatemia*, and is the result of an increase in the production of pyruvate without a defect in tissue oxygenation or oxygen utilization (10). The lactate elevation in severe sepsis and septic shock is usually associated with increased lactate:pyruvate ratios and a decrease in plasma pH.

Thiamine Deficiency

The manifestations of thiamine deficiency include high-output heart failure (wet beriberi), Wernicke's encephalopathy, peripheral neuropathy (dry beriberi), and lactic acidosis. The lactic acidosis can be severe (17), and is caused by a deficiency in thiamine pyrophosphate, which serves as a co-factor for pyruvate dehydrogenase (see Figure 32.1). Thiamine deficiency may be more common than suspected in critically ill patients, and should be considered in all cases of unexplained lactic acidosis. (See Chapter 47 for a more detailed description of thiamine deficiency.)

Pharmaceutical Agents

A variety of drugs can produce hyperlactatemia, including metformin, antiretroviral agents, epinephrine, nitroprusside, and linezolid. Most cases (except epinephrine) are due to an impairment of oxidative metabolism, and can be lethal if left undetected. The hyperlactatemia produced by epinephrine is due to an increase in pyruvate production, and is not associated with a derangement in oxidative metabolism.

METFORMIN: Metformin is an oral hypoglycemic agent that can produce lactic acidosis during therapeutic dosing. The mechanism for the lactic acidosis is unclear, but it occurs primarily in patients with renal insufficiency, and has a mortality rate in excess of 45% (18,19). Plasma metformin levels are not routinely available, and the diagnosis is based on excluding other causes of lactic acidosis. The preferred treatment is hemodialysis (18,19), which removes both metformin and lactate.

ANTIRETROVIRAL AGENTS: Hyperlactatemia is reported in 8–18% of patients receiving antiretroviral therapy for HIV infection (20). The responsible drugs are the nucleoside analogues (e.g., didanosine, stavudine), and the presumed mechanism is inhibition of mitochondrial DNA polymerase (21). In most cases, the hyperlactatemia is mild and not associated with acidemia, but lactate levels above 10 mmol/L have a reported mortality rate of 33–57% (21).

LINEZOLID: Lactic acidosis has been reported during therapy with linezolid (22,23). Most cases are mild and without adverse consequences, but lactate levels as high as 10 mmol/L have been reported (23). The mechanism is unknown, and lactate levels normalize after discontinuing the drug.

Non-Pharmaceutical Toxidromes

Lactic acidosis can be the result of intoxications with cyanide, carbon monoxide, and propylene glycol. The latter agent is used as a solvent for intravenous drugs, and can be overlooked as a cause of lactic acidosis.

PROPYLENE GLYCOL: The intravenous drugs that use propylene glycol as a solvent include lorazepam, diazepam, esmolol, nitroglycerin, and phenytoin. About 55–75% of propylene glycol is metabolized by the liver and the primary metabolites are lactate and pyruvate (24). Propylene glycol toxicity (i.e., agitation, coma, seizures, hypotension, and lactic acidosis) has been reported in 19% to 66% of *patients receiving high-dose intravenous lorazepam for more than 2 days* (24,25). If suspected, the drug infusion should be stopped and another sedative agent selected (midazolam and propofol do not use propylene glycol as a solvent). An assay for propylene glycol in blood is available, but the acceptable range has not been determined.

Lactic Alkalosis

Severe alkalosis (respiratory or metabolic) can raise blood lactate levels as a result of increased activity of pH-dependent enzymes in the glycolytic pathway (26). When liver function is normal, the liver clears the extra lactate generated during alkalosis, and *lactic alkalosis* becomes evident only when the blood pH is 7.6 or higher. However, in patients with impaired liver function, hyperlactatemia can be seen with less severe degrees of alkalemia.

Other Causes

Other possible causes of hyperlactatemia in ICU patients include *generalized seizures* (from hypermetabolism) (27), *hepatic insufficiency* (from reduced lactate clearance) (28), *acute asthma* (from enhanced lactate production by the respiratory muscles) (29), and *hematologic malignancies* (rare) (30). Hyperlactatemia associated with hepatic insufficiency is often mild (28). Hyperlactatemia that accompanies generalized seizures can be severe (with lactate levels of 15 mmol/L) but is transient (27).

Diagnostic Considerations

The normal lactate concentration in blood is ≤ 2 mmol/L, but increases in lactate concentration do not have prognostic value until they reach 4 mmol/L (1), so a higher threshold of 4 mmol/L is used to define"clinically significant" hyperlactatemia. Measurements can be obtained on arterial or venous blood samples. If immediate measurements are unavailable, the blood should be placed on ice to retard lactate production by red blood cells.

The anion gap (described on pages 594–596) should be elevated in lactic acidosis, but there are numerous reports of a normal anion gap in patients with lactic acidosis (31). As a result, *the anion gap should not be used as a screening test for lactic acidosis.*

D-Lactic Acidosis

The lactate produced by mammalian tissues is a levo-isomer (l-lactate), whereas a dextro-isomer of lactate (d-lactate) is produced by certain strains of bacteria that can populate the bowel (32). D-lactate generated by bacterial fermentation in the bowel can gain access to the systemic circulation and produce a metabolic acidosis, often combined with a metabolic encephalopathy (33). Most cases of d-lactic acidosis have been reported after extensive small bowel resection or after jejunoileal bypass for morbid obesity (32–34).

DIAGNOSIS: D-lactic acidosis can produce an elevated anion gap, but the standard laboratory assay for blood lactate measures only l-lactate. If d-lactic acidosis is suspected, you must request the laboratory to perform a d-lactate assay.

ALKALI THERAPY

The primary goal of therapy in lactic acidosis is to correct the underlying metabolic abnormality. Alkali therapy aimed at correcting the pH is of questionable value (35). The following is a brief summary of the pertinent issues regarding alkali therapy for lactic acidosis.

Acidosis Is Not Harmful

The principal fear from acidosis is the risk of impaired myocardial contractility (36). However, in the intact organism, *acidemia is often accompanied by an increase in cardiac output* (37). This is explained by the ability of acidosis to stimulate catecholamine release from the adrenals and to produce vasodilation. Therefore, impaired contractility from acidosis is less of a concern in the intact organism. In addition, acidosis may have a protective role in the setting of clinical shock. For example, extracellular acidosis has been shown to protect energy-depleted cells from cell death (38).

Bicarbonate Is Not an Effective Buffer

Sodium bicarbonate is the standard buffer used for lactic acidosis, but has limited success in raising the serum pH (39). This can be explained by the titration curve for the carbonic acid-bicarbonate buffer system, which is shown in Figure 32.2. The HCO_3 buffer pool is generated by the dissociation of carbonic acid (H_2CO_3):

$$CO_2 + H_2O \Leftrightarrow H_2CO_3 \Leftrightarrow H^+ + HCO_3^- \qquad (32.4)$$

The dissociation constant (pK) for carbonic acid (i.e., the pH at which the acid is 50% dissociated) is 6.1, as indicated on the titration curve. Buffers are most effective within 1 pH unit on either side of the pK (40), so the effective range of the bicarbonate buffer system should be an extracellular pH between 5.1 and 7.1 pH units (indicated by the shaded area on the titration curve). Therefore, *bicarbonate is not expected to be an effective buffer in the usual pH range of extracellular fluid.* Bicarbonate is not really a buffer; rather, it is a transport form of carbon dioxide in blood.

Bicarbonate Can be Harmful

A number of undesirable effects are associated with sodium bicarbonate therapy. One of these is the ability of bicarbonate to generate CO_2, which can actually lower the intracellular pH and cerebrospinal fluid pH (41,42). In fact, considering that *the PCO_2 is 200 mm Hg in standard bicarbonate solutions* (see Table 32.1), bicarbonate is really a CO_2 burden (an acid load!) that must be removed by the lungs.

Finally, *bicarbonate infusions can increase blood lactate levels* (42). Although this effect is attributed to alkalosis-induced augmentation of lactate production, it is not a desirable effect for a therapy of lactic acidosis.

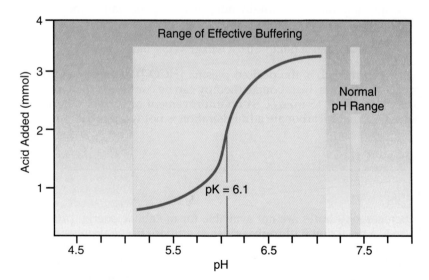

FIGURE 32.2 The titration curve for the carbonic acid-bicarbonate buffer system. The large, shaded area indicates the effective pH range for the bicarbonate buffer system, which does not coincide with the physiological pH range of extracellular fluid. Adapted from Reference 40.

Carbicarb

Carbicarb is a commercially available buffer solution that is a 1:1 mixture of sodium bicarbonate and disodium carbonate. As shown in Table 32.1, carbicarb has less bicarbonate and a much lower PCO_2 than the standard 7.5% sodium bicarbonate solution. As a result, carbicarb does not produce the increase in PCO_2 seen with sodium bicarbonate infusions (41).

Table 32.1	Bicarbonate-Containing Buffer Solutions	
	7.5% NaHCO₃	**Carbicarb**
Sodium	0.9 mEq/mL	0.9 mEq/mL
Bicarbonate	0.9 mEq/mL	0.3 mEq/mL
Dicarbonate	—	0.3 mEq/mL
PCO₂	>200 mm Hg	3 mm Hg
Osmolality	1461 mOsm/kg	1667 mOsm/kg
pH (25°C)	8.0	9.6

Recommendation

Alkali therapy has no role in the routine management of metabolic acidosis. However, when patients are deteriorating rapidly in the setting of a severe acidemia (pH < 7.0), a trial infusion of bicarbonate can be attempted as a desperation measure by administering one-half of the estimated HCO_3 deficit (42).

$$HCO_3 \text{ deficit (mEq)} = 0.6 \times wt(kg) \times (15 - \text{measured } HCO_3) \qquad (32.5)$$

(where 15 mEq/L is the desired plasma $[HCO_3]$). If cardiovascular improvement occurs, bicarbonate therapy can be continued to maintain the plasma HCO_3 at 15 mEq/L. If no improvement or further deterioration occurs, further bicarbonate administration is not warranted.

KETOACIDS

Ketogenesis

When carbohydrates are not available for metabolic energy production, there is a breakdown of triglycerides in adipose tissue (lipolysis) to generate fatty acids, which are transported to the liver and metabolized to form 3 ketone bodies; i.e., acetoacetate, β-hydroxybutyrate, and acetone. This is illustrated in Figure 32.3. These ketones are released from the liver and can be used as oxidative fuels by vital organs such as the heart and central nervous system. The oxidative metabolism of ketones yields 4 kcal/g, which is slightly in excess of the energy yield from the oxidative metabolism of glucose (3.7 kcal/g).

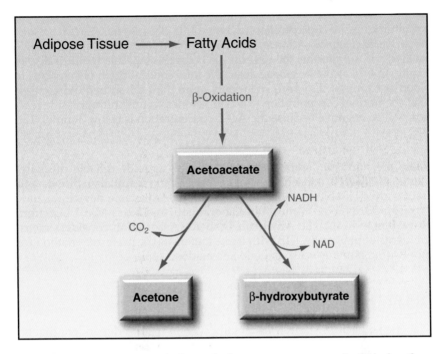

FIGURE 32.3 Ketogenesis in the liver, which occurs in response to diminished availability of glucose. Acetone is a ketone, but is not a ketoacid.

Ketoacids in Blood

The normal concentration of ketones in the blood is negligible (0.1 mmol/L), but blood ketone levels increase tenfold (to 1 mmol/L) after just 3 days of starvation. Acetone is not a ketoacid, but is responsible for the "fruity" odor of breath in patients with ketoacidosis. Acetoacetate (AcAc) and β-hydroxybutyrate (β-OHB) are strong acids (i.e., readily dissociate), and they promote a decrease in plasma pH when their plasma concentrations reach 3 mmol/L (43). The balance of AcAc and β-OHB in blood is determined by the following redox reaction (see Figure 32.3):

$$\text{AcAc} + \text{NADH} \Leftrightarrow \beta\text{-OHB} + \text{NAD} \qquad (32.6)$$

The balance of this reaction favors the formation of β-OHB. In conditions of enhanced ketone production, the β-OHB:AcAc ratio ranges from 3:1 in diabetic ketoacidosis, to as high as 8:1 in alcoholic ketoacidosis. The concentration of ketoacids in the blood in diabetic and alcoholic ketoacidosis is shown in Figure 32.4. Note the preponderance of β-OHB in both conditions. Because of this preponderance, ketoacidosis is more accurately called β-*hydroxybutyric acidosis*.

The Nitroprusside Reaction

The nitroprusside reaction is a colorimetric method for detecting AcAc and acetone in blood and urine. The test can be performed with tablets (Acetest) or reagent strips (Ketostix, Labstix, Multistix). A detectable reaction requires a minimum AcAc concentration of 3 mmol/L. Because *this reaction does not detect the predominant ketoacid, β-hydroxybutyrate* (43), it is an insensitive method for monitoring the severity of ketoacidosis. This is illustrated in Figure 32.4. In alcoholic ketoacidosis, the total concentration of ketoacids in blood is 13 mmol/L, which represents more than a hundredfold increase over the normal concentration of blood ketones, yet the nitroprusside reaction will be negative because the AcAc concentration is below 3 mmol/L.

β-hydroxybutyrate Testing

There are portable "ketone meters" that can provide reliable measurements of β-OHB concentrations in fingerstick (capillary) blood, and results are available in about 10 seconds (44). (Available devices include Precision Xtra meter from Abbot Laboratories and Nova Max PLUS from Nova Biomedical.) The American Diabetes Association considers measurements of plasma β-OHB with these meters as the preferred method for monitoring patients with diabetic ketoacidosis (45).

DIABETIC KETOACIDOSIS

Diabetic ketoacidosis (DKA) is usually seen in insulin-dependent diabetic patients, but there is no previous history of diabetes mellitus in 27–37% of cases (46). The most common precipitating factors in DKA are inappropriate insulin dosing and concurrent illness (e.g., infection). The mortality rate of DKA is 1–5% (46).

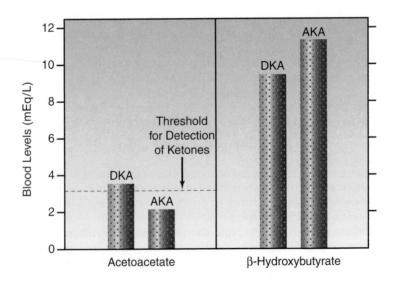

FIGURE 32.4 The concentrations of acetoacetate and ß-hydroxybutyrate in the blood in diabetic ketoacidosis (DKA) and alcoholic ketoacidosis (AKA). The horizontal hatched line represents the minimum concentration of acetoacetate required to produce a positive nitroprusside reaction.

Clinical Features

The definition of DKA proposed by the American Diabetes Association includes a blood glucose > 250 mg/dL, plasma [HCO_3] < 18 mEq/L, plasma pH ≤ 7.30, an elevated anion gap, and evidence of ketones in blood or urine (45). However, there are exceptions:

1. The blood glucose is only mildly elevated (< 250 mg/dL) in about 20% of cases of DKA(47).

2. The anion gap can be normal in DKA (48). The renal excretion of ketones is accompanied by an increase in chloride reabsorption in the renal tubules, and the resulting hyperchloremia limits the increase in the anion gap.

Additional clinical features of interest in DKA are summarized below.

1. Leukocytosis is not a reliable marker of infection in DKA because ketonemia produces a leukocytosis, which is proportional to the concentration of ketones in plasma (45). However, an increase in immature neutrophils (band forms) can be a reliable marker of infection in patients with DKA (49).

2. Elevated troponin I levels without evidence of an acute coronary event has been reported in 27% of patients with DKA (50).

3. Dehydration is almost universal in DKA, but this may not be reflected in the plasma sodium concentration because hyperglycemia has a dilutional effect on plasma sodium; i.e., the plasma sodium concentration decreases by 1.6–2 mEq/L for every 100 mg/dL increase in the plasma glucose concentration (51,52).

Management

The management of DKA is summarized in Table 32.2. The following are some of the details.

Intravenous Fluids

Volume deficits in DKA average 50–100 mL/kg (4–8 L for an 80 kg adult) (45). Volume resuscitation begins with isotonic (0.9%) saline infused at a rate of 1 liter per hour (or 15–20 mL/kg/hr) (45). When the patient stabilizes (e.g., blood pressure returns to normal), the infusion rate can be decreased to 250–500 mL/hr (4–14 mL/kg/hr). When the blood glucose falls to 250 mg/dL, change the intravenous fluid to 5% dextrose in 0.45% saline and decrease the infusion rate to 150–250 mL/hr.

Insulin

Insulin therapy is started with regular insulin given intravenously, starting with a bolus dose of 0.15 units per kilogram body weight and followed with a continuous infusion at 0.1 units/kg/hr. Because insulin adsorbs to intravenous tubing, the initial 50 mL of infusate should be run through the IV setup before the insulin drip is started. The blood glucose levels should decrease by 50 to 75 mg/dL per hour (46), and the insulin infusion should be adjusted to achieve this goal. When the blood glucose level falls to 200 mg/dL, the insulin infusion should be decreased to 0.05 to 0.1 units/kg/hr, and dextrose should be added to the intravenous fluids. Thereafter, the blood glucose levels should be maintained between 150–200 mg/dL (45,46). Achieving euglycemia is not recommended because of the risk of hypoglycemia.

Table 32.2	Management of Diabetic Ketoacidosis

I. Intravenous Fluids

1. Start with isotonic saline at 1 L/hr (15–20 mL/kg/hr). When BP normalizes, decrease rate to 250–500 mL/hr.
2. When blood glucose falls to 250 mg/dL, change to 5% dextrose in 0.45% saline and infuse at 150–250 mL/hr.
3. Volume deficit in DKA is usually 50–100 mL/kg (4–8 L in 80 kg adult).

II. Insulin

1. Regular insulin: 0.15 units/kg as an IV bolus, then infuse at 0.1 units/kg/hr.
2. Adjust infusion so that blood glucose decreases by 50–75 mg/dL per hour.
3. When blood glucose reaches 250 mg/dL, decrease infusion rate to 0.1–0.5 units/kg/hr, and maintain blood glucose at 150–200 mg/dL.
4. Begin SC insulin when DKA resolves (pH 7.3) and oral fluids are tolerated, but continue IV insulin for a few hours after starting SC insulin.

III. Potassium

1. If initial serum $[K^+]$ is <3.3 mEq/L, hold the insulin infusion and give 40 mEq K^+ per hour until the $[K^+]$ is ≥3.3 mEq/L.
2. If initial serum $[K^+]$ is 3.3–4.9 mEq/L, give 20–30 mEq K^+ in each liter of IV fluid to keep serum $[K^+]$ at 4–5 mEq/L.
3. If initial serum $[K^+]$ is ≥5 mEq/L, do not give K+, but check serum $[K^+]$ every 2 hours.
4. Average K^+ deficit in DKA is 3–5 mEq/kg.

From the American Diabetes Association guidelines in Reference 45.

AFTER DKA RESOLVES: When DKA has resolved (i.e., glucose < 200 mg/dL, plasma $[HCO_3]$ > 18 mEq/L, plasma pH > 7.3) and the patient can tolerate oral fluids, subcutaneous insulin can be started. Patients who were insulin-dependent prior to admission can be placed on their usual outpatient regimen. Patients who are new to insulin should receive 0.5–0.8 Units/kg per day in divided doses (46).

Potassium

Potassium depletion is universal in DKA, and the average deficit is 3 to 5 mEq/kg (47). However, the initial serum K^+ is often normal (74% of patients) or even elevated (22% of patients) (47). The serum K^+ can fall dramatically during insulin therapy (transcellular shift), so if the initial serum K^+ is low (< 3.3 mEq/L), the insulin should be withheld until the serum K^+ can be normalized (by giving 40 mEq KCL hourly). If the serum K^+ is high (≥ 5 mEq/L), no potassium is given initially, and when the serum K^+ is normal, 20 – 30 mEq of KCL should be added to each liter of IV fluid (45). Regardless of the initial potassium regimen, the serum K^+ should be checked every 1 – 2 hours for the first 4 – 6 hours.

Phosphate

Phosphate depletion is also common in DKA, and serum phosphate levels are typically 1–1.5 mmol/kg (47). However, phosphate replacement has no documented benefit in DKA, and is not recommended unless the hypophosphatemia is severe (45–47). If the serum PO_4 is < 1 mg/dL, give 20 – 30 mEq potassium phosphate with each liter of IV fluid (45).

Bicarbonate

Bicarbonate therapy does not improve the outcome in DKA, and is not recommended as a routine measure (45–47). However, in patients who are *in extremis* with a pH < 7.0, the bicarbonate regimen presented earlier can be used as a desperation measure.

Monitoring Acid-Base Status

The serum [HCO_3] is not a reliable measurement for following the acid-base status during the management of DKA because the isotonic saline produces a hyperchloremic acidosis that prevents the bicarbonate from rising despite a resolving ketoacidosis. In this situation, monitoring *the gap-gap ratio* is more informative. The gap-gap ratio is the ratio of the anion gap excess to the bicarbonate deficit, and is described at the end of the last chapter (see pages 596 – 597). This ratio is unity (1.0) in pure ketoacidosis, and it decreases as the ketoacidosis resolves and is replaced by the hyperchloremic acidosis. When the ketones have been cleared from the bloodstream, the ratio approaches zero.

ALCOHOLIC KETOACIDOSIS

Alcoholic ketoacidosis (AKA) is a complex acid-base disorder that occurs in chronic alcoholics and usually appears 1 to 3 days after a period of heavy binge drinking (53,54). Several mechanisms are involved, including reduced nutrient intake (which initiates enhanced ketone production), hepatic oxidation of ethanol (which generates NADH and enhances β-hydroxybutyrate formation), and dehydration (which impairs ketone excretion in the urine).

Clinical Features

Patients with AKA tend to be chronically ill and have several comorbid conditions. The presentation usually includes nausea, vomiting, and abdominal pain (53). Electrolyte abnormalities are common, particularly the *hypos* (e.g., hyponatremia, hypokalemia, hypophosphatemia, hypomagnesemia, hypoglycemia). Mixed acid-base disorders are also common in AKA. More than half the patients can have lactic acidosis (caused by other conditions), and metabolic alkalosis occurs in patients with protracted vomiting.

Diagnosis

The diagnosis of AKA is suggested by the clinical setting (i.e., after a period of binge drinking), an elevated anion gap, and the presence of ketones in the blood or urine. However, *the nitroprusside reaction for detecting ketones can be negative in AKA*. This is shown in Figure 32.4. The oxidation of ethanol in the liver generates NADH, and this favors the conversion of acetoacetate to β-hydroxybutyrate, and results in a low concentration of acetoacetate blood and urine. Even though most cases of AKA have a positive nitroprusside reaction for ketones (53), the severity of the ketoacidosis is significantly underestimated.

Management

The management of AKA is notable for its simplicity; i.e., infusion of dextrose-containing saline solutions is usually all that is required. The glucose infusion slows hepatic ketone production, while the infused volume promotes the renal clearance of ketones. The ketoacidosis usually resolves within 24 hours. Other electrolyte deficiencies are corrected as needed, and thiamine supplementation is recommended because glucose infusions can deplete marginal thiamine reserves.

A FINAL WORD

It's Not the Acidosis

One of the important messages in this chapter is the fact that the clinical problem created by lactic acidosis or diabetic ketoacidosis is not because of the acidosis, but because of the underlying metabolic derangement. The same degree of acidosis can be associated with diabetic ketoacidosis and lactic acidosis, but the survival is much better with ketoacidosis because the underlying problem is an exaggeration of an adaptive response to intracellular glucose deprivation, while the problem with lactic acidosis is a generalized derangement in cellular energy metabolism.

The other point that deserves emphasis is the fact that bicarbonate is not much of a buffer in the physiological pH range. In fact, bicarbonate can be viewed as a consequence of the accumulation of CO_2, the principal volatile acid in the human body.

REFERENCES

Lactic Acidosis—Reviews

1. Okorie ON, Dellinger P. Lactate: biomarker and potential therapeutic target. Crit Care Clin 2011; 27:299–326.

2. Vernon C, LeTourneau JL. Lactic acidosis: Recognition, kinetics, and associated prognosis. Crit Care Clin 2010; 26:255–283.

Lactate Metabolism

3. Borregaard N, Herlin T. Energy metabolism of human neutrophils during phagocytosis. J Clin Invest 1982; 70:550–557.

4. De Backer D, Creteur J, Zhang H, et al. Lactate production by the lungs in acute lung injury. Am J Respir Crit Care Med 1997; 156:1099–1104.

5. Lehninger AL. Bioenergetics. New York: WA Benjamin, 1965; 16.

6. Brooks GA. Lactate production under fully aerobic conditions: the lactate shuttle during rest and exercise. Fed Proc 1986; 45:2924–2929.

7. Gladden LB. Lactate metabolism: a new paradigm for the third millennium. J Physiol 2004; 558.1:5–30.

8. Dhainaut J-F, Huyghebaert M-F, Monsallier JF, et al. Coronary hemodynamics and myocardial metabolism of lactate, free fatty acids, glucose, and ketones in patients with septic shock. Circulation 1987; 75:533–541.

Lactate as a Biomarker

9. Gore DC, Jahoor F, Hibbert JM, DeMaria EJ. Lactic acidosis during sepsis is related to increased pyruvate production, not deficits in tissue oxygen availability. Ann Surg 1996; 224:97–102.

10. Fink MP. Cytopathic hypoxia. Crit Care Clin 2001; 17:219–238.

11. Vary TC, O'Neill P, Cooney RN, et al. Chronic infusion of interleukin-1 induces hyperlactatemia and altered regulation of lactate metabolism in skeletal muscle. J Parenter Ent Nutr 1999; 23:213–217.

12. Thomas GW, Mains CW, Slone DS, et al. Potential dysregulation of the pyruvate dehydrogenase complex by bacterial toxins and insulin. J Trauma 2009; 67:628–633.

13. Stewart PA. Modern quantitative acid-base chemistry. Can J Physiol Pharmacol 1983; 61:1444–1461.

14. Stewart PA. Strong ions and the strong ion difference. In Kellum JA, Elbers PWG, eds. Stewart's Textbook of Acid Base 2009: Amsterdam; Acidbase.org:55–70.

15. Adrogue HJ, Gennari J, Gala JH, Madias NE. Assessing acid-base disorders. Kidney Int 2009; 76:1239–1247.

Causes of Hyperlactatemia

16. Mizock BA. Metabolic derangements in sepsis and septic shock. Crit Care Clin 2000; 16:319–336.

17. Campbell CH. The severe lactic acidosis of thiamine deficiency: acute, pernicious or fulminating beriberi. Lancet 1984; 1:446–449.

18. Seidowsky A, Nseir S, Houdret N, Fourrier F. Metformin-associated lactic acidosis: a prognostic and therapeutic study. Crit Care Med 2009; 37:2191–2196.

19. Perrone J, Phillips C, Gaieski D. Occult metformin toxicity in three patients with profound lactic acidosis. J Emerg Med 2011; 40:271–275.

20. Ogedegbe AO, Thomas DL, Diehl AM. Hyperlactatemia syndromes associated with HIV therapy. Lancet Infect Dis 2003; 3:329–337.

21. Falco V, Rodriguez D, Ribera E, et al. Severe nucleoside-associated lactic acidosis in human immunodeficiency virus-infected patients: report of 12 cases and review of the literature. Clin Infect Dis 2002; 34:838–846.

22. Gould FK. Linezolid: safety and efficacy in special populations. J Antimicrob Chemoth 2011; 66(Suppl 4):iv3–iv6.

23. Apodaca AA, Rakita RM. Linezolid-induced lactic acidosis. New Engl J Med 2003; 348:86–87.

24. Wilson KC, Reardon C, Theodore AC, Farber HW. Propylene glycol toxicity: a severe iatrogenic illness in ICU patients receiving IV benzodiazepines. Chest 2005; 128:1674–1681.

25. Arroglia A, Shehab N, McCarthy K, Gonzales JP. Relationship of continuous infusion lorazepam to serum propylene glycol concentration in critically ill adults. Crit Care Med 2004; 32:1709–1714.

26. Bersin RM, Arieff AI. Primary lactic alkalosis. Am J Med 1988; 85:867–871.

27. Orringer CE, Eusace JC, Wunsch CD, Gardner LB. Natural history of lactic acidosis after grand-mal seizures. A model for the study of anion-gap acidoses not associated with hyperkalemia. N Engl J Med 1977; 297:796–781.

28. Kruse JA, Zaidi SAJ, Carlson RW. Significance of blood lactate levels in critically ill patients with liver disease. Am J Med 1987; 83:77–82.

29. Mountain RD, Heffner JE, Brackett NC, Sahn SA. Acid-base disturbances in acute asthma. Chest 1990; 98:651–655.

30. Friedenberg AS, Brnadoff DE, Schiffman FJ. Type B lactic acidosis as a severe metabolic complication of lymphoma and leukemia: a case series from a single institution and literature review. Medicine (Baltimore) 2007; 86:225–232.

Diagnostic Considerations

31. Iberti TS, Liebowitz AB, Papadakos PJ, et al. Low sensitivity of the anion gap as a screen to detect hyperlactatemia in critically ill patients. Crit Care Med 1990; 18:275–277.

32. Anonymous. The colon, the rumen, and d-lactic acidosis. Lancet 1990; 336:599–600 (editorial).

33. Thurn JR, Pierpoint GL, Ludvigsen CW, Eckfeldt JH. D-lactate encephalopathy. Am J Med 1985; 79:717–720.

34. Bustos D, Ponse S, Pernas JC et al. Fecal lactate and the short bowel syndrome. Dig Dis Sci 1994; 39:2315–2319.

Alkali Therapy

35. Forsythe SM, Schmidt GA. Sodium bicarbonate for the treatment of lactic acidosis. Chest 2000; 117:260–267.

36. Sonnett J, Pagani FD, Baker LS, et al. Correction of intramyocardial hypercarbic acidosis with sodium bicarbonate. Circ Shock 1994; 42:163–173.

37. Mehta PM, Kloner RA. Effects of acid-base disturbance, septic shock, and calcium and phosphorous abnormalities on cardiovascular function. Crit Care Clin 1987; 3:747–758.

38. Gores GJ, Nieminen AL, Fleischman KE, et al. Extracellular acidosis delays onset of cell death in ATP-depleted hepatocytes. Am J Physiol 1988; 255:C315–C322.

39. Graf H, Arieff AI. The use of sodium bicarbonate in the therapy of organic acidoses. Intensive Care Med 1986; 12:286–288.

40. Comroe JH. Physiology of respiration. Chicago: Yearbook Medical Publishers, 1974; 203.

41. Rhee KY, Toro LO, McDonald GG, et al. Carbicarb, sodium bicarbonate, and sodium chloride in hypoxic lactic acidosis. Chest 1993; 104:913–918.

42. Rose BD. Clinical physiology of acid-base and electrolyte disorders. 4th ed. New York: McGraw-Hill, 1994; 590.

Ketoacids

43. Cartwright MM, Hajja W, Al-Khatib S, et al. Toxigenic and metabolic causes of ketosis and ketoacidotic syndromes. Crit Care Clin 2012; 601–631.

44. Plüdderman A, Hemeghan C, Price C, et al. Point-of-care blood test for ketones in patients with diabetes: primary care diagnostic technology update. Br J Clin Pract 2011; 61:530–531.

45. American Diabetes Association. Hyperglycemic crisis in diabetes. Diabetes Care 2004; 27(Suppl):S94–S102.

Diabetic Ketoacidosis

46. Westerberg DP. Diabetic ketoacidosis: evaluation and treatment. Am Fam Physician 2013; 87:337–346.

47. Charfen MA, Fernandez-Frackelton M. Diabetic ketoacidosis. Emerg Med Clin N Am 2005; 23:609–628.

48. Gamblin GT, Ashburn RW, Kemp DG, Beuttel SC. Diabetic ketoacidosis presenting with a normal anion gap. Am J Med 1986; 80:758–760.

49. Slovis CM, Mork VG, Slovis RJ, Brain RP. Diabetic ketoacidosis and infection: leukocyte count and differential as early predictors of serious infection. Am J Emerg Med 1987; 5:1–5.

50. AlMallah M, Zuberi O, Arida M, Kim HE. Positive troponin in diabetic ketoacidosis without evident acute coronary syndrome predicts adverse cardiac events. Clin Cardiol 2008; 31:67–71.

51. Rose BD, Post TW. Hyperosmolal states: hyperglycemia. In: Clinical physiology of acid-base and electrolyte disorders. 5th ed. New York, NY: McGraw-Hill, 2001; 794–821.

52. Moran SM, Jamison RL. The variable hyponatremic response to hyperglycemia. West J Med 1985; 142:49–53.

Alcoholic Ketoacidosis

53. Wrenn KD, Slovis CM, Minion GE, Rutkowsli R. The syndrome of alcoholic ketoacidosis. Am J Med 1991; 91:119–128.

54. McGuire LC, Cruickshank AM, Munro PT. Alcoholic ketoacidosis. Emerg Med J 2006; 23:417–420.

Chapter 33

METABOLIC ALKALOSIS

To do common things perfectly is far better worth our endeavor,
than to do uncommon things respectably.

Harriet Beecher Stowe
1864

Although the spotlight usually falls on metabolic acidosis, the most common acid-base disturbance in hospitalized patients is metabolic *alkalosis* (1–3). The prevalence of metabolic alkalosis can be attributed to three factors: (a) common predisposing conditions (e.g., diuretic therapy), (b) the ability of the alkalosis to sustain itself (thanks to chloride), and (c) the tendency for the condition to go unnoticed and untreated. The latter factor reveals that metabolic alkalosis is not just a common disorder, it is a common and often untreated disorder.

PATHOGENESIS

Metabolic alkalosis is defined as an increase in the bicarbonate (HCO_3) concentration in extracellular fluid (> 26 mEq/L) that is not an adaptive response to hypercapnia. This condition can be the result of any of the following: (a) loss of hydrogen ions (H^+) from extracellular fluid, (b) a gain in bicarbonate ions in extracellular fluid, or (c) a decrease in extracellular volume. Once developed, metabolic alkalosis is sustained by a decrease in HCO_3 excretion in the urine, which is the result of both an increase in HCO_3 reabsorption and a decrease in HCO_3 secretion in the distal nephron. These renal adjustments are promoted by chloride depletion, hypokalemia, and aldosterone, as explained next.

Renal Mechanisms

The kidneys play a major role in the maintenance of metabolic alkalosis by decreasing HCO_3 excretion in the urine, as just mentioned. The following is a description of the mechanisms involved.

Bicarbonate Reabsorption

Bicarbonate is readily filtered at the glomerulus, and is almost entirely reabsorbed in the renal tubules. Most (90%) of the filtered HCO_3 is reabsorbed in the proximal tubules, and the remainder is reabsorbed by specialized cells in the collecting ducts. The distal site is the principal site of increased HCO_3 reabsorption in metabolic alkalosis (4). The mechanism of HCO_3 reabsorption in the collecting ducts is shown in Figure 33.1 A membrane ATPase pump moves H^+ into the tubular lumen, where it reacts with HCO_3 to form carbonic acid, which dissociates to form CO_2 and H_2O. The CO_2 moves into the tubular cell and is hydrated to regenerate HCO_3 and H^+. The HCO_3 moves into the bloodstream and the H^+ is

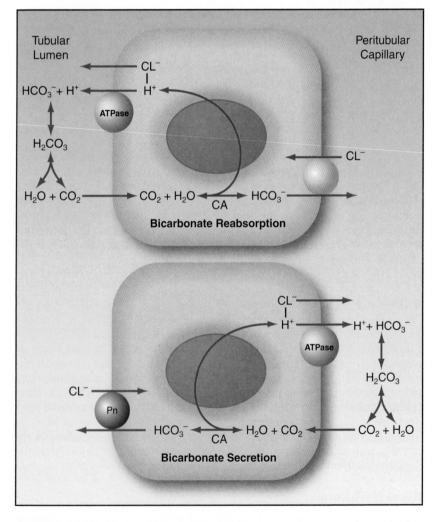

FIGURE 33.1 Mechanisms of bicarbonate reabsorption and secretion in the renal collecting tubules. CA = carbonic anhydrase, Pn = pendrin (the chloride-bicarbonate exchanger). See text for explanation.

transported back into the tubular lumen for another go-round. Chloride (CL^-) moves out of the peritubular capillaries in exchange for HCO_3.

Bicarbonate Secretion

Bicarbonate can also be secreted from specialized cells in the collecting ducts. This does not occur normally, but appears when there is excess HCO_3 in plasma (i.e., metabolic alkalosis). The mechanism for HCO_3 secretion is the reverse of HCO_3 reabsorption, with the H^+ pump on the capillary side of the tubular cells (see Figure 33.1). The principal difference is the presence of a chloride-bicarbonate exchange protein, called *pendrin*, on the luminal surface of the cells. This anion exchange protein has an important role in HCO_3 secretion (5–8). The pendrin gene is up-regulated in metabolic alkalosis (6), and pendrin activity is directly related to the luminal chloride concentration (7).

Chloride Depletion

Chloride depletion plays a major role in promoting metabolic alkalosis by increasing HCO_3 reabsorption and inhibiting HCO_3 secretion. Both effects are mediated by a decrease in luminal chloride concentration in the distal nephron, which: (a) increases HCO_3 reabsorption by promoting the movement of chloride and H^+ into the tubular lumen, and (b) impairs HCO_3 secretion by reducing the activity of the anion exchange protein, pendrin. The effects of luminal chloride on HCO_3 secretion are considered the principal mechanism for the ability of chloride depletion to promote metabolic alkalosis, and for the ability of chloride replacement to correct metabolic alkalosis (5).

Hypokalemia

Like chloride depletion, hypokalemia promotes metabolic alkalosis by increasing HCO_3 reabsorption and decreasing HCO_3 secretion in the distal nephron. The increase in HCO_3 reabsorption is caused by the simultaneous movement of K^+ out of cells and H^+ into cells, and the resulting decrease in intracellular pH promotes HCO_3 reabsorption in the distal nephron (4). The decrease in HCO_3 secretion in hypokalemia is attributed to a decrease in pendrin activity (8).

Aldosterone

Aldosterone (a mineralocorticoid produced in the adrenal cortex) promotes HCO_3 reabsorption in the distal nephron by stimulating the membrane H^+ pump on the luminal surface of acid-secreting renal tubular cells (9).

Predisposing Conditions

The three principal causes of sustained metabolic alkalosis are chloride depletion, hypokalemia, and mineralocorticoid excess. The clinical conditions that produce these derangements in ICU patients are described next.

Volume Loss

A decrease in extracellular volume promotes metabolic alkalosis. Early descriptions of this effect led to the term "contraction alkalosis," but this term is misleading because the underlying mechanism is chloride depletion (i.e., the alkalosis is not corrected by replacing the volume deficit without chloride replacement, but it is corrected with chloride replacement without correcting the volume deficit) (5).

Loss of Gastric Acid

Nasogastric suction results in loss of gastric secretions, which are rich in H^+ (50–100 mEq/L), CL^- (120–160 mEq/L), and to a lesser degree, K^+ (10–15 mEq/L)(10). Loss of H^+ will initiate a metabolic alkalosis, while loss of CL^- and K^+ will sustain the alkalosis.

Diuretics

Thiazide diuretics and "loop" diuretics like furosemide promote metabolic alkalosis via chloride and potassium depletion. The principal action of these diuretics is to increase sodium loss in urine (natriuresis), and an equivalent amount of chloride is also lost in urine (chloruresis) because urinary chloride excretion usually matches urinary sodium excretion.

The increased luminal sodium also promote potassium loss in urine via the Na^+- K^+ exchange pump on the luminal surface of specialized cells in the distal renal tubules.

CLINICAL MANIFESTATIONS

Metabolic alkalosis has no apparent deleterious effects in most patients. In one case report, an elderly patient with protracted vomiting and a plasma [HCO_3] of 151 mEq/L showed no signs of an immediate threat to life, and recovered fully after correction of the alkalosis (11). The lack of clinical consequences raises questions about the value of recognition and management of metabolic alkalosis.

Neurologic Manifestations

The neurologic manifestations attributed to alkalosis include depressed consciousness, generalized seizures, paresthesias, and carpopedal spasms. However, these manifestations are usually associated with *respiratory alkalosis*, not metabolic alkalosis. This is traditionally explained by the greater tendency for respiratory alkalosis to influence intracellular and central nervous system pH.

Neurologic manifestations seem to be more prominent in cases of metabolic alkalosis due to baking soda (sodium bicarbonate) ingestion (12), but this condition is accompanied by other electrolyte abnormalities (particularly hypercalcemia) that could be the responsible factor.

Hypoventilation

The ventilatory response to metabolic alkalosis is hypoventilation, with a subsequent rise in arterial PCO_2. However, this is not a vigorous response, and a considerable rise in plasma HCO_3 may be necessary before significant hypoventilation is evident (13). The ventilatory response to metabolic alkalosis is described by the following equation (14).

$$\Delta PaCO_2 = 0.7 \times \Delta HCO_3 \qquad (33.1)$$

($PaCO_2$ is the arterial PCO_2 and HCO_3 is the plasma bicarbonate concentration.) This equation was used to construct the curve in Figure 33.2 that shows the relationship between $PaCO_2$ and plasma HCO_3 in progressive metabolic alkalosis. (A normal $PaCO_2$ of 40 mm Hg and a normal plasma HCO_3 of 24 mEq/L were used in constructing this curve.) Note that hypercapnia (i.e., $PaCO_2 > 46$ mm Hg) does not occur until the plasma HCO_3 increases from 24 to 32 mEq/L, which represents a 40% increase in plasma HCO_3. In patients who have an increased ventilatory drive from an acute pulmonary process (e.g., pneumonia), even greater increases in plasma HCO_3 will be necessary to produce significant hypoventilation.

Oxyhemoglobin Dissociation Curve

Alkalosis shifts the oxyhemoglobin dissociation curve to the left (Bohr effect), which results in a decreased tendency for hemoglobin to release oxygen into the tissues. When the O_2 extraction from capillary blood is constant, a leftward shift of the oxyhemoglobin dissociation curve results

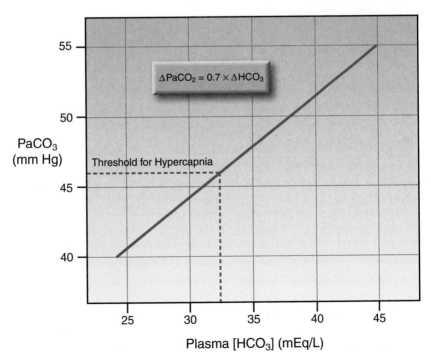

FIGURE 33.2 The relationship between plasma bicarbonate (HCO_3) and arterial PCO_2 ($PaCO_2$) in metabolic alkalosis, as predicted by the equation shown at the top of the graph (using a normal $PaCO_2$ of 40 mm Hg and a normal plasma [HCO_3] of 24 mEq/L).

in a decrease in venous PO_2 (15), which typically indicates a decrease in tissue PO_2. However, there is no evidence of inadequate tissue oxygenation (e.g., lactate accumulation) from this effect.

EVALUATION

The likely source(s) of metabolic alkalosis in ICU patients are loss of gastric secretions, diuretics, volume depletion, and hypokalemia, and these are readily apparent. In the rare case of uncertainty, the urinary chloride concentration can be informative, as described next.

Classification

The urinary chloride concentration is used to classify metabolic alkalosis as *chloride-responsive* or *chloride-resistant*, and the conditions associated with each category are listed in Table 33.1.

Chloride-Responsive Alkalosis

A chloride-responsive metabolic alkalosis is characterized by a low urinary chloride concentration (i.e., <15 mEq/L), indicating chloride depletion. The principal conditions that produce this type of metabolic alkalosis include loss of gastric secretions, therapy with chloruretic diuretics (i.e., diuretics that promote urinary chloride excretion), and volume depletion. In cases of metabolic alkalosis due to *chloruretic* diuretics (e.g., thiazides or furosemide), the urinary chloride may be inappropriately high when the drug is active, but this effect is lost when the drug effect dissipates.

Table 33.1	Classification of Metabolic Alkalosis	
Category	**Criteria**	**Conditions**
Chloride-Responsive	Urine [CL⁻] <15 mEq/L	Vomiting
		Nasogastric suction
		Choluretic diuretics
		Volume depletion
		Laxative abuse
Chloride-Resistant	Urine [CL⁻] >25 mEq/L	Primary aldosteronism
		Licorice ingestion
		Severe hypokalemia (plasma K⁺ <2 mEq/L)

Chloride-responsive metabolic alkalosis is typically accompanied by volume depletion, and improves with infusion of isotonic saline. Almost all cases of metabolic alkalosis in ICU patients are chloride-responsive.

LAXATIVE ABUSE: Diarrhea usually produces a hyperchloremic metabolic acidosis from bicarbonate losses in stool, but the diarrhea associated with chronic laxative abuse is rich in potassium and chloride (70–90 mEq/L), and it typically results in hypokalemia and a saline (chloride)-responsive metabolic alkalosis (16). The diagnosis can be elusive because patients often deny both laxative abuse and diarrhea.

Chloride-Resistant Alkalosis

A chloride-resistant metabolic alkalosis is characterized by an elevated urinary chloride concentration (i.e., > 25 mEq/L). Most cases of chloride-resistant alkalosis are caused by primary mineralocorticoid excess (e.g., primary aldosteronism). Whereas volume depletion is common in chloride-responsive metabolic alkalosis, volume expansion is common in chloride-resistant metabolic alkalosis. As a result, this type of metabolic alkalosis does not improve with infusions of isotonic saline. This type of metabolic alkalosis is infrequent in ICU patients.

SEVERE K+ DEPLETION: Mineralocorticoid excess promotes urinary potassium loss, so hypokalemia is common in chloride-resistant metabolic alkalosis. However, a chloride-resistant metabolic alkalosis has been reported in patients with hypokalemia that is not caused by mineralocorticoid excess (17). The hypokalemia is typically severe (plasma K^+ <2 mEq/L), and the proposed mechanism is diminished chloride reabsorption is the distal renal tubules. This condition is saline-resistant, but it can be corrected with potassium repletion (17).

MANAGEMENT

Since maintenance of a metabolic alkalosis is primarily the result of chloride and potassium depletion, these ions must be replenished to correct the alkalosis. This is accomplished with isotonic saline (0.9% NaCL) and potassium chloride.

Saline Infusion

Because volume depletion is common in chloride-responsive metabolic alkalosis, infusion of isotonic saline will help to correct the alkalosis. The volume of isotonic saline needed to correct the alkalosis can be estimated by first estimating the chloride (CL^-) deficit, as shown below (2,18):

$$CL^- \text{ deficit (mEq)} = 0.2 \times wt \text{ (kg)} \times (100 - \text{plasma } [CL^-]) \qquad (33.2)$$

(wt is lean body weight in kg, and 100 is the desired plasma chloride concentration). The required volume of isotonic saline (in liters) is then estimated as follows:

$$\text{Volume of isotonic saline (L)} = CL^- \text{ deficit } /154 \qquad (33.3)$$

(154 is the chloride concentration in mEq/L in isotonic saline). This method is summarized in Table 33.2. If the patient is not hemodynamically compromised, rapid saline infusion is not necessary, and a rate of 100–125 mL/hr above total hourly fluid losses (including insensible loss) is appropriate.

Table 33.2	Saline Infusions for Metabolic Alkalosis

Step 1. Estimate the chloride deficit:

$$CL^- \text{ deficit (mEq)} = 0.2 \times wt \text{ (kg)} \times (100 - \text{plasma } [CL^-])$$

Step 2. Determine the replacement volume of saline:

$$\text{Volume of 0.9\% NaCL (L)} = \frac{CL^- \text{ deficit}}{154}$$

Step 3: Rate of replacement: 100 mL/hr > hourly fluid losses.

From References 2 and 18.

EXAMPLE: A 70 kg adult with protracted vomiting has a metabolic alkalosis with a plasma chloride of 80 mEq/L. The chloride deficit in this case (using a normal plasma [CL$^-$] of 100 mEq/L) is $0.2 \times 70 \times (100 - 80) = 280$ mEq. The volume of isotonic saline needed to correct this deficit is 280/154 = 1.8 liters.

Edematous States

Isotonic saline infusion is contraindicated in edematous states because crystalloid fluids are distributed primarily in the interstitial fluid compartment. For every liter of isotonic saline infused, 825 mL will be added to the interstitial edema fluid (see Figure 12.2 on page 220) (19). Metabolic alkalosis in edematous states is often accompanied by hypokalemia, so potassium chloride replacement therapy can be used to treat the alkalosis.

Potassium Chloride

Potassium replacement is used to correct hypokalemia, and is always given as KCL, to take advantage of chloride replacement for correcting metabolic alkalosis. It is important to emphasize that *diuretic-induced hypokalemia can be resistant to potassium replacement if there is concurrent magnesium depletion* (20). Since magnesium depletion is also common during diuretic therapy, the plasma magnesium level should be checked at the outset of K$^+$ replacement. (The evaluation of magnesium depletion is described in Chapter 37.)

Saline-Resistant Alkalosis

Alkalosis from mineralocorticoid excess (primary or secondary) is associated with an increased extracellular volume (which may be apparent as peripheral edema), and saline infusions will be counterproductive. Hypokalemia is common in this type of metabolic alkalosis, so K$^+$

replacement (as KCL) helps in correcting the alkalosis. However, corrective therapy may require one of the following measures.

Acetazolamide

Acetazolamide (Diamox) inhibits carbonic anhydrase, the enzyme involved in HCO_3 reabsorption and secretion (see Figure 33.1). The major effect of acetazolamide is inhibition of HCO_3 reabsorption (proximal and distal sites) and an increase in urinary HCO_3 excretion (the urine pH should rise to 7 or higher during acetazolamide therapy). The in-crease in HCO_3 excretion is accompanied by an increase in sodium excretion, so acetazolamide provides the dual benefit of diuresis and correction of the metabolic alkalosis. The recommended dose is 5 to 10 mg/kg IV (or PO), and the maximum effect occurs after an average of 15 hours (21).

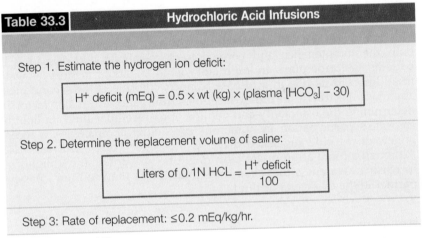

Table 33.3	Hydrochloric Acid Infusions

Step 1. Estimate the hydrogen ion deficit:

$$H^+ \text{ deficit (mEq)} = 0.5 \times \text{wt (kg)} \times (\text{plasma } [HCO_3] - 30)$$

Step 2. Determine the replacement volume of saline:

$$\text{Liters of 0.1N HCL} = \frac{H^+ \text{ deficit}}{100}$$

Step 3: Rate of replacement: ≤0.2 mEq/kg/hr.

From References 2 and 18.

Hydrochloric Acid Infusion

Alkalosis that is not corrected with K^+ replacement and acetazolamide can be treated with an infusion of dilute hydrochloric acid (HCL), but this can be risky, and is reserved only for severe alkalemia (plasma pH > 7.5).

METHOD: The "dose" of HCL is determined by estimating the hydrogen ion (H^+) deficit with the equation below (see also Table 33.3).

$$H^+ \text{ deficit (mEq)} = 0.5 \times \text{wt (kg)} \times (\text{plasma } [HCO_3] - 30) \qquad (33.4)$$

(wt is the lean body weight in kg, and 30 is the desired plasma $[HCO_3]$, which is higher than normal because the goal is to curb the alkalosis and not correct it). The preferred HCL solution for intravenous use is 0.1N HCL, which contains 100 mEq H^+ and 100 mEq CL in one liter of distilled water. The volume of 0.1N HCL (in liters) needed to correct the H^+ deficit is determined by the ratio (H^+ deficit/100), as shown in Table 33.3. Because HCL solutions are corrosive, they *should be infused through a large, central vein* (22). and *the infusion rate should not exceed 0.2 mEq/kg/hr* (18).

EXAMPLE: Consider a lean, 70 kg adult with a severe, refractory metabolic alkalosis resulting in a plasma HCO_3 of 40 meq/L and an arterial pH of 7.57. The H^+ deficit is $0.5 \times 70 \times (40 - 30) = 350$ meq. The corresponding volume of 0.1N HCL is $350/100 = 3.5$ L, and the maximum infusion rate is $(0.2 \times 70) = 0.14$ L/hour (2.3 mL/minute).

ADVERSE EFFECTS: The major concern with HCL infusions is the corrosive effect on blood vessels. Extravasation of HCL solutions can produce severe tissue necrosis (and a fatal outcome), even when the solution is infused through a central vein (23).

A FINAL WORD

It's Chloride

The final word in metabolic alkalosis is *chloride*, the principal element in both the maintenance and correction of metabolic alkalosis in ICU patients. Chloride plays an important role in metabolic acidosis as well. In addition to its role in acid-base balance, chloride is the second most abundant electrolyte in the extracellular fluid, and is a major factor in determining the osmolality and volume of extracellular fluid. In light of chloride's participation in numerous physiological processes, a recent review of chloride suggested that it is the "queen of electrolytes" (24). Although a more appropriate term might be warranted, it highlights an increasing awareness that chloride is much more than sodium's passive partner in the extracellular fluid.

REFERENCES

Reviews

1. Laski ME, Sabitini S. Metabolic alkalosis, bedside and bench. Semin Nephrol 2006; 26:404–421.

2. Khanna A, Kurtzman NA. Metabolic alkalosis. Respir Care 2001; 46:354–365.

3. Galla JH. Metabolic alkalosis. J Am Soc Nephrol 2000; 11:360–375.

Pathogenesis

4. Rose BD, Post TW. Regulation of acid-base balance. In: Clinical Physiology of Acid-Base and Electrolyte Disorders. 5th ed. New York: McGraw-Hill, 2001:325–371.

5. Luke RG, Galla JH. It is chloride depletion alkalosis, not contraction alkalosis. J Am Soc Nephrol 2012; 23:204–207.

6. Adler L, Efrati E, Zelikovic I. Molecular mechanisms of epithelial cell-specific expression and regulation of the human anion exchanger (pendrin) gene. Am J Physiol Cell Physiol 2008; 294L:C1261–C1276.

7. Vallet M, Picard N, Loffling-Cueni D, et al. Pendrin regulation in mouse kidney primarily is chloride-dependent. J Am Soc Nephrol 2006; 17:2153–2163.

8. Wagner CA, Finberg KE, Stehberger PA, et al. Regulation of the expression of the CL/anion exchanger pendrin in mouse kidney by acid-base status. Kidney Int 2002; 62:2109–2117.

9. Winter C, Kampik NB, Vedovelli L, et al. Aldosterone stimulates vacuolar (H+-ATPase activity in acid-secreting intercalated cells mainly via a protein kinase C-dependent pathway. Am J Physiol Cell Physiol 2011; 1:C1251–C1261.

10. Gennari FJ, Weise WJ. Acid-base disturbances in gastrointestinal disease. Clin J Am Soc Nephrol 2008; 3:1861–1868.

Clinical Manifestations

11. Giovanni I, Greco F, Chiarla C, et al. Exceptional nonfatal metabolic alkalosis (blood base excess + 48 mEq/L). Intensive Care Med 2005; 31:166–167.

12. Fitzgibbons LJ, Snoey ER. Severe metabolic alkalosis due to baking soda ingestion: case reports of two patients with unsuspected antacid overdose. J Emerg Med 1999; 17:57–61.

13. Javaheri S, Kazemi H. Metabolic alkalosis and hypoventilation in humans. Am Rev Respir Dis 1987; 136:1011–1016.

14. Adrogue HJ, Madias NE. Secondary responses to altered acid-base status: The rules of engagement. J Am Soc Nephrol 2010; 21:920–923.

15. Nunn JF. Nunn's Applied Respiratory Physiology. 4th ed. Oxford: Butterworth-Heinemann Ltd, 1993:275–276.

Evaluation

16. Roerig JL, Steffen KJ, Mitchell JE, Zunker C. Laxative abuse. Epidemiology, diagnosis, and management. Drugs 2010; 70:1487–1503.

17. Garella S, Chazan JA, Cohen JJ. Saline-resistant metabolic alkalosis or "chloride-wasting nephropathy". Report of four patients with severe potassium depletion. Ann Intern Med 1970; 73:31–38.

Management

18. Androgue HJ, Madias N. Management of life-threatening acid-base disorders. Part 2. N Engl J Med 1998; 338:107–111.

19. Imm A, Carlson RW. Fluid resuscitation in circulatory shock. Crit Care Clin 1993; 9:313-333.

20. Whang R, Flink EB, Dyckner T, et al. Mg depletion as a cause of refractory potassium depletion. Arch Intern Med 1985; 145:1686–1689.

21. Marik PE, Kussman BD, Lipman J, Kraus P. Acetazolamide in the treatment of metabolic alkalosis in critically ill patients. Heart Lung 1991; 20:455–458.

22. Brimioulle S, Vincent JL, Dufaye P, et al. Hydrochloric acid infusion for treatment of metabolic alkalosis: effects on acid-base balance and oxygenation. Crit Care Med 1985; 13:738–742.

23. Buchanan IB, Campbell BT, Peck MD, Cairns BA. Chest wall necrosis and death secondary to hydrochloric acid infusion for metabolic alkalosis. South Med J 2005; 98:822.

A Final Word

24. Berend K, van Hulsteijn LH, Gans RO. Chloride: the queen of electrolytes? Eur J Intern Med 2012; 23:203–211.

RENAL AND ELECTROLYTE DISORDERS

A man is a bundle of relations.

Ralph Waldo Emerson
Essays
1841

Chapter 34

ACUTE KIDNEY INJURY

> *You can never solve all difficulties at once.*
>
> Paul A.M. Dirac
> (1903–1984)

As many as 70% of ICU patients have some degree of renal dysfunction, and about 5% of ICU patients require renal replacement therapy (1–3). The renal dysfunction that occurs in critically ill patients is now called *acute kidney injury*. This condition is similar to the acute respiratory distress syndrome (ARDS) because it typically occurs as part of multiorgan failure in patients with progressive systemic inflammation (1). Patients with acute kidney injury who require hemodialysis have a mortality rate of 50–70% (3), which has not changed over the last 30 years (4). The inability of hemodialysis to curb the mortality rate in acute renal failure has apparently escaped the notice of the "evidence-based medicine" junkies, who preach that an intervention should be discarded if it does not improve mortality.

DIAGNOSTIC CRITERIA

The term "acute kidney injury" (AKI) was introduced over a decade ago to include the spectrum of renal dysfunction that occurs in critically ill patients. Also introduced was a classification system for severity of illness and outcome. The intent is to standardize the description of renal dysfunction in critically ill patients, but the reality (as will be presented) is a system of competing criteria that seems to complicate rather than simplify the approach to renal dysfunction in critically ill patients.

The RIFLE Criteria

In 2002, a group of experts known as the Acute Dialysis Quality Initiative (ADQI) proposed a classification system to define the progressive states of acute kidney injury (AKI). This system included 5 categories, and was given the name RIFLE, which is an acronym for Risk, Injury, Failure, Loss, and End-stage renal disease. The RIFLE criteria are shown in Table 34.1. There are 3 severity categories and 2 clinical outcome categories. The severity categories are defined by the serum creatinine and the urine output. The first (Risk) category identifies the minimum requirements for the diagnosis of AKI: i.e., a 50% increase in the serum creatinine concentration and a decrease in urine output to 0.5 mL/kg/hr (the definition of oliguria) for at least a 6-hour time period. If the creatinine and urine output criteria don't match, the "worst" measurement is used to determine the category).

The RIFLE criteria have 2 limitations: (a) there is no defined time period for the change in serum creatinine, and (b) the minimum change in serum creatinine required for the diagnosis of AKI is considered too large.

Table 34.1	RIFLE and AKIN Criteria for Acute Kidney Injury	
Categories	**Serum Creatinine Criteria**	**Urine Output Criteria†**
RIFLE:		
Risk	↑ in SCr to 1.5–<2 × baseline	UO: <0.5 mL/kg/hr for 6 hrs
Injury	↑ in SCr to 2–<3 × baseline	UO: <0.5 mL/kg/hr for 12 hrs
Failure	↑ in SCr to ≥3 × baseline	UO: <0.3 mL/kg/hr for 24 hrs or anuria for 12 hrs
Loss	Loss of kidney function for >4 wks	
ESRD	Loss of kidney function for >3 mos	
AKIN*:		
Stage 1	↑ in SCr to ≥0.3 mg/dL or to 1.5–2 × baseline	UO: <0.5 mL/kg/hr for >8 hrs
Stage 2	↑ in SCr to >2–3 × baseline	UO: <0.5 mL/kg/hr for >12 hrs
Stage 3	↑ in SCr to >3 × baseline or SCr ≥4 mg/dL with an acute increase of ≥0.5 mg/dL	UO: <0.5 mL/kg/hr for 24 hrs or anuria for 12 hrs

*The AKIN criteria require the increase in serum creatinine to occur within 48 hrs.
†Ideal body weight is recommended for urine output determinations.
From References 1 and 2. ESRD=end-stage renal disease; SCr=serum creatinine; UO=urine output.

AKIN Criteria

Because of the limitations of the RIFLE criteria just mentioned, revised criteria were introduced by the Acute Kidney Injury Network (AKIN), and these criteria are shown at the bottom of Table 34.1. The AKIN criteria require a smaller change in creatinine (≥0.3 mg/dL) for the diagnosis of AKI, and a time limit of 48 hours is imposed on the change in serum creatinine. Unfortunately, the RIFLE criteria were not abandoned after introduction of the AKIN criteria, so there are two competing systems for the diagnosis and classification of AKI at the present time.

What Now?

So, which criteria should be used to diagnose and stage AKI? The AKIN criteria seem to be favored in published reviews, but comparison studies have not demonstrated a difference between the RIFLE and AKIN criteria for predicting outcomes. This is demonstrated in Figure 34.1, which shows that the two sets of criteria are equivalent for predicting mortality rates (5).

Sources of Confusion

Despite the intent of simplifying the approach to renal failure in critically ill patients, the newly minted condition known as acute kidney injury has created the following sources of confusion:

1. The diagnosis of AKI includes prerenal conditions (e.g., hypovolemia) where there is no "injury" in the kidneys.

2. Oliguria (i.e., urine output < 0.5 mL/kg/hr) is required for the diagnosis of AKI, which neglects cases of nonoliguric acute renal failure (e.g., interstitialnephritis, myoglobinuric renal failure).

3. There is a lack of agreement about the minimum increase in serum creatinine required for the diagnosis of AKI.

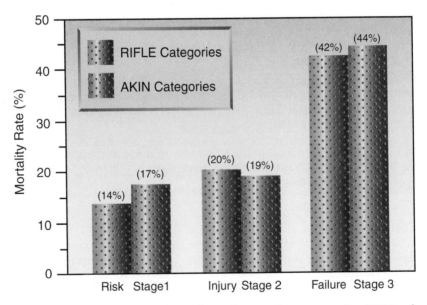

FIGURE 34.1 Comparison of in-hospital mortality rates for corresponding RIFLE and AKIN criteria in 291 patients with AKI. There is no difference between the classification systems for predicting mortality. Data from Reference 5.

DIAGNOSTIC CONSIDERATIONS

Categories

The clinical disorders that promote AKI can be categorized according to the location of the insult; i.e., prerenal, intrarenal, or postrenal.

Prerenal Disorders

The insult in prerenal disorders is a decrease in renal blood flow. Prerenal disorders are responsible for 30–40% of cases of AKI (6), and most cases are the result of hypovolemia and low-output heart failure. Prerenal AKI typically responds to interventions that augment systemic blood flow (e.g., volume resuscitation), but the response can be lost when the low-flow state is severe (e.g., hypovolemic shock).

Renal Disorders

The intrarenal conditions that produce AKI are acute tubular necrosis (ATN) and acute interstitial nephritis (AIN).

ATN: ATN is responsible for over 50% of cases of AKI (6). This condition was originally considered to be the result of renal hypoperfusion, but there is now convincing evidence that the pathologic process is inflammatory (oxidative) injury in the epithelial cell lining of the renal tubules (7). The damaged cells are sloughed into the lumen of the renal tubules, where they create an obstruction (see Figure 34.2). The luminal obstruction creates a back pressure on the luminal side of the glomerulus, and this decreases the net filtration pressure across the glomerulus, which reduces the glomerular filtration rate (GFR). This process is called *tubuloglomerular feedback* (8).

ATN is not a primary renal disease, and is typically a manifestation of one of the following disorders: severe sepsis and septic shock, radiocontrast dye, nephrotoxic drugs (e.g., aminoglycoside), or rhabdomyolysis with myoglobinuric renal injury.

AIN: AIN is also the result of inflammatory injury, but the injury is located in the renal interstitium rather than the renal tubules. AIN is described later in the chapter.

Postrenal Obstruction

Obstruction distal to the renal parenchyma is responsible for only about 10% of cases of AKI (6). The obstruction can involve the most distal portion of the renal collecting ducts (papillary necrosis), the ureters (extraluminal obstruction from a retroperitoneal mass), or the urethra (strictures). Ureteral obstruction from stones does not cause AKI unless there is a solitary functional kidney.

Common Sources of AKI

Most cases of AKI are caused by one of the clinical disorders in Table 34.2.

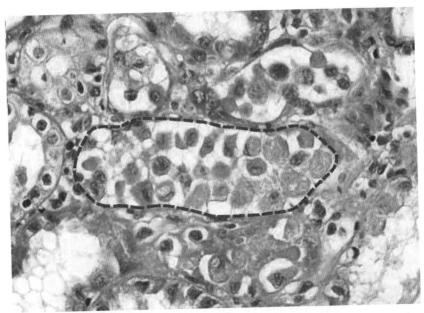

FIGURE 34.2 Photomicrograph of acute tubular necrosis (ATN) showing a proximal tubule (outlined by the dotted line) filled with exfoliated renal tubular cells.

The most common causes of AKI are listed in the left column. Sepsis (i.e., infection plus systemic inflammation) is the most common offender, and accounts for up to 50% of cases of AKI (3,9). AKI has been reported in up to 40% of postoperative patients following major surgery, particularly cardiopulmonary bypass surgery (3). AKI has also been reported in 30% of major trauma victims (3), and rhabdomyolysis is responsible for 30% of these cases (3). Nephrotoxic drugs and radiocontrast dye are implicated in about 20% of cases of AKI (9). Increased abdominal pressure is emerging as a common, and often overlooked, source of AKI. This condition is described later in the chapter.

Table 34.2	Common Causes of Acute Kidney Injury
Most Common Causes†	**Other Common Causes**
Sepsis*	Increased Abdominal Pressure
Major Surgery	Cardiopulmonary Bypass
Hypovolemia	Trauma
Low Cardiac Output	Rhabdomyolysis
Nephrotoxic Agents	

†From Reference 9.
*The leading cause of acute kidney injury.

Diagnostic Evaluation

The evaluation of AKI begins with a bedside ultrasound evaluation of the kidneys for evidence of postrenal obstruction. If there is no obstruction, the remaining evaluation is aimed at determining if the problem is a prerenal disorder (e.g., hypovolemia or a reduced cardiac output) or an intrinsic renal disorder (e.g., ATN or AIN). The measurements in Table 34.3 can help to distinguish prerenal from renal disorders, but only in patients with oliguria.

Spot Urine Sodium

In prerenal disorders, the renal hypoperfusion is accompanied by an increase in sodium reabsorption in the renal tubules and a subsequent decrease in urine sodium concentration. In contrast, renal "tubulopathies" like ATN are characterized by impaired sodium reabsorption and increased urinary sodium losses. Therefore, when a random urine sample (spot urine) is obtained in a patient with AKI, a urine sodium < 20 mEq/L is used as evidence of a prerenal disorder, while a urine sodium > 40 mEq/L is used as evidence of an intrinsic renal disorder (10).

EXCEPTIONS: A prerenal disorder can be associated with a high urine sodium (> 40 mEq/L) if there is ongoing diuretic therapy, or the patient has chronic renal disease (where there is "obligatory" sodium loss in the urine).

Table 34.3	Urinary Measurements for the Evaluation of AKI	
Measurement	**Prerenal Disorder**	**Renal Disorder**
Spot Urine Sodium	< 20 mEq/L	> 40 mEq/L
Fractional Excretion of Na	< 1%	> 2%
Fractional Excretion of Urea	< 35%	> 50%
Urine Osmolality	> 500 mOsm/kg	300–400 mOsm/kg
U/P Osmolality	> 1.5	1–1.3

Fractional Excretion of Sodium

The fractional excretion of sodium (FENa) is considered a more accurate measure of renal tubular function than the spot urine sodium concentration. The FENa is equivalent to the fractional sodium clearance divided by the fractional creatinine clearance, as expressed by the following equation:

$$\text{FENa}(\%) = \frac{U/P\,[\text{Na}]}{U/P\,[\text{Cr}]} \qquad (34.1)$$

(U/P is the urine-to-plasma ratio for sodium and creatinine concentrations.) In euvolemic patients with normal renal function, the FENa is 1%

(i.e., only 1% of the filtered sodium is excreted in the urine). In prerenal disorders like hypovolemia, the FENa is < 1% (reflecting sodium conservation), and in intrinsic renal disorders like ATN, the FENa is typically > 2% (reflecting an increase in urinary sodium excretion) (11).

EXCEPTIONS: Like the spot urine sodium, the FENa can be falsely elevated (> 1%) by diuretic therapy and chronic renal insufficiency (11). In addition, the FENa can be falsely low (< 1%) in patients with renal failure due to sepsis (12), radiocontrast dyes (13), and hemoglobinuria or myoglobinuria (14).

Fractional Excretion of Urea

The fractional excretion of urea (FEU) is conceptually similar to the FENa, and is equivalent to the fractional urea clearance divided by the fractional creatinine clearance, as expressed by the following equation:

$$FEU\,(\%) = \frac{U/P\,[Urea]}{U/P\,[Cr]} \qquad (34.2)$$

(U/P is the urine-to-plasma ratio for urea and creatinine concentrations.) The FEU is low (< 35%) in prerenal disorders like hypovolemia, and high (> 50%) in renal disorders like ATN. However, *the FEU is not influenced by diuretics* (15), which is the major advantage of the FEU over FENa.

Uncertainty

Distinguishing between prerenal and intrarenal causes of AKI can be difficult, and often a fluid challenge is necessary to distinguish between these two conditions (see next section).

INITIAL MANAGEMENT

The early management of AKI should include the following: (a) volume infusion to promote renal blood flow, (b) discontinuing any nephrotoxic drugs, and (c) treating any conditions that predispose to AKI (e.g., sepsis).

Fluid Challenges

If a prerenal source of AKI has not been ruled out, prompt volume infusion is warranted. Delays in correcting renal hypoperfusion can lead to intrarenal damage, so prompt attention to volume resuscitation is mandatory. Fluid challenges can be given in 500 ml to 1,000 mL aliquots for crystalloid fluids and 300 mL to 500 mL aliquots for colloid fluids, infused over 30 minutes (16). The fluid challenges are continued until there is a response (i.e., an increase in urine output), or until you are concerned about volume overload. (Remember that only 20–25% of infused crystalloid fluids remain in the intravascular space, so 500 mL of infused crystalloid fluid will increase the plasma volume by only 100–125 mL.

Therefore, fluid challenges with crystalloid fluids should not stop if a volume of 500 ml does not produce a favorable response.) *Diuretics should never be used to increase urine output until the possibility of a prerenal condition has been eliminated.*

Hydroxyethyl Starch:

Several studies have shown an association between hydroxyethyl starch solutions and AKI (see page 231). Therefore, it is wise to avoid starch solutions for fluid challenges in AKI.

Intrarenal Disorders

The following considerations are relevant in patients with AKI due to intrarenal disorders (i.e., ATN and AIN). Unfortunately, the only early option available for halting or reversing the course of AKI is to discontinue possible offending drugs.

Furosemide

Despite its popularity in AKI, *intravenous furosemide does not improve renal function in AKI, and does not convert oliguric to non-oliguric renal failure* (3,17). Furosemide can increase urine output during the recovery phase of AKI (18), and a trial of furosemide is reasonable during this period to relieve fluid accumulation.

Low-Dose Dopamine

Low-dose dopamine (2 μg/kg/min) can act as a renal vasodilator, but it does not improve renal function in patients with AKI (19,20). Furthermore, low-dose dopamine can have deleterious effects on hemodynamics (decreased splanchnic blood flow) immune function (inhibition of T-cell lymphocyte function) and endocrine function (inhibition of thyroid-stimulating hormone release from the pituitary) (20). Because of the lack of benefit combined with the risk of harm, the use of low-dose dopamine in patients with AKI is considered *bad medicine* (borrowing the title from Reference 20).

Nephrotoxic Agents

As mentioned, discontinuing possible offending drugs is the most effective early measure for halting or reversing the course of AKI. A variety of drugs can be responsible for AKI, as indicated in Table 34.4.

SPECIFIC CONDITIONS

Contrast-Induced Renal Injury

Iodinated contrast agents can damage the kidneys in several ways, including direct renal tubular injury, renal vasoconstriction, and the generation of toxic oxygen metabolites (21). Using the AKIN criteria for the diagnosis of

AKI, the incidence of AKI after contrast studies is 8–9% (22). The AKI usually appears within 72 hours after the contrast study. The incidence is greater in patients with multiorgan failure, chronic renal insufficiency, or during therapy with other nephrotoxic agents (23). Most cases resolve within two weeks, and few require renal replacement therapy (24).

Prevention

INTRAVENOUS HYDRATION: The most effective preventive measure for contrast-induced nephropathy in high-risk patients is intravenous hydration (if permitted). The recommended regimen is *isotonic saline at 100–150 mL/hr started 3 to 12 hours before the procedure and continued for 6–24 hours after the procedure* (23). For emergency procedures, at least 300–500 mL isotonic saline should be infused just prior to the procedure.

Table 34.4	Drugs Most Often Implicated in Acute Kidney Injury	
Mechanism	**Offending Drugs**	
Intrarenal Hemodynamics	Most Frequent:	Nonsteroidal anti-inflammatory agents (NSAIDs)
	Others:	ACE inhibitors, angiotensin receptor-blocking drugs, cyclosporine, tacrolimus
Osmotic Nephropathy	Most Frequent:	Hydroxyethyl starches
	Others:	Mannitol, intravenous immunoglobulins
Renal Tubular Injury	Most Frequent:	Aminoglycosides
	Others:	Amphotericin B, antiretrovirals, cisplatin
Interstitial Nephritis	Most Frequent:	Antimicrobials (penicillins, cephalosporins, sulfonamides, vancomycin, macrolides, tetracyclines, rifampin)
	Others:	Anticonvulsants (phenytoin, valproic acid), H_2 blockers, NSAIDs, proton pump inhibitors

Adapted from Reference 26.

N-ACETYLCYSTEINE: N-acetylcysteine (NAC) is a glutathione surrogate with antioxidant actions that has had mixed results as a protective agent for contrast-induced nephropathy (3). However, an analysis of 16 studies using high-dose NAC (exceeding 1,200 mg daily) showed a 50% risk-reduction for contrast-induced nephropathy (24). The high-dose NAC regimen is 1,200 mg orally twice daily for 48 hours, beginning the night before the contrast procedure. For emergency procedures, the first 1,200 mg dose should be given just prior to the procedure. Despite continuing debate, NAC is a popular preventive agent because of its low cost and safety.

Acute Interstitial Nephritis (AIN)

AIN is an inflammatory condition that involves the renal interstitium and presents as acute renal failure. However, oliguria is not always a feature of AIN (25), which means that AIN does not always qualify for the diagnosis of AKI. Most cases of AIN are the result of a hypersensitivity drug reaction, but infections (usually viral or atypical pathogens) can also be involved. The drugs most often implicated in AIN are listed in Table 34.4 (26). Antibiotics are the most common offenders, particularly the penicillins.

Drug-induced AIN is often (but not always) accompanied by signs of a hypersensitivity reaction; i.e., fever, rash, and eosinophilia. The onset of renal injury usually appears several weeks after the first exposure (26), but can appear within a few days after a second exposure. Sterile pyuria and eosinophiluria are common manifestations (26). A renal biopsy can secure the diagnosis, but these are rarely performed. AIN usually resolves spontaneously after the offending agent is discontinued, but recovery can take months

Myoglobinuric Renal Failure

Acute renal failure develops in about one-third of patients with diffuse muscle injury (rhabdomyolysis) (27,28). The culprit is myoglobin, which is released by the injured muscle and is capable of damaging the renal tubular epithelial cells. The source of cell injury may be the iron moiety in heme (29), which is capable of oxidative cell injury via the production of hydroxyl radicals (see Figure 22.6 on page 437). This would explain why hemoglobin is also capable of producing renal tubular injury.

The diagnosis of AKI can be difficult in the setting of rhabdomyolysis because the injured muscle releases creatine, which is measured as creatinine, and falsely elevates the serum creatinine concentration (29).

Myoglobin in Urine

Myoglobin can be detected in urine with the orthotoluidine dipstick reaction (Hemastix), which is used to detect occult blood in urine. If the test is positive, the urine should be centrifuged (to separate erythrocytes) and the supernatant should be passed through a micropore filter (to remove hemoglobin). A persistently positive test after these measures is evidence of myoglobin in urine. An alternative approach is to inspect the urine sediment for red blood cells; i.e., a positive dipstick test for blood without red blood cells in the urine sediment can be used as evidence of myoglobinuria.

The presence of myoglobin in urine does not ensure the diagnosis of AKI, but *the absence of myoglobin in urine can be used to exclude the diagnosis of myoglobinuric renal injury* (28).

Management

Aggressive *volume resuscitation* to promote renal blood flow is the most effective measure for preventing or limiting the renal injury in rhabdomyolysis. Alkalinizing the urine can also help to limit the renal injury, but this is difficult to accomplish, and is often not necessary. The potassium and phosphate levels in plasma must be monitored closely in rhabdomyolysis because these electrolytes are released by injured skeletal muscle, and their concentrations in plasma can increase dramatically, especially when renal function is impaired. About 30% of patients who develop myoglobinuric renal injury will require dialysis (28).

Abdominal Compartment Syndrome

Abdominal compartment syndrome (ACS) is the condition where an increase in abdominal pressure leads to dysfunction in one or more vital organs (30,31). This organ dysfunction usually involves the bowel (splanchnic ischemia), the kidneys (AKI), and cardiovascular system (reduced cardiac output).

Definitions

The pertinent definitions related to ACS are shown in Table 34.5 (30). The intraabdominal pressure (IAP) is normally 5–7 mm Hg in the supine position (the IAP measurement is described later), and intraabdominal hypertension (IAH) is defined as a sustained increase in IAP to ≥ 12 mm Hg. ACS occurs when the IAP rises above 20 mm Hg and there is evidence of a newly-developed organ dysfunction.

Table 34.5	Definitions Related to Intraabdominal Pressure

Intraabdominal Pressure (IAP)

The pressure in the abdominal cavity, which is normally 5–7 mm Hg in the supine position.

Intraabdominal Hypertension (IAH)

A sustained increase in IAP to ≥ 12 mm Hg in the supine position.

Abdominal Compartment Syndrome (ACS)

A sustained increase in IAP to ≥ 20 mm Hg in the supine position that is accompanied by newly-developed organ dysfunction.

Abdominal Perfusion Pressure (APP)

A measure of visceral perfusion pressure, equivalent to the difference between the mean arterial pressure and the intraabdominal pressure: APP = MAP − IAP. The desired APP is ≥ 60 mm Hg.

Filtration Gradient (FG)

The mechanical force across the glomerulus, equivalent to the difference between the glomerular filtration pressure (or MAP − IAP) and the proximal tubular pressure (or IAP): FG = MAP − (IAP × 2).

From Reference 30.

Predisposing Conditions

ACS is traditionally associated with abdominal trauma, but several conditions can raise the IAP and predispose to ACS, including gastric distension, bowel obstruction, ileus, peritoneal hemorrhage, ascites, bowel wall edema, hepatomegaly, positive-pressure breathing, upright body position, and obesity (31). Several of these factors can co-exist in critically ill patients, which explains why *IAH is discovered in as many as 60% of patients in medical and surgical ICUs* (32).

LARGE VOLUME RESUSCITATION: One of the more common and unrecognized causes of IAH is large volume resuscitation, which can raise the IAP by promoting edema in the abdominal organs (particularly the bowel). In one report of ICU patients with a net positive fluid balance > 5 liters over 24 hours, ICH was discovered in 85% of the patients, and ACS was diagnosed in 25% of the patients (33). This observation adds to the growing consensus that avoiding a positive fluid balance will reduce morbidity and mortality in ICU patients (see page 457).

Renal Dysfunction

An increase in IAP can affect virtually every organ (by decreasing venous return and subsequently decreasing cardiac output), but the kidneys are most frequently affected. The influence of IAP on renal function can be explained by the two variables described next.

ABDOMINAL PERFUSION PRESSURE: The driving pressure for renal blood flow is the difference between the mean arterial pressure (MAP) and the mean pressure in the renal veins. When the IAP exceeds the renal venous pressure, the driving pressure for renal blood flow is the difference between MAP and IAP. This pressure difference is called the *abdominal perfusion pressure* (APP):

$$APP = MAP - IAP \qquad (34.3)$$

In patients with IAH, the APP is equivalent to the *renal perfusion pressure*, and thus an increase in IAP will reduce renal blood flow by decreasing the APP. The APP needed to preserve renal blood flow is not known, but in studies of IAH and ACS, maintaining an APP > 60 mm Hg is associated with improved survival (30).

FILTRATION GRADIENT: The filtration gradient (FG) is the pressure gradient across the glomerulus, and is equivalent to the difference between the glomerular filtration pressure (GFP) and the proximal tubular pressure (PTP) (30):

$$FG = GFP - PTP \qquad (34.4)$$

In patients with IAH, GFP is considered equivalent to MAP − IAP, and PTP is considered equivalent to IAP, so equation 34.4 can be rewritten as:

$$FG = MAP - (IAP \times 2) \qquad (34.5)$$

According to this relationship, an increase in IAP will have a greater impact on glomerular filtration (and urine flow) than an equivalent decrease in MAP. This might explain why oliguria is one of the first signs of IAH (30).

Measuring Intraabdominal Pressure

Patients with AKI and a predisposing condition for ACS (which includes most ICU patients) should have a measurement of IAP. The physical examination is insensitive for detecting an increase in IAP (34), so the IAP must be measured. The standard measure of IAP is the pressure in a decompressed urinary bladder (intravesicular method). Specialized bladder drainage catheters are available for measuring IAP (e.g., from Bard Medical, Covington, GA). The following conditions are required for each measurement (30): (a) the patient must be in the supine position, with the pressure transducer zeroed along the mid-axillary line, (b) a small volume (25 mL) of isotonic saline in injected into the bladder 30–60 seconds prior to each measurement, and (c) the IAP is measured only at the end of expiration, and only when there is no evidence of abdominal muscle contractions. The IAP is measured in mm Hg, not cm H_2O (1 mm Hg = 1.36 cm H_2O).

Management

General measures for reducing IAP include sedation (to reduce abdominal muscle contractions), avoiding elevation of the head more than 20° above the horizontal plane (35), and avoiding a positive fluid balance. Specific measures are dictated by the source of the elevated IAP, and can include decompression of the stomach, small bowel, or colon, percutaneous drainage of peritoneal fluid, or surgery (e.g., for abdominal injuries or bowel obstruction). As mentioned earlier, efforts to maintain an APP > 60 mm Hg (with vasopressors to increase MAP, if necessary) is associated with improved outcomes in ACS.

Surgical decompression is recommended for patients with ACS when the IAP cannot be reduced by conventional measures (35). However, this procedure has considerable risks (e.g., the abdomen is often left open for continued drainage), and these risks must be weighed against the risks of not performing the procedure.

RENAL REPLACEMENT THERAPY

About 70% of patients with acute renal failure will require some form of renal replacement therapy (RRT). The usual indications for RRT in acute renal failure include (a) volume overload, (b) life-threatening hyperkalemia or metabolic acidosis that is refractory to conventional measures, and (c) removal of toxins (e.g., ethylene glycol). Otherwise, the optimal timing for RRT in acute renal failure is unclear (36).

There is a growing body of RRT techniques, which includes not only hemodialysis and hemofiltration, but also hemodiafiltration, high flux dialysis, and plasmafiltration. The descriptions that follow are limited to hemodialysis and hemofiltration. The mechanisms of fluid and solute removal by each of these techniques is shown in Figure 34.3.

Hemodialysis

Hemodialysis removes solutes by diffusion, which is driven by the concentration gradient of solutes across a semipermeable membrane. To maintain this concentration gradient, a technique called *countercurrent exchange* is used, where blood and dialysis fluid are driven in opposite directions across the dialysis membrane. A blood pump is used to move blood in one direction across the dialysis membrane at a rate of 200–300 mL/min. The dialysis fluid on the other side of the membrane moves about twice as fast, at a rate of 500 to 800 mL/min (37). Large-bore, double lumen catheters are required for acute hemodialysis, and these catheters are described in Chapter 1 (see Table 1.5 on page 13, and Figure 1.6 on page 14).

Advantages and Disadvantages

The principal benefit of hemodialysis is rapid clearance of small solutes. Only a few hours of hemodialysis is needed to clear life-threatening accumulations of potassium or organic acids, or to remove a day's worth of accumulated nitrogenous waste. The disadvantages of hemodialysis include (a) limited removal of large molecules (e.g., inflammatory cytokines), and (b) the need to maintain a blood flow of 200–300 mL/min through the dialysis chamber. This latter requirement creates a risk of hypotension, which occurs in about one-third of hemodialysis treatments (37).

Hemofiltration

Hemofiltration removes solutes by convection, where a hydrostatic pressure gradient is used to move a solute-containing fluid across a semipermeable membrane. Since the bulk movement of fluid "drags" the solute across the membrane, this method of solute removal is also known as *solvent drag* (37).

Hemofiltration can remove large volumes of fluid (up to 3 liters per hour), but the rate of solute clearance is much slower than during hemodialysis. Therefore, hemofiltration must be performed continuously to provide effective solute clearance. Because solutes are cleared with water, the plasma concentration of these solutes (e.g., urea) does not decrease during hemofiltration unless a solute-free intravenous fluid is infused to replace some of the ultrafiltrate that is lost (this is often necessary because of the large volumes removed during hemofiltration).

Methods

Hemofiltration was originally performed by cannulating an artery (radial, brachial, or femoral) and a large vein (internal jugular or femoral). This method of *continuous arteriovenous hemofiltration* (CAVH) uses the mean arterial pressure as the filtration pressure, and does not require a

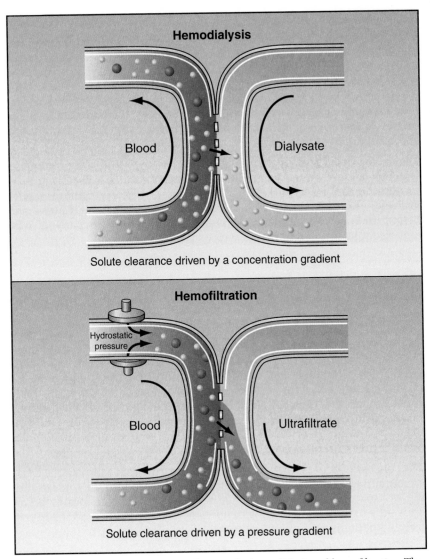

FIGURE 34.3 Mechanisms of solute clearance by hemodialysis and hemofiltration. The smaller particles represent small solutes (e.g., urea), which can be cleared by both techniques, while the larger particles represent larger molecules (e.g., inflammatory cytokines) that can be cleared by hemofiltration, but not by hemodialysis.

pump in the circuit. However, it is not well suited for patients with labile blood pressures.

The more popular method at present is *continuous venovenous hemofiltration* (CVVH), where venous blood is removed and returned through large-bore, double-lumen catheters like the ones used for hemodialysis. This method does not require cannulation of an artery, but a pump in the circuit is required to create an effective filtration pressure.

Advantages and Disadvantages

There are two major advantages with hemofiltration. First, hemofiltration allows more gradual fluid removal than hemodialysis, and thus is less likely to produce hemodynamic compromise. Secondly, hemofiltration removes larger molecules than hemodialysis, which makes it the preferred method for removing toxins such as ethylene glycol. This feature also allows for the removal of inflammatory mediators, which can provide a therapeutic advantage in patients with systemic inflammation and multiorgan failure (38).

The major disadvantage of hemofiltration is the slow solute removal, which is not well suited when rapid removal of solutes is necessary (e.g., for life-threatening hyperkalemia or acidosis). A newer method of RRT known as *hemodiafiltration* (which combines the features of dialysis and hemofiltration) is more suitable than hemofiltration for patients who require rapid solute removal as well as volume removal.

A FINAL WORD

The Dirac Equation & Acute Kidney Injury

The author of the introductory quote, Paul Dirac, was a prominent (and eccentric) theoretical physicist who introduced the concept of antimatter (39). His quote refers to his equation (the Dirac equation) for describing the behavior of electrons, which was later shown to have some limitations. Like the Dirac equation, the concept of acute kidney injury has not achieved its intent to describe the spectrum of renal failure experienced by critically ill patients. The sources of confusion created by the concept of acute kidney injury are described on page 635.

The concept of acute kidney injury has one feature that is unlike the Dirac equation; i.e., the Dirac equation added considerably to the understanding of how electrons behave, while the concept of acute kidney injury adds little to the understanding of how or why renal failure occurs in critically ill patients.

REFERENCES

Clinical Practice Guidelines

1. Fliser D, Laville M, Covic A, et al. A European Renal Best Practice (ERBP) Position Statement on Kidney Disease Improving Global Outcomes (KDIGO) clinical practice guidelines on acute kidney injury. Nephrol Dial Transplant 2012; 27:4263–4272.

2. Brochard L, Abroug F, Brenner M, et al. An official ATS/ERS/ESICM/SCCM/ SRLF statement: Prevention and management of acute renal failure in the ICU patient. Am J Respir Crit Care Med 2010; 1126–1155.

Diagnostic Criteria

3. Dennen P, Douglas IS, Anderson R. Acute kidney injury in the intensive care unit: an update and primer for the intensivist. Crit Care Med 2010; 38:261–275.

4. Ympa YP, Sakr Y, Reinhart K, et al. Has mortality from acute renal failure decreased? A systematic review of the literature. Am J Med 2005; 118:827–832.

5. Chang C-H, Lin C-Y, Tian Y-C, et al. Acute kidney injury classification: comparison of AKIN and RIFLE criteria. Shock 2010; 33:247–252.

Diagnostic Evaluation

6. Abernathy VE, Lieberthal W. Acute renal failure in the critically ill patient. Crit Care Clin 2002; 18:203–222.

7. Wang Z, Holthoff JH, Seely KA, et al. Development of oxidative stress in the peritubular capillary microenvironment mediates sepsis-induced renal microcirculatory failure and acute kidney injury. Am J Pathol 2012; 180:505–516.

8. Blantz RC, Pelayo JC. A functional role for the tubuloglomerular feedback mechanism. Kidney Int 1984; 25:739–746.

9. Uchino S, Kellum JA, Bellomo R, et al. Acute renal failure in critically ill patients. A multinational, multicenter study. JAMA 2005; 294:813–818.

10. Subramanian S, Ziedalski TM. Oliguria, volume overload, Na$^+$ balance, and diuretics. Crit Care Clin 2005; 21:291–303.

11. Steiner RW. Interpreting the fractional excretion of sodium. Am J Med 1984; 77:699–702.

12. Vaz AJ. Low fractional excretion of urine sodium in acute renal failure due to sepsis. Arch Intern Med 1983; 143:738–739.

13. Fang LST, Sirota RA, Ebert TH, Lichtenstein NS. Low fractional excretion of sodium with contrast media-induced acute renal failure Arch Intern Med 1980; 140:531–533.

14. Corwin HL, Schreiber MJ, Fang LST. Low fractional excretion of sodium. Occurrence with hemoglobinuric- and myoglobinuric-induced acute renal failure. Arch Intern Med 1984; 144:981–982.

15. Gottfried J, Wiesen J, Raina R, Nally JV Jr. Finding the cause of acute kidney injury: which index of fractional excretion is better? Clev Clin J Med 2012; 79:121–126.

Initial Management

16. Vincent J-L, Gerlach H. Fluid resuscitation in severe sepsis and septic shock: an evidence-based review. Crit Care Med 2004; 32(Suppl):S451–S454.

17. Venkataram R, Kellum JA. The role of diuretic agents in the management of acute renal failure. Contrib Nephrol 2001; 132:158–170.

18. van der Voort PH, Boerma EC, Koopmans M, et al. Furosemide does not improve renal recovery after hemofiltration for acute renal failure in critically ill patients. A double blind randomized controlled trial. Crit Care Med 2009; 37:533–538.

19. Kellum JA, Decker JM. Use of dopamine in acute renal failure: a meta-analysis. Crit Care Med 2001; 29:1526–1531.

20. Holmes CL, Walley KR. Bad medicine. Low-dose dopamine in the ICU. Chest 2003; 123:1266–1275.

Contrast-Induced Renal Injury

21. Pierson PB, Hansell P, Lias P. Pathophysiology of contrast medium-induced nephropathy. Kidney Int 2005; 68:14–22.

22. Ehrmann S, Badin J, Savath L, et al. Acute kidney injury in the critically ill: Is iodinated contrast medium really harmful? Crit Care Med 2013; 41:1017–1025.

23. McCullough PA, Soman S. Acute kidney injury with iodinated contrast. Crit Care Med 2008; 36(Suppl):S204–S211.

24. Triverdi H, daram S, Szabo A, et al. High-dose N-acetylcysteine for the prevention of contrast-induced nephropathy. Am J Med 2009; 122:874.e9–15.

Acute Interstitial Nephritis

25. Ten RM, Torres VE, Millner DS, et al. Acute interstitial nephritis. Mayo Clin Proc 1988; 3:921–930.

26. Bentley ML, Corwin HL, Dasta J. Drug-induced acute kidney injury in the critically ill adult: Recognition and prevention strategies. Crit Care Med 2010; 38(Suppl): S169–S174.

Myoglobinuric Renal Injury

27. Beetham R. Biochemical investigation of suspected rhabdomyolysis. Ann Clin Biochem 2000; 2000:37:581–587.

28. Sharp LS, Rozycki GS, Feliciano DV. Rhabdomyolysis and secondary renal failure in critically ill surgical patients. Am J Surg 2004; 188:801–806.

29. Visweswaran P, Guntupalli J. Rhabdomyolysis. Crit Care Clin 1999; 15:415–428.

Abdominal Compartment Syndrome

30. Malbrain ML, Cheatham ML, Kirkpatrick A, et al. Results from the International Conference of Experts on Intra-abdominal Hypertension and Abdominal Compartment Syndrome. I. Definitions. Intensive Care Med 2006; 32:1722–1723.

31. Al-Mufarrej F, Abell LM, Chawla LS. Understanding intra-abdominal hypertension: from bench to bedside. J Intensive Care Med 2012; 27:145–160.

32. Malbrain ML, Chiumello D, Pelosi P, et al. Prevalence of intra-abdominal hypertension in critically ill patients: A multicenter epidemiological study. Intensive Care Med 2004; 30:822–829.

33. Daugherty EL, Hongyan L, Taichman D, et al. Abdominal compartment syndrome is common in medical ICU patients receiving large-volume resuscitation. J Intensive Care Med 2007; 22:294–299.

34. Sugrue M, Bauman A, Jones F, et al. Clinical examination is an inaccurate predictor of intraabdominal pressure. World J Surg 2002; 26:1428–1431.

35. Cheatham ML, Malbrain ML, Kirkpatrick A, et al. Results from the International Conference of Experts on Intra-abdominal Hypertension and Abdominal Compartment Syndrome. II. Recommendations. Intensive Care Med 2007; 33:951–962.

Renal Replacement Therapy

36. Pannu N, Klarenbach S, Wiebe N, et al. Renal replacement therapy in patients with acute renal failure. A systematic review. JAMA 2008; 299:793–805.

37. O'Reilly P, Tolwani A. Renal replacement therapy III. IHD, CRRT, SLED. Crit Care Clin 2005; 21:367–378.

38. Morgera S, Haase M, Kuss T, et al. Pilot study on the effects of high cutoff hemofiltration on the need for norepinephrine in septic patients with acute renal failure. Crit Care Med 2006; 34:2099–2104.

A Final Word

39. Farmelo G. The Strangest Man. The Hidden Life of Paul Dirac, Mystic of the Atom. New York: Basic Books, 2009.

Chapter 35

OSMOTIC
DISORDERS

*In dealing with any subject matter, find out what entities
are undeniably involved, and state everything in terms of
these entities.*

Bertrand Russell
1914

As many as 40% of ICU patients have a disorder involving the osmotic balance between intracellular and extracellular fluids, and in many cases, the problem is acquired after admission to the ICU (1). The presenting feature of these disorders is a change in the plasma sodium concentration (i.e., hypernatremia or hyponatremia), but the pathological problem is a change in cell volume, which is most apparent in the central nervous system.

This chapter presents a simple approach to osmotic disorders based on a single variable: the extracellular volume. The first part of the chapter is a brief review of osmotic forces and how they influence the distribution of total body water.

OSMOTIC ACTIVITY

The movement of water between fluid compartments is determined by a property of fluids known as *osmotic activity*, which is a reflection of *the number of solute particles* per unit volume of solvent. Osmotic activity is a *colligative property*, and depends only on the number of solute particles in a fluid, and not on the electrical charge, size, or chemical behavior of the solutes. The total osmotic activity of a solution is the summed osmotic activity of all the solute particles in the solution.

Relative Osmotic Activity

When two fluid compartments are separated by a membrane that is permeable to solutes and water, the solutes in each fluid compartment will equilibrate across the membrane, and the osmotic activity will be equivalent in both fluid compartments. Since water movement follows solute movement, the volume in both fluid compartments will be equivalent. This is illustrated in the panel on the left in Figure 35.1. In this situation, the two fluids are described as *isotonic* (i.e., the term "tonicity" refers to the relative osmotic activity of two fluids).

Effective Osmotic Activity

When two fluid compartments are separated by a membrane that is permeable to water but is not freely permeable to solutes, the solutes will not distribute evenly in the fluid compartments, and the osmotic activity will be different in each fluid. In this situation, water moves from the fluid with the lower osmotic activity to the fluid with the higher osmotic activity, as demonstrated in the panel on the right in Figure 35.1. The difference in osmotic activity between the fluid compartments is called the *effective osmotic activity,* and it is the force that drives the movement of water between fluids with different osmotic activities. This force is also called the *osmotic pressure.* The fluid with the higher osmotic activity is described as *hypertonic,* and the fluid with the lower osmotic activity is described as *hypotonic.*

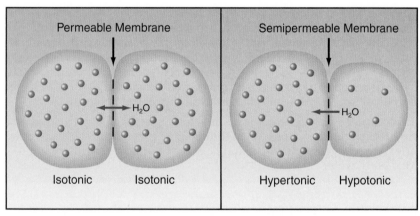

FIGURE 35.1 Illustration of the relationship between osmotic activity and the movement of water between fluid compartments. See text for explanation.

Summary

The following statements summarize the relationship between osmotic activity and the transcellular shift of water.

1. A change in the relative osmotic activity of extracellular fluid produces a transcellular water shift.

2. When the extracellular fluid is hypertonic, water will move out of cells.

3. When the extracellular fluid is hypotonic, water will move into cells.

Units of Osmotic Activity

The unit of measurement for osmotic activity is the osmole (osm), which is defined as one gram molecular weight (one mole) of a nondissociable substance, and is equivalent to 6×10^{23} particles (Avogadro's Number). Osmotic activity can be expressed in relation to the volume of water in a solution, or the total volume of the solution (3,4).

1. Osmotic activity per volume of solution is called *osmolarity*, and is expressed as milliosmoles per liter (mosm/L).

2. Osmotic activity per volume of water is called *osmolality*, and is expressed as milliosmoles per kilogram of H_2O (mosm/kg H_2O, or mosm/kg).

Plasma is mostly (93%) water, so the osmotic activity of plasma solutes is typically expressed as osmolality (mosm/kg H_2O). However, there is little difference between the osmolality and osmolarity of extracellular fluid, and the two terms are often used interchangeably (4).

Conversion Factors

The following formulas (where n is the number of nondissociable particles) can be used to convert plasma solute concentrations to units of osmolality:

1. For solute concentrations expressed in mEq/L:

$$\frac{mEq/L}{valence} \times n = mosm/kg\ H_2O \qquad (35.1)$$

Thus, for univalent ions like Na^+, the plasma concentration in mEq/L is equivalent to the osmotic activity in mosm/kg H_2O.

2. For solute concentrations expressed in mg/dL:

$$\frac{mg/dL \times 10}{mol\ wt} \times n = mosm/kg\ H_2O \qquad (35.2)$$

where mol wt is molecular weight, and the factor 10 is used to convert deciliters (dL) to liters. For example, glucose has a molecular weight of 180, so a plasma glucose concentration of 90 mg/dL is equivalent to $(90 \times 10/180) \times 1 = 5$ mosm/kg H_2O.

Plasma Osmolality

The osmotic activity of plasma can be measured or calculated.

Measured Plasma Osmolality

The standard method for measuring plasma osmolality is the *freezing point depression* method. Solute-free water freezes at 0°C, and this freezing point decreases by 1.86°C for each osmole of solute that is added to one kilogram of water. Therefore, depression of the freezing point of plasma is proportional to the osmotic activity in plasma.

Calculated Plasma Osmolality

Plasma osmolality can also be calculated using the concentrations of the principal solutes in plasma (sodium, chloride, glucose, and urea) (3); i.e.,

$$\text{Posm} = (2 \times [\text{Na}^+]) + \frac{[\text{glucose}]}{18} + \frac{\text{BUN}}{2.8} \tag{35.3}$$

where Posm is the plasma osmolality in mosm/kg H_2O, [Na] is the plasma sodium concentration in mEq/L, [glucose] and BUN are the glucose and urea concentrations in plasma in mg/dL, and the factors 18 and 2.8 are the molecular weights of glucose and urea divided by 10, respectively, to express their concentrations in mosm/kg H_2O (analogous to Equation 35.2). The [Na^+] is doubled to include the osmotic activity of chloride.

EXAMPLE: Using normal plasma concentrations of Na^+ (140 mEq/L), glucose (90 mg/dL), and BUN (14 mg/dL), the plasma osmolality is: (2 × 140) + 90/18 + 14/2.8 = 290 mosm/kg H_2O.

EFFECTIVE PLASMA OSMOLALITY: Urea readily crosses cell membranes, so an increase in blood urea nitrogen (BUN) will not increase the relative osmotic activity of plasma (i.e., *azotemia is a hyperosmotic, but not a hypertonic, condition*). Therefore, the calculation of effective plasma osmolality does not include the BUN; i.e.,

$$\text{Effective Posm} = (2 \times [\text{Na}^+]) + \frac{[\text{glucose}]}{18} \tag{35.4}$$

Using normal plasma concentrations of Na^+ (140 mEq/L) and glucose (90 mg/dL) yields an effective plasma osmolarity of (2 × 140) + 90/18 = 285 mosm/kg H_2O. Note the following:

1. There is only a minor difference (5 mosm/kg H_2O) between the total and effective plasma osmolarity.

2. Plasma sodium accounts for 98% (280 of 285 mosm/kg H_2O) of the effective osmotic activity of the extracellular fluid. This highlights the fact that *the sodium concentration in extracellular fluid is the principal determinant of the distribution of total body water in the intracellular and extracellular fluid compartments.*

Osmolal Gap

Because solutes other than sodium, glucose, and urea are present in the extracellular fluid, the measured plasma osmolality will be greater than the calculated osmolality. This *osmolal gap* (i.e., the difference between measured and calculated plasma osmolality) is normally ≤ 10 mosm/kg H_2O (3,5). Accumulation of a nondiffusable solute (like an exogenous toxin) will increase the osmolal gap, and this has led to the use of the osmolal gap to detect the presence of ingested toxins that are not easily measured (6).

HYPERNATREMIA

The normal plasma [Na⁺] is 135–145 mEq/L, and thus hypernatremia is defined as a plasma [Na⁺] > 145 mEq/L. This condition is reported in as many as 25% of ICU patients (1), and *is acquired in the ICU in most cases* (1,7).

Approach to Hypernatremia

Hypernatremia can be the result of 3 conditions: (a) Loss of sodium and water, with water loss > sodium loss (i.e., hypotonic fluid loss), (b) free water loss, and (c) gain of sodium and free water, with sodium gain > free water gain (i.e., gain of hypertonic fluid) (8).

Extracellular Volume

Each of the conditions responsible for hypernatremia is associated with a different extracellular volume (ECV); i.e., hypotonic fluid loss is associated with a low ECV, free water loss is associated with a normal ECV, and hypertonic fluid gain is associated with a high ECV. Therefore, assessment

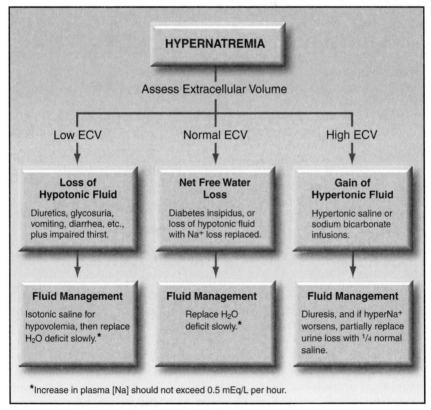

FIGURE 35.2 Flow diagram for the approach to hypernatremia based on the extracellular volume (ECV).

of the extracellular volume (ECV) can be used to identify the condition responsible for hypernatremia. The approach to hypernatremia based on the ECV is shown in Figure 35.2. (Assessment of the extracellular volume is not presented here. See Chapter 11 for the evaluation of hypovolemia.)

Hypertonicity

The principal consequence of hypernatremia is an increase in the effective osmolality (tonicity) of the extracellular fluid, which draws water out of cells. This is most evident in the central nervous system.

Hypernatremic Encephalopathy

The clinical manifestations of hypernatremic encephalopathy range from agitation and lethargy to coma and generalized or focal seizures (1). Encephalopathy is more likely to occur with a rapid rise in plasma Na^+, and possible mechanisms include shrinkage of neuronal cell bodies (9) and osmotic demyelination (10). The presence of encephalopathy is a poor prognostic sign in hypernatremia, and carries a mortality rate as high as 50% (9).

HYPOVOLEMIC HYPERNATREMIA

Hypernatremia associated with a low extracellular volume (ECV) is the result of loss of hypotonic fluids (i.e., fluids with a $[Na^+] < 135$ mEq/L). This is the most common cause of community-acquired (but not ICU-acquired) hypernatremia (1).

Hypotonic Fluid Loss

The average sodium concentration in fluids that can be lost is shown in Table 35.1 (11–13). Note the following:

1. All fluid losses involve the loss of sodium, which promotes a decrease in ECV.
2. All lost fluids are hypotonic to plasma (i.e., have a sodium concentration < 135 mEq/L), and will eventually result in hypernatremia if not replaced.

Common sources of hypotonic fluid loss include (a) excessive diuresis (osmotic or drug-induced), (b) excessive sweat loss in heat-related illnesses, and (c) normal or accentuated fluid losses in elderly, debilitated patients, particularly those with sepsis.

Impaired Thirst

The normal response to hypotonic fluid loss is an increase in the sensation of thirst, which promotes water ingestion to limit the rise in plasma osmolality. Patients who develop symptomatic hypernatremia often have an impaired sensation of thirst from a debilitating or chronic illness, or advanced age. For this reason, symptomatic hypernatremia from hypotonic fluid loss can be a sign of a more serious condition; i.e., "failure to thrive."

Table 35.1	Average Sodium Concentration in Lost Fluids		
GI Fluids	**[Na⁺] (mEq/L)**	**Other Fluids**	**[Na⁺] (mEq/L)**
Normal Stool	25	Normal Urine	<10*
Vomitus/NG Drainage	60	Diuretic Urine	80
Ileostomy Drainage	125		
Inflammatory Diarrhea	75	Sweat	65
Secretory Diarrhea	90		

From References 11–13.
*Dependent on sodium intake.

Plasma Volume

Hypotonic fluid loss has less of an effect on plasma volume than ECV because the accentuated loss of free water increases the *colloid osmotic pressure* in plasma (i.e., the osmotic pressure generated by plasma proteins, principally albumin, that do not move readily into the interstitial fluid), and this draws fluid from the interstitial fluid and helps to maintain the plasma volume. The influence of hypotonic fluid loss on plasma volume is determined by the severity of sodium losses; i.e., the greater the sodium loss, the greater the likelihood of a significant decrease in plasma volume (and a subsequent decrease in cardiac output).

Management

Management is aimed at the two consequences of hypotonic fluid loss: (a) loss of sodium, which reduces the ECV and threatens the plasma volume (and cardiac output), and (b) loss of water in excess of sodium (the *free water deficit*), which increases the plasma osmolality.

Volume Resuscitation

The most immediate concern with sodium loss is a decrease in plasma volume, which can decrease cardiac output and impair tissue perfusion. Therefore, any signs of a low flow state (e.g., cold extremities, a decrease in blood pressure or urine output) should prompt immediate volume resuscitation with isotonic saline. Fortunately, loss of hypotonic fluids carries a low risk of hypovolemic shock.

Free Water Replacement

When hypovolemia has been corrected, the next step is to replace the free water deficit. The calculation of free water deficit is based on the assumption that the product of total body water (TBW) and plasma sodium concentration [PNa] is always constant (8).

$$\text{Current TBW} \times \text{Current [PNa]} = \text{Normal TBW} \times \text{Normal [PNa]} \qquad (35.5)$$

Substituting 140 mEq/L for a normal [PNa] and rearranging terms yields the following relationship:

$$\text{Current TBW} = \text{Normal TBW} \times (140/\text{Current [PNa]}) \qquad (35.6)$$

1. The normal TBW (in liters) is usually 60% of *lean* body weight (in kg) in men and 50% of lean body weight in women, but a 10% reduction in the normal TBW has been suggested for hypernatremic patients who are water depleted (14)

2. In patients who are hyperglycemic, *the plasma sodium should be corrected for the dilutional effect of hyperglycemia.* This effect averages 2 mEq/L for every 100 mg/dL increase in plasma glucose. (See the section on "Hypertonic Hyperglycemia" for more on this correction factor.)

3. Once the current TBW is calculated, the free water deficit is the difference between the normal and current TBW.

$$\text{H}_2\text{O Deficit (L)} = \text{Normal TBW} - \text{Current TBW} \qquad (35.7)$$

EXAMPLE: For an adult male with a lean body weight of 70 kg and a plasma [Na] of 160 mEq/L, the normal TBW is $0.5 \times 70 = 35$ L, the current TBW is $35 \times (140/160) = 30.5$ L, and the H$_2$O deficit is $35 - 30.5 = 4.5$ L.

REPLACEMENT VOLUME: Free water deficits are corrected with sodium-containing fluids such as 0.45% NaCL (to correct sodium deficits and ongoing sodium losses). The volume needed to correct the H$_2$O deficit is a function of the [Na] in the replacement fluid and the desired plasma [Na] (15). The following equation uses 140 mEq/L as the desired plasma [Na]:

$$\text{Volume (L)} = \text{H}_2\text{O Deficit} \times (140/[\text{Na] in IV Fluid}) \qquad (35.8)$$

EXAMPLE: Using the H$_2$O deficit of 4.5 L from the prior example, if the replacement fluid is 0.45% NaCL ([Na$^+$] = 77 mEq/L), the replacement volume is $4.5 \times (140/77) = 8.1$ liters.

RATE OF REPLACEMENT: Neuronal cells initially shrink in response to hypertonic extracellular fluid, but cell volume is restored within hours; an effect attributed to the generation of osmotically active substances within brain cells, called *idiogenic osmoles* (8). Once the cell volume is restored to normal, aggressive replacement of free water deficits can produce cell swelling and cerebral edema. To limit the risk of cerebral edema, *the decrease in plasma [Na$^+$] should not exceed 0.5 mEq/L per hour during free water replacement* (1,8,9).

EXAMPLE: Using the prior examples, where the plasma [Na$^+$] is 160 mEq/L, the H$_2$O deficit is 4.5 L, and the replacement volume is 8.1 L using 0.45% NaCL, the time needed to reduce the plasma [Na$^+$] to 140 mEq/L at a rate of 0.5 mEq/L/hr is $(160 - 140)/0.5 = 40$ hours, and the infusion rate of the half-normal saline will be 8.1 L/40 hrs = 200 mL/hr.

VARIABILITY: The calculations for free water deficit and replacement are estimates, and do not account for ongoing sodium and free water losses, so fluid management based on these calculations can produce variable results (1). Therefore, it is important to monitor the plasma [Na⁺]fre-quently and make appropriate adjustments. *About half of the free water deficit can be replaced in the first 12 to 24 hours* of replacement (1).

HYPERNATREMIA WITHOUT HYPOVOLEMIA

Hypernatremia with a normal ECV is the result of free water loss with no net sodium loss. This condition is common in ICU patients with hyper-natremia (1), and usually occurs when sodium losses are replaced, leav-ing a net free water deficit. The condition described next is the best exam-ple of a free water deficit.

Diabetes Insipidus

Diabetes insipidus (DI), is a disorder of renal water conservation, and is characterized by loss of urine that is largely devoid of solute (i.e., like pure water) (16,17). The underlying problem in DI is a defect related to antidiuretic hormone (ADH), a polypeptide released by the posterior pituitary gland that promotes water reabsorption in the distal renal tubules. DI can involve two distinct defects related to ADH:

1. *Central DI* is characterized by failure of ADH release from the posteri-or pituitary (18). Common causes include traumatic brain injury, anox-ic encephalopathy, meningitis, and brain death. The onset is heralded by polyuria that usually is evident within 24 hours of the inciting event.

2. *Nephrogenic DI* is characterized by impaired end-organ responsiveness to ADH. Possible causes of nephrogenic DI include amphotericin, aminoglycosides, radiocontrast dyes, dopamine, lithium, hypokalemia, and the recovery (polyuric) phase of ATN (17,19). The defect in renal concentrating ability is less severe in nephrogenic DI than in central DI.

Diagnosis

The hallmark of DI is a dilute urine in the face of hypertonic plasma. In central DI, the urine osmolarity is often below 200 mosm/L, whereas in nephrogenic DI, the urine osmolarity is usually between 200 and 500 mosm/L (20). The diagnosis of DI is confirmed by noting the urinary response to fluid restriction. Failure of the urine osmolarity to increase more than 30 mosm/L in the first few hours of complete fluid restriction is diagnostic of DI. The fluid losses can be excessive during fluid restric-tion in DI (particularly central DI), and thus fluid restriction must be monitored carefully.

Once the diagnosis of DI is confirmed, the response to vasopressin (5 Units intravenously) will differentiate central from nephrogenic DI. In central DI, the urine osmolality increases by at least 50% almost immedi-ately after vasopressin administration, whereas in nephrogenic DI, the urine osmolality is unchanged after vasopressin.

Management

The fluid loss in DI is almost pure water, so the replacement strategy is aimed at replacing free water deficits using Equations 35.6–35.9 and limiting the rate of sodium correction to ≤ 0.5 mEq/L per hour (1,8,9).

VASOPRESSIN: In central DI, vasopressin administration is also required to prevent ongoing free water losses. The usual dose is *2 to 5 Units of aqueous vasopressin given subcutaneously every 4 to 6 hours* (17). The serum sodium must be monitored carefully during vasopressin therapy because water intoxication and hyponatremia can occur if the central DI begins to resolve.

Hypervolemic Hypernatremia

Hypernatremia with a high ECV is uncommon, and is usually the result of sodium bicarbonate infusions for metabolic acidosis, or aggressive use of hypertonic saline to treat increased intracranial pressure. Excessive ingestion of table salt (often in females with a psychiatric disorder) should also be considered in patients admitted with hypervolemic hypernatremia (21).

Management

In patients with normal renal function, excess sodium and water are excreted rapidly. When renal sodium excretion is impaired, it might be necessary to increase renal sodium excretion with a diuretic (e.g., furosemide). Because the urinary sodium concentration during furosemide diuresis (~ 80 mEq/L) is less than the plasma sodium concentration, diuresis can aggravate the hypernatremia. If this occurs, urine losses should be partially replaced with a fluid that is hypotonic to urine (e.g., quarter-normal saline).

HYPERTONIC HYPERGLYCEMIA

Although normoglycemia has little osmotic impact, severe hyperglycemia has a considerable influence on plasma osmolality (e.g., a plasma glucose level of 600 mg/dL is equivalent to $600/18 = 40$ mosm/kg H_2O).

Non-Ketotic Hyperglycemia

The syndrome of *non-ketotic hyperglycemia* (NKH) is characterized by severe hyperglycemia without ketoacidosis. This condition typically occurs in elderly patients with type 2 diabetes (who have enough endogenous insulin to prevent ketogenesis), and is precipitated by a physiological stress (e.g., infection, trauma). Blood glucose levels are typically > 600 mg/dL, and can reach levels in excess of 1,000 mg/dL. Glycosuria is marked, and the resulting osmotic diuresis results in hypovolemia. The combination of hyperglycemia and hypotonic fluid loss produces a considerable increase in plasma osmolality. The mortality rate in NKH (5–20%) is higher than in diabetic ketoacidosis (1–5%) (22).

Clinical Manifestations

The manifestations of NKH include severe hyperglycemia (plasma glucose levels typically >600 mg/dL), absent (or mild) ketosis, signs of encephalopathy (e.g., depressed consciousness), and evidence of hypovolemia (22).

ENCEPHALOPATHY: Mental status changes begin when the plasma osmolality rises to 320 mosm/kg H_2O, and coma can develop at a plasma osmolality of 340 mosm/kg H_2O (22). Both generalized and focal seizures can appear, and there are several reports of involuntary movements (chorea and hemiballismus) associated with hyperglycemic encephalopathy (23).

Fluid Management

VOLUME INFUSION: Volume deficits can be profound in NKH, and aggressive volume infusion with isotonic fluids (1–2 liters in the first hour) is often necessary. Thereafter, volume infusion should be guided by signs of hypovolemia (e.g., decreased blood pressure). The initial volume infusion will also ameliorate the hyperosmolar condition, which will reduce insulin resistance. The plasma [Na] is an unreliable marker of extracellular volume in NKH because of the dilutional effect of hyperglycemia.

HYPERGLYCEMIA AND PLASMA [NA⁺]: Hyperglycemia draws water from the intracellular space and creates a dilutional effect on the plasma [Na]. There is some disagreement about the extent of the dilutional effect, which ranges from 1.6 to 2.4 mEq/L for each 100 mg/dL increment in plasma glucose above 100 mg/dL (24,25). In other words, *for every 100 mg/dL increment in plasma glucose above 100 mg/dL, the plasma [Na] will decrease 1.6–2.4 mEq/L (or about 2 mEq/L).*

EXAMPLE: Using a correction factor of 2 mEq/L per 100 mg/dL increase in plasma glucose above 100 mg/dL, then if the plasma [Na] is 125 mEq/L and the plasma glucose is 800 mg/dL, the corrected plasma [Na] is (7 × 2) + 125 = 139 mEq/L.

Insulin Therapy

Because insulin drives both glucose and water into cells, insulin therapy can aggravate hypovolemia. Therefore, in patients who are hypovolemic, *insulin should be withheld until the vascular volume is restored.* Once this is accomplished, insulin is started using the same regimen recommended for diabetic ketoacidosis (see pages 610–613). However, *the insulin requirement will diminish as the hypertonic condition is corrected* (because hypertonicity promotes insulin resistance), so plasma glucose levels should be monitored frequently during insulin infusions to prevent hypoglycemia.

HYPONATREMIA

Hyponatremia (plasma [Na] < 135 mEq/L) (26), is reported in 40–50% of ICU patients (26,27), and is particularly prevalent in neurosurgical patients (27). Although hyponatremia is typically a hypotonic condition, there are instances of isotonic hyponatremia (e.g., pseudohyponatremia) and hypertonic hyponatremia (i.e., non-ketotic hyperglycemia, described in the last section).

Pseudohyponatremia

The traditional method of measuring the plasma [Na] (flame photometry) includes both aqueous and nonaqueous phases of plasma, while sodium is restricted to the aqueous phase of plasma. Therefore, the measured plasma [Na]can be lower than the actual (aqueous phase) plasma [Na]. Plasma is about 93% water, so the difference between measured and actual plasma [Na] is small (about 7%).

Marked increases in lipid or protein levels in plasma will add to the nonaqueous phase of plasma, and this can significantly lower the measured plasma [Na] without affecting the actual (aqueous phase) plasma [Na]. This condition is called *pseudohyponatremia* (28). It usually does not occur until the plasma lipid levels rise above 1,500 mg/dL or the plasma protein levels rise above 12–15 g/dL (28). The influence of hypertriglyceridemia on the measured plasma [Na] is described by the following equation (28):

$$\% \text{ decrease in [Na]} = 2.1 \times \text{triglycerides (g/dL)} - 0.6 \qquad (35.9)$$

Diagnosis

The diagnosis of pseudohyponatremia can be confirmed or eliminated by measuring the plasma osmolality, which will be normal in pseudohyponatremia, and reduced in "true" or hypotonic hyponatremia. An alternative method involves measuring the plasma [Na] with an ion-specific electrode. These electrodes measure the [Na] in the aqueous phase of plasma, and the plasma [Na] will be normal in cases of pseudohyponatremia.

Hypotonic Hyponatremia

Hypotonic hyponatremia is the result of excess free water relative to sodium in the extracellular fluid. Most cases involve loss of the normal control mechanisms for antidiuretic hormone (ADH) release.

Nonosmotic ADH Release

Antidiuretic hormone (ADH) is released by the posterior pituitary in response to an increase in the osmolality of extracellular fluid, and it helps to curb the hyperosmolar condition by promoting water reabsorption in the distal renal tubules. ADH release is normally suppressed at a plasma [Na] ≤ 135 mEq/L (1). ADH is also released in response to nonosmotic factors like a decrease in blood pressure (via baroreceptors) or "physiological stress" (i.e., the same stimulus for ACTH release from the anterior pituitary).

When nonosmotic stimuli for ADH release are active, ADH release persists despite a plasma [Na] ≤ 135 mEq/L, and the resulting water reabsorption in the kidneys aggravates the hyponatremia. Therefore, *nonosmotic or "inappropriate" release of ADH is an important factor in the development of severe and sustained hyponatremia* (29).

Clinical Features

ENCEPHALOPATHY: The principal consequence of hypotonic hyponatremia is a life-threatening encephalopathy characterized by cerebral edema, increased intracranial pressure, and the risk of brain herniation (29,30). Symptoms range from headache, nausea and vomiting to seizures, coma, and brain death. The risk and severity of encephalopathy are greater with acute (< 48 hrs) hyponatremia (29,30).

EXTRACELLULAR VOLUME: Like hypernatremia, the extracellular volume can be low, normal, and high in hyponatremia, and the approach can be organized according to the extracellular volume (ECV). This is shown in Figure 35.3.

Hypovolemic Hyponatremia

Hyponatremia with a low ECV is the result of sodium loss with excess free water retention. The sodium loss decreases the ECV, and the excess free water retention decreases the extracellular [Na]. The excess free water retention is due to baroreceptor-mediated (nonosmotic) ADH release (29) combined with free water intake (oral intake or infusion of a fluid that is hypotonic to the fluid lost).

Etiologies

The principal conditions associated with hypovolemic hyponatremia are shown in Table 35.2. Thiazide diuretics are common offenders, probably because they impair renal diluting ability. Other conditions in critically ill patients are primary adrenal insufficiency and cerebral salt wasting.

PRIMARY ADRENAL INSUFFICIENCY: Primary adrenal insufficiency is accompanied by mineralocorticoid deficiency, which results in renal sodium wasting. In contrast, secondary (hypothalamic) adrenal insufficiency is primarily a glucocorticoid deficiency, and does not promote renal sodium loss.

CEREBRAL SALT WASTING: Cerebral salt wasting is a syndrome that occurs with traumatic brain injury, subarachnoid hemorrhage, and neurosurgery (27). The mechanism for the renal sodium loss is unclear (29).

Diagnostic Considerations

The source of Na$^+$ loss is usually apparent. If this is unclear, the spot urine

[Na] can help to distinguish renal from extrarenal losses; i.e., a high urine [Na] (> 20 mEq/L) suggests a renal source of sodium loss, while a low urine [Na] (< 20 mEq/L) suggests an extrarenal source (see Figure 35.3).

Table 35.2	Predisposing Conditions for Hyponatremia	
Low ECV*	**Normal ECV**	**High ECV**
Renal NA+ Loss	*ADH-Related*	Cirrhosis
Diuretics	SIADH	Heart Failure
Cerebral Salt Wasting	Physiological Stress	Renal Failure
Primary Adrenal Insufficiency	Hypothyroidism	
Extrarenal NA+ Loss	*Not ADH-Related*	
GI Losses	Primary Polydipsia	

*Must be combined with water retention to produce hyponatremia.

Euvolemic Hyponatremia

Euvolemic hyponatremia is the result of excess water intake or excess water retention from nonosmotic ADH release.

Etiologies

The leading cause of euvolemic hyponatremia is the *syndrome of inappropriate ADH* (SIADH) (29). Other notable conditions include nonosmotic ADH release during physiological stress (often in postoperative patients), hypothyroidism (usually severe), and excessive water intake in primary polydipsia (usually in schizophrenics).

SIADH: SIADH is a condition of nonosmotic ADH release associated with a variety of malignancies, infections, and drugs. The hallmark of SIADH is the combination of euvolemia, hypotonic plasma, inappropriately concentrated urine (urine osmolality > 100 mosm/kg H_2O) and a high urine sodium (> 20 mEq/L) (29).

Diagnostic Considerations

Disorders of ADH release are associated with a urine osmolality > 100 mosm/kg H_2O, while excess water intake is associated with a urine osmolality < 100 mosm/kg H_2O (29).

Hypervolemic Hyponatremia

Hypervolemic hyponatremia is the result of Na^+ and H_2O retention, with H_2O retention exceeding Na^+ retention. This condition occurs in advanced heart failure, cirrhosis, and renal failure. Renal failure is associated with a high urine [Na^+] (> 20 mEq/L), while the urine [Na^+] is low (< 20 mEq/L) in heart failure and cirrhosis, except during diuretic therapy when the drug is active.

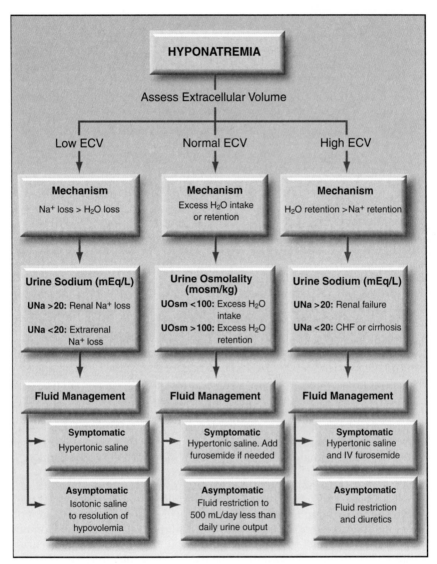

FIGURE 35.3 Flow diagram for the approach to hyponatremia based on the extracellular volume (ECV).

Fluid Management

The management of hyponatremia is determined by the ECV and the presence or absence of neurological symptoms. Symptomatic hyponatremia (which usually occurs when the plasma [Na] falls below 120 mEq/L) requires a more rapid increase in the plasma [Na] than asymptomatic cases, and this is accomplished with hypertonic saline (3% NaCL). However, correction that is too rapid can be deleterious, as described next.

Rate of Correction

Rapid correction of the plasma [Na] (i.e., > 10–12 mEq/L in 24 hrs) can produce an osmotic demyelinating syndrome (sometimes called *central pontine myelinolysis*) characterized by dysarthria, quadriparesis, and loss of consciousness (27,29). Chronic hyponatremia poses a greater risk for this complication than acute (within 48 hrs) hyponatremia. The following measures are recommended for avoiding osmotic demyelination:

1. For chronic hyponatremia, the plasma [Na] should not rise faster than 0.5 mEq/L per hour (or 10–12 mEq/L in 24 hours), and the rapid correction phase should stop when the plasma [Na] reaches 120 mEq/L (29).

2. For acute hyponatremia, the plasma [Na] can be increased by 4–6 mEq/L in the first 1–2 hrs (27). However, the final plasma [Na] should not exceed 120 mEq/L.

INFUSION RATE FOR HYPERTONIC SALINE: The initial infusion rate of hypertonic saline (3% NaCL) can be estimated by multiplying the patients body weight (in kg) by the desired rate of increase in plasma [Na] (29). For example, if the patient weighs 70 kg and the desired rate of rise in plasma [Na] is 0.5 mEq/L per hour, the initial infusion rate of hypertonic saline is $70 \times 0.5 = 35$ mL/hr. The plasma [Na] is monitored periodically to determine when the target plasma [Na] (120 mEq/L) is achieved.

Strategies:

The following are some general strategies for fluid management based on the ECV. (These strategies are also summarized in Figure 35.3.)

LOW ECV: For symptomatic patients, infuse hypertonic saline (3% NaCL) using the rapid correction guidelines in the prior section. For asymptomatic patients, infuse isotonic saline until there are no signs of hypovolemia.

NORMAL ECV: For symptomatic patients, infuse hypertonic saline (3% NaCL) using the rapid correction guidelines in the prior section. Intravenous furosemide (20–40 mg) is advised if there is a concern for volume overload (i.e., in patients with heart failure) (29). For asymptomatic patients, fluid restrict to an intake that is 500 mL/ below the daily urine output (29). If fluid restriction is ineffective or intolerable, consider the drug therapies described later.

HIGH ECV: There are no guidelines for treating hypervolemic hyponatremia. Hypertonic saline could be used for severely symptomatic patients, but should be combined with furosemide diuresis (29). For asymptomatic patients, fluid restriction and furosemide diuresis are the standard measures.

Pharmacotherapy

Demeclocycline

Demeclocycline is a tetracycline derivative that blocks the effects of ADH in the renal tubules. It is used primarily in patients with SIADH and chronic hyponatremia who do not tolerate fluid restriction. The drug is given orally, and the dose is 600–1200 mg daily in divided doses (29). Maximum effect takes several days, and success is variable. Demeclocycline can be nephrotoxic, so monitoring renal function is advised while using the drug.

Vasopressin Antagonists

Since 2005, two drugs have been introduced that block receptors for arginine vasopressin (the other term for antidiuretic hormone). These drugs, *conivaptan* and *tolvaptan* (the "vaptans") can be used as an alternative to fluid restriction in patients with euvolemic or hypervolemic hyponatremia (except renal failure). At the present time, their principal use is in patients with SIADH-related hyponatremia. These drugs are contraindicated in hypovolemic hyponatremia because of their *aquaretic* effects.

CONIVAPTAN: Conivaptan is the original vaptan, and blocks vasopressin effects in the kidneys and elsewhere. It is given intravenously with a loading dose of 20 mg, followed by a continuous infusion of 40 mg/day for 96 hours. The effect of this dosing regimen on the plasma [Na] is shown in Figure 35.4 (32). Note the 6–7 mEq/L increase in plasma [Na] in the first 24 hours of drug infusion, which is maintained for the 96-hour infusion period.

TOLVAPTAN: Tolvaptan is more selective than conivaptan, and blocks only vasopressin receptors in the kidneys. The drug is given orally, starting at a dose of 15 mg once daily, and increasing the dose, if necessary, to a maximum of 60 mg daily. Increases in plasma [Na] of 6–7 mEq/L have been

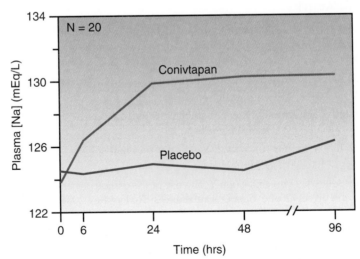

FIGURE 35.4 Effect of intravenous conivaptan (using the same dosing regimen described in the text) on the plasma sodium concentration in patients with euvolemic and hypervolemic hyponatremia. N is the number of study patients. Data from Reference 32.

observed in the first 4 days of tolvaptan therapy (31), which is the time to maximal drug effect.

COMMENT: The vaptans have not gained widespread acceptance, although they may have a role as an alternative to fluid restriction in SIADH-related hyponatremia. However, these agents offer no apparent advantages for the acute management of symptomatic hyponatremia in critically ill patients.

A FINAL WORD

The following points from this chapter deserve emphasis:

1. Sodium is the principal determinant of the distribution of total body water in the intracellular and extracellular fluids.

2. An abnormal plasma sodium concentration is not about sodium, it's about cell volume.

3. A single variable (the extracellular volume), can be used to understand, identify, and correct the osmotic impact of hypernatremia and hyponatremia. (Bertrand Russell would be proud.)

REFERENCES

Introduction

1. Pokaharel M, Block CA. Dysnatremia in the ICU. Curr Opin Crit Care 2011; 17:581–593.

Osmotic Activity

2. Rose BD, Post TW. The total body water and the plasma sodium concentration. In: Clinical physiology of acid-base and electrolyte disorders. 5th ed. New York, NY: McGraw-Hill, 2001; 241–257.

3. Gennari FJ. Current concepts. Serum osmolality. Uses and limitations. N Engl J Med 1984; 310:102–105.

4. Erstad BL. Osmolality and osmolarity: narrowing the terminology gap. Pharmacother 2003; 23:1085–1086.

5. Turchin A, Seifter JL, Seely EW. Clinical problem-solving. Mind the gap. N Engl J Med 2003; 349:1465–1469.

6. Purssell RA, Lynd LD, Koga Y. The use of the osmole gap as a screening test for the presence of exogenous substances. Toxicol Rev 2004; 23:189–202.

Hypernatremia

7. Darmon N, Timsit JF, Fancais A, et al. Association between hypernatremia acquired in the ICU and mortality: a cohort study. Nephrol Dial Transplant 2010; 25:2510–2515.

8. Adrogue HJ, Madias NE. Hypernatremia. N Engl J Med 2000; 342:1493–1499.

9. Arieff AI, Ayus JC. Strategies for diagnosing and managing hypernatremic encephalopathy. J Crit Illness 1996; 11:720–727.

10. Naik KR, Saroja AO. Seasonal postpartum hypernatremic encephalopathy with osmotic extrapontine myelinolysis and rhabdomyolysis. J Neurol Sci 2010; 291:5–11.

11. Gennari FJ, Weise WJ. Acid-base disturbances in gastrointestinal disease. Clin J Am Soc Nephrol 2008; 3:1861–1868.

12. Bates GP,, Miller VS. Sweat rate and sodium loss during work in the heat. J Occup Med Toxicol 2008; 3:4 (open access article).

13. Stason WB, Cannon PJ, Heinemann HO, Laragh JH. Furosemide: A clinical evaluation of its diuretic action. Circulation 1966; 34:910–920.

14. Rose BD, Post TW. Hyperosmolal states: hypernatremia. In: Clinical physiology of acid-base and electrolyte disorders. 5th ed. New York, NY: McGraw-Hill, 2001; 746–792.

15. Marino PL, Krasner J, O'Moore P Fluid and electrolyte expert, Philadelphia, PA: WB Saunders, 1987.

16. Makaryus AN, McFarlane SI. Diabetes insipidus: diagnosis and treatment of a complex disease. Cleve Clin J Med 2006; 73:65–71.

17. Blevins LS, Jr., Wand GS. Diabetes insipidus. Crit Care Med 1992; 20:69–79.

18. Ghirardello S, Malattia C, Scagnelli P, et al. Current perspective on the pathogenesis of central diabetes insipidus. J Pediatr Endocrinol Metab 2005; 18:631–645.

19. Garofeanu CG, Weir M, Rosas-Arellano MP, et al. Causes of reversible nephrogenic diabetes insipidus: a systematic review. Am J Kidney Dis 2005; 45:626–637.

20. Geheb MA. Clinical approach to the hyperosmolar patient. Crit Care Clin 1987; 3:797–815.

21. Ofran Y, Lavi D, Opher D, et al. Fatal voluntary salt intake resulting in the highest ever documented sodium plasma level in adults (255 mmol/L): a disorder linked to female gender and psychiatric disorders. J Intern Med 2004; 256:525–528.

Hypertonic Hyperglycemia

22. Chaithongdi N, Subauste JS, Koch CA, Geraci SA. Diagnosis and management of hyperglycemic emergencies. Hormones 2011; 10:250–260.

23. Awasthi D, Tiwari AK, Upadhyaya A, et al. Ketotic hyperglycemia with movement disorder. J Emerg Trauma Shock 2012; 5:90–91.

24. Moran SM, Jamison RL. The variable hyponatremic response to hyperglycemia. West J Med 1985; 142:49–53.

25. Hiller TA, Abbott RD, Barrett EJ. Hyponatremia: evaluating the correction factor for hyperglycemia. Am J Med 1999; 106:399–403.

Hyponatremia

26. Hoorn EJ, Lindemans J, Zietse R. Development of severe hyponatremia in hospitalized patients: treatment-related risk factors and inadequate management. Nephrol Dial Transplant 2006; 21:70–76.

27. Upadhyay UM, Gormley WB. Etiology and management of hyponatremia in neurosurgical patients. J Intensive Care Med 2012; 27:139–144.

28. Aw TC, Kiechle FL. Am J Emerg Med 1985; 3:236–239.

29. Verbalis JG, Goldsmith SR, Greenberg A, et al. Hyponatremia treatment guidelines 2007: Expert panel recommendations. Am J Med 2007; 120(Suppl): S1–S21.

30. Arieff AI, Ayus JC. Pathogenesis of hyponatremic encephalopathy. Current concepts. Chest 1993; 103:607–610.

31. Lehrich RW, Greenberg A. Hyponatremia and the use of vasopressin receptor antagonists in critically ill patients. J Intensive Care Med 2012; 27:207-218.

32. Zeltser D, Rosansky S, van Rensburg H, et al. Assessment of efficacy and safety of intravenous conivaptan in euvolemic and hypervolemic hyponatremia. Am J Nephrol 2007; 27:447–457.

Chapter 36

POTASSIUM

No stream can rise higher than its source.

Frank Lloyd Wright
1875

The earliest sea-living organisms showed a preference for intracellular potassium and a disdain for intracellular sodium, and this behavior eventually changed the composition of the oceans from a potassium salt solution to a sodium salt solution. The same preferences are found in the human organism, where 98% of the total body potassium is located inside cells, and only 2% remains in the extracellular fluid (1–3). As a result, monitoring the plasma (extracellular) potassium level as an index of total body potassium is like evaluating the size of an iceberg by its tip. With this limitation in mind, this chapter describes the causes and consequences of abnormalities in the plasma potassium concentration.

BASICS

Potassium Distribution

The intracellular preponderance of potassium is the result of a sodium-potassium (Na^+- K^+) exchange pump on cell membranes that moves Na^+ out of cells and moves K^+ into cells in a 3:2 ratio (1). One of the major roles of this pump is to create a voltage gradient across cell membranes in "excitable" tissues (i.e., nerves and muscle), which allows for the transmission of electrical impulses in these tissues.

The small fraction of total body K^+ that is present outside cells is illustrated in Figure 36.1. The total body potassium in healthy adults is about 50–55 mEq per kg body weight (1). Using the conservative estimate of 50 mEq/kg in a 70 kg adult yields a total body potassium of 3,500 mEq, with 70 mEq (2%) in extracellular fluid. Because the plasma accounts for about 20% of the extracellular fluid, *the potassium content of plasma* will be about 15 mEq, which *is only 0.4% of the total body potassium*. This emphasizes the limited size of the K^+ pool that is available for evaluating total body potassium.

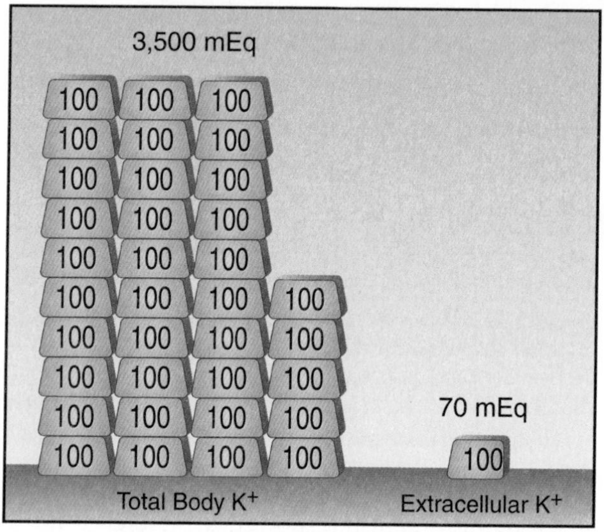

FIGURE 36.1 Illustration of the small fraction of total body K+ that is present outside cells. This example pertains to a 70 kg adult with an estimated total body K+ of 50 mEq/kg body weight. Each gold bar represents 100 mEq of K+.

Serum Potassium

The relationship between total body K+ and serum (plasma) K+ is shown in Figure 36.2 (4,5). Note the curvilinear shape of the curve, with the flat portion of the curve in the region of potassium deficiency. In an aver-aged-size adult with a normal serum K+ of 4 mEq/L, a total body K+ deficit of 200–400 mEq is required to produce a decrease in plasma K+ of 1 mEq/L, while a total body K+ excess of 100–200 mEq is required to produce a similar (1 mEq/L) increase in plasma K (5). Therefore, *for a given change in serum K+, the change in total body K+ is twofold greater with K+ depletion (hypokalemia) than with K+ excess (hyperkalemia)*. The larger deficit associated with hypokalemia is due to the large pool of intracellu-lar K+ that can replenish extracellular K+ (and help to maintain serum K+) when K+ is lost.

Potassium Excretion

Small amounts of K+ are lost in stool (5–10 mEq/day) and sweat (0–10 mEq/day), but the majority of K+ loss is in urine (40–120 mEq/day, depending on K+ intake) (1).

Renal Excretion

Most of the K+ that is filtered at the glomerulus is passively reabsorbed in the proximal tubules (along with sodium and water), and K+ is then secreted in the distal tubules and collecting ducts (1). Potassium excre-tion in urine is primarily a function of K+ secretion in the distal nephron,

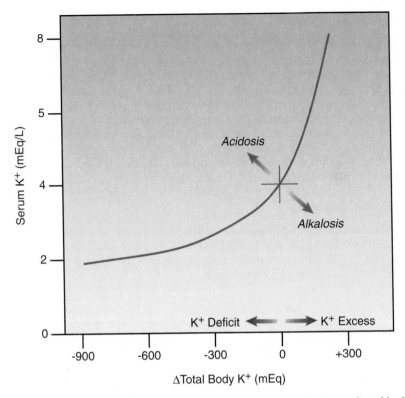

FIGURE 36.2 Relationship between the serum potassium concentration and total body potassium. Redrawn from Reference 4.

which is controlled by plasma K^+ and (primarily by) aldosterone. When renal function is normal, the capacity for renal K^+ excretion is great enough to prevent a sustained rise in serum K^+ in response to an increased K^+ load (1).

ALDOSTERONE: Aldosterone is a mineralocorticoid that is released by the adrenal cortex in response to an increase in plasma K^+ (and angiotensin II), and it increases K^+ excretion in the urine by stimulating K^+ secretion in the distal nephron. Potassium secretion is linked to sodium reabsorption, so aldosterone also promotes sodium and water retention. The diuretic *spironolactone* acts by blocking the actions of aldosterone in the kidneys. As a result, spironolactone is a *potassium-sparing diuretic.*

HYPOKALEMIA

Hypokalemia (serum $K^+ < 3.5$ mEq/L) can be the result of K^+ movement into cells (transcellular shift), or a decrease in total body K^+ (K^+ depletion) (3–6).

Transcellular Shift

The movement of K^+ into cells is facilitated by stimulation of β_2 adrenergic receptors on cell membranes in muscle, and this explains the decrease in serum K^+ associated with *inhaled β_2-agonist bronchodilators* (e.g., albuterol) (7). This effect is mild (≤ 0.5 mEq/L) in the usual therapeutic doses (7), but is more significant when inhaled β_2-agonists are used in combination with diuretics (8). Other conditions that promote K^+ movement into cells include *alkalosis* (respiratory or metabolic), *hypothermia* (accidental or induced), and *insulin*. Alkalosis has a variable and unpredictable effect on serum K^+ (9). Hypothermia causes a transient drop in serum K^+ that resolves on rewarming (10).

Potassium Depletion

Potassium depletion can be the result of K^+ loss via the kidneys or gastrointestinal tract. The site of K^+ loss (renal or extrarenal) is usually obvious, but can be identified by measuring the urinary K^+ and chloride concentrations, as shown in Figure 36.3.

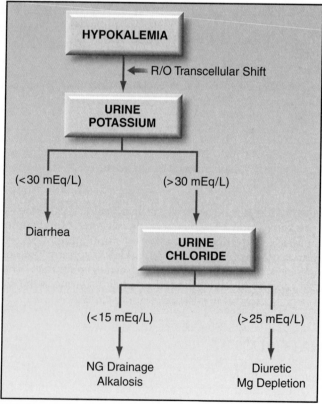

FIGURE 36.3 Diagnostic approach to hypokalemia.

Renal Potassium Loss

The leading cause of renal K^+ loss is diuretic therapy. Other causes likely to be seen in the ICU include nasogastric drainage, alkalosis, and magnesium depletion. Nasogastric drainage has a low concentration of K^+ (10–15 mEq/L), but the resulting loss of volume and H^+ promotes K^+ loss in the urine. The urine chloride is low (< 15 mEq/L) with nasogastric drainage and alkalosis, and it is high (> 25 mEq/L) with diuretic therapy and magnesium depletion. *Magnesium depletion* impairs K^+ reabsorption in the renal tubules and *may play a very important role in promoting K^+ depletion in critically ill patients*, particularly those receiving diuretics (12).

Extrarenal Potassium Loss

The major cause of extrarenal K^+ loss is diarrhea. Normal K^+ loss in stool is only 5–10 mEq daily. In secretory and inflammatory diarrhea, the concentration of K^+ in stool is 15–40 mEq/L, and the daily stool volume can reach 10 liters in severe cases. Therefore, K^+ losses can reach 400 mEq daily in severe cases of inflammatory or secretory diarrhea (11).

Clinical Manifestations

Severe hypokalemia (serum K^+ < 2.5 mEq/L) can be associated with diffuse muscle weakness (3), but in most cases, hypokalemia is asymptomatic. Abnormalities in the ECG are the major manifestation of hypokalemia, and can be present in 50% of cases (13). The ECG abnormalities include prominent U waves (more than 1 mm in height), flattening and inversion of T waves, and prolongation of the QT interval. However, these changes are not specific for hypokalemia; i.e., the T wave changes and U waves can be seen with digitalis or left ventricular hypertrophy, and QT prolongation can be the result of drugs, hypocalcemia, or hypomagnesemia.

Arrhythmias

Contrary to popular belief, *hypokalemia alone is not a risk for serious arrhythmias* (3,13). However, hypokalemia can add to the risk of serious arrhythmias from other conditions (e.g., myocardial ischemia) (3).

Management of Hypokalemia

The first concern in hypokalemia is to eliminate or treat any condition that promotes transcellular potassium shifts (e.g., alkalosis) (3). If the hypokalemia is due to K^+ depletion, proceed as described next.

Estimate Potassium Deficits

About 10% of total body K^+ is lost for every 1 mEq/L decrease in serum K^+ (14). For a 70 kg adult with a normal total body K^+ of 50 mEq/kg, the estimated K^+ deficits associated with progressive hypokalemia are shown in Table 36.1. Note that even mild hypokalemia (serum K^+ = 3 mEq/L) is associated with a considerable K^+ deficit (175 mEq).

Table 36.1	Potassium Deficits in Hypokalemia*	
Serum Potassium (mEq/L)	**Potassium Deficit**	
	mEq	**% Total Body K**
3.0	175	5
2.5	350	10
2.0	470	15
1.5	700	20
1.0	875	25

*Estimated deficits are for a 70 kg adult with a total body potassium of 50 mEq/kg.

Potassium Replacement

FLUIDS: The usual replacement fluid is potassium chloride, which is available as a concentrated solution (1–2 mEq/mL) in ampules containing 10, 20, 30, and 40 mEq of potassium. These solutions are extremely hyperosmotic (the 2 mEq/mL solution has an osmolality of 4,000 mosm/kg H_2O) and must be diluted (15). A potassium phosphate solution is also available that contains 4.5 mEq potassium and 3 mmol phosphate per mL, and this solution is preferred by some for potassium replacement in diabetic ketoacidosis (because of the phosphate depletion in diabetic ketoacidosis).

RATE OF REPLACEMENT: The standard method of intravenous K^+ replacement is to add 20 mEq of K^+ to 100 mL of isotonic saline and infuse this mixture over 1 hour (16). The *maximum rate* of intravenous potassium replacement is usually set at *20 mEq/hr* (16), but dose rates of 40 mEq/hour may be necessary (e.g., serum K^+ < 1.5 mEq/L or serious arrhythmias), and *dose rates as high as 100 mEq/hour have been used safely* (17). Infusion through a large, central vein is preferred, if possible, because of the irritating properties of the hyperosmotic KCL solutions. However, delivery into the superior vena cava is not recommended if the desired rate of replacement exceeds 20 mEq/hr because there is a (poorly documented) risk of an abrupt rise in plasma K^+ in the right heart chambers severe enough to produce asystole.

RESPONSE: The serum K^+ may be slow to rise initially, as predicted by the flat portion of the curve in Figure 36.2. If the hypokalemia is resistant or refractory to K^+ replacement, magnesium depletion should be considered. Magnesium depletion promotes urinary K^+ loss (as described earlier), and *in patients who are magnesium deficient, hypokalemia is often refractory to K^+ replacement until the magnesium is repleted* (18). Magnesium deficiency may play an important role in diuretic-induced hypokalemia, as described in the next chapter.

HYPERKALEMIA

While hypokalemia is often well tolerated, hyperkalemia (serum $K^+ > 5.5$ mEq/L) can be a life-threatening condition (2,3,19,20).

Etiology

Hyperkalemia can be the result of potassium release from cells (transcellular shift), or impaired renal excretion of potassium. If the source of the hyperkalemia is unclear, a spot urine K^+ can be useful. A high urine K^+ (> 30 mEq/L) suggests a transcellular shift, and a low urine K^+ (< 30 mEq/L) indicates impaired renal excretion. If the hyperkalemia is unexpected, the condition described next should be considered.

Pseudohyperkalemia

Hyperkalemia that is present *ex vivo* (in the blood sample), but not *in vivo*, is known as *pseudohyperkalemia*. The leading cause of this condition is potassium release from traumatic hemolysis during the venipuncture. This is more common than suspected, and has been reported in 20% of blood samples with hyperkalemia (21). Other sources of pseudohyperkalemia include: (a) K^+ release from muscles during fist clenching (22), and (b) potassium release from clot formation in the blood collection tube in patients with severe leukocytosis ($> 50,000/mm^3$) or severe thrombocytosis (platelet count > 1 million/mm^3). When pseudohyperkalemia is suspected, a repeat blood sample should be obtained using precautions to mitigate the suspected problem (e.g., minimize suction when withdrawing blood).

Transcellular Shift

The conditions associated with K^+ movement out of cells include acidosis, rhabdomyolysis, tumor lysis syndrome, drugs, and blood transfusions.

ACIDOSIS: The presumed mechanism for the relationship between acidosis and hyperkalemia is competition between H^+ and K^+ for the same site on the membrane pump that moves K^+ into cells. However, a causal link between acidosis and hyperkalemia is being questioned because *the organic acidoses* (lactic acidosis and ketoacidosis) *are not associated with hyperkalemia* (9), and respiratory acidosis has an inconsistent and unpredictable association with hyperkalemia (9).

TUMOR LYSIS SYNDROME: Tumor lysis syndrome is an acute, life-threatening condition that appears within 7 days after the initiation of cytotoxic therapy for selected malignancies (e.g., non-Hodgkins lymphoma). Characteristic features include the combination of hyperkalemia, hyperphosphatemia, hypocalcemia, and hyperuricemia, often accompanied by acute kidney injury (23). Hyperkalemia is the most immediate threat to life.

DRUGS: The drugs that promote K^+ movement out of cells are listed in Table 36.2. Digitalis inhibits the membrane Na^+-K^+ exchange pump, but hyperkalemia occurs only with acute (not chronic) *digitalis toxicity* (24). *Succinylcholine* is an ultra short-acting neuromuscular blocking agent that also inhibits the membrane Na^+- K^+ exchange pump (a depolarizing effect), and this effect is associated with a minor increase in serum K^+ (< 1 mEq/L) that lasts only 5–10 minutes (25). Life-threatening increases in serum K^+ have been reported when succinylcholine is used in patients with "denervation injury"of skeletal muscle (e.g., spinal cord injury). This is attributed to a an exaggerated response to depolarizing signals following denervation (denervation hypsersensitivity).

Table 36.2	Drugs That Promote Hyperkalemia in the ICU
Promote Transcellular Shift	**Impair Renal K^+ Excretion**
β-blockers	ACE Inhibitors
Digitalis	Angiotensin-receptor blockers
Succinylcholine	K^+- sparing diuretics
	NSAIDS
	Heparin
	Trimethoprim-sulfamethoxazole

Impaired Renal Excretion

As mentioned earlier in the chapter, when renal function is normal, the capacity for urinary K^+ excretion is great enough to prevent a sustained increase in serum K^+ in response to a K^+ load (1). As a result, *hyperkalemia always involves a defect in renal K^+ excretion.* The common causes of impaired renal K^+ excretion include renal failure, adrenal insufficiency, and drugs. In renal failure, hyperkalemia usually doesn't occur until the GFR drops below 10 mL/min, but it can appear earlier when renal failure is the result of interstitial nephritis. Adrenal insufficiency impairs renal potassium excretion, but *hyperkalemia is seen only in chronic adrenal insufficiency.*

DRUGS: Drugs that impair renal potassium excretion represent a common source of hyperkalemia. A list of common offenders is shown in Table 36.2 (25–29). The drugs most often implicated are angiotensin-converting enzyme inhibitors, angiotensin receptor blockers, potassium sparing diuretics, and nonsteroidal antiinflammatory drugs. All of these agents promote hyperkalemia by inhibiting the renin–angiotensin–aldosterone system. The hyperkalemia from these drugs often occurs in combination with K^+ supplements or renal insufficiency.

Blood Transfusion

Hyperkalemia is a recognized (but inconsistent) complication of massive blood transfusion (i.e., blood replacement equivalent to the blood volume). The temperature used to store red blood cells (4°C) shuts off the

Na$^+$- K$^+$ exchange pump in the erythrocyte cell membrane, and this results in a steady leakage of K$^+$ from the cells (30). The K$^+$ concentration in the supernatant increases steadily as the storage time increases. After 18 days of storage (the average time that blood is stored), the potassium load in one unit of packed red blood cells is 2 to 3 mEq (30), so massive transfusion (usually at least 6 units of red blood cells) represents a K$^+$ load of at least 12–18 mEq. This is a considerable load, considering that plasma contains about 9–10 mEq of K$^+$ in an average-sized adult.

The K$^+$ load in transfused blood is normally cleared by the kidneys, but when systemic blood flow is compromised (which applies to most patients who need massive blood transfusions), renal K$^+$ excretion is impaired, and the K$^+$ infused in blood transfusions will accumulate. The transfusion volume needed to produce hyperkalemia will vary, but one study has shown that hyperkalemia begins to appear after transfusion of 7 units of red blood cells (31).

Cautopyreiophagia

In 1985, a case report was published describing a patient with severe hyperkalemia who was discovered to be ingesting 1,500 burnt match heads daily (a pica) (32). It turns out that burnt match heads are rich in potassium chlorate, and the habit of eating burnt match heads is known as *cautopyreiophagia*. This case is mentioned to demonstrate that anything is possible in medicine, and that there is a name for everything.

Clinical Consequences

The principal threat of hyperkalemia is slowed impulse transmission in the heart (from depolarization of cardiac muscle), which can progress to heart block and bradycardic cardiac arrest.

ECG Abnormalities

The ECG changes in progressive hyperkalemia are shown in Figure 36.4. The earliest change is the appearance of a tall, tapering (tented) T wave that is most evident in precordial leads V$_2$ and V$_3$. As the hyperkalemia progresses, the P wave amplitude decreases and the PR interval lengthens. The P waves eventually disappear and the QRS complex widens. The final event is ventricular fibrillation or asystole.

ECG changes usually begin to appear when the serum K$^+$ reaches 7 mEq/L (33), but the threshold for ECG changes can vary widely. This is demonstrated by one case report that showed no ECG abnormalities at a serum K$^+$ of 14 mEq/L (!) (34). Because of the variable relationship between the serum K$^+$ and the ECG, both are used for management decisions in hyperkalemia.

Management of Severe Hyperkalemia

Severe hyperkalemia is defined as a serum K$^+$ > 6.5 mEq/L, or any serum K$^+$ associated with ECG changes (33). The management of this condition

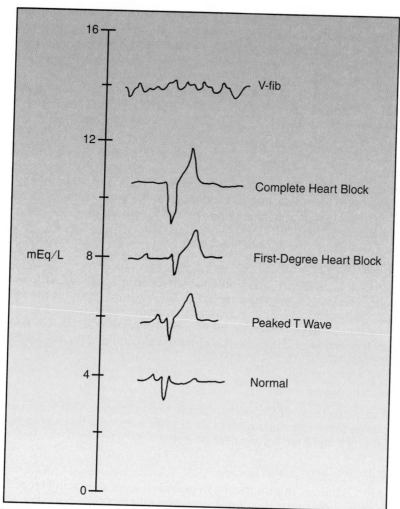

FIGURE 36.4 ECG abnormalities in progressive hyperkalemia.

has 3 goals: (a) antagonism of the cardiac effects of hyperkalemia, (b) transcellular shift of K+ into cells, and (c) removal of excess K+ from the body. The methods used to achieve these goals are described next, and are summarized in Table 36.3.

Membrane Antagonism

Calcium increases the electrical charge difference across myocardial cell membranes and opposes the depolarization produced by hyperkalemia (35). The preferred calcium preparation is calcium gluconate, which is given in the dosing regimen shown in Table 36.3. The response to calcium is short-lived (20–30 minutes) and it does not reduce the serum K^+, so other measures (e.g., insulin-glucose) should be initiated to reduce serum K^+ levels. Calcium must be used cautiously in patients receiving digitalis because hypercalcemia aggravates digitalis cardiotoxicity. For patients receiving digitalis, calcium gluconate can be added to 100 mL of isotonic saline and infused over 20 to 30 minutes. *Calcium is contraindicated if the hyperkalemia is a manifestation of digitalis toxicity.*

Table 36.3	Management of Severe Hyperkalemia
Goal	**Treatment Regimen**
Antagonize Cardiac Effects	• 10% calcium gluconate; 10 mLs IV over 3 min, and repeat after 5 min, if necessary • Use calcium chloride for circulatory shock. • Effect lasts 30–60 min. • Do NOT use calcium for digitalis toxicity.
Transcellular Shift	• Regular insulin: 10 units as IV bolus + 50% dextrose: 50 mLs as IV bolus • Start dextrose infusion • Peak effect at 30–60 min
Potassium Removal	• Kayexalate (oral): 30 g in 20% sorbitol (50 mL) (rectal): 50 g in 20% sorbitol (200 mL) • Slow-acting (onset at 2 hrs, peak at 6 hrs) • Small risk of bowel necrosis

When hyperkalemia is associated with circulatory shock or cardiac arrest, calcium chloride is preferred to calcium gluconate. One ampule (10 mL) of 10% calcium chloride has three times the elemental calcium in one ampule of 10% calcium gluconate (270 mg vs. 90 mg, respectively), and the extra calcium has a potential advantage by promoting cardiac output and preserving peripheral vascular tone. The osmolality of calcium chloride is 2,000 mosm/kg H_2O, so administration through a free-flowing central venous catheter is strongly advised.

Transcellular Shift

INSULIN-DEXTROSE: Insulin drives K^+ into skeletal muscle cells by activating the membrane Na^+- K^+ exchange pump (36), and the insulin-dextrose regimen in Table 36.3 will decrease the serum K^+ by at least 0.6 mEq/L (33). A dextrose infusion is advised after insulin-dextrose (unless the patient is hyperglycemic) because there is a risk of hypoglycemia at one hour (33). In the setting of hyperglycemia, insulin should be used without dextrose (33). The insulin effect is temporary (peak effect at 30–60 min), so measures that promote K^+ removal should be started.

β_2-AGONISTS: The dose of inhaled β_2- agonists (e.g., albuterol) needed to produce a significant (0.5 – 1 mEq/L) drop in serum K^+ is at least 4 times the therapeutic dose (33), and this can produce unwanted side effects (e.g., tachycardia). Therefore, these agents are not advised for severe hyperkalemia.

BICARBONATE: There are two reasons to avoid bicarbonate for the management of severe hyperkalemia: (a) short-term infusions of bicarbonate (up to four hours) have no effect on serum K^+ levels (33), and (b) bicarbonate can form complexes with calcium, which is counterproductive when calcium is used to antagonize the membrane effects of hyperkalemia.

Potassium Removal

Excess K^+ can be removed via the bowel (with a cation-exchange resin) or directly from the bloodstream (with hemodialysis).

CATION EXCHANGE RESIN: Sodium polystyrene sulfonate (Kayexalate) is a cation exchange resin that promotes K^+ clearance across the bowel mucosa. It can be given orally (preferred) or by retention enema, using the doses shown in Table 36.3. Kayexalate is usually mixed with sorbitol to prevent concretions. Each gram of resin binds 0.65 mEq of K^+, and at least 6 hours is required for maximum effect (33). There are several case reports of necrotic lesions in the bowel linked to Kayexalate (37). Although this is an uncommon complication, the mortality rate is high (33%) (37).

HEMODIALYSIS: The most effective method of potassium removal is hemodialysis, which can produce a 1 mEq/L drop in serum K^+ after one hour, and a 2 mEq/L drop after 3 hours (33).

A FINAL WORD

The following points in this chapter deserve emphasis.

1. Plasma K^+ is only the "tip of the iceberg" in terms of evaluating total body potassium.

2. Potassium deficits are often larger than suspected in hypokalemia, even in mild cases (see Table 36.1).

3. Hypokalemia is remarkably well tolerated, and is not a risk for serious arrhythmias unless combined with another arrhythmogenic condition (e.g., acute coronary syndrome).

4. When hypokalemia is resistant or refractory to K^+ replacement, magnesium deficiency is the likely culprit.

5. When using calcium to antagonize the cardiac effects of hyperkalemia, make sure to decrease the serum K^+ (insulin-glucose is best), and begin measures to remove excess K^+ (e.g., Kayexalate).

REFERENCES

Basics

1. Rose BD, Post TW. Potassium homeostasis. In: Clinical physiology of acid-base and electrolyte disorders. 5th ed. New York, NY: McGraw-Hill, 2001; 372–402.

2. Alfonzo AVM, Isles C, Geddes C, Deighan C. Potassium disorders—clinical spectrum and emergency management. Resusc 2006; 70:10–25.

3. Schaefer TJ, Wolford RW. Disorders of potassium. Emerg Med Clin North Am 2005; 23:723–747, viii–ix.

4. Brown RS. Extrarenal potassium homeostasis. Kidney Int 1986; 30:116–127.

5. Sterns RH, Cox M, Feig PU, et al. Internal potassium balance and the control of the plasma potassium concentration. Medicine 1981; 60:339–354.

Hypokalemia

6. Glover P. Hypokalaemia. Crit Care Resusc 1999; 1:239–251.

7. Allon M, Copkney C. Albuterol and insulin for treatment of hyperkalemia in hemodialysis patients. Kidney Int 1990; 38:869–872.

8. Lipworth BJ, McDevitt DG, Struthers AD. Prior treatment with diuretic augments the hypokalemic and electrocardiographic effects of inhaled albuterol. Am J Med 1989; 86:653–657.

9. Adrogue HJ, Madias NE. Changes in plasma potassium concentration during acute acid-base disturbances. Am J Med 1981; 71:456–467.

10. Bernard SA, Buist M. Induced hypothermia in critical care medicine: a review. Crit Care Med 2003; 31:2041–2051.

11. Gennari FJ, Weise WJ. Acid-base disturbances in gastrointestinal disease. Clin J Am Soc Nephrol 2008; 3:1861–1868.

12. Salem M, Munoz R, Chernow B. Hypomagnesemia in critical illness. A common and clinically important problem. Crit Care Clin 1991; 7:225–252.

13. Flakeb G, Villarread D, Chapman D. Is hypokalemia a cause of ventricular arrhythmias? J Crit Illness 1986; 1:66–74.

14. Stanaszek WF, Romankiewicz JA. Current approaches to management of potassium deficiency. Drug Intell Clin Pharm 1985; 19:176–184.

15. Trissel LA. Handbook on Injectable Drugs. 13th ed. Bethesda, MD: Amer Soc Health System Pharmcists, 2005; 1230.

16. Kruse JA, Carlson RW. Rapid correction of hypokalemia using concentrated intravenous potassium chloride infusions. Arch Intern Med 1990; 150: 613–617.

17. Kim GH, Han JS. Therapeutic approach to hypokalemia. Nephron 2002; 92 Suppl 1:28–32.

18. Whang R, Flink EB, Dyckner T, et al. Magnesium depletion as a cause of refractory potassium repletion. Arch Intern Med 1985; 145:1686–1689.

Hyperkalemia

19. Williams ME. Endocrine crises. Hyperkalemia. Crit Care Clin 1991; 7:155–174.

20. Evans KJ, Greenberg A. Hyperkalemia: a review. J Intensive Care Med 2005; 20:272–290.

21. Rimmer JM, Horn JF, Gennari FJ. Hyperkalemia as a complication of drug therapy. Arch Intern Med 1987; 147:867–869.

22. Don BR, Sebastian A, Cheitlin M, et al. Pseudohyperkalemia caused by fist clenching during phlebotomy. N Engl J Med 1990; 322:1290–1292.

23. Howard SC, Jones DP, Pui C-H. The tumor lysis syndrome. N Engl J Med 2012; 364:1844–1854.

24. Krisanda TJ. Digitalis toxicity. Postgrad Med 1992; 91:273–284.

25. Ponce SP, Jennings AE, Madias N, Harington JT. Drug-induced hyperkalemia. Medicine 1985; 64:357–370.

26. Perazella MA. Drug-induced hyperkalemia: old culprits and new offenders. Am J Med 2000; 109:307–314.

27. Palmer BF. Managing hyperkalemia caused by inhibitors of the renin-angiotensin-aldosterone system. N Engl J Med 2004; 351:585–592.

28. Oster JR, Singer I, Fishman LM. Heparin-induced aldosterone suppression and hyperkalemia. Am J Med 1995; 98:575–586.

29. Greenberg S, Reiser IW, Chou SY, et al. Trimethoprim-sulfamethoxazole induces reversible hyperkalemia. Ann Intern Med 1993; 119:291–295.

30. Vraets A, Lin Y, Callum JL. Transfusion-associated hyperkalemia. Transfus Med Rev 2011; 25:184–196.

31. Aboudara MC, Hurst FP, Abbott KC, et al. Hyperkalemia after packed red blood cell transfusion in trauma patients. J Trauma 2008; 64:S86–S91.

32. Abu-Hamden DK, Sondheimer JH, Mahajan SK. Cautopyeiophagia: cause of life-threatening hyperkalemia in a patient undergoing hemodialysis. Am J Med 1985; 79:517–519.

33. Weisberg L. Management of severe hyperkalemia. Crit Care Med 2008; 36:3246–3251.

34. Tran HA. Extreme hyperkalemia. South Med J 2005; 98:729–732.

35. Bosnjak ZJ, Lynch C, 3rd. Cardiac Electrophysiology. In: Yaksh T, et al., eds. Anesthesia: Biologic Foundations. New York: Lippincott-Raven, 1998; 1001–1040.

36. Clausen T, Everts ME. Regulation of the Na, K-pump in skeletal muscle. Kidney Int 1989; 35:1–13.

37. Harel Z, Harel S, Shah PS, et al. Gastrointestinal adverse events with sodium polystyrene sulfonate (Kayexalate) use: a systematic review. Am J Med 2013; 126:264.e9–264.e24.

Chapter 37

MAGNESIUM

You can know the name of a bird in all the languages of the world,
but you'll know absolutely nothing about the bird. So let's look at
the bird and see what it's doing — that's what counts.

Richard Feynman
The Physics Teacher
1969

Magnesium is an essential element for the utilization of energy in the organic world. In green plants, magnesium is the heart of the chlorophyll molecule that captures the energy in sunlight in order to produce oxygen and carbohydrates (i.e., photosynthesis). Aerobic organisms then use the oxygen to release the energy stored in organic nutrients (including carbohydrates), and this energy is stored as adenosine triphosphate (ATP). The release of energy from ATP requires magnesium, which is an essential cofactor for the ATPase enzymes that hydrolyze ATP. Therefore, magnesium is essential for providing us with energy, and for allowing us to utilize this energy to sustain life. Now that's an element.

More specific roles of magnesium include the proper functioning of the Na^+-K^+ exchange pump (which is a magnesium-dependent ATPase) that generates the electrical gradient across cell membranes. As a result, magnesium plays an important role in the activity of electrically excitable tissues (1–4). Magnesium also regulates the movement of calcium into smooth muscle cells, which gives it a pivotal role in the maintenance of cardiac contractile strength and peripheral vascular tone (4).

MAGNESIUM BASICS

Distribution

The distribution of magnesium (Mg) in the human body is shown in Table 37.1 (5). The average-sized adult contains approximately 24 g (1 mole, or 2,000 mEq) of magnesium; a little over half is located in bone, whereas *less than 1% is located in plasma*. This lack of representation in the plasma limits the value of the plasma Mg as an index of total body magnesium (similar to plasma potassium). This is particularly true in patients with magnesium deficiency, in whom *plasma Mg levels can be normal in the face of total body magnesium depletion* (5,6).

Table 37.1	Magnesium Distribution in Adults		
Tissue	Wet Weight (kg)	Mg Content (mEq)	Total Body Mg (%)
Bone	12	1060	53
Muscle	30	540	27
Soft Tissue	23	384	19
RBC	2	10	0.7
Plasma	3	6	0.3
Total	70 kg	2,000 mEq	100%

From Reference 5.

Serum Magnesium

Serum is favored over plasma for magnesium assays because the anticoagulant used for plasma samples can be contaminated with citrate or other anions that bind magnesium (5). The reference range for serum Mg depends on the daily magnesium intake, which varies according to geographic region. The normal range of serum Mg for healthy adults in the United States is shown in Table 37.2 (7).

Note: The clinical laboratory typically reports the serum Mg concentration in mg/dL (because Mg is partially bound to plasma proteins), while the medical literature typically uses mEq/L for the serum Mg concentration. The conversion is as follows:

$$mEq/L = \frac{mg/dL \times 10}{mol\,wt} \times valence \qquad (37.1)$$

where mol wt is the molecular weight (atomic weight in the case of magnesium) and valence is the number of charges on the atom or molecule. Magnesium has an atomic weight of 24 and a valence of 2, so a serum Mg concentration of 1.7 mg/dL is equivalent to $(1.7 \times 10)/24 \times 2 = 1.4$ mEq/L.

Ionized Magnesium

About 67% of the magnesium in plasma is in the ionized (active) form, and the remaining 33% is either bound to plasma proteins (19% of the total) or chelated with divalent anions such as phosphate and sulfate (14% of the total) (8). The standard assay for magnesium (i.e., spectrophotometry) measures all three fractions. Therefore, when the serum Mg is abnormally low, it is not possible to determine if the problem is a decrease in the ionized (active) fraction, or a decrease in the bound fractions (e.g., hypoproteinemia) (9). The level of ionized Mg can be measured with an ion-specific electrode (10), but this is not routinely available. However, because only a small amount of magnesium resides in plasma, the difference between the ionized and bound magnesium *content* may not be large enough to be clinically relevant.

Table 37.2	Reference Ranges for Magnesium	
Fluid	**Traditional Units**	**SI Units**
Serum Magnesium:		
Total	1.7–2.4 mg/dL 1.4–2.0 mEq/L	0.7–1.0 mmol/L
Ionized	0.8–1.1 mEq/L	0.4–0.6 mmol/L
Urinary Magnesium:	5–15 mEq/24 hr	2.5–7.5 mmol/24 hr

Pertains to healthy adults residing in the United States. From Reference 7.

Conversions: mEq/L = [(mg/dL × 10)/24] × 2; MEq/L = mmol/L × 2.

Urinary Magnesium

The normal range for urinary Mg excretion is shown in Table 37.2. Under normal circumstances, only small quantities of magnesium are excreted in the urine (3). When magnesium intake is deficient, the kidneys conserve magnesium, and urinary magnesium excretion falls to negligible levels. This is shown in Figure 37.1. Note that the serum Mg remains in the normal range one week after starting a Mg-3 diet, while the urinary Mg excretion has dropped to negligible levels. This illustrates the relative

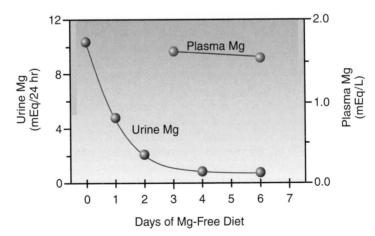

FIGURE 37.1 Urinary magnesium excretion and plasma magnesium levels in a healthy volunteer placed on a magnesium-free diet. Solid bars on the vertical axes indicate the normal range for each variable. Adapted from Shils ME. Experimental human magnesium deficiency. Medicine 1969;48:61–82.

value of urinary magnesium excretion in the detection of magnesium deficiency.

MAGNESIUM DEFICIENCY

Hypomagnesemia is reported in as many as 65% of patients in ICU's (1–3). Because magnesium depletion may not be accompanied by hypomagnesemia, the incidence of magnesium depletion is probably higher. In fact, *magnesium depletion has been described as "the most underdiagnosed electrolyte abnormality in current medical practice"* (11).

Predisposing Conditions

Because serum Mg levels have a limited ability to detect magnesium depletion, recognizing the conditions that predispose to magnesium depletion may be the only clue of an underlying electrolyte imbalance. The common predisposing conditions for magnesium depletion are listed in Table 37.3.

Table 37.3	Markers of Possible Magnesium Depletion
Predisposing Conditions	**Clinical Findings**

Drug Therapy:*
   Furosemide (50%)
   Aminoglycosides (30%)
   Amphotericin, pentamidine
   Digitalis (20%)
   Cisplatin, cyclosporine
	Electrolyte abnormalities:
	   Hypokalemia (40%)
	   Hypophosphatemia (30%)
	   Hyponatremia (27%)
	   Hypocalcemia (22%)

Diarrhea (secretory)	Cardiac manifestations: Ischemia
Alcohol abuse (chronic)	Arrhythmias Digitalis toxicity
Diabetes mellitus	
Acute MI	Hyperactive CNS Syndrome

*Numbers in parentheses indicate incidence of associated hypomagnesemia.

Diuretic Therapy

Diuretics are the leading cause of magnesium deficiency. Diuretic-induced inhibition of sodium reabsorption also interferes with magnesium reabsorption, and the resultant urinary magnesium losses can parallel urinary sodium losses. Urinary magnesium excretion is most pronounced with the loop diuretics (furosemide and ethacrynic acid). *Magnesium deficiency has been reported in 50% of patients receiving chronic therapy with furosemide* (12). The thiazide diuretics show a similar tendency for magnesium depletion, but only in elderly patients (13). Magnesium depletion does not occur with "potassium-sparing" diuretics (14).

Antibiotic Therapy

The antibiotics that promote magnesium depletion are the aminoglycosides, amphotericin and pentamidine (15,16). The aminoglycosides block magnesium reabsorption in the ascending loop of Henley, and hypomagnesemia has been reported in 30% of patients receiving aminoglycoside therapy (16).

Other Drugs

There are several case reports indicating that prolonged use of proton pump inhibitors (14 days to 13 years) can be associated with severe hypomagnesemia (17), possibly due to diminished magnesium absorption in the GI tract. Other drugs associated with magnesium depletion include digitalis, epinephrine, and the chemotherapeutic agents cisplatin and cyclosporine (15,18). The first two agents shift magnesium into cells, whereas the latter two promote renal magnesium excretion.

Alcohol-Related Illness

Hypomagnesemia is reported in 30% of hospital admissions for alcohol abuse, and in 85% of admissions for delirium tremens (19,20). The magnesium depletion is due to a number of factors, including generalized malnutrition and chronic diarrhea. In addition, there is an association between magnesium deficiency and thiamine deficiency (21). Magnesium is required for the transformation of thiamine into thiamine pyrophosphate, so *magnesium deficiency can promote thiamine deficiency in the face of adequate thiamine intake*. For this reason, the magnesium status should be monitored periodically in patients receiving daily thiamine supplements.

Secretory Diarrhea

Secretions from the lower GI tract are rich in magnesium (10–14 mEq/L) (22), and secretory diarrhea can be accompanied by profound magnesium depletion (20). Upper GI tract secretions are not rich in magnesium (1–2 mEq/L), so vomiting does not pose a risk for magnesium depletion.

Diabetes Mellitus

Magnesium depletion is common in insulin-dependent diabetic patients, probably as a result of urinary Mg losses that accompany glycosuria (23). Hypomagnesemia is reported in only 7% of admissions for diabetic ketoacidosis, but the incidence increases to 50% over the first 12 hours after admission (24), probably as a result of insulin-induced movement of magnesium into cells.

Acute Myocardial Infarction

Hypomagnesemia is reported in as many as 80% of patients with acute myocardial infarction (25). The mechanism is unclear, but may be due to an intracellular shift of Mg from excess catecholamines.

Clinical Manifestations

There are no specific clinical manifestations of magnesium deficiency, but the following clinical findings can suggest an underlying magnesium deficiency.

Other Electrolyte Abnormalities

Magnesium depletion is often accompanied by depletion of potassium, phosphate, and calcium (see Table 37.3) (26).

HYPOKALEMIA: Hypokalemia is reported in 40% of cases of magnesium depletion (26). Furthermore, *the hypokalemia that accompanies magnesium depletion can be refractory to potassium replacement therapy*, and magnesium replacement is often necessary before the hypokalemia can be corrected (27).

HYPOCALCEMIA: Magnesium depletion can cause hypocalcemia as a result of impaired parathormone release (28) combined with an impaired end-organ response to parathormone (29). As with the hypokalemia, *the hypocalcemia from magnesium depletion is difficult to correct unless magnesium deficits are corrected.*

HYPOPHOSPHATEMIA: Phosphate depletion is a cause rather than effect of magnesium depletion. The mechanism is enhanced renal magnesium excretion (30).

Arrhythmias

As mentioned earlier, magnesium is required for proper function of the membrane pump on cardiac cell membranes. Magnesium depletion will depolarize cardiac cells and promote tachyarrhythmias. Because both digitalis and magnesium deficiency act to inhibit the membrane pump, magnesium deficiency will magnify the digitalis effect and promote digitalis cardiotoxicity. Intravenous magnesium can suppress digitalis-toxic arrhythmias, even when serum Mg levels are normal (31). Intravenous magnesium can also abolish refractory arrhythmias (i.e., unresponsive to traditional antiarrhythmic agents) in the absence of hypomagnesemia (32). This effect may be due to a membrane-stabilizing effect of magnesium that is unrelated to magnesium repletion.

One of the serious arrhythmias associated with magnesium depletion is *torsade de pointes* (see Figure 15.8). The role of magnesium in this arrhythmia is discussed in Chapter 15.

Neurologic Findings

The neurologic manifestations of magnesium deficiency include altered mentation, generalized seizures, tremors, and hyperreflexia. All are uncommon, nonspecific, and have little diagnostic value.

A neurologic syndrome described recently that can abate with magnesium therapy deserves mention. The clinical presentation is characterized by ataxia, slurred speech, metabolic acidosis, excessive salivation, diffuse muscle spasms, generalized seizures, and progressive obtundation (33). The clinical features are often brought out by loud noises or bodily contact, and thus the term reactive central nervous system magnesium deficiency has been used to describe this disorder. This syndrome is associated with reduced magnesium levels in cerebrospinal fluid, and it resolves with magnesium infusion. The prevalence of this disorder is unknown at present.

Diagnosis

As mentioned several times, the serum Mg level is an insensitive marker of magnesium depletion. When magnesium depletion is due to nonrenal factors (e.g., diarrhea), the urinary magnesium excretion is a more sensitive test for magnesium depletion (34). However, most cases of magnesium depletion are due to enhanced renal magnesium excretion, so the diagnostic value of urinary magnesium excretion is limited.

Magnesium Retention Test

In the absence of renal magnesium wasting, the urinary excretion of magnesium in response to a magnesium load may be the most sensitive index of total body magnesium stores (35,36). This method is outlined in Table 37.4. The normal rate of magnesium reabsorption is close to the maximum rate (T_{max}), so most of an infused magnesium load will be excreted in the urine when magnesium stores are normal. However, when magnesium stores are deficient, the magnesium reabsorption rate is much lower than the T_{max}, so more of the infused magnesium will be reabsorbed and less will be excreted in the urine. *Magnesium deficiency is likely when less than 50% of the infused Mg is recovered in the urine, and is unlikely when more than 80% of the infused Mg is excreted in the urine.* This test can be also be valuable for identifying the end-point of magnesium replacement therapy (see later). It is important to emphasize that this test will be unreliable in patients with impaired renal function or when there is ongoing renal magnesium wasting.

Table 37.4	Renal Magnesium Retention Test

Indications:
  1. For suspected Mg deficiency when serum Mg is normal
  2. For identifying the end-point of Mg replacement therapy

Contraindications:
  1. Renal failure or ongoing renal magnesium wasting

Protocol:
  1. Add 24 mmol of magnesium (6g of $MgSO_4$) to 250 mL of isotonic saline and infuse over 1 hour.
  2. Collect urine for 24 hrs, beginning at the onset of the magnesium infusion.

Results:
  1. Urinary Mg excretion <12 mmol (24 mEq) in 24 hrs (i.e., less than 50% of the infused Mg) is evidence of Mg depletion.
  2. Urinary Mg excretion >19 mmol (38 mEq) in 24 hrs (i.e., more than 80% of the infused Mg) is evidence against Mg depletion.

From Reference 35.

Magnesium Replacement

The magnesium preparations available for oral and parenteral use are listed in Table 37.5 (37,38). The oral preparations can be used for daily maintenance therapy (5 mg/kg in normal subjects). However, because intestinal absorption of oral magnesium is erratic, parenteral magnesium is advised for managing hypomagnesemia.

The standard intravenous magnesium preparation is magnesium sulfate ($MgSO_4$). *Each gram of $MgSO_4$ has 8 mEq (4 mmol) of elemental magnesium* (4). A 50% magnesium sulfate solution (500 mg/mL) has an osmolarity of 4,000 mosm/L (43), so it must be diluted to a 10% (100 mg/mL) or 20% (200 mg/mL) solution for intravenous use. Ringer's solutions should not be used as the diluent for $MgSO_4$ because the calcium in Ringer's solutions will counteract the actions of the infused magnesium.

Table 37.5	Oral and Parenteral Magnesium Preparations	
Preparation	**Elemental Mg**
Oral Preparations:	
Magnesium chloride enteric coated tablets	64 mg (5.3 mEq)
Magnesium oxide tablets (400 mg)	241 mg (19.8 mEq)
Magnesium oxide tablets (140 mg)	85 mg (6.9 mEq)
Magnesium gloconate tablets (500 mg)	27 mg (2.3 mEq)
Parenteral solutions	
Magnesium sulfate (50%)*	500 mg/dL (4 mEq/L)
Magnesium sulfate (12.5%)	120 mg/dL (1 mEq/L)

*Should be diluted to a 20% solution for intravenous injection.

The following magnesium replacement protocols are recommended for patients with normal renal function (39).

Mild, Asymptomatic Hypomagnesemia

The following guidelines can be used for a serum Mg of 1–1.4 mEq/L with no apparent complications (44):

1. Assume a total magnesium deficit of 1–2 mEq/kg.

2. Because 50% of the infused magnesium can be lost in the urine, assume that the total magnesium requirement is twice the magnesium deficit.

3. Replace 1 mEq/kg for the first 24 hours, and 0.5 mEq/kg daily for the next 3–5 days.

Moderate Hypomagnesemia

The following protocol is recommended for a serum Mg < 1 mEq/L, or for a low serum Mg that is accompanied by other electrolyte abnormalities:

1. Add 6 g $MgSO_4$ (48 mEq of Mg) to 250 or 500 mL isotonic saline and infuse over 3 hours.
2. Follow with 5 g $MgSO_4$ (40 mEq of Mg) in 250 or 500 mL isotonic saline infused over the next 6 hours.
3. Continue with 5 g $MgSO_4$ every 12 hours (by continuous infusion) for the next 5 days.

Life-Threatening Hypomagnesemia

The following is recommended for hypomagnesemia associated with serious cardiac arrhythmias (e.g., torsade de pointes) or generalized seizures:

1. Infuse 2 g $MgSO_4$ (16 mEq of Mg) intravenously over 2–5 minutes.
2. Follow with 5 g $MgSO_4$ (40 mEq of Mg) in 250 or 500 mL isotonic saline infused over the next 6 hours.
3. Continue with 5 g $MgSO_4$ every 12 hours (by continuous infusion) for the next 5 days.

Monitoring Replacement Therapy

Serum Mg levels will rise after the initial magnesium bolus, but will begin to fall after 15 minutes. Therefore, it is important to follow the bolus dose with a continuous magnesium infusion. Serum Mg levels may normalize after 1 to 2 days, but it will take several days to replenish the total body magnesium stores.

The *magnesium retention test* in Table 37.4 can be valuable for identifying the end-point of potassium replacement therapy; i.e., magnesium replacement is continued until urinary magnesium excretion is ≥80% of the infused magnesium load.

Hypomagnesemia and Renal Insufficiency

Hypomagnesemia is not common in renal insufficiency but can occur when severe or chronic diarrhea is present and the creatinine clearance is >30 mL/minute. When magnesium is replaced in the setting of renal insufficiency, no more than 50% of the magnesium in the standard replacement protocols should be administered (39), and the serum Mg should be monitored carefully.

MAGNESIUM EXCESS

Magnesium accumulation occurs much less frequently than magnesium depletion. In one survey, hypermagnesemia (i.e., serum Mg >2 mEq/L) was observed in 5% of hospitalized patients (40).

Predisposing Conditions

Renal Insufficiency

Most cases of hypermagnesemia are the result of impaired renal magnesium excretion, which occurs when the creatinine clearance falls below 30 mL/minute (41). However, hypermagnesemia is not a prominent feature of renal insufficiency unless magnesium intake is increased.

Hemolysis

The Mg concentration in erythrocytes is approximately three times greater than in serum (42), so hemolysis can increase the serum Mg. The serum Mg is expected to rise by 0.1 mEq/L for every 250 mL of erythrocytes that lyse completely (46), so hypermagnesemia is expected only with massive hemolysis.

Other Conditions

Other conditions that can predispose to mild hypermagnesemia are diabetic ketoacidosis (transient), adrenal insufficiency, hyperparathyroidism, and lithium intoxication (41).

Clinical Features

The clinical consequences of progressive hypermagnesemia are listed below (42).

Threshold Serum Mg	*Manifestation*
>4 mEq/L	Hyporeflexia
>5 mEq/L	1st° AV Block
>10 mEq/L	Complete Heart Block
>13 mEq/L	Cardiac Arrest

Magnesium has been described as *nature's physiologic calcium blocker* (43), and most of the serious consequences of hypermagnesemia are due to calcium antagonism in the cardiovascular system. Most of the cardiovascular depression is the result of cardiac conduction delays. Depressed contractility and vasodilation are not prominent.

Management

Hemodialysis is the treatment of choice for severe hypermagnesemia. Intravenous calcium gluconate (1 g IV over 2 to 3 minutes) can be used to antagonize the cardiovascular effects of hypermagnesemia *temporarily*, until dialysis is started (44). If fluids are permissible and some renal function is preserved, aggressive volume infusion combined with furosemide may be effective in reducing the serum magnesium levels in less advanced cases of hypermagnesemia.

A FINAL WORD

Magnesium often takes a back seat to sodium and potassium, but as mentioned in the introduction to this chapter, magnesium is required for the release of energy stored in ATP, and is also required for the proper functioning of the membrane Na-K exchange pump that allows the transmission of electrical impulses in excitable tissues. Therefore, magnesium deserves more attention that it receives.

The following are some specific points about magnesium that warrant emphasis:

1. The serum Mg can be normal in patients who are magnesium depleted.

2. Hypomagnesemia is reported in over 50% of ICU patients, and the frequency of magnesium depletion is likely to be even higher. Diuretic therapy with furosemide is the leading cause of magnesium depletion in ICUs.

3. Magnesium depletion should be suspected in any patient with diuretic-induced hypokalemia, and especially when hypokalemia is refractory to potassium replacement.

4. Magnesium replacement will correct the serum Mg before total body stores of magnesium are replenished. The best indicator of magnesium repletion is the urinary retention test (see Table 37.4)

REFERENCES

Introduction

1. Noronha JL, Matuschak GM. Magnesium in critical illness: metabolism, assessment, and treatment. Intensive Care Med 2002; 28:667–679.

2. Tong GM, Rude RK. Magnesium deficiency in critical illness. J Intensive Care Med 2005; 20:3–17.

3. Martin KJ, Gonzalez EA, Slatpolsky E. Clinical consequences and management of hypomagnesemia. J Am Soc Nephrol 2009; 20:2291–2295.

4. White RE, Hartzell HC. Magnesium ions in cardiac function. Regulator of ion channels and second messengers. Biochem Pharmacol 1989; 38:859–867.

Magnesium Balance

5. Elin RJ. Assessment of magnesium status. Clin Chem 1987; 33:1965–1970.

6. Reinhart RA. Magnesium metabolism. A review with special reference to the relationship between intracellular content and serum levels. Arch Intern Med 1988; 148:2415–2420.

7. Lowenstein FW, Stanton MF. Serum magnesium levels in the United States, 1971-1974. J Am Coll Nutr 1986; 5:399–414.

8. Altura BT, Altura BM. A method for distinguishing ionized, complexed and protein-bound Mg in normal and diseased subjects. Scand J Clin Lab Invest 1994; 217:83–87.

9. Kroll MH, Elin RJ. Relationships between magnesium and protein concentrations in serum. Clin Chem 1985; 31:244–246.

10. Alvarez-Leefmans FJ, Giraldez F, Gamino SM. Intracellular free magnesium in excitable cells: its measurement and its biologic significance. Can J Physiol Pharmacol 1987; 65:915–925.

Magnesuim Depletion

11. Whang R. Magnesium deficiency: pathogenesis, prevalence, and clinical implications. Am J Med 1987; 82:24–29.

12. Dyckner T, Wester PO. Potassium/magnesium depletion in patients with cardiovascular disease. Am J Med 1987; 82:11–17.

13. Hollifield JW. Thiazide treatment of systemic hypertension: effects on serum magnesium and ventricular ectopic activity. Am J Cardiol 1989; 63:22G–25G.

14. Ryan MP. Diuretics and potassium/magnesium depletion. Directions for treatment. Am J Med 1987; 82:38–47.

15. Atsmon J, Dolev E. Drug-induced hypomagnesaemia: scope and management. Drug Safety 2005; 28:763–788.

16. Zaloga GP, Chernow B, Pock A, et al. Hypomagnesemia is a common complication of aminoglycoside therapy. Surg Gynecol Obstet 1984; 158:561–565.

17. Hess MW, Hoenderop JG, Bindeis RJ, Drenth JP. Systematic review: hypomagnesemia induced by proton pump inhibition. Ailement Pharmacol Ther 2012; 36:415–413.

18. Whang R, Oei TO, Watanabe A. Frequency of hypomagnesemia in hospitalized patients receiving digitalis. Arch Intern Med 1985; 145:655–656.

19. Balesteri FJ. Magnesium metabolism in the critically ill. Crit Care Clin 1985; 5:217–226.

20. Martin HE. Clinical magnesium deficiency. Ann N Y Acad Sci 1969; 162:891–900.

21. Dyckner T, Ek B, Nyhlin H, et al. Aggravation of thiamine deficiency by magnesium depletion. A case report. Acta Med Scand 1985; 218:129–131.

22. Kassirer J, Hricik D, Cohen J. Repairing Body Fluids: Principles and Practice. 1st ed. Philadelphia, PA: WB Saunders, 1989; 118–129.

23. Sjogren A, Floren CH, Nilsson A. Magnesium deficiency in IDDM related to level of glycosylated hemoglobin. Diabetes 1986; 35:459–463.

24. Lau K. Magnesium metabolism: normal and abnormal. In: Arieff AI, DeFronzo RA, eds. Fluids, electrolytes, and acid base disorders. New York, NY: Churchill Livingstone, 1985; 575–623.

25. Abraham AS, Rosenmann D, Kramer M, et al. Magnesium in the prevention of lethal arrhythmias in acute myocardial infarction. Arch Intern Med 1987; 147:753–755.

Clinical Manifestations

26. Whang R, Oei TO, Aikawa JK, et al. Predictors of clinical hypomagnesemia. Hypokalemia, hypophosphatemia, hyponatremia, and hypocalcemia. Arch Intern Med 1984; 144:1794–1796.

27. Whang R, Flink EB, Dyckner T, et al. Magnesium depletion as a cause of refractory potassium repletion. Arch Intern Med 1985; 145:1686–1689.

28. Anast CS, Winnacker JL, Forte LR, et al. Impaired release of parathyroid hormone in magnesium deficiency. J Clin Endocrinol Metab 1976; 42:707–717.

29. Rude RK, Oldham SB, Singer FR. Functional hypoparathyroidism and parathyroid hormone end-organ resistance in human magnesium deficiency. Clin Endocrinol 1976; 5:209–224.

30. Dominguez JH, Gray RW, Lemann J, Jr. Dietary phosphate deprivation in women and men: effects on mineral and acid balances, parathyroid hormone and the metabolism of 25-OH-vitamin D. J Clin Endocrinol Metab 1976; 43:1056–1068.

31. Cohen L, Kitzes R. Magnesium sulfate and digitalis-toxic arrhythmias. JAMA 1983; 249:2808–2810.

32. Tzivoni D, Keren A. Suppression of ventricular arrhythmias by magnesium. Am J Cardiol 1990; 65:1397–1399.

33. Langley WF, Mann D. Central nervous system magnesium deficiency. Arch Intern Med 1991; 151:593–596.

34. Fleming CR, George L, Stoner GL, et al. The importance of urinary magnesium values in patients with gut failure. Mayo Clin Proc 1996; 71:21–24.

35. Clague JE, Edwards RH, Jackson MJ. Intravenous magnesium loading in chronic fatigue syndrome. Lancet 1992; 340:124–125.

36. Hebert P, Mehta N, Wang J, et al. Functional magnesium deficiency in critically ill patients identified using a magnesium-loading test. Crit Care Med 1997; 25:749–755.

Magnesium Replacement Therapy

37. DiPalma JR. Magnesium replacement therapy. Am Fam Physician 1990; 42:173–176.

38. Trissel LA. Handbook on injectable drugs. 13th ed. Bethesda, MD: Amer Soc Health System Pharmcists, 2005.

39. Oster JR, Epstein M. Management of magnesium depletion. Am J Nephrol 1988; 8:349–354.

Magnesium Excess

40. Whang R, Ryder KW. Frequency of hypomagnesemia and hypermagnesemia. Requested vs routine. JAMA 1990; 263:3063–3064.

41. Van Hook JW. Hypermagnesemia. Crit Care Clin 1991; 7:215–223.

42. Elin RJ. Magnesium metabolism in health and disease. Dis Mon 1988; 34:161–218.

43. Iseri LT, French JH. Magnesium: nature's physiologic calcium blocker. Am Heart J 1984; 108:188–193.

44. Mordes JP, Wacker WE. Excess magnesium. Pharmacol Rev 1977; 29:273–300.

Chapter 38

CALCIUM AND PHOSPHORUS

*Nature never deceives us, it is always we
who deceive ourselves.*

Jean Jacques Rousseau
1754

Calcium and phosphorus are responsible for much of the structural integrity of the bony skeleton. Although neither is found in abundance in the soft tissues, both have an important role in vital cell functions. Phosphorus participates in aerobic energy production, whereas calcium participates in blood coagulation, neuromuscular transmission, and smooth muscle contraction. Considering the important functions of these electrolytes, it is surprising that abnormalities in calcium and phosphorus balance are so well tolerated.

CALCIUM IN PLASMA

Calcium is the most abundant electrolyte in the human body (the average adult has more than half a kilogram of calcium), but 99% is in bone (1,2). In the soft tissues, calcium is 10,000 times more concentrated than in the extracellular fluids (2,3).

Plasma Calcium

The calcium in plasma is present in three forms, as depicted in Figure 38.1. Approximately half of the calcium is ionized (biologically active) and the remainder is complexed (biologically inactive) (1). About 80% of the bound calcium is bound to albumin, while 20% is complexed to plasma anions such as proteins and sulfates. The concentration of total and ionized calcium in plasma is shown in Table 38.1. These values may vary slightly in different clinical laboratories.

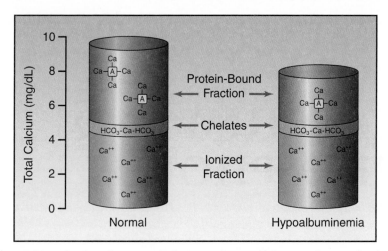

FIGURE 38.1 The three fractions of calcium in plasma and the contribution of each to the total calcium concentration. The column on the right shows how a decrease in plasma albumin can reduce the total plasma calcium without affecting the ionized calcium.

Total vs. Ionized Calcium

The calcium assay used by most clinical laboratories measures all three fractions of calcium, which can be misleading. This is demonstrated in the column on the right in Figure 38.1, which shows that a decrease in the plasma albumin concentration will decrease the total calcium concentration in plasma without affecting the ionized (biologically active) calcium concentration.

A variety of correction factors have been proposed for adjusting the plasma calcium concentration in patients with hypoalbuminemia. However, none of these correction factors are reliable (4,5), and *the only reliable method of determining the concentration of ionized calcium is to measure it with ion-specific electrodes.*

Table 38.1	Normal Ranges for Calcium and Phosphate in Blood		
Serum Electrolyte	Traditional Units (mg/dL)	Conversion Factor*	SI Units (mmol/L)
Total Calcium	9.0–10.0	0.25	2.25–2.50
Ionized Calcium	4.6–5.0	0.25	1.15–1.25
Phosphorus	2.5–5.0	0.32	0.8–1.6

*Multiply traditional units by conversion factor to derive SI Units or divide SI units by conversion factor to derive traditional units.

Ionized Calcium Measurement

Ionized calcium can be measured in whole blood, plasma, or serum with ion-specific electrodes that are now available in most clinical laboratories.

BLOOD COLLECTION Some precautions are necessary when collecting blood samples for an ionized calcium measurement (7). Loss of carbon dioxide from a blood sample could falsely lower the ionized calcium (by increasing calcium binding to albumin), so it is important to avoid gas bubbles in the blood sample. Anticoagulants (e.g., heparin, citrate, and EDTA) can bind calcium, so blood samples should not be placed in collection tubes that contain these anticoagulants. Tubes with red stoppers ("red top" tubes) contain silicone, and are adequate for measuring ionized calcium in serum samples.

IONIZED HYPOCALCEMIA

In a large, multicenter survey that included over 7,000 ICU patients, 88% of the patients had at least one episode of mild ionized hypocalcemia (0.9–1.14 mmol/L), and 3.3% of patients had at least one episode of severe ionized hypocalcemia (< 0.8 mmol/L) (7). The common disorders associated with ionized hypocalcemia in ICU patients are listed in Table 38.2. Hypoparathyroidism is a leading cause of hypocalcemia in outpatients, but is not a consideration in the ICU unless a patient has had recent neck surgery.

Table 38.2	Causes of Ionized Hypocalcemia in the ICU	
Alkalosis	Fat Embolism
Blood Transfusions (15%)	Magnesium Depletion (70%)
Drugs:	Pancreatitis
Aminoglycosides (40%)	Renal Insufficiency (50%)
Heparin (10%)	Sepsis (30%)

Numbers in parentheses show the frequency of ionized hypocalcemia reported in each condition.

Predisposing Conditions

Magnesium Depletion

Magnesium depletion promotes hypocalcemia by inhibiting parathormone secretion and reducing end-organ responsiveness to parathormone (see Chapter 37 for references). Hypocalcemia from magnesium depletion is refractory to calcium replacement therapy, and magnesium replacement often corrects the hypocalcemia.

Sepsis

Sepsis is a common cause of hypocalcemia in the ICU (8,9), but the mechanism is unclear. Hypocalcemia is independent of the systemic vasodilation that accompanies sepsis (9), so the clinical significance of the hypocalcemia is unclear.

Alkalosis

Alkalosis promotes the binding of calcium to albumin, which reduces the concentration of ionized calcium in blood. Symptomatic hypocalcemia is more common with respiratory alkalosis than with metabolic alkalosis. Infusions of sodium bicarbonate can also produce ionized hypocalcemia because calcium directly binds to the infused bicarbonate.

Blood Transfusions

Ionized hypocalcemia has been reported in 20% of patients receiving blood transfusions (8). The mechanism is calcium binding by the citrate anticoagulant in banked blood. Hypocalcemia from blood transfusions is usually transient, and resolves when the infused citrate is metabolized by the liver and kidneys (8). In patients with renal or hepatic failure, a more prolonged hypocalcemia can result. The hypocalcemia associated with blood transfusions does not impede blood coagulation; as a result, calcium infusions are not necessary in massive blood transfusions.

Drugs

A number of drugs can bind calcium and promote ionized hypocalcemia (8). The ones most often used in the ICU are aminoglycosides and heparin.

Renal Failure

Ionized hypocalcemia can accompany renal failure as a result of phosphate retention and impaired conversion of vitamin D to its active form in the kidneys. The treatment is aimed at lowering the phosphate levels in blood with antacids that block phosphorus absorption in the small bowel. However, the value of this practice is unproven. The acidosis in renal failure can decrease the binding of calcium to albumin, so hypocalcemia in renal failure does not imply ionized hypocalcemia.

Pancreatitis

Severe pancreatitis can produce ionized hypocalcemia through several mechanisms. The prognosis is adversely affected by the appearance of hypocalcemia (10), although a causal relationship between hypocalcemia and fatal outcomes has not been proven.

Clinical Manifestations

The major consequences of hypocalcemia are enhanced cardiac and neuromuscular excitability, and reduced contractile force in cardiac muscle and vascular smooth muscle. However, most cases of ionized hypocalcemia in the ICU have no apparent adverse consequences (7).

Neuromuscular

Hypocalcemia can be accompanied by tetany (of peripheral or laryngeal muscles), hyperreflexia, paresthesias, and seizures (11). Chvostek's and

Trousseau's signs are often listed as manifestations of hypocalcemia, but *Chvostek's sign is nonspecific* (it is present in 25% of normal adults), and *Trousseau's sign is insensitive* (it can be absent in at least 30% of patients with hypocalcemia) (12).

Cardiovascular

The cardiovascular complications of hypocalcemia include hypotension, decreased cardiac output, and ventricular ectopic activity. However, these complications are reported only in cases of extreme ionized hypocalcemia (< 0.65 mmol/L) (8).

Calcium Replacement Therapy

The treatment of ionized hypocalcemia should be directed at the underlying cause of the problem. If calcium replacement is needed, the intravenous calcium solutions and a recommended dosing regimen are shown in Table 38.3.

Table 38.3	Intravenous Calcium Replacement Therapy		
Solution	**Elemental Ca**	**Unit Volume**	**Osmolarity**
10% Calcium chloride	27 mg/mL	10 mL ampules	2,000 mosm/L
10% Calcium gluconate	9 mg/mL	10 mL ampules	680 mosm/L

For symptomatic hypocalcemia:
1. Give a bolus dose of 200 mg elemental calcium (e.g., 22 mL of 10% calcium gluconate) in 100 mL isotonic saline over 10 minutes.
2. Follow with a continuous infusion of 1–2 mg/kg per hour for 6–12 hrs.
3. Monitor ionized calcium levels hourly for the first few hours.

Calcium Salt Solutions

The calcium solutions available for intravenous use are 10% calcium chloride and 10% calcium gluconate. *Calcium chloride contains three times more elemental calcium than calcium gluconate*, but calcium gluconate is usually preferred because it has a lower osmolarity, and is less irritating when injected. However, both calcium solutions are hyperosmolar, and should be given via a large central vein, if possible.

Dosing Regimen

A bolus dose of 200 mg elemental calcium (diluted in 100 mL isotonic saline and given over 5–10 minutes) should raise the total serum calcium by 0.5 mg/dL, but levels will begin to fall after 30 minutes (8). Therefore, the bolus dose of calcium should be followed by a continuous infusion at a dose rate of 1–2 mg/kg/hr (elemental calcium) for at least 6 hours. Individual responses will vary, so calcium dosing should be guided by the level of ionized calcium in blood (8).

CAUTION: Intravenous calcium can be risky in select patient populations. Calcium infusions can promote vasoconstriction and ischemia in any of the vital organs (13). The risk of calcium-induced ischemia should be particularly high in patients with low cardiac output who are already vasoconstricted. In addition, aggressive calcium replacement can promote intracellular calcium overload, which can produce lethal cell injury (14), particularly in patients with circulatory shock. Because of these risks, it is wise to avoid correcting ionized hypocalcemia with intravenous calcium unless there is evidence of a serious complication linked to the hypocalcemia.

Maintenance Therapy

The daily maintenance dose of calcium is 2–4 g in adults. This can be administered orally using calcium carbonate (e.g., Oscal) or calcium gluconate tablets (500 mg calcium per tablet).

IONIZED HYPERCALCEMIA

In the large survey of ionized calcium levels mentioned previously (7), 23% of ICU patients had at least one episode of mild ionized hypercalcemia (1.26–1.35 mmol/L), and 17% of patients had at least one episode of ionized hypercalcemia *and* ionized hypocalcemia. The source of ionized hypercalcemia in ICU patients has not been adequately studied, but common causes of hypercalcemia outside the ICU are hyperparathyroidism and malignancy (15–17).

Clinical Manifestations

The manifestations of hypercalcemia are nonspecific, and can be categorized as follows (16):

1. *Gastrointestinal:* nausea, vomiting, constipation, ileus, and pancreatitis
2. *Cardiovascular:* hypovolemia, hypotension, and shortened QT interval
3. *Renal:* polyuria and nephrocalcinosis
4. *Neurologic:* confusion and depressed consciousness, including coma

These manifestations can become evident when the total serum calcium is > 12 mg/dL (or the ionized calcium is > 3.0 mmol/L), and they are almost always present when the serum calcium is > 14 mg/dL (or the ionized calcium is > 3.5 mmol/L) (17). Manifestations are more likely with rapid rises in serum calcium.

Management

Treatment is indicated when the hypercalcemia is associated with adverse effects, or when the serum calcium is greater than 14 mg/dL (or ionized calcium > 3.5 mmol/L). Most cases of severe, symptomatic hypercalcemia (*hypercalcemic crisis*) are cancer-related, and the treatment is summarized in Table 38.4 (1,15–17).

Table 38.4	Management of Severe Hypercalcemia
Agent Drugs	**Dosing Regimen and Comments**
Isotonic Saline	Dosing: 200–500 mL/hr, to maintain a urine output of 100–150 mL/hr.
	Comment: Volume infusion does not usually correct the serum calcium.
Furosemide	Dosing: 40–80 mg IV every 2 hrs, to maintain urine output of 100–150 mL/hr.
	Comment: Promotes calcuria, but is counterproductive to volume infusion, and is recommended only for evidence of volume overload.
Calcitonin	Dosing: 4 units/kg by subcutaneous or intramuscular injection every 12 hrs.
	Comment: Rapid onset of action (2 hrs) but only modest effect. Tachyphylaxis is common.
Glucocorticoids	Dosing: Oral prednisone (20–100 mg daily) or IV hydrocortisone (200–400 mg daily) for 3–5 days.
	Comment: Useful in lymphoma and myeloma. Effects may not be evident for 4 days.
Biphosphonates	Dosing: Zoledronate (4–8 mg IV over 15 min) or pamidronate (90 mg IV over 2 hrs). Can be repeated in 10 days.
	Comment: First line drugs, but effect is not apparent for 2 days. Zoledronate is more effective than pamidronate, but the higher dose can be nephrotoxic.

Isotonic Saline Infusion

Hypercalcemia usually is accompanied by hypercalciuria, which produces an osmotic diuresis. This eventually leads to hypovolemia, which reduces calcium excretion in the urine and precipitates a rapid rise in the serum calcium. Therefore, *volume infusion to correct hypovolemia and promote renal calcium excretion is the first goal of management* for hypercalcemia. Isotonic saline (200–500 mL/hr) is recommended for the volume infusion (16) because natriuresis promotes renal calcium excretion. The goal is a urine output of 100–150 mL/hr (15–17).

Furosemide

Saline infusion does not correct hypercalcemia in over 70% of cases (15), and furosemide is often recommended (40 to 80 mg IV every 2 hours) to further promote urinary calcium excretion. However, this can be counterproductive because it promotes hypovolemia, so *furosemide is recommended only in cases of volume overload* (15,17).

Calcitonin

Calcitonin is a naturally occurring hormone that inhibits bone resorption. It is available as salmon calcitonin, which is given subcutaneously or intramuscularly in a dose of 4 U/kg every 12 hours. The response is rapid (onset within a few hours), but the effect is mild (the maximum drop in serum calcium is 0.5 mmol/L) and tachyphylaxis is common (15). As a result, calcitonin has largely been abandoned for the treatment of severe hypercalcemia (15).

Glucocorticoids

Glucocorticoids have several effects that can decrease the serum calcium, including increased renal excretion of calcium, decreased osteoclast activity in bone, and decreased extrarenal production of calcitriol in lymphoma and myeloma (15). Glucocorticoid regimens include oral prednisone (40–100 mg daily) or intravenous hydrocortisone (200–400 mg daily) for 3–5 days. On the negative side, glucocorticoid effects may not be evident for 4 days, and they can precipitate tumor lysis syndrome (15).

Bisphosphonates

The biphosphonates are potent inhibitors of osteoclast activity. Two drugs in this class, *zoledronate* (4 or 8 mg IV over 15 min) and *pamidronate* (90 mg IV over 2 hours) are considered first line agents in the treatment of severe hypercalcemia (15). Zoledronate is the more effective agent, but the higher dose carries a risk of renal injury. Both drugs have a delayed onset of action (2–4 days). The peak effect is at 4–7 days, and the effect lasts 1–4 weeks (15).

Dialysis

Dialysis (hemodialysis or peritoneal dialysis) is effective in removing calcium in patients with renal failure.

HYPOPHOSPHATEMIA

Unlike calcium, inorganic phosphate (PO_4) is predominantly intracellular in location, where it participates in glycolysis and high energy phosphate (ATP) production. The normal concentration of PO_4 in plasma is shown in Table 38.1 (18).

Hypophosphatemia (serum PO_4 < 2.5 mg/dL or < 0.8 mmol/L) is reported in 17–28% of critically ill patients (19,20), and can be the result of an intracellular shift of phosphorus, an increase in the renal excretion of phosphorus, or a decrease in phosphorus absorption from the GI tract. Most cases of hypophosphatemia are due to movement of PO_4 into cells.

Predisposing Conditions

Glucose Loading

The movement of glucose into cells is accompanied by a similar move-

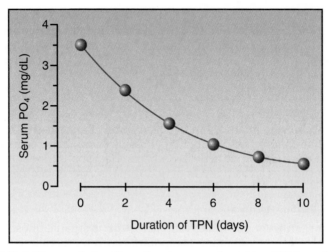

FIGURE 38.2 The cumulative effect of total parenteral nutrition (TPN) on the serum phosphate level. Data from Reference 21.

ment of PO_4 into cells, and this can lead to hypophosphatemia if extracellular PO_4 levels are marginal. *Glucose loading is the most common cause of hypophosphatemia in hospitalized patients* (19,21,22), and typically occurs during refeeding in alcoholic, malnourished, or debilitated patients. The influence of parenteral nutrition on serum PO_4 levels is shown in Figure 38.2. Note the gradual decline in the serum PO_4 and the severe degree of hypophosphatemia (serum PO_4 < 1 mg/dL) after 7 days of intravenous nutrition. The risk of hypophosphatemia is one of the reasons why parenteral nutrition regimens are advanced gradually for the first few days.

Prolonged Hyperglycemia

A phenomenon similar to glucose loading is seen in patients with prolonged hyperglycemia who receive insulin. The hyperglycemia produces an osmotic diuresis (from glycosuria), which promotes urinary PO_4 losses, but the hypophosphatemia appears only when insulin is given (which drives PO_4 into cells). An example of this phenomenon is the hypophosphatemia that appears during the treatment of diabetic ketoacidosis (see page 613).

Respiratory Alkalosis

Respiratory alkalosis can increase intracellular pH, and this accelerates glycolysis. The increase in glucose utilization is accompanied by an increase in glucose and phosphorus movement into cells (23). This may be an important source of hypophosphatemia in ventilator-dependent patients because overventilation and respiratory alkalosis are common in these patients.

β-Receptor Agonists

Stimulation of β-adrenergic receptors can move PO_4 into cells and promote hypophosphatemia. This effect is evident in patients treated with β-agonist bronchodilators. In one study of patients with acute asthma who were treated aggressively with nebulized albuterol (2.5 mg every 30 minutes), the serum PO_4 decreased by 1.25 mg/dL (0.4 mmol/L) 3 hours after the onset of therapy (24).

Systemic Inflammation

There is an inverse relationship between serum PO_4 and circulating levels of inflammatory cytokines (25). Possible explanations include increased PO_4 utilization by activated neutrophils, and a transcellular shift of PO_4 caused by elevated levels of endogenous catecholamines.

Phosphate Binding Agents

Aluminum can form insoluble complexes with inorganic phosphates. As a result, aluminum-containing compounds such as sucralfate (Carafate) can impede the absorption of phosphate in the upper GI tract and promote phosphate depletion (26).

Clinical Manifestations

Hypophosphatemia is often clinically silent, even when the serum PO_4 falls to extremely low levels. In one study of patients with severe hypophosphatemia (i.e., serum $PO_4 < 1$ mg/dL), none of the patients showed evidence of harm (27). Despite the apparent lack of harm, phosphate depletion creates a risk for impaired energy metabolism.

Energy Metabolism

Phosphate depletion has several effects that could impair energy metabolism. These are summarized below, and indicated in Figure 38.3.

1. *Cardiac Output:* Phosphate depletion can impair myocardial contractility and reduce cardiac output. Hypophosphatemic patients with heart failure have shown improved cardiac performance after phosphate supplementation (28).

2. *Erythrocytes:* Reduction of high energy phosphate production from glycolysis in erythrocytes can reduce the deformability of red cells. This may explain why severe hypophosphatemia can be accompanied by a hemolytic anemia (26).

3. *Oxyhemoglobin Dissociation:* Phosphate depletion is accompanied by depletion of 2,3-diphosphoglycerate, and this shifts the oxyhemoglobin dissociation curve to the left. When this occurs, hemoglobin is less likely to release oxygen to the tissues.

4. *Energy Availability:* Phosphate depletion can reduce the availability of cellular energy by impeding the production of high-energy phosphate compounds (ATP).

Muscle Weakness

There is one report of respiratory muscle weakness and failure to wean from mechanical ventilation in patients with severe hypophosphatemia (29). However, other studies have not shown significant respiratory muscle weakness associated with hypophosphatemia (30). At present, *there is little evidence of a link between phosphate depletion and clinically apparent muscle weakness.*

Phosphate Replacement

Intravenous phosphate replacement is recommended for all patients with severe hypophosphatemia (i.e., serum PO_4 <1.0 mg/dL or 0.3 mmol/L), and for patients with hypophosphatemia of any degree who also have cardiac dysfunction, respiratory failure, muscle weakness, or impaired tissue oxygenation. The phosphate solutions and dosing regimen are shown in Table 38.5 (31).

Maintenance Therapy

The normal daily maintenance dose of phosphorus is 1,200 mg if given orally (32). The IV maintenance dose of PO_4 is lower, at 800 mg/day, because only 70% of orally administered phosphate is absorbed from the GI tract.

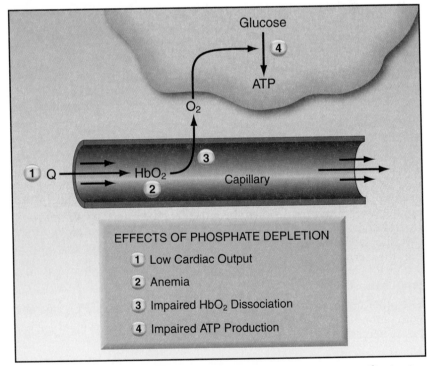

FIGURE 38.3 The effects of phosphate depletion that can impair energy utilization in cells. See text for explanation.

Table 38.5	Phosphate Replacement Therapy	
Solution	**PO₄ Content**	**Other Content**
Sodium Phosphate	93 mg (3 mmol)/mL	Na^+: 4.0 mEq
Potassium Phosphate	93 mg (3 mmol)/mL	K^+: 4.3 mEq

PO₄ Replacement IV by Body Weight†			
Serum PO₄ (mg/dL)	40–60 kg	61–80 kg	81–120 kg
<1	30 mmol	40 mmol	50 mmol
1–1.7	20 mmol	30 mmol	40 mmol
1.8–2.5	10 mmol	15 mmol	20 mmol

†If the plasma K^+ is ≥4 mEq/L, use sodium phosphate, and if the plasma K^+ is <4 mEq/L, use potassium phosphate. Infusion time is 6 hrs. From Reference 31.

HYPERPHOSPHATEMIA

Most cases of hyperphosphatemia in the ICU are the result of impaired PO_4 excretion from renal insufficiency, or PO_4 release from disrupted cells (e.g., rhabdomyolysis or tumor lysis).

Clinical Manifestations

The clinical manifestations of hyperphosphatemia include: (a) the formation of insoluble calcium–phosphate complexes (with deposition into soft tissues), and (b) acute hypocalcemia (with tetany) (11). There is little information about the prevalence or significance of these manifestations in ICU patients.

Management

There are two approaches to hyperphosphatemia. The first is to promote PO_4 binding in the upper GI tract, which can lower serum PO_4 levels, even in the absence of any oral intake of phosphate (i.e., GI dialysis). Sucralfate or aluminum-containing antacids can be used for this purpose. In patients with significant hypocalcemia, calcium acetate tablets (PhosLo, Braintree Labs) can help raise the serum calcium while lowering the serum PO_4. Each calcium acetate tablet (667 mg) contains 8.45 mEq elemental calcium. The recommended dose is 2 tablets three times a day (33,34).

The other approach to hyperphosphatemia is to enhance PO_4 clearance with hemodialysis. This is reserved for patients with renal failure, and is rarely necessary.

A FINAL WORD

Despite the potential for harm, disorders of calcium and phosphorus are notable for the lack of apparent adverse consequences. It may be that abnormal plasma levels of calcium and phosphorus are markers of illness more than abnormalities that warrant correction. Otherwise, the following points about calcium and phosphorus deserve emphasis.

For calcium:

1. For patients with hypoalbuminemia, do not use any of the correction factors proposed for adjusting the plasma calcium concentration (because they are unreliable). You must measure the ionized calcium in these patients.

2. Magnesium depletion, which is common in ICU patients, should always be considered as a possible cause of hypocalcemia.

3. Because calcium infusions can be damaging, intravenous calcium should be reserved for cases of symptomatic hypocalcemia (which is uncommon, as mentioned).

For phosphorus:

1. Watch the plasma PO_4 levels carefully when starting parenteral nutrition because of the risk for hypophosphatemia. This also applies to the use of continuous insulin infusions for tight glycemic control.

2. Watch for hypophosphatemia in patients receiving sucralfate for prophylaxis of stress ulcer bleeding.

REFERENCES

Calcium Reviews

1. Bushinsky DA, Monk RD. Electrolyte quintet: Calcium. Lancet 1998; 352:306–311.

2. Baker SB, Worthley LI. The essentials of calcium, magnesium and phosphate metabolism: part I. Physiology. Crit Care Resusc 2002; 4:301–306.

3. Weaver CM, Heaney RP. Calcium. In: Shils ME, et al., eds. Modern nutrition in health and disease. 10th ed. Philadelphia, PA: Lippincott, Williams & Wilkins, 2006; 194–210.

Plasma Calcium

4. Slomp J, van der Voort PH, Gerritsen RT, et al. Albumin-adjusted calcium is not suitable for diagnosis of hyper- and hypocalcemia in the critically ill. Crit Care Med 2003; 31:1389–1393.

5. Byrnes MC, Huynh K, Helmer SD, et al. A comparison of corrected serum calcium levels to ionized calcium levels among critically ill surgical patients. Am J Surg 2005; 189:310–314.

6. Forman DT, Lorenzo L. Ionized calcium: its significance and clinical usefulness. Ann Clin Lab Sci 1991; 21:297–304.

Ionized Hypocalcemia

7. Moritoki E, Kim I, Nichol A, et al. Ionized calcium concentration and outcome in critical illness. Crit Care Med 2011; 39:314–321.

8. Zaloga GP. Hypocalcemia in critically ill patients. Crit Care Med 1992; 20:251–262.

9. Burchard KW, Simms HH, Robinson A, et al. Hypocalcemia during sepsis. Relationship to resuscitation and hemodynamics. Arch Surg 1992; 127:265–272.

10. Steinberg W, Tenner S. Acute pancreatitis. N Engl J Med 1994; 330:1198–1210.

11. Baker SB, Worthley LI. The essentials of calcium, magnesium and phosphate metabolism: part II. Disorders. Crit Care Resusc 2002; 4:307–315.

12. Zaloga G. Divalent cations: calcium, magnesium, and phosphorus. In: Chernow B., ed. The pharmacologic approach to the critically ill patient. Baltimore: Williams & Wilkins, 1994.

13. Shapiro MJ, Mistry B. Calcium regulation and nonprotective properties of calcium in surgical ischemia. New Horiz 1996; 4:134–138.

14. Trump BF, Berezesky IK. Calcium-mediated cell injury and cell death. FASEB J 1995; 9:219–228.

Ionized Hypercalcemia

15. McCurdy MT, Shanholtz CB. Oncologic emergencies. Crit Care Med 2012; 40:2212–2222.

16. Stewart AF. Clinical practice. Hypercalcemia associated with cancer. N Engl J Med 2005; 352:373–379.

17. Body JJ. Hypercalcemia of malignancy. Semin Nephrol 2004; 24:48–54.

Hypophosphatemia

18. Geerse DA, Bindels AJ, Kuiper MA, et al. Treatment of hypophosphatemia in the intensive care unit: a review. Crit Care 2010; 14:R147. (An open access journal).

19. French C, Bellomo R. A rapid intravenous phosphate replacement protocol for critically ill patients. Critical Care Resusc 2004; 6:175–179.

20. Fiaccadori E, Coffrini E, Fracchia C, et al. Hypophosphatemia and phosphorus depletion in respiratory and peripheral muscles of patients with respiratory failure due to COPD. Chest 1994; 105:1392–1398.

21. Knochel JP. The pathophysiology and clinical characteristics of severe hypophosphatemia. Arch Intern Med 1977; 137:203–220.

22. Marinella MA. Refeeding syndrome and hypophosphatemia. J Intensive Care Med 2005; 20:155–159.

23. Paleologos M, Stone E, Braude S. Persistent, progressive hypophosphataemia after voluntary hyperventilation. Clin Sci 2000; 98:619–625.

24. Bodenhamer J, Bergstrom R, Brown D, et al. Frequently nebulized beta-agonists for asthma: effects on serum electrolytes. Ann Emerg Med 1992; 21:1337–1342.

25. Barak V, Schwartz A, Kalickman I, et al. Prevalence of hypophosphatemia in sepsis and infection: the role of cytokines. Am J Med 1998; 104:40–47.

26. Miller SJ, Simpson J. Medication-nutrient interactions: hypophosphatemia associated with sucralfate in the intensive care unit. Nutr Clin Pract 1991; 6:199–201.

27. King AL, Sica DA, Miller G, et al. Severe hypophosphatemia in a general hospital population. South Med J 1987; 80:831–835.

28. Davis SV, Olichwier KK, Chakko SC. Reversible depression of myocardial performance in hypophosphatemia. Am J Med Sci 1988; 295:183–187.

29. Agusti AG, Torres A, Estopa R, et al. Hypophosphatemia as a cause of failed weaning: the importance of metabolic factors. Crit Care Med 1984; 12:142–143.

30. Gravelyn TR, Brophy N, Siegert C, et al. Hypophosphatemia-associated respiratory muscle weakness in a general inpatient population. Am J Med 1988; 84:870–876.

31. Taylor BE, Huey WY, Buchman TG, et al. Treatment of hypophosphatemia using a protocol based on patient weight and serum phosphorus level in a surgical intensive care unit. J Am Coll Surg 2004; 198:198–204.

32. Knochel JP. Phosphorous. In: Shils ME, et al., eds. Modern nutrition in health and disease. 10th ed. Philadelphia, PA: Lippincott, Williams & Wilkins, 2006; 211–222.

Hyperphosphatemia

33. Kraft MD, Btaiche IF, Sacks GS, et al. Treatment of electrolyte disorders in adult patients in the intensive care unit. Am J Health Syst Pharm 2005; 62:1663–1682.

34. Lorenzo Sellares V, Torres Ramirez A. Management of hyperphosphataemia in dialysis patients: role of phosphate binders in the elderly. Drugs Aging 2004; 21:153–165.

THE ABDOMEN & PELVIS

Obscurity is painful to the mind, as well as the eye.

David Hume

Chapter 39

PANCREATITIS & LIVER FAILURE

Medicine is a science that hath been more labored than advanced.
I find much iteration, but small addition.

Sir Francis Bacon
1605

The conditions described in this chapter (i.e., necrotizing pancreatitis and liver failure) share the following features: (a) both are associated with injury in multiple organs, (b) both are plagued by infections from pathogens that reside in the bowel, (c) the management of both conditions is mostly supportive care, and (d) mortality rates are high, and have not changed in recent memory. The management of patients with liver failure is a particular challenge because of the enormous number of life-supporting functions (including the production of over 20,000 proteins) that are lost when the liver fails.

ACUTE PANCREATITIS

Acute pancreatitis is an inflammatory condition of the pancreas that is characterized by abdominal pain and elevated levels of pancreatic enzymes (amylase, lipase) in blood. Two types of pancreatitis are identified (1):

1. *Edematous Pancreatitis* is the most common form of pancreatitis, and is characterized by inflammatory infiltration of the pancreas without involvement of other organs. The clinical presentation is usually a self-limited period of abdominal pain, nausea, and vomiting. The mortality rate is low (< 2%) (2), and management rarely requires ICU-level care.

2. *Necrotizing Pancreatitis* occurs in 10–15% of cases (1), and is characterized by areas of necrotic destruction in the pancreas, usually accompanied by progressive systemic inflammation and inflammatory injury in one or more extraabdominal organs (e.g., lungs, kidneys, and circulatory system). The mortality rate can be as high as 40% (2), and management usually requires ICU-level care.

Etiologies

Pancreatitis can have a variety of etiologies, as shown in Table 39.1. About 90% of cases are related to gallstones (40% of cases), alcohol abuse (30% of cases), or are idiopathic (20% of cases) (2,4,5). Less common causes include abdominal trauma, severe hypertriglyceridemia (serum levels >1,000 mg/dL), drugs (e.g., acetaminophen, pentamidine, tri-methoprim-sulfamethoxazole, omeprazole, furosemide), infections (e.g., HIV, cytomegalovirus, mycoplasma, *Legionella*), and vasculitides (lupus and polyarteritis nodosa).

Table 39.1	Etiology of Acute Pancreatitis
Leading Causes	**Less Common Causes**
Gallstones (40%)	Abdominal trauma
Alcohol (30%)	Hypertriglyceridemia
Idiopathic (20%)	Drugs†
	Infections§
	Vasculitis

Reported prevalence indicated in parentheses.

†Includes acetaminophen, omeprazole, metronidazole, trimethoprim-sulfamethoxazole, furosemide and valproic acid.

§Includes HIV, cytomegalovirus, mycoplasma, and *Legionella*.

Diagnosis

The diagnosis of acute pancreatitis requires: (a) an increase in serum levels of pancreatic enzymes (amylase and lipase) to at least 3 times the upper limit of normal, and (b) evidence of pancreatitis on contrast-enhanced computed tomography (1).

Pancreatic Enzymes

AMYLASE: Amylase is an enzyme that cleaves starch into smaller polysaccharides. The principal sources of amylase are the pancreas, salivary glands, and fallopian tubes. Serum amylase levels begin to rise 6–12 hours after the onset of acute pancreatitis, and they return to normal in 3–5 days. An increase in serum amylase levels to 3 times the upper limit of normal (the threshold for the diagnosis of acute pancreatitis) has a high sensitivity (> 90%) but a low specificity (as low as 70%) for the diagnosis of acute pancreatitis (6).

The low specificity of serum amylase is a reflection of the numerous conditions that can elevate serum amylase levels. These are listed in Table 39.2 (7). About 25% of the nonpancreatic conditions in this table can result in serum amylase levels that overlap those seen in acute pancreatitis (8). The ones that deserve mention include parotitis, ruptured ectopic pregnancy, and acute alcohol intoxication. Of particular note, *hyperamy-*

lasemia of salivary origin is reported in 40% of cases of acute alcohol intoxication (6). (*Note:* The reference range for serum amylase is not mentioned because it often varies in different clinical laboratories.)

Table 39.2	Sources of Elevated Serum Amylase and Lipase Levels	
Conditions	**Drugs and Other Agents[t]**
Pancreatitis	*Amylase:*
Cholecystitis	Ethanol intoxication
Renal Failure	Hydroxyethyl starch
	Histamine H_2 blockers
Parotitis (amylase)	Metaclopramide
Peptic Ulcer Disease	Opiates
Bowel Obstruction or Infarction	
	Lipase:
Liver Disease	Lipid infusions:
Ruptured Ectopic Pregnancy (amylase)	Methylprednisone
Diabetic Ketoacidosis	Opiates

[t]Includes only substances that are likely to be encountered in ICU patients. For a more complete list, see Reference 7.

LIPASE: Lipase is an enzyme that hydrolyses triglycerides to form glycerol and free fatty acids. The principal sources of lipase are the tongue, pancreas, liver, intestine, and circulating lipoproteins. In acute pancreatitis, serum lipase levels begin to rise earlier than serum amylase (at 4 to 8 hours), and the serum levels remain elevated longer than serum amylase (for 8 to 14 days).

Like amylase, there are several nonpancreatic conditions that can elevate serum lipase levels, as shown in Table 39.2. However, unlike amylase, nonpancreatic conditions rarely raise serum lipase levels high enough to overlap with the levels seen in acute pancreatitis (8). Therefore, *serum lipase is considered more specific than serum amylase for the diagnosis of acute pancreatitis.* An increase in serum lipase to three times the upper limit of normal has a sensitivity and specificity of 80–100% for acute pancreatitis (6).

RECOMMENDATION: *The serum lipase can be used alone for the diagnostic evaluation of pancreatitis.* Adding the serum amylase assay does not increase diagnostic accuracy (6). However, pancreatic enzyme assays cannot be used to evaluate the severity of illness (6).

Computed Tomography

Contrast-enhanced computed tomography (CT) is the most reliable diagnostic test for acute pancreatitis, and can identify the type of pancreatitis (edematous vs. necrotizing) as well as localized complications (e.g., infection). Figure 39.1 shows a contrast-enhanced CT image of edematous pancreatitis. The pancreas is thickened and enhances completely, and the

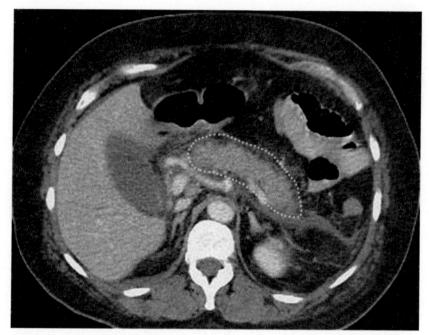

FIGURE 39.1 Contrast-enhanced CT image showing edematous pancreatitis. The pancreas (outlined by the dotted line) is enlarged and enhances completely. There is also blurring of the pancreatic border, which is characteristic of edema formation. Image digitally enhanced.

border of the pancreas is blurred, which is characteristic of pancreatic edema. Compare this with the image in Figure 39.2, which shows a large area that is not contrast-enhanced in the region of the neck and body of the pancreas. This represents pancreatic necrosis, and identifies the condition as necrotizing pancreatitis. *The full extent of pancreatic necrosis may not be evident on CT imaging for the first week after the onset of symptoms* (1), so repeat imaging is advised in patients with persistent symptoms or severe pancreatitis.

When IV contrast cannot be administered (because of a dye allergy or a serum creatinine above 1.5 mg/dL) CT imaging is less likely to distinguish between edematous and necrotizing pancreatitis.

Biliary Evaluation

Since gallstones are the leading cause of acute pancreatitis in the United States (4), an evaluation of the gall bladder and biliary tree is advised in all cases of confirmed acute pancreatitis. Contrast-enhanced CT images may suffice for this evaluation, but in cases where a CT scan is inconclusive, or has not been performed, ultrasonography is recommended.

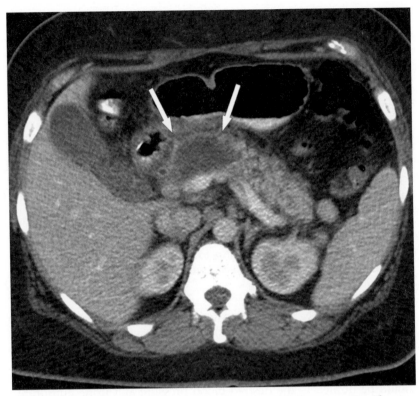

FIGURE 39.2 Contrast-enhanced CT image showing necrotizing pancreatitis. The area that is not contrast-enhanced (indicated by the arrows) represents necrosis in the neck and body of the pancreas. Image from Reference 1.

SEVERE PANCREATITIS

Severe pancreatitis is defined as acute (usually necrotizing) pancreatitis that is associated with persistent (> 48 hrs) injury in at least one other organ system (1). The cause of the extrapancreatic organ injury is progressive systemic inflammation (similar to severe sepsis and septic shock), and the organs that are typically involved include the lungs (acute respiratory distress syndrome, or ARDS), the kidneys (acute kidney injury), and the circulatory system (hypotension and circulatory shock). Pancreatic enzymes and CT images have a poor correlation with the clinical severity of this condition

The management of severe pancreatitis is best conducted in an ICU setting, and includes the following measures: (a) removing the precipitating condition (e.g., obstructing gallstones), (b) providing supportive care for the extrapancreatic organ injuries (e.g., mechanical ventilation for ARDS), (c) early nutritional support with enteral tube feedings, and (d) managing intraabdominal complications (e.g., infection).

Circulatory Support

Circulatory support includes volume resuscitation and vasopressor drugs, if necessary.

Fluid Therapy

Severe pancreatitis is associated with loss of intravascular fluid through leaky systemic capillaries, and the resulting hypovolemia can produce additional pancreatic necrosis. For this reason, aggressive fluid therapy has been recommended early in the course of severe pancreatitis (9). There is no agreement on which type of fluid (colloid or crystalloid) is best, but crystalloid fluids are currently the popular choice. The initial regimen for volume resuscitation is summarized as follows:

1. For crystalloid fluids, infuse 20 mL/kg (about 1.5 liters) over 60 to 90 minutes.

2. Follow with an infusion rate up to 250 mL/hr for the next 24–48 hours, to maintain a mean arterial pressure ≥ 65 mm Hg, and a urine output ≥ 0.5 mL/kg/hr.

CAUTION: Aggressive volume infusion has not been shown to improve outcomes in severe pancreatitis (10), and this practice can be deleterious by promoting edema formation, which can aggravate conditions like ARDS, and increases the risk of abdominal compartment syndrome. Therefore, after the initial volume infusion of 20 mL/kg, the infusion rate should be titrated to the desired blood pressure and urine output, but should not exceed 250 mL/hr. If volume infusion does not achieve the desired hemodynamic goals, vasopressor therapy should be initiated.

Vasopressor Therapy

There are no official recommendations regarding vasopressor therapy in severe pancreatitis, but norepinephrine is an appropriate choice. The initial infusion rate is 0.1 µg/kg/hr, which is then titrated to maintain a mean arterial pressure ≥ 65 mm Hg. All vasoconstrictor drugs can reduce splanchnic blood flow (especially phenylephrine), and could aggravate pancreatic necrosis, so careful titration of infusion rates (and avoiding phenylephrine) is advised.

Prophylactic Antibiotics

About one-third of patients with necrotizing pancreatitis develop infections in the necrotic areas of the pancreas (11). The pathogens are almost always Gram-negative enteric organisms, and the infections typically appear 7–10 days after the onset of illness. These infections are difficult to eradicate, and they are associated with increased mortality rates (11). Unfortunately, antibiotic prophylaxis does not reduce the incidence of pancreatic infections, and does not influence the mortality rate in severe pancreatitis (12). As a result, *prophylactic antibiotics are not recommended in necrotizing pancreatitis* (11).

Nutrition Support

Nutrition support should be started early (within 48 hours after the onset of illness) using enteral tube feedings, if possible (13).

Enteral Nutrition

The preference for enteral nutrition is based on the ability of tube feedings to exert a trophic effect on the bowel mucosa. This helps to maintain the structural and functional integrity of the bowel mucosa, and thereby reduce the risk of bacterial translocation across the bowel wall (which is considered the major route leading to pancreatic infections). Clinical studies have shown that *enteral nutrition is associated with fewer infections, less multiorgan failure, and a lower mortality rate than total parenteral nutrition* in patients with severe pancreatitis (14). (The effect of enteral feedings on the bowel mucosa is described in more detail in Chapter 48.)

FEEDING SITE: Tube feedings should be infused into the jejunum using long feeding tubes that can be placed with fluoroscopic or endoscopic guidance. Alternately, a feeding jejunostomy can be created in patients who require laparotomy for pancreatic debridement. Nasogastric feedings are not currently recommended, although one small study has shown no apparent harm from nasogastric feedings in severe pancreatitis (15).

FEEDING REGIMEN: The jejunum does not have the reservoir capacity of the stomach, so jejunal feedings should be advanced more slowly than gastric feedings. The diluting effect of gastric secretions is also lost in the jejunum, so isotonic feeding formulas are preferred to hypertonic formulas. Standard (polymeric) tube feedings can be used for jejunal feedings (13), but in patients with diarrhea, elemental feeding formulas may be preferred. (Elemental formulas are low in fat, and the protein is available as individual amino acids, which are presumably easier to digest.)

Abdominal Complications

Pancreatic Infection

The appearance of infection in necrotizing pancreatitis is often heralded by reappearance, persistence, or progression of systemic inflammation and multiorgan failure at 7–10 days after the onset of illness. A contrast-enhanced CT scan may show gas bubbles in the necrotic areas of the pancreas, as shown in Figure 39.3. If infection is suspected but gas bubbles are not evident on CT imaging, cultures must be obtained from the necrotic areas of the pancreas (using CT-guided needle aspiration). The treatment of choice for infected pancreatic necrosis is surgical debridement *(necrosectomy)* (11).

Abdominal Compartment Syndrome

There are several sources of increased intraabdominal pressure in severe pancreatitis, including peripancreatic fluid collections, ascites, and edema of the bowel wall (which is exaggerated by aggressive volume

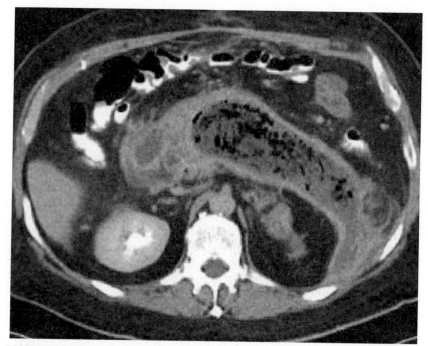

FIGURE 39.3 Contrast-enhanced CT image showing extensive necrosis of the pancreas with numerous gas bubbles, indicating infection.

infusion). Abdominal compartment syndrome (ACS) has been reported in as many as 55% of patients with severe pancreatitis (16), but this may be an exaggeration because it is based on studies that used a relatively low abdominal pressures (15–20 mm Hg) for the diagnosis of ACS. Nevertheless, ACS is more common than suspected in severe pancreatitis, and measurements of abdominal pressure are warranted in any patient with acute pancreatitis who develops acute oliguric renal failure. (See Chapter 34 for more information on ACS.)

Gallstone Pancreatitis

When acute pancreatitis is associated with gallstones, early endoscopic retrograde cholangio-pancreatography (ERCP) is indicated for biliary obstruction or evidence of cholangitis (i.e., fever and increasing liver enzymes) (17).

LIVER FAILURE

Types of Liver Failure

There are two types of liver failure that can appear in the ICU: (a) acute liver failure, and (b) acute-on-chronic liver failure.

Acute Liver Failure

Acute liver failure is an abrupt and rapid deterioration in liver function that occurs *de novo*, without prior liver disease. This is an uncommon condition with an annual incidence of 1 to 6 cases per million people in developed countries (18). Most cases are the result of viral hepatitis or drug-induced liver injury, and the principal clinical manifestation is severe hepatic encephalopathy. The leading cause of acute liver failure in the United States is acetaminophen overdose. (See Chapter 54 for a description of acetaminophen hepatotoxicity.)

Acute-on-Chronic Liver Failure

Most cases of liver failure involve patients with chronic liver disease (cirrhosis) who develop an abrupt deterioration in liver function as a result of a precipitating condition, usually an infection or variceal hemorrhage (19). The clinical manifestations often include signs of systemic inflammation (fever, leukocytosis, etc.), worsening ascites, mental status changes (hepatic encephalopathy), and a deterioration in renal function. The evaluation and management of this group of patients is described in the following text. The mortality rate in these patients is considerable, and ranges from 35% to 70% (19,20).

Spontaneous Bacterial Peritonitis

In patients with acute-on-chronic liver failure and ascites, 10% to 27% have evidence of infection in the ascitic fluid without an apparent primary site of infection (21). This condition is called *spontaneous bacterial peritonitis* (SBP), and the presumed mechanism is translocation of enteric pathogens across the bowel mucosa and into the peritoneal fluid. Cirrhosis predisposes to SBP because it impairs the normal function of the liver in eradicating enteric pathogens that translocate across the bowel wall. A single organism is isolated in most cases of SBP, and the isolates are Gram-negative aerobic bacilli (especially *Escherichia coli)* in 75% of cases, and Gram-positive aerobic cocci (especially streptococcal species) in 25% of cases (21).

Clinical Features

Fever, abdominal pain, and rebound tenderness are present in at least 50% of cases of SBP, but the condition can be asymptomatic in one-third of cases (21).

Diagnostic Approach

A diagnostic paracentesis should be performed on all patients with cirrhosis and ascites who are admitted for acute-on-chronic liver failure. An absolute neutrophil count ≥250 cells/mm^3 in the ascitic fluid is presumptive evidence of infection, and is an indication to begin empiric antimicrobial therapy. *Culture samples of ascitic fluid should be injected directly into blood culture bottles at the bedside* because standard culture methods have a diagnostic yield of only 50% in cases of probable SBP (22).

Management

The preferred antibiotic for suspected SBP is cefotaxime (2 grams IV every 8 hours), or another third-generation cephalosporin (21–23). Unfortunately, the mortality rate in SBP is 30 to 40% despite adequate antibiotic coverage (22); this may be explained by the fact that *30% of patients with SBP develop hepatorenal syndrome* (23), which has a mortality rate in excess of 50% (see later for a description of this syndrome).

ALBUMIN INFUSIONS: Because renal hypoperfusion plays an important role in the pathogenesis of hepatorenal syndrome (see later), clinical studies have evaluated the role of albumin infusions in SBP. The results of these studies indicate that infusions of albumin can reduce the incidence of hepatorenal syndrome in SBP, but only in high-risk patients; i.e., those with a BUN > 30 mg/dL, creatinine > 1 mg/dL and bilirubin > 4 mg/dL (24). The recommended albumin infusion regimen is as follows (24):

Day 1: 1.5 g /kg body weight, infused within 6 hours of the diagnosis of SBP.

Day 3: 1.0 g/kg body weight.

It is unclear at this time if the benefit from albumin is a volume effect, or is related to some other effect (e.g., albumin has antioxidant activity, and can also bind cytokines).

Management of Ascites

The formation of ascites in patients with cirrhosis is partly the result of sodium retention by the kidneys in response to activation of the renin-angiotensin-aldosterone system. The management of ascites is aimed at counteracting this sodium retention using diuretics (furosemide and spironolactone) and restricted sodium intake.

Sodium Restriction

Daily intake of sodium should be restricted to 2 grams (88 mEq), if possible (22). This is often an unrealistic goal in hospitalized patients (who require saline or Ringer's lactate infusions for a variety of reasons), but higher sodium intakes can be tolerated when urinary sodium losses exceed 88 mEq daily (i.e., during diuretic therapy). Fluid restriction is not necessary unless it is needed for symptomatic hyponatremia.

Spironolactone

The actions of aldosterone to promote sodium retention in cirrhotic patients can be antagonized by spironolactone. The drug is given orally (or via feeding tube) at an initial dose of 100 mg once daily. The daily dose can be increased in 100 mg increments, if needed, to a maximum daily dose of 400 mg. The use of spironolactone alone is not advised because of the risk of hyperkalemia (22).

Furosemide

Diuretic therapy with furosemide promotes urinary sodium loss, and also reduces the risk of hyperkalemia from spironolactone. The initial dose is 40 mg (oral or intravenous) daily, and this can be increased gradually, in 40 mg increments, to a maximum daily dose of 160 mg, if necessary. Furosemide should not be used alone because it is less effective than spironolactone for treating cirrhosis-related ascites (22).

Large-Volume Paracentesis

Patients with tense ascites can receive immediate relief from large-volume paracentesis. A volume of 5 liters can be removed at one "sitting" without adverse hemodynamic consequences (25). If larger volumes are removed, albumin can be infused at a dose of 8.5 mg/kg for each liter of fluid removed (23).

End-Points

There is no ceiling for daily weight loss in cirrhotic patients with edema and ascites (22). Fluid loss is permitted until the baseline or premorbid body weight is achieved, or until there is evidence of prerenal azotemia. An increase in serum creatinine to 2 mg/dL is an indication to discontinue diuretic therapy. Avoiding excessive diuresis is an important consideration for limiting the risk of hepatorenal syndrome (see later).

About 10% of patients with cirrhosis and ascites are resistant to diuretic therapy (22). The prognosis in this situation is poor, and liver transplantation should be considered.

Hepatorenal Syndrome

Hepatorenal syndrome (HRS) is a functional renal failure (i.e., occurs without intrinsic renal disease) that occurs in patients with advanced cirrhosis, especially those with spontaneous bacterial peritonitis or sepsis from another source (26).

Pathogenesis

HRS is the result of hemodynamic alterations in the splanchnic and renal circulations. Cirrhosis is associated with splanchnic vasodilation, and the neurohumoral (renin system) response to this vasodilation results in vasoconstriction in other organs, including the kidneys (26). The renal vasoconstriction creates a situation where the glomerular filtration rate is vulnerable to small decrements in cardiac output. Sepsis is also associated with splanchnic vasodilation, which could explain the association between sepsis and HRS.

Diagnosis

The diagnostic criteria for HRS are shown in Table 39.3. The criteria include renal impairment (serum creatinine > 1.5 mg/dL) that does not respond to albumin infusions, and no other likely source of renal dysfunction (i.e., nephrotoxic drugs, shock, or parenchymal kidney disease).

Table 39.3	Clinical Approach to Hepatorenal Syndrome
Diagnostic Criteria	**Management**
1. Cirrhosis with ascites	1. Terlipressin: 1–2 mg IV every 4–6 hr
2. Serum creatinine >1.5 mg/dL	Albumin: 1 g/kg (to 100 mg) on day 1, then 20–40 g daily.†
3. No improvement in renal function after 2 days of albumin infusions and no diuretics	
4. No evidence of shock	2. TIPS: If response to #1 is suboptimal.
5. No nephrotoxic drugs	3. Liver transplant: Optimal
6. No evidence of parenchymal kidney disease	

†Discontinue if serum albumin >4.5 g/dL.
From Reference 26.

Management

The management of HRS is designed to correct the hemodynamic changes that are responsible for HRS. First-line therapy includes a splanchnic vaso-constrictor (terlipressin, a vasopressin analogue) and a volume expander (albumin). An effective dosing regimen is shown in Table 39.3. Over 50% of patients with HRS will show improvement in renal function with this regimen (26,27). However, *HRS often relapses after drug therapy is discontinued*, and long-term survival requires liver transplantation (26). Transjugular intrahepatic portosystemic stent-shunt (TIPS) can improve renal function in HRS (26), but this procedure promotes hepatic encephalopathy, so it is reserved for transplant candidates that are unresponsive to pharmacotherapy.

HEPATIC ENCEPHALOPATHY

Liver failure produces an encephalopathy that is characterized by cerebral edema, disordered thinking, and altered consciousness. Hepatic encephalopathy is the dominant manifestation in acute liver failure, whereas in acute-on-chronic liver failure, the encephalopathy is usually preceded by an acute insult (e.g., variceal hemorrhage). Ammonia has been identified as a key factor in the pathogenesis of hepatic encephalopathy (28).

Pathogenesis

Ammonia (NH_3) is a byproduct of protein degradation, and is produced primarily in the bowel (and to a lesser degree in skeletal muscle and kidneys). The liver plays a major role in clearing ammonia by converting it to urea in the urea cycle. This clearance mechanism is impaired or lost in liver failure, resulting in a progressive rise in ammonia levels in blood. Ammonia eventually crosses the blood-brain barrier and is taken up by astrocytes, which use the ammonia to convert glutamate to glutamine; i.e.,

$$glutamate + NH_3 + ATP \rightarrow glutamine + ADP$$

(Astrocytes normally provide glutamine for neurons, which use the glutamine as a substrate for the production of glutamate, a neurotransmitter.) The ammonia load in astrocytes leads to accumulation of glutamine, and this creates an osmotic force that draws water into the astrocytes. The result is cerebral edema, astrocyte damage, and impaired synaptic transmission in the brain.

Clinical Features

The principal features of progressive hepatic encephalopathy are shown in Table 39.4 (29). Agitation and disorientation are prominent in the early stages, while depressed consciousness is the dominant feature in the late stages. The cranial nerves are not affected, but dysarthria can be present (30). Involuntary movements like tremors or asterixis (clonic movements during wrist extension) can appear, while sensation is intact. Focal neurological deficits are considered evidence of an alternative diagnosis (30).

Table 39.4	Progressive Stages of Hepatic Encephalopathy
Stage	**Features**
Stage 0	• No encephalopathy
Stage 1	• Short attention span • Euphoria or depression • Asterixis may be present
Stage 2	• Lethargy or apathy • Disorientation • Asterixis usually present
Stage 3	• Somnolent, but responsive to verbal commands • Severe disorientation • Asterixis absent
Stage 4	• Coma

The "West Haven Criteria," from Reference 29.

Diagnostic Evaluation

The diagnosis of hepatic encephalopathy is usually made by excluding other causes of altered mentation. Other conditions that should be considered in patients with cirrhotic liver failure include drug overdose, subdural hematoma, and Wernicke's encephalopathy (from thiamine deficiency). Neuroimaging studies are performed to eliminate other diagnoses. The only diagnostic test that can help to identify hepatic enceph-alopathy is the serum ammonia level.

Serum Ammonia

Considering the role played by ammonia in the pathogenesis of hepatic encephalopathy, it is no surprise that serum ammonia levels are typically elevated in patients with hepatic encephalopathy. This is demonstrated in Figure 39.4, which shows the relationship between ammonia levels in blood (arterial and venous) and the presence and severity of hepatic encephalopathy (31). Although the ammonia levels are mildly elevated in the absence of hepatic encephalopathy (stage 0), the levels are higher in the presence of hepatic encephalopathy, and the degree of elevation

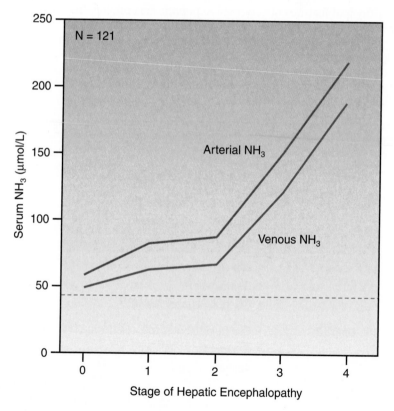

FIGURE 39.4 Relationship between arterial and venous ammonia (NH_3) and the presence and severity of hepatic encephalopathy. The stages of encephalopathy correspond to those in Table 39.3. The horizontal dotted line represents the upper limit of the normal range for serum ammonia (47 µmol/L) at the study hospital. N indicates number of patients studied. Data from Reference 31.

corresponds to the severity of the condition. Note that the ammonia levels are higher in arterial blood. Although the difference between arterial and venous ammonia levels was not statistically significant in this study (31), arterial blood seems optimal for identifying hepatic encephalopathy in the early stages of the condition.

Treatment

The treatment of hepatic encephalopathy is aimed at reducing the ammonia burden in the central nervous system. The most effective strategy is to impair ammonia production in the bowel with lactulose (first-line therapy) and nonabsorbable antibiotics (second-line therapy).

Lactulose

Lactulose is a nonabsorbable disaccharide that is metabolized by "lactic acid bacteria" (e.g., *Lactobacillus acidophilus*) in the bowel (32). This promotes the formation of short-chain fatty acids, and the resulting acidification of the bowel lumen reduces the ammonia burden from the bowel in two ways: (a) by eradicating ammoniagenic microorganisms (mostly Gram-negative aerobic bacilli), and (b) by reducing ammonia absorption from the bowel. (The bactericidal actions of an acid pH are illustrated in Figure 5.3.) The dosing recommendations for lactulose in acute hepatic encephalopathy are as follows (29):

1. *Oral or Nasogastric Route:* Start with 45 mL lactulose every hour until evacuation occurs, then reduce dose to 30 mL every 8–12 hours. This is the preferred route.

2. *Retention Enema:* Mix 300 mL lactulose in one liter of tap water. Administer by high rectal enema, and retain for one hour with the patient in the Trendelenburg position.

Lactulose can promote an osmotic diarrhea, and the dosage should be reduced (or temporarily halted) if diarrhea appears. In patients with diarrhea at the outset, lower doses of lactulose can be combined with a nonabsorbable antibiotic.

Nonabsorbable Antibiotics:

Nonabsorbable antibiotics are used to eradicate ammonia-generating organisms (i.e., Gram-negative aerobic bacilli). The following are 2 regimens that can be used in acute hepatic encephalopathy:

1. *Neomycin:* The oral (nasogastric) dose is 3 to 6 grams daily in 3 divided doses, and continued for 1 to 2 weeks (23).

2. *Rifaximin:* A regimen with proven success is 1,200 mg daily (400 mg by mouth or nasogastric tube every 8 hours) for 10–21 days (33).

Neomycin is the traditional choice (and is devoid of oto- and nephrotoxic effects when used in short-term therapy), while rifaximin (a rifampin analogue with broad-spectrum activity and little toxicity) is rapidly gaining in popularity. There is currently no evidence of superiority with either drug regimen.

Nutrition Support

Protein restriction (which would reduce the ammonia burden from the bowel) is not recommended for patients with hepatic encephalopathy because these patients have increased rates of protein catabolism, and restricting protein intake would promote a negative nitrogen balance (34). The recommended protein intake in critically ill patients is 1.2 to 1.5 g/kg/day (see Chapter 47), so staying at the low end of this range (1.2 g/kg/day) might be the best choice in patients with hepatic encephalopathy.

A FINAL WORD

Back to the Bowel

One of the recurring themes in this book is the importance of the bowel as a source of infection in critically ill patients (see Chapters 5 and 40). Two observations in this chapter demonstrate the normal defense mechanisms that prevent infections of bowel origin.

The first observation is the ability of enteral tube feedings to reduce the incidence of sepsis and multiorgan failure in patients with severe pancreatitis. This highlights the trophic effect of bulk nutrients on the structural and functional integrity of the mucosal barrier in the gut; i.e., the "non-nutritive" function of enteral feeding. (See Chapter 48 for more information on this topic.)

The second observation is the occurrence of spontaneous bacterial peritonitis in patients with cirrhosis and ascites. This is a classic example of an infection that is caused by the translocation of enteric pathogens across the bowel mucosa, and it highlights the importance of the reticuloendothelial system in the bowel (mostly represented by the liver) in defending against the spread of enteric pathogens.

REFERENCES

Pancreatitis

1. Banks PA, Bollen TL, Dervenis C, et al. Classification of acute pancreatitis – 2012: revision of the Atlanta classification and definitions by international consensus. Gut 2012; 62:102–111.

2. Cavallini G, Frulloni L, Bassi C, et al. Prospective multicentre survey on acute pancreatitis in Italy (Proinf-AISP). Dig Liver Dis 2004; 36:205–211.

3. Greer SE, Burchard KW. Acute pancreatitis and critical illness. A pancreatic tale of hypoperfusion and inflammation. Chest 2009; 136:1413–1419.

4. Forsmark CE, Baille J. AGA Institute technical review on acute pancreatitis. Gastroenterol 2007; 132:2022–2044.

5. Yang AL, Vadhavkar S, Singh G, Omary MB. Epidemiology of alcohol-related liver and pancreatic disease in the United States. Arch Intern Med 2008; 168:649–656.

6. Yadav D, Agarwal N, Pitchumoni CS. A critical evaluation of laboratory tests in acute pancreatitis. Am J Gastroenterol 2002; 97:1309–1318.

7. Gelrud D, Gress FG. Elevated serum amylase and lipase. UpToDate (accessed on May 30, 2013).

8. Gumaste VV, Roditis N, Mehta D, Dave PB. Serum lipase levels in nonpancreatic abdominal pain versus acute pancreatitis. Am J Gastroenterol 1993; 88:2051–2055.

Severe Pancreatitis

9. Tenner S. Initial management of acute pancreatitis: critical issues in the first 72 hours. Am J Gastroenterol 2004; 99:2489–2494.

10. Haydock MD, Mittal A, Wilms HR, et al. Fluid therapy in acute pancreatitis: anybody's guess. Ann Surg 2013; 257:182–188.

11. Banks PA, Freeman ML, Practice Parameters Committee of the American College of Gastroenterology. Practice guidelines in acute pancreatitis. Am J Gastroenterol 2006; 101:2379–2400.

12. Hart PA, Bechtold ML, Marshall JB, et al. Prophylactic antibiotics in necrotizing pancreatitis: a meta-analysis. South Med J 2008; 101:1126–1131.

13. Parrish CR, Krenitsky J, McClave SA. Pancreatitis. 2012 A.S.P.E.N. Nutrition Support Core Curriculum. Silver Spring, MD: American Society of Parenteral and Enteral Nutrition, 2012:472–490.

14. Al-Omran M, AlBalawi ZH, Tashkandi MF, Al-Ansary LA. Enteral versus parenteral nutrition for acute pancreatitis. Cochrane Database Syst Rev 2010:CD002837.

15. Eatock FC, Chong P, Menezes N, et al. A randomized study of early nasogastric versus nasojejunal feeding in severe acute pancreatitis. Am J Gastroenterol 2005; 100:432–439.

16. Al-Bahrani AZ, Abid GH, Holt A. et al. Clinical relevance of intra-abdominal hypertension in patients with severe acute pancreatitis. Pancreas 2008; 36:39–43.

17. Nathens AB, Curtis JR, Beale RJ, et al. Management of the critically ill patient with severe acute pancreatitis. Crit Care Med 2004; 32:2524–2536.

Liver Failure

18. Bernal W, Auzinger G, Dhawan A, Wendon J. Acute liver failure. Lancet 2010; 376:190–201.

19. Olson JC, Kamath PS. Acute-on-chronic liver failure: concept, natural history, and prognosis. Curr Opin Crit Care 2011; 17:165–169.

20. Saliba F, Ichai P, Levesque E, Samuel D. Cirrhotic patients in the ICU: prognostic markers and outcome. Curr Opin Crit Care 2013; 19:154–160.

Ascites

21. Gilbert JA, Kamath PS. Spontaneous bacterial peritonitis: an update. Mayo Clin Proc 1995; 70:365–370.

22. Runyon BA. Management of adult patients with ascites caused by cirrhosis. Hepatology 1998; 27:264–272.

23. Moore CM, van Thiel DH. Cirrhotic ascites review: pathophysiology, diagnosis, and management. World J Hepatol 2013; 5:251–263.

24. Narula N, Tsoi K, Marshall JK. Should albumin be used in all patients with spontaneous bacterial peritonitis? Can J Gastroenterol 2011; 25:373–376.

25. Peltekian KM, Wong F, Liu PP, et al. Cardiovascular, renal, and neurohumoral responses to single large-volume paracentesis in cirrhotic patients with diuretic resistant ascites. Am J Gastroenterol 1997; 92:394–399.

Hepatorenal Syndrome

26. Dalerno F, Gerbes A, Gines P, et al. Diagnosis, prevention and treatment of hepatorenal syndrome in cirrhosis. Gut 20071 56:131–1318.

27. Rajekar H, Chawla Y. Terlipressin in hepatorenal syndrome: evidence for present indications. J Gastroenterol Hepatol 2011; 26(Suppl):109–114.

Hepatic Encephalopathy

28. Clay AS, Hainline BE. Hyperammonemia in the ICU. Chest 2007; 132: 1368–1378.

29. Blei AT, Cordoba J, and the Practice Parameters Committee of the American College of Gastroenterology. Hepatic encephalopathy. Am J Gastroenterol 2001; 96:1968–1976.

30. Ferenci P, Lockwood A, Mullen K, et al. Hepatic encephalopathy – definition,nomenclature, diagnosis and quantification: Final report of the Working Party at the 11th World Congress of Gastroenterology, Vienna, 1998. Hepatol 2002; 55:716–721.

31. Ong JP, Aggarwal A, Krieger D, et al. Correlation between ammonia levels and the severity of hepatic encephalopathy. Am J Med 2003; 114:188–193.

32. Salminen S, Salminen E. Lactulose, lactic acid bacterial, intestinal microecology, and mucosal protection. Scand J Gastroenterol 1997; 222(Suppl):45–48.

33. Lawrence KR, Klee JA. Rifaximin for the treatment of hepatic encephalopathy. Pharmacotherapy 2008; 28:1019–1032.

34. Nutrition in end-stage liver disease: principles and practice. Gastroenterology 2008; 134:1729–1740.

Chapter 40

ABDOMINAL INFECTIONS IN THE ICU

If you know your enemies and know yourself,
you will not be imperiled in a hundred battles.

Sun Tzu
The Art of War

The concept of the bowel as noxious reservoir first appeared in the early years of the twentieth century, when a Scottish surgeon William Arbuthnot-Lane began performing total colectomies in patients with chronic constipation, to prevent "autointoxication" from toxic bowel contents (1). This practice was abandoned (along with the surgeon), but the concept of autointoxication has been revived, and the bowel is now recognized as a leading source of morbidity and mortality in critically ill patients.

This chapter describes abdominal infections that occur in the ICU, including infections of the biliary tree (acalculous cholecystitis), bowel (*Clostridium diffcile* enterocolitis), and peritoneal cavity (postoperative infections) (2,3).

ACALCULOUS CHOLECYSTITIS

Acalculous cholecystitis accounts for only 5–15% of cases of acute cholecystitis (4), but it is more common in critically ill patients, and has a mortality rate (about 45%) that rivals that of septic shock (4,5).

Pathogenesis

Common conditions associated with acalculous cholecystitis include the postoperative period (especially following cardiopulmonary bypass surgery), trauma, circulatory shock, and multiorgan failure (4,5). Prolonged

737

bowel rest (i.e., during total parenteral nutrition) predisposes to acalculous cholecystitis by promoting cholestasis, but as much as 4 weeks of bowel rest may be required before acalculous cholecystitis is a risk (6), which is longer than the ICU stay of most patients.

Possible underlying mechanisms for acalculous cholecystitis include hypoperfusion, gallbladder distension from diminished contractions, and a change in the composition of bile. The latter mechanism may have an important role, because biliary "sludge" (i.e., echogenic matter in the gallbladder associated with acalculous cholecystitis) contains small crystals called "microliths" that can produce cholecystitis (5).

Clinical Features

Most cases of acalculous cholecystitis are not discovered until complications arise (e.g., gangrenous cholecystitis or gallbladder perforation), so the clinical manifestations reported for acalculous cholecystitis are often those of advanced, complicated cholecystitis. The diagnosis of acalculous cholecystitis is often delayed because *pain and tenderness in the right upper quadrant can be absent in one-third of patients with acalculous cholecystitis* (2). Fever (100%), elevated bilirubin (90%), hypotension (90%), and multiorgan failure (65–80%) are common but nonspecific findings (4,5). Blood cultures are positive in 90% of cases (2) and Gram-negative aerobic bacilli are isolated in almost all cases.

Diagnosis

Ultrasound is the favored diagnostic test for acalculous cholecystitis because it can be performed at the bedside. Gallbladder distension and sludge are suggestive findings, but are nonspecific. The ultrasound image in Figure 40.1 shows more specific findings; i.e., marked thickness of the gallbladder wall and sloughed mucosa in the lumen of the gallbladder. The diagnostic yield from ultrasound varies widely in different reports (4,8), and may be operator-specific. If ultrasound is not helpful, the next step is a hepatobiliary scan, which is the "gold standard" method for the diagnosis of acute cholecystitis (but requires a functional liver to move the tracer into the bile ducts).

Management

Prompt intervention is mandatory. Cholecystectomy is the procedure of choice, but for patients who are too unstable for surgery, percutaneous drainage of the gallbladder is a suitable alternative. Empiric antibiotic therapy should be started as soon as the diagnosis is confirmed. The recommended antibiotics are piperacillin-tazobactam, or a carbapenem (imipenem or meropenem) (2).

COLONIZATION OF THE GI TRACT

The microbial landscape in the GI tract is altered in critically ill patients,

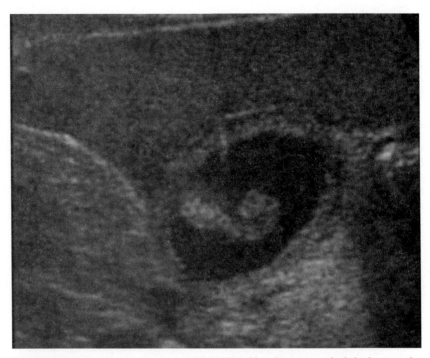

FIGURE 40.1 Transverse sonogram of the gallbladder showing marked thickening of the gallbladder wall and an echogenic mass projecting into the lumen of the gallbladder. This mass represents sloughed mucosa, and is characteristic of gangrenous cholecystitis.

and the infections that can appear as a result of this change are described in this section.

Gastric Colonization

Because bacteria do not thrive in an acid environment (see Figure 5.3 on page 81), gastric acidity maintains a sterile environment in the stomach. Loss of gastric acidity (from acid-suppressing drugs used to prevent stress ulcer bleeding) promotes colonization of the stomach, and the following observations indicate that gastric colonization increases the risk of nosocomial infections.

1. The use of acid-suppressing drugs for stress ulcer prophylaxis is associated with an increased incidence of nosocomial pneumonia (9).

2. Translocation of organisms has been documented in 15% of cases of gastric colonization, and about half of the cases of translocation resulted in a nosocomial infection (10).

3. The organisms isolated most often from the stomach are the same as the organisms isolated most often in nosocomial infections (11). This is shown in Figure 40.2.

Corrective Measures

There are two measures that could reduce colonization of the stomach: (a) avoiding the use of gastric acid-suppressing drugs for prophylaxis of stress ulcer bleeding, and (b) selective digestive decontamination with nonabsorbable antibiotics. Both of these measures are presented in Chapter 5.

Clostridium difficile

Clostridium difficile is a spore-forming, Gram-positive anaerobic bacillus that does not inhabit the bowel in healthy subjects, but is able to colonize and proliferate in the bowel when the normal microflora has been altered by antibiotic therapy (12). The typical host for *C. difficile* colonization is an elderly or debilitated patient or nursing home resident who has received antibiotics at some time in the last 2 weeks. Colonization is uncommon in healthy subjects who live in the community (although this may change).

Pathogenesis

C. difficile is transmitted from patient to patient via the fecal-oral route. There is a dormant (spore) form that can survive on environmental

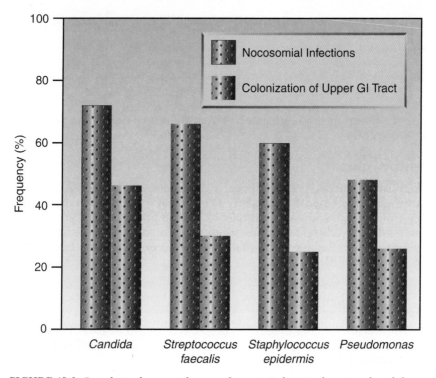

FIGURE 40.2 Correlation between the most frequent isolates in the stomach and the most frequent isolates in nosocomial infections in critically ill patients. Data from Reference 4.

surfaces for months, but patient-to-patient transmission usually occurs via the hands of hospital personnel (13). As a result, strict adherence to the use of disposable gloves can significantly reduce transmission (14).

C. difficile is not an invasive organism, but releases cytotoxins that damage the bowel mucosa. This leads to inflammatory infiltration of the bowel wall and symptomatic disease. Severe inflammation is accompanied by raised, plaque-like lesions on the mucosal surface known as "pseudomembranes." The presence of these lesions (pseudomembranous colitis) is evidence of severe disease.

GASTRIC ACID SUPPRESSION: There are several reports showing that use of acid-suppressing drugs, particularly proton pump inhibitors, is associated with an increased risk of *C. difficile* infection (15–17). The risk of other enteric infections (e.g., salmonellosis) is also increased by loss of gastric acidity (18), and this effect is further evidence of the role of gastric acid as an antimicrobial defense mechanism.

The protective effect of gastric acid on *C. difficile* infections has important implications because of the escalating and excessive use of gastric acid-suppressing drugs, particularly proton pump inhibitors, in hospitalized patients. In fact, there has been a marked increase in the frequency and severity of *C. difficile* infections in recent years (19), and this coincides with the marked increase in the use of proton pump inhibitors for prophylaxis of stress ulcer bleeding. Therefore, *it is possible that the recent surge in C. difficile infections is a reflection of the escalating (and unnecessary) use of proton pump inhibitors* in hospitalized patients (20).

Clinical Features

The principal manifestation of *Clostridium difficile* infection (CDI) is a watery diarrhea, which can occur alone (in mild cases) or in combination with fever and leukocytosis (in more severe cases), and can progress to circulatory shock and multiorgan failure. The feared (but uncommon) complication of CDI is toxic megacolon, which presents with abdominal distension, circulatory shock, and an x-ray that looks like Figure 40.3.

Diagnostic Evaluation

The diagnosis of CDI requires evidence of *C. difficile* cytotoxins in stool. Stool cultures for *C. difficile* are unreliable because they do not distinguish toxigenic from nontoxigenic strains of the organism. Most laboratories use an ELISA (Enzyme-Linked Immunosorbent Assay) method to detect cytotoxins. The sensitivity of this test is about 85% for one stool specimen and up to 95% for 2 stool specimens (12,21,22). Therefore, *the cytotoxin assay will miss 15% of diagnoses if one stool specimen is tested, and only misses 5% of diagnoses if two stool specimens are tested.* The specificity of this test is up to 98% (21), so false-positive results are uncommon.

COLONOSCOPY: Direct visualization of the bowel mucosa is reserved for the occasional case where there is a high clinical suspicion of *C. difficile* infection that is not confirmed by cytotoxin assays. The presence of pseudomembranes confirms the diagnosis of *C. difficile* infection. Colonoscopy is preferred to proctosigmoidoscopy for optimal results.

Antibiotic Treatment

The first step in treating CDI is to discontinue any predisposing drugs (antibiotics and proton pump inhibitors), if possible. Antiperistaltic agents should also be discontinued because *reduced peristalsis can prolong the exposure to C. difficile cytotoxins* (12). The recommended antibiotic regimens for CDI are shown in Table 40.1. Treatment is organized by the clinical condition (mild, severe, or relapsed CDI), and by the ability to give PO (or nasogastric) medications.

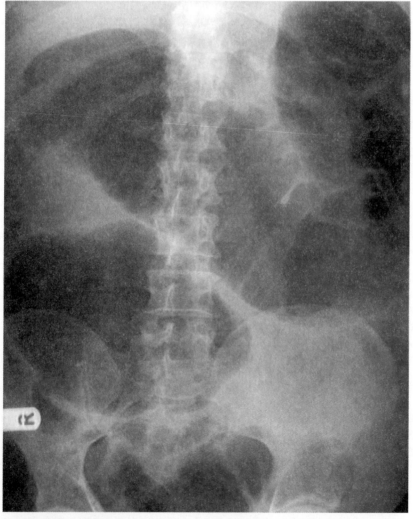

FIGURE 40.3 Radiographic appearance of toxic megacolon in a patient with *C. difficile* enterocolitis.

Table 40.1	Antibiotic Therapy for *Clostridium difficile* Infections (CDI)	
Condition	**Category**	**Drug Regimen†**
Mild CDI • Temp ≤101°F • WBC ≤15,000	Preferred	Metronidazole: 500 mg PO every 8 hrs
	Alternate (PO)	Vancomycin: 125 mg PO every 6 hrs or Fidaxomicin: 200 mg PO every 12 hrs
	Alternate (IV)	Metronidazole: 500 mg IV every 8 hrs
Severe CDI	Preferred	Vancomycin: 125 mg PO every 6 hrs
	Alternate (IV)	Metronidazole: 500 mg IV every 8 hrs
Life-Threatening CDI	Preferred	Vancomycin: 500 mg every 6 hrs via NG tube or by enema, plus Metronidazole: 500 mg IV every 8 hrs
Relapsed CDI	Preferred	Same regimens as in first episode
	Alternate (PO)	Fidaxomicin: 200 mg PO every 12 hrs

†Duration of therapy is 10–14 days.
From References 19, 23–25.

MILD CDI: Mild CDI is defined as cytotoxin-positive diarrhea with a body temperature no higher than 101°F and a blood leukocyte count no higher than 15,000/mm³ (19,23,24). *The preferred treatment is oral metronidazole* (500 mg every 8 hrs) for 10–14 days (23,24). Oral vancomycin (125 mg every 6 hrs) is equally effective, but is used as a second-line agent to limit proliferation of vancomycin-resistant enterococci. Fidaxomicin is a recently-introduced antibiotic that is equivalent to vancomycin for treating an acute episode of CDI, and has 50% fewer relapses (25).

SEVERE CDI: Severe CDI is defined as cytotoxin-positive diarrhea with any of the following: (a) a body temperature above 101°F and a blood leukocyte count above 15,000/mm³, (b) the presence of pseudomembranes, or (c) a complication of CDI (e.g., toxic megacolon, renal failure, septic shock). *The treatment of choice for severe CDI is oral vancomycin* (125 mg every 6 hrs), which is more effective than oral metronidazole (24). For patients who are critically ill from CDI, the recommended treatment is vancomycin in a dose 500 mg (via NG tube or enema) plus IV metronidazole (500 mg every 8 hrs) (23).

RESPONSE: In most cases, the fever resolves in 24–48 hrs, and the diarrhea resolves in 4–5 days (12). Treatment is continued for 10–14 days. Persistence of symptomatic disease occurs with complications like toxic megacolon, peritonitis, or progressive sepsis and multiorgan failure, which often require surgical intervention (26). The procedure of choice is subtotal colectomy.

RELAPSES: Relapses (usually within 3 weeks) are reported in 25% of cases treated with metronidazole or vancomycin (12,24), and 13% of cases treated with fidaxomicin (24). Repeat therapy using the same antibiotic is successful in about 75% of relapses, and another relapse is expected in about 25% of cases (27). Fewer relapses are reported with fidaxomicin (25), which may become the preferred treatment for recurrent CDI. About 5% of patients experience more than 6 relapses (12).

Microbial Therapy

Microbial therapy is used for recurrent CDI, and is an attempt to restore the normal microflora of the bowel to antagonize or prevent colonization with *C. difficile.*

PROBIOTICS: Probiotics are non-pathogenic organisms (*Saccharomyces boulardii* or *Lactobacillus* species) that bind to epithelial cells and prevent the attachment of *C. difficile.* Probiotic therapy with *S. boulardii* (1 g/day, started with antimicrobial therapy and continued for 4 weeks), but not *Lactobacillus*, can reduce the incidence of recurrent CDI (23). Therefore, probiotic therapy with *S. boulardii* can be used as adjunctive therapy for CDI to prevent recurrences (23).

FECAL TRANSPLANTATION: Instillation of liquid preparations of stool from healthy donors (via nasogastric tube or enemas) has proven successful in treating recurrent CDI in 70–100% of cases (23,28). (For a description of the fecal transplantation process, including donor screening, see Reference 28.)

POSTOPERATIVE INFECTIONS

Postoperative abdominal infections are located in the peritoneal cavity, and are the result of peritoneal seeding during the procedure, or leakage of bowel contents from an anastomotic site or undetected injury to the bowel wall. These infections can present as diffuse peritonitis or an abdominal abscess.

Peritonitis

Generalized peritonitis is not a common presentation for postoperative infection, and is usually the result of an undetected tear in the bowel wall during the procedure.

Clinical Features

Small tears often present with non-specific abdominal pain initially, and the first sign of a tear may be the presence of air under the diaphragm, as shown in Figure 40.4. As little as 1 mL of gas can be detected under the right hemidiaphragm in the upright position (29). The presence of air under the diaphragm may not, however, be a useful finding soon after a laparoscopic procedure, because the instillation of CO_2 during laparoscopy can result in residual air under the diaphragm for days.

A persistent leak through a tear in the bowel wall will eventually produce signs of peritoneal irritation (i.e., involuntary guarding and rebound tenderness) and a systemic inflammatory response (fever, leukocytosis, etc.). Progression to circulatory shock (e.g., hypotension, change in mental status) can be rapid.

Management

Signs of diffuse peritonitis merit immediate surgical exploration. The initial management should include the following measures.

FLUIDS: Peritonitis is often accompanied by considerable fluid loss into the peritoneal cavity, so signs of circulatory compromise (i.e., a decrease in urine output or blood pressure) should prompt aggressive volume resuscitation. Avoiding vasopressor therapy is advised, whenever possible, because vasopressors promote splanchnic vasoconstriction and can aggravate an underlying ischemic condition in the bowel.

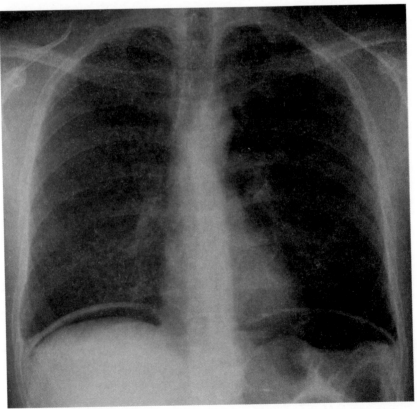

FIGURE 40.4 Abdominal x-ray in the upright position showing free air under both hemidiaphragms. In the absence of a recent laparoscopy, this finding is evidence of a perforated hollow viscus.

ANTIBIOTICS: Antibiotic therapy should be started as soon as possible using antibiotics that are active against the frequent isolates as presented in Table 40.2. Single-agent antibiotic coverage using piperacillin-tazobactam, or a carbapenem (imipenem-cilastatin, meropenem, or doripenem) is recommended (2). In patients who may be colonized by *Candida* species (e.g., patients who have received antibiotics recently), additional empiric coverage with an antifungal agent (e.g., fluconazole) seems wise.

Table 40.2	Organisms Isolated in 1,237 Patients With Complicated Abdominal Infections	
Organism		**Patients (%)**
Gram-negative aerobic bacilli		
Escherichia coli		71
Klebsiella spp		14
Pseudomonas aeruginosa		14
Proteus mirabilis		5
Enterobacter spp		5
Anaerobic organisms		
Bacteroides fragilis		35
Other *Bacteroides spp*		71
Clostridium spp		29
Other anaerobes		55
Gram-positive aerobic cocci		
Streptococcus spp		38
Enterococcus spp		23
Staphylococcus aureus		4

From Reference 2.

Abdominal Abscess

Abdominal abscesses typically serve as an occult source of sepsis, and are difficult to detect with routine clinical evaluations.

Clinical Features

Fever is almost always present (30), but localized abdominal tenderness can be absent in 60% of cases, and a palpable abdominal mass is evident in less than 10% of cases (30,31). Abdominal x-rays can show extraluminal air, but this occurs in less than 15% of cases (31).

Computed Tomography

Computed tomography (CT) of the abdomen is the most reliable diagnostic method of detection for abdominal abscesses, with a sensitivity

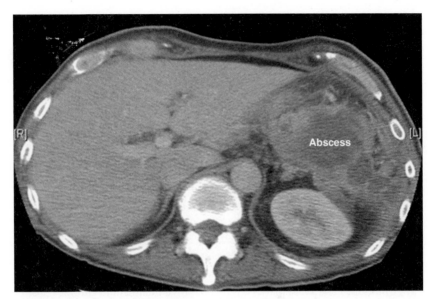

FIGURE 40.5 Abdominal CT scan showing a multiloculated abscess in the left upper quadrant in a post-splenectomy patient.

and specificity of 90% or higher (31). However, CT imaging in the early postoperative period can be misleading because collections of blood or irrigant solutions in the peritoneal cavity can be misread as an abscess. CT scans are most reliable when performed after the first postoperative week (when peritoneal fluid collections have resorbed) (31). The CT appearance of an abdominal abscess is shown in Figure 40.5.

Management

Immediate drainage is advised for postoperative abdominal abscesses. Precise localization with CT imaging allows many abscesses to be drained percutaneously with CT-guided drainage catheters (30). Empiric antibiotic therapy should be started while awaiting the results of abscess fluid cultures. The empiric antibiotic regimen is the same as described for peritonitis.

A FINAL WORD

Spotlight on Gastric Acid

As mentioned often in this book, the role of gastric acid as an antimicrobial defense mechanism has not received the attention it deserves. This is particularly true regarding the observation that suppression of gastric acidity with proton pump inhibitors promotes the transmission of *Clostridium difficile* infections. In fact, the recent surge in the incidence and severity of *C. difficile* infections may be a reflection of the escalating (and unnecessary) use of proton pump inhibitors for prophylaxis of stress ulcer bleeding (20).

The following observation should help you to avoid proton pump inhibitors for stress ulcer prophylaxis.

1. Proton pump inhibitors are not more effective than H_2 blockers (e.g., ranitidine) for preventing stress ulcer bleeding (33).

And the following observation should help you to avoid any type of gastric acid-suppressing drug for stress ulcer prophylaxis.

2. When patients are receiving enteral tube feedings for full nutritional support, there is no added benefit from gastric acid-suppressing drugs for the prevention of stress ulcer bleeding (34).

REFERENCES

Introduction

1. Arbuthnot-Lane W. Remarks on the operative treatment of chronic constipation. Reprinted in Dis Colon & Rectum 1985; 28:750–757.

Reviews

2. Solomkin JS, Mazuski JE, Bradley JS, et al. Diagnosis and management of complicated intra-abdominal infection in adults and children: guidelines by the Surgical Infection Society and the Infectious Disease Society of America. Clin Infect Dis 2010; 50:133–164.

3. Sarteli M, Viale P, Catena F, et al. 2013 WSES guidelines for the management of intra-abdominal infections. World J Emerg Surg 2013; 8:3.

Acalculous Cholecystitis

4. McChesney JA, Northrup PG, Bickston SJ. Acute acalculous cholecystitis associated with systemic sepsis and visceral arterial hypoperfusion. A case series and review of pathophysiology. Dig Dis Sci 2003; 48:1960–1967.

5. Laurila J, Syrjälä H, Laurila PA, et al. Acute acalculous cholecystitis in critically ill patients. Acta Anesthesiol Scand 2004; 48:986–991.

6. Messing B, Bories C, Kuntslinger C. Does parenteral nutrition induce gallbladder sludge formation and lithiasis? Gastroenterology 2983; 84:1012–1019.

7. Jüngst C, Killack-Ublick GA, Jüngst D. Gallstone disease: microlithiasis and sludge. Best Prect Res Clin Gastroenterol 2006; 20:1053–1062.

8. Puc MM, Tran HS, Wry PW, Ross SE. Ultrasound is not a useful screening tool for acalculous cholecystitis in critically ill trauma patients. Am Surg 2002; 68:65–69.

Gastric Colonization

9. Huang J, Cao Y, Liao C, et al. Effect of histamine-2-receptor antagonists versus sucralfate on stress ulcer prophylaxis in mechanically ventilated patients: A meta-analysis of 10 randomized controlled trials. Crit Care 2010; 14:R194–R204.

10. MacFie J, Reddy BS, Gatt M, et al. Bacterial translocation studied in 927 patients over 13 years. Br J Surg 2006; 93:87–93.

11. Marshall JC, Christou NV, Meakins JL. The gastrointestinal tract: the "undrained abscess" of multiple organ failure. Ann Surg 1993; 218:111–119.

Clostridium difficile Infections

12. Bartlett JG. Antibiotic-associated diarrhea. N Engl J Med 2002; 346:334–339.

13. Samore MH, Venkataraman L, DeGirolami, et al. Clinical and molecular epidemiology of sporadic and clustered cases of nosocomial *Clostridium difficile* diarrhea. Am J Med 1996; 100:32–40.

14. Johnson S, Gerding DN, Olson MM, et al. Prospective, controlled study of vinyl glove use to interrupt *Clostridium difficile* nosocomial transmission. Am J Med 1990; 88:137–140.

15. Dial S, Alrasadi K, Manoukian C, et al. Risk of *Clostridium-difficile* diarrhea among hospitalized patients prescribed proton pump inhibitors: cohort and case-control studies. Canad Med Assoc J 2004; 171:33–38.

16. Dial S, Delaney JA, Barkun AN, Suissa S. Use of gastric acid-suppressing agents and the risk of community-acquired *Clostridium difficile*-associated disease. JAMA 2005; 294:2989–2995.

17. Aseri M, Schroeder T, Kramer J, Kackula R. Gastric acid suppression by proton pump inhibitors as a risk factor for *Clostridium difficile*-associated diarrhea in hospitalized patients. Am J Gastroenterol 2008; 103:2308–2313.

18. Cook GC. Infective gastroenteritis and its relationship to reduced gastric acidity. Scand J Gastroenterol 1985; 20(Suppl 111):17–21.

19. Kelly CP, LaMont JT. *Clostridium difficile* – more difficult than ever. N Engl J Med 2008; 359:1932–1940.

20. Cunningham R, Dial S. Is over-use of proton pump inhibitors fuelling the current epidemic of *Clostridium-difficile*-associated diarrhea? J Hosp Infect 2008; 70:1–6.

21. Mylonakis E, Ryan ET, Calderwood SB. *Clostridium difficile*-associated diarrhea. Arch Intern Med 2001; 161:525–533.

22. Yassin SF, Young-Fadok TM, Zein NN, Pardi DS. *Clostridium difficile*- associated diarrhea and colitis. Mayo Clin Proc 2001; 76:725–730.

23. van Nispen tot Pannerden CMF, Verbon A, Kuipers E. Recurrent *Clostridium difficile* infection. What are the treatment options. Drugs 2011; 71:853–868.

24. Zar FA, Bakkanagari SR, Moorthi KM, Davis MB. A comparison of vancomycin and metronidazole for the treatment of *Clostridium difficile*-associated diarrhea, stratified by disease severity. Clin Infect Dis 2007; 45:302–307.

25. Louie TJ, Miller MA, Mullane KM, et al. Fidaxomicin versus vancomycin for *Clostridium difficile* infection. N Engl J Med 2011; 364:422–431.

26. Lipsett PA, Samantaray DK, Tam ML, et al. Pseudomembranous colitis: a surgical disease? Surgery 1994; 116:491–496.

27. Aslam S, Hamill RJ, Musher DM. Treatment of *Clostridium difficile*-associated disease: old therapies and new strategies. Lancet Infect Dis 2005; 5:549–557.

28. Aas J, Gessert CE, Bakken JS. Recurrent *Clostridium difficile* colitis: case series involving 18 patients treated with donor stool administered via nasogastric tube. Clin Infect Dis 2003; 36:580–585.

Complicated Abdominal Infections

29. Miller RE, Nelson SW. The roentgenologic demonstration of tiny amounts of free intraperitoneal gas: experimental and clinical studies. AJR Am J Roentgenol 1971; 112:574–585.

30. Khurrum Baig M, Hua Zao R, Batista O, et al. Percutaneous postoperative intra-abdominal abscess drainage after elective colorectal surgery. Tech Coloproctol 2002; 6:159–164.

31. Fry DE. Noninvasive imaging tests in the diagnosis and treatment of intra-abdominal abscesses in the postoperative patient. Surg Clin North Am 1994; 74:693–709.

A Final Word

32. Lin P-C, Chang C-H, Hsu P-I, et al. The efficacy and safety of proton pump inhibitors vs. histamine-2 receptor antagonists for stress ulcer bleeding prophylaxis among critical care patients: A meta-analysis. Crit Care Med 2010; 38:1197–1205.

33. Marik PE, Vasu T, Hirani A, Pachinburavan M. Stress ulcer prophylaxis in the new millennium: a systematic review and meta-analysis. Crit Care Med 2010; 38:2222–2228.

Chapter 41

URINARY TRACT INFECTIONS IN THE ICU

Throughout nature, infection without disease
is the rule rather than the exception.

René Dubois
Man Adapting
1966

Urethral catheters are commonplace in critically ill patients, and surveys indicate that catheter-associated urinary tract infections account for 40% of all hospital-acquired infections in the United States (1). However, these surveys are misleading, because a majority of the catheter-associated infections represent asymptomatic bacteriuria (*infection without disease,* according to Dubois), and do not require antimicrobial therapy. This chapter describes the current recommendations for the diagnosis and treatment of catheter-associated *symptomatic* urinary tract infection.

PATHOGENESIS

The presence of a urethral catheter is associated with a 3–8% incidence of bacteriuria ($\geq 10^5$ colony forming units/mL) *per day* (1). This is assumed to be the result of bacterial migration along the outer surface of the catheter and into the bladder. Bacteria also form biofilms on the inner and outer surface of urethral catheters (2), and these biofilms can serve as a source of continued microbial colonization in the bladder. However, this is not the full story, because *direct injection of pathogens into the bladder of healthy subjects does not result in a urinary tract infection* (3). Furthermore, the continuous flow of urine that is allowed by bladder drainage catheters should wash away microbes that migrate up the urethra.

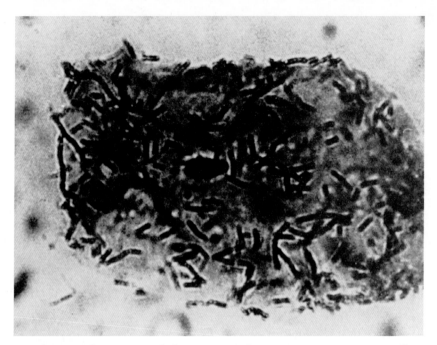

FIGURE 41.1 Photomicrograph showing non-pathogenic *Lactobacillus* organisms adhering to a bladder epithelial cell. From Reference 3. Image has been digitally enhanced.

Bacterial Adherence

The missing piece of the puzzle is the ability of pathogenic organisms to adhere to the bladder epithelium. The epithelial cells of the bladder are normally coated with non-pathogenic organisms, as shown in Figure 41.1 (4); this prevents the attachment of pathogenic organisms, which is the precipitating event that leads to infections of the lower urinary tract (5). This is the same phenomenon that occurs in colonization of the oral mucosa with pathogenic Gram-negative aerobic bacilli (see Figure 5.5), which serves as a prelude to nosocomial pneumonia. The link between bladder catheters and the change in bacterial adherence is unclear. However, it is possible that an increase in severity of illness is responsible for both the change in bacterial adherence and the need for a bladder catheter. (For more on the role of bacterial adherence in nosocomial infections, see "A Final Word" at the end of the chapter.)

Microbiology

The pathogens isolated in catheter-associated bacteriuria are shown in Table 41.1 (6). The predominant organisms are Gram-negative aerobic bacilli (especially *Escherichia coli*), enterococci, and *Candida* species, while staphylococci are infrequent isolates. A single organism predominates in bacteriuria associated with short-term catheterization (< 30 days), whereas bacteriuria is often polymicrobial in long-term catheterization (≥ 30 days).

Table 41.1	Pathogens Isolated in Catheter-Associated Bacteriuria	
Pathogen	**% of Infections**	
	Hospital	**ICU**
Escherichia coli	21.4	22.3
Enterococci	15.5	15.8
Candida albicans	14.5	15.3
Other *Candida* species	6.5	9.5
Pseudomonas aeruginosa	10.0	13.3
Klebsiella pneumoniae	7.7	7.5
Enterobacter species	4.1	5.5
Coag-neg. staphylococci	2.5	4.6
Staphylococcus aureus	2.2	2.5
Acinetobacter baumannii	1.2	1.5

Adapted from Reference 6. Some of the percentages represent median values.

Prevention

The risk of catheter-associated infection is determined primarily by the duration of catheterization (1), so *removing catheters when they are no longer necessary is the single most effective prophylactic measure* for catheter-associated infections. Other observations about prevention are summarized below.

1. Cleansing of catheter insertion sites (with antiseptic solutions, antibiotic creams, or soap and water) is NOT recommended because this practice can increase the risk of bacteriuria (1).

2. Prophylaxis with systemic antibiotics is not recommended for preventing infections of the urinary tract (1).

3. Antimicrobial-impregnated urinary catheters (i.e., with silver alloy or nitrofurazone) can reduce the incidence of asymptomatic bacteriuria in short-term catheterization (< 1 week) (7), but the benefit in preventing symptomatic urinary tract infections is not clear (1).

DIAGNOSIS AND TREATMENT

The recommendations in this section are taken from the most recent guidelines developed by the Infectious Disease Society of America (1).

Diagnosis

1. In patients with short-term catheters (< 30 days), urine specimens for culture can be obtained by sampling through the catheter port or catheter tubing. For patients with long-term catheters (≥ 30 days), the catheter should be replaced before collecting the urine specimen.

2. Significant bacteriuria in catheterized patients is defined as a urine culture that grows ≥ 10^5 colony forming units (cfu) per mL. However, over 90% of patients with significant bacteriuria have no other evidence of infection (*asymptomatic bacteriuria*) (8).

3. Catheter-associated urinary tract infection (CA-UTI) is defined as a urine culture that grows > 10^3 cfu/mL in a patient with clinical signs of a symptomatic UTI. These can include:

   a. Bacteremia with the same organism isolated in blood and urine.

   b. New costovertebral tenderness.

   c. Rigors.

   d. New onset of delirium or depressed consciousness.

   e. Increased spasticity in patients with spinal cord injuries.

   Common symptoms of UTI such as dysuria and frequency are not relevant in catheterized patients, and the usual signs of infection (fever, leukocytosis) can lack specificity in catheterized patients (see next).

4. The following findings are NOT reliable for the diagnosis of CA-UTI:

   a. The presence of fever or leukocytosis.

   b. Cloudy urine.

   c. The presence of white blood cells in urine (pyuria).

   The problem with fever and leukocytosis is that catheterized patients often have another infection that could explain these findings. Furthermore, in one study comparing patients with suspected CA-UTI to patients without CA-UTI where there was no other apparent infection, the incidence of fever and leukocytosis was the same in the two groups of patients (8). The presence of white blood cells in urine (pyuria) does not differentiate between asymptomatic bacteriuria and CA-UTI, but *the absence of pyuria can be used as evidence against the diagnosis of CA-UTI* (1).

Treatment

1. Screening for, or antibiotic treatment of, asymptomatic bacteriuria is NOT advised unless the patient is scheduled for a urologic procedure that is associated with mucosal bleeding (e.g., transurethral resection of the prostate) (9). These recommendations are based on the following observations: (a) few cases of asymptomatic bacteriuria progress to CA-UTI, (b) antibiotic therapy does not reduce the incidence of CA-UTI, and (3) antibiotic therapy promotes the emergence of resistant organisms.

2. Empiric antibiotics are recommended for patients with suspected CA-UTI. Single agent therapy with *piperacillin-tazobactam or a carbapenem* (imipenem or meropenem) is recommended, while levofloxacin (750 mg IV once daily) is a second-line agent (10).

3. If the diagnosis of CA-UTI is confirmed by urine culture, antibiotic therapy should be adjusted according to the organism isolated and the reported sensitivities. Catheters that have been in place for > 2 weeks should be replaced.

4. The duration of antibiotic therapy for CA-UTI should be 7 days for patients who respond promptly, and 10–14 days for patients with a delayed response.

CANDIDURIA

The presence of *Candida* species in urine usually represents colonization in patients with indwelling urethral catheters, but candiduria can also be a sign of disseminated candidiasis (i.e., the candiduria being the result, not the cause, of the disseminated candidiasis). Disseminated candidiasis can be an elusive diagnosis because blood cultures are unrevealing in more than 50% of cases (11), and *candiduria may be the only evidence of disseminated disease*. The clinical condition of the patient becomes an important factor in the approach to candiduria in the ICU.

Microbiology

In cases of candiduria, the colony count has no predictive value for identifying renal or disseminated candidiasis (11). The most frequent isolate is *Candida albicans* (about 50% of cases), followed by *Candida glabrata* (about 15% of cases) (11). The latter organism is notable for resistance to the antifungal agent fluconazole.

Asymptomatic Candiduria

Asymptomatic candiduria does not require treatment unless the patient is neutropenic (12,13). Removal of the catheter is always advised, when possible, because this can eradicate candiduria in 40% of cases (13). Repeat urine cultures are recommended, and persistent candiduria in high-risk (immunosuppressed) patients should be investigated with blood cultures and imaging studies of the kidneys.

In neutropenic patients with asymptomatic candiduria, the recommended prophylaxis includes *caspofungin*: 70 mg IV as a loading dose, followed by 50 mg IV daily (12).

Symptomatic Candiduria

Candiduria that is associated with fever, suprapubic tenderness, or costovertebral tenderness requires antifungal therapy as well as blood cultures and imaging studies of the kidneys (with ultrasound or computed tomography) to search for renal abscesses or evidence of urinary tract obstruction. Renal candidiasis is usually a consequence of disseminated candidiasis (11).

The treatment for symptomatic candiduria is summarized below.

1. The recommended treatment for *Candida* cystitis and pyelonephritis is *fluconazole* (PO or IV): 400 mg daily for 2 weeks (14). This regimen can eradicate infections caused by organisms that are resistant to fluconazole (i.e., *C. glabrata* and *C. krusei*) because fluconazole is concentrated in the urine. Decreasing the dose of fluconazole in renal insufficiency (which is normally recommended) is not advised for *Candida* UTIs because this would decrease urinary concentrations of fluconazole to subtherapeutic levels (14).

2. *Candida* UTIs that do not respond to fluconazole can be treated with oral *flucytosine:* 25 mg/kg every 6 hours (with adjustments for renal insufficiency) for 7–10 days (14). The duration of treatment is limited with this drug because it causes bone marrow suppression and mucosal injury in the GI tract.

3. For candiduria that is associated with hemodynamic instability or progressive multiorgan dysfunction (i.e., when disseminated candidiasis is suspected) the recommended treatment is IV fluconazole in a loading dose of 800 mg followed by 400 mg daily (14).

A FINAL WORD

Bacterial Adherence

The unifying feature in nosocomial infections that involve the gastrointestinal, respiratory, and urinary tracts is a change in the character of microbes that adhere to epithelial surfaces. In healthy subjects, the epithelial surfaces in the mouth, GI tract, and urinary tract are covered by harmless, commensal organisms, but in patients who develop severe or chronic illness, these surfaces are covered with pathogenic organisms, and this serves as a prelude to nosocomial infections. Of interest in this regard is a study conducted in patients with spinal cord injuries and long-term urinary catheters, where *injection of non-pathogenic E. coli into the bladder was associated with 50% fewer urinary tract infections* (15).

However, the population of epithelial surfaces is not just a matter of "territorial imperative" (where one population takes over, or defends, a territory) but is the result of receptors on epithelial cells that bind to specific groups of microorganisms. A change in the configuration of these receptors allows pathogens to bind to epithelial surfaces, and this is the precipitating event that leads to nosocomial infections. As such, we need to study how microbes bind to epithelial surfaces if we want to eliminate the threat of nosocomial infections.

REFERENCES

1. Hooton TM, Bradley SF, Cardenas DD, et al. Diagnosis, prevention, and treatment of catheter-associated urinary tract infections in adults: 2009 international clinical practice guidelines from the Infectious Disease Society of America. Clin Infect Dis 2010; 50:625–663.

2. Ganderton L, Chawla J, Winters C, et al. Scanning electron microscopy of bacterial biofilms on indwelling bladder catheters. Eur J Clin Microbiol Infect Dis 1992; 11:789–796.

3. Howard RJ. Host defense against infection – Part 1. Curr Probl Surg 1980; 27:267–316.

4. Sobel JD. Pathogenesis of urinary tract infections: host defenses. Infect Dis Clin North Am 1987; 1:751–772.

5. Daifuku R, Stamm WE. Bacterial adherence to bladder uroepithelial cells in catheter-associated urinary tract infection. N Engl J Med 1986; 314:1208–1213.

6. Shuman EK, Chenoweth CE. Recognition and prevention of healthcare-associated urinary tract infections in the intensive care unit. Crit Care Med 2010; 38(Suppl):S373–S379.

7. Schumm K, Lam TB. Types of urethral catheters for management of short-term voiding problems in hospitalized adults. Cochrane Database Syst Rev 2008:CD004013.

8. Tambyah PA, Maki DG. Catheter-associated urinary tract infection is rarely symptomatic. Arch Intern Med 2000; 160:678–682.

9. Nicolle LE, Bradley S, Colgan R, et al. Infectious Disease Society of America guidelines for the diagnosis and treatment of asymptomatic bacteriuria in adults. Clin Infect Dis 2005; 40:643–654.

10. Gilbert DN, Moellering RC, Eliopoulis, et al, eds. The Sanford guide to antimicrobial therapy, 2009. 39th ed. Sperryville, VA: Antimicrobial Therapy, Inc, 2009:31.

11. Hollenbach E. To treat or not to treat – critically ill patients with candiduria. Mycoses 2008; 51(Suppl 2):12–24.

12. Pappas PG, Kauffman CA, Andes D, et al. Clinical practice guidelines for the management of candidiasis: 2009 update by the Infectious Disease Society of America. Clin Infect Dis 2009; 48:503–525.

13. Sobel JD, Kauffman CA, McKinsey D, et al. Candiduria: a randomized double-blind study of treatment with fluconazole or placebo. Clin Infect Dis 2000; 30:19–24.

14. Fisher JF, Sobel JD, Kauffman CA, Newman CA. Candida urinary tract infections – treatment. Clin Infect Dis 2011; 52(Suppl 6):S457–S466.

15. Darouiche RO, Thornby JI, Cerra-Stewart C, et al. Bacterial interference for prevention of urinary tract infection: a prospective, randomized, placebo-controlled, double-blind pilot trial. Clin Infect Dis 2005; 41:1531–1534.

DISORDERS OF BODY TEMPERATURE

*There is no possibility of escaping the entropic doom
imposed on all natural phenomena.*

Aharon Katchalsky
1965

Chapter 42

HYPERTHERMIA & HYPOTHERMIA

Heat not a furnace for your foe so hot that you singe yourself.

William Shakespeare

Henry VIII

The human body is a metabolic furnace that generates enough heat to raise the body temperature by 1°C every hour, even at rest (1). Fortunately, the external surface of the body acts like a radiator, and discharges excess heat into the surrounding environment. The behavior of this radiator is guided by a thermostat (the thermoregulatory system) that limits the daily variation in body temperature to ±0.6°C (2). This chapter describes what happens when this thermostat fails, and allows the body temperature to rise or fall to life-threatening levels.

HEAT-RELATED ILLNESS

Hyperthermia vs. Fever

The distinction between hyperthermia and fever deserves mention at the outset. Both conditions are characterized by an elevated body temperature, but hyperthermia is the result of a defect in temperature regulation, while fever is the result of a normal thermoregulatory system operating at a higher set point. The elevations in body temperature in this chapter represent hyperthermia, not fever. Because the underlying mechanisms involved in the production of hyperthermia and fever are different, *the antipyretic agents used to treat fever (e.g., acetaminophen) are ineffective in hyperthermia.*

Response to Thermal Stress

The maintenance of body temperature in conditions of thermal stress (e.g., hot weather, strenuous exercise) is primarily achieved by enhanced blood flow to the skin (convective heat loss) and the loss of sweat (evaporative heat loss).

Convective Heat Loss

When heat is lost from the skin, it warms the air just above the skin surface, and the increase in surface temperature limits the further loss of body heat by conduction. However, when an air current (e.g., from a fan or gust of wind) is passed across the skin, it displaces the warm layer of air above the skin and replaces it with cooler air, and this process facilitates the continued loss of body heat by conduction. The same effect is produced by increases in blood flow just underneath the skin. The action of currents (air and blood) that promotes heat loss is known as *convection*.

Evaporative Heat Loss

The transformation of water from a liquid to a gas requires heat (called the 'latent heat of vaporization'), and the heat required for the evaporation of sweat from the skin is provided by body heat. The evaporation of one liter of sweat from the skin is accompanied by the loss of 580 kilocalories (kcal) of heat from the body (3). This is about one-quarter of the daily heat production by an average-sized adult at rest. Thermal sweating (as opposed to "nervous sweating") can achieve rates of 1–2 liters per hour (3), which means that over 1,000 kcal of heat can be lost in one hour during profuse sweating. It is important to emphasize that *sweat must evaporate to ensure loss of body heat*. Wiping sweat off the skin will not result in heat loss, so this practice should be discouraged during strenuous exercise.

Syndromes

Heat-related illnesses are conditions where the thermoregulatory system is no longer able to maintain a constant body temperature in response to thermal stress. There are a number of minor heat-related illnesses, such as heat cramps and heat rash (prickly heat), but the following descriptions are limited to the major heat-related illnesses: *heat exhaustion* and *heat stroke*. The comparative features of these conditions are shown in Table 42.1

Table 42.1	Comparative Features of Heat Exhaustion and Heat Stroke	
Feature	**Heat Exhaustion**	**Heat Stroke**
Body Temperature	<39°C	≥41°C
CNS Dysfunction	Mild	Severe
Sweat Production	Yes	Minimal
Dehydration	Yes	Yes
Multiorgan Involvement	No	Yes

Heat Exhaustion

Heat exhaustion is the most common form of heat-related illness. Patients with heat exhaustion experience flu-like symptoms that include hyperthermia (usually < 39°C or 102°F), muscle cramps, nausea, and malaise. The hallmark of this condition is *volume depletion* without signs of hemodynamic compromise. The volume loss can be accompanied by hypernatremia (from sweat loss) or hyponatremia (when sweat loss is partly replaced with water intake). There is no evidence of significant neurologic impairment.

The management of heat exhaustion includes volume repletion and other general supportive measures. Cooling measures to reduce body temperature are not necessary.

Heat Stroke

Heat stroke is a life-threatening condition characterized by extreme elevations in body temperature (≥ 41°C or 106°F), severe neurologic dysfunction (e.g., delirium, coma, and seizures), severe volume depletion with hypotension, and multiorgan involvement that includes rhabdomyolysis, acute kidney injury, disseminated intravascular coagulopathy (DIC), and marked elevation in serum transaminases, presumably from liver. The inability to produce sweat (anhidrosis) is a typical, but not universal, feature of heat stroke (4).

There are two types of heat stroke: (a) *classic heat stroke*, which is related to environmental temperatures, and (b) *exertional heat stroke*, which is related to strenuous exercise. Exertional heat stroke tends to be more severe, with a higher incidence of multiorgan dysfunction.

Management

The management of heat stroke includes volume resuscitation and body cooling to reduce the body temperature to 38°C (100.4°F).

EXTERNAL COOLING: External cooling is the easiest and quickest way to reduce the body temperature. This is accomplished by placing ice packs in the groin and axilla, and covering the upper thorax and neck with ice. Cooling blankets are then placed over the entire length of the body. The major drawback of external cooling is the risk of shivering, which is counterproductive because it raises the body temperature. Shivering occurs when the skin temperature falls below 30°C (86°F) (5).

The most effective external cooling method is *evaporative cooling*, which involves spraying the skin with cool water (at 15°C or 59°F) and then fanning the skin to promote evaporation of the water. This method can reduce the body temperature at a rate of 0.3°C (0.6°F) per minute (6). Evaporative cooling is used mostly in the field, and is particularly effective when the weather is hot and dry (which enhances evaporation from the skin).

INTERNAL COOLING: Internal cooling can be achieved with cold water lavage of the stomach, bladder, or rectum. These methods produce a more rapid reduction in body temperature than external cooling, but they are more labor-intensive. Internal cooling is usually reserved for cases where external cooling is ineffective or produces unwanted shivering.

Rhabdomyolysis

Skeletal muscle injury (rhabdomyolysis) is a common complication of hyperthermia syndromes, including heat stroke (particularly the exertional type) and drug-induced hyperthermia (described later in the chapter). Disruption of myocytes in skeletal muscle leads to the release of creatine kinase (CK) into the bloodstream, and the measurement of CK levels in plasma is used to determine the presence and severity of rhabdomyolysis. There is no standard CK level for the diagnosis of rhabdomyolysis, but CK levels that are five times higher than normal (or about 1,000 Units/liter) have been used to identify rhabdomyolysis in clinical studies (7). Plasma CK levels above 15,000 Units/L indicate severe rhabdomyolysis and an increased risk of acute renal failure from myoglobin released by disrupted myocytes (7).

Myoglobinuric Renal Failure

Renal tubular injury from myoglobin results in acute renal failure in about one-third of patients with rhabdomyolysis (8). This condition is described in Chapter 34.

DRUG-INDUCED HYPERTHERMIA

The heat-related illnesses just described are triggered by thermal stress in the environment. The source of the thermal stress in the following conditions is drug-induced metabolic heat production.

Malignant Hyperthermia

Malignant hyperthermia (MH) is an uncommon disorder that occurs once every 15,000 exposures to inhalational anesthesia, and affects approximately 1 in 50,000 adults (9). It is an inherited disorder with an autosomal dominant pattern, and is characterized by excessive release of calcium from the sarcoplasmic reticulum in skeletal muscle in response to halogenated inhalational anesthetic agents (e.g., halothane, isoflurane, servoflurane, and desflurane) and depolarizing neuromuscular blockers (e.g., succinylcholine) (9). The calcium release leads to uncoupling of oxidative phosphorylation and a marked rise in metabolic rate.

Clinical Manifestations

The clinical manifestations of MH include muscle rigidity, hyperthermia, depressed consciousness, and autonomic instability. The first sign of MH may be a sudden and unexpected rise in end-tidal PCO_2 (reflecting the underlying hypermetabolism) in the operating room (9,10). This is followed (within minutes to a few hours) by generalized muscle rigidity, which can progress rapidly to widespread myonecrosis (rhabdomyolysis) and subsequent myoglobinuric renal failure. The heat generated by the muscle rigidity is responsible for the marked rise in body temperature (often above 40°C or 104°F) in MH. The altered mental status in MH can range from agitation to coma. Autonomic instability can lead to cardiac arrhythmias, fluctuating blood pressure, or persistent hypotension.

Management

The first suspicion of MH should prompt immediate discontinuation of the offending anesthetic agent.

DANTROLENE: Specific treatment for the muscle rigidity is available with dantrolene sodium, a muscle relaxant that blocks the release of calcium from the sarcoplasmic reticulum. When given early in the course of MH, dantrolene can reduce the mortality rate from 70% or higher (in untreated cases) to 10% or less (9,10). The dosing regimen for dantrolene in MH is as follows:

Regimen: 1–2 mg/kg as IV bolus, and repeat every 15 minutes if needed to a total dose of 10 mg/kg. Follow the initial dosing regimen with a dose of 1 mg/kg IV or 2 mg/kg orally four times daily for 3 days.

Treatment is extended to 3 days to prevent recurrences. The most common side effect of dantrolene is muscle weakness, particularly grip strength, which usually resolves in 2–4 days after the drug is discontinued (11). The most troublesome side effect of dantrolene is hepatocellular injury, which is more common when the daily dose exceeds 10 mg/kg (9). Active hepatitis and cirrhosis are contraindications to dantrolene therapy (11) but in light of the high mortality in MH if left untreated, these contraindications should not be absolute.

Prevention

All patients who survive an episode of MH should be given a medical bracelet that identifies their susceptibility to MH. In addition, because MH is a genetic disorder with an known inheritance pattern (autosomal dominant), immediate family members should be informed of their possible susceptibility to MH. A test is available to identify the responsible gene for MH in family members (10).

Neuroleptic Malignant Syndrome

The neuroleptic malignant syndrome (NMS) is strikingly similar to malignant hyperthermia in that it is a drug-induced disorder characterized by hyperthermia, muscle rigidity, altered mental status, and autonomic instability (12).

Pathogenesis

NMS is associated with drugs that influence dopamine-mediated synaptic transmission in the brain. A decrease in dopaminergic transmission in the basal ganglia and hypothalamic-pituitary axis may be responsible for many of the clinical manifestations of NMS (12). As indicated in Table 42.2, NMS can be the result of therapy with drugs that inhibit dopaminergic transmission (most cases), or can be triggered by discontinuing drugs that facilitate dopaminergic transmission. (Note that not all drugs associated with NMS are neuroleptic drugs.) The drugs most frequently implicated in NMS are *haloperidol* and *fluphenazine* (12). The incidence of NMS during therapy with neuroleptic agents is reported at 0.2–1.9% (13).

Table 42.2	Drugs Implicated in Neuroleptic Malignant Syndrome
I. Drugs That Inhibit Dopaminergic Transmission	
Antipsychotic agents	Butyrophenones (e.g., haloperidol), phenothiazines, clozapine, olanzapine, respiradone
Antiemetic agents	Metaclopramide, droperidol, prochlorperazine
CNS stimulants	Amphetamines, cocaine
Other	Lithium, tricyclic antidepressants (overdose)
II. Drugs That Facilitate Dopaminergic Transmission†	
Dopaminergic drugs	Amantidine, bromocriptine, levodopa

†Discontinuing these drugs can trigger the neuroleptic malignant syndrome.

There is no relationship between the intensity or duration of drug therapy and the risk of NMS (12), so NMS is an idiosyncratic drug reaction and not a manifestation of drug toxicity. There is some evidence of a familial tendency, but a genetic pattern of transmission has not been identified (14).

Clinical Features

Most cases of NMS begin to appear 24–72 hours after the onset of drug therapy, and almost all cases are apparent in the first 2 weeks of drug therapy. The onset is usually gradual, and can take days to fully develop. In 80% of cases, the initial manifestation is muscle rigidity or altered mental status (12). The muscle rigidity has been described as *lead-pipe rigidity* to distinguish it from the rigidity associated with tremulousness (cogwheel rigidity). The change in mental status can range from agitation to coma. Hyperthermia (body temperature can exceed 41°C) is required for the diagnosis of NMS (12), but the increase in body temperature can be delayed for 8–10 hours after the appearance of muscle rigidity (15). Autonomic instability can produce cardiac arrhythmias, labile blood pressure, or persistent hypotension.

Laboratory Studies

Dystonic reactions to neuroleptic agents may be difficult to distinguish from the muscle rigidity in NMS. This is particularly relevant in the early stage of NMS, when muscle rigidity may be the only manifestation. The serum CK level can help in this regard because serum CK levels are only mildly elevated in dystonic reactions, but are higher than 1,000 Units/L in NMS (13).

The leukocyte count in blood can increase to 40,000/µL with a leftward shift in NMS (12), so the clinical presentation of NMS (fever, leukocytosis, altered mental status) can be mistaken as sepsis. The serum CK level can help to distinguish NMS from sepsis.

Management

The single most important measure in the management of NMS is *immediate* removal of the offending drug. If NMS is caused by discontinuation of dopaminergic drugs, the drug should be restarted immediately, with gradual reduction of the drug dosage at a later time. General measures for NMS include volume resuscitation (for rhabdomyolysis or hypotension).

DANTROLENE: Dantrolene sodium (the same muscle relaxant used in the treatment of MH) can be given intravenously for severe cases of muscle rigidity. The optimal dose is not clearly defined, but one suggestion is shown below (12,16):

> Regimen: 2–3 mg/kg as IV bolus, and repeat every few hours if needed to a total dose of 10 mg/kg. Follow with oral dantrolene in doses of 50–200 mg daily (given in divided doses every 6–8 hrs).

BROMOCRIPTINE: Bromocriptine mesylate is a dopamine agonist that has been successful in treating NMS when given orally in a dose of 2.5–10 mg three times daily (16). Some improvement in muscle rigidity can be seen within hours after the start of therapy, but the *full response often takes days to develop*. Hypotension is a troublesome side effect. *There is no advantage with bromocriptine over dantrolene*, except in patients with advanced liver disease (where dantrolene is not advised).

Treatment of NMS should continue for about 10 days after clinical resolution because of delayed clearance of many neuroleptics (when depot preparations are implicated, therapy should continue for 2–3 weeks after clinical resolution) (12). There is a heightened risk of venous thromboembolism during NMS (12), so heparin prophylaxis is recommended. The mortality rate in NMS is about 20% (13), and it is unclear if dantrolene or bromocriptine has a favorable effect on mortality (12,13).

Serotonin Syndrome

Overstimulation of serotonin receptors in the central nervous system produces a combination of mental status changes, autonomic hyperactivity, and neuromuscular abnormalities that is known as the *serotonin syndrome* (SS) (17). The recent growth in popularity of seritonergic drugs such as selective serotonin reuptake inhibitors (SSRIs) has led to a marked increase in the prevalence of SS in recent years. The severity of illness can vary widely, and the most severe cases can be confused with the other drug-induced hyperthermia syndromes.

Pathogenesis

Serotonin is a neurotransmitter that participates in sleep–wakefulness cycles, mood, and thermoregulation. A variety of drugs can enhance serotonin neurotransmission and produce SS, and a list of these drugs is shown in Table 42.3. Many of these drugs work in combination to produce SS, although single-drug therapy can also result in SS. Many of the drugs involved in SS are mood enhancers, including illegal substances like "ecstasy," an amphetamine derivative implicated in life-threatening cases of SS (18).

Table 42.3	Drugs That Can Produce Serotonin Syndrome[†]
Mechanism of Action	**Drugs**
Increased serotonin synthesis	L-tryptophan
Decreased serotonin breakdown	MAOIs (including linezolid), ritonavir
Increased serotonin release	Amphetamines, MDMA (ecstasy), cocaine, fenfluramine
Decreased serotonin reuptake	SSRIs, TCAs, dextromethorphan, meperidine, fentanyl, tramadol
Serotonin receptor agonists	Lithium, sumitriptan, buspirone, LSD

[†]See Reference 17 for a comprehensive list of drugs. Abbreviations: MAOIs = monoamine oxidase inhibitors; MDMA = methylenedioxy-methamphetamine; SSRIs = selective serotonin reuptake inhibitors; TCAs = tricyclic antidepressants.

Clinical Manifestations

The onset of SS is usually abrupt (in contrast to NMS, where the full syndrome can take days to develop), and over half of the cases are evident within 6 hours after ingestion of the responsible drug(s) (17). The clinical findings include mental status changes (e.g., confusion, delirium, coma), hyperthermia, autonomic hyperactivity (e.g., mydriasis, tachycardia, hypertension), and neuromuscular abnormalities (e.g., hyperkinesis, hyperactive deep tendon reflexes, clonus, and muscle rigidity). The clinical presentation can vary markedly (17). Mild cases may include only hyperkinesis, hyperreflexia, tachycardia, diaphoresis, and mydriasis. Moderate cases often have additional findings of hyperthermia (temperature > 38°C) and clonus. The clonus is most obvious in the patellar deep-tendon reflexes, and horizontal ocular clonus may also be present. Severe cases of SS often present with delirium, hyperpyrexia (temperature > 40°C), widespread muscle rigidity, and spontaneous clonus. Life-threatening cases are marked by rhabdomyolysis, renal failure, metabolic acidosis, and hypotension.

A useful worksheet for the diagnosis of SS is shown in Table 42.4. The first step in the diagnostic evaluation is to establish recent ingestion of seritonergic drugs. Although the worksheet in Table 42.2 indicates drug ingestion in the past five weeks, most cases of SS follow within hours of drug ingestion (17). Hyperthermia and muscle rigidity can be absent in mild cases of the illness. *The features that most distinguish SS from other drug-induced hyperthermia syndromes are hyperkinesis, hyperreflexia, and clonus.* However, muscle rigidity can mask these clinical findings in severe cases of SS.

Table 43.4	Diagnostic Worksheet for Serotonin Syndrome*
Diagnostic	

Answer the following questions:	YES	NO
Has the patient received a serotinergic drug in the past 5 wks?	☑	☐

If the answer is YES, proceed to the questions below.

Does the patient have any of the following?	YES	NO
Tremor + hyperreflexia	☑	☐
Spontaneous clonus	☑	☐
Rigidity + Temp >38°C + ocular or inducible clonus	☑	☐
Ocular clonus + agitation or diaphoresis	☑	☐
Inducible clonus + agitation or diaphoresis	☑	☐

> If the answer is YES to ANY of the above conditions, the patient has Serotonin Syndrome.

*Adapted from Reference 17.

Management

As in other drug-induced hyperthermia syndromes, removal of the precipitating drug(s) is the single most important task in the management of SS. The remainder of the management includes measures to control agitation and hyperthermia, and the use of serotonin antagonists. Many cases of SS will resolve within 24 hours after initiation of therapy, but seritonergic drugs with long elimination half-lives can produce more prolonged symptomatology.

Sedation with *benzodiazepines* is important for controlling agitation in SS. *Physical restraints should be avoided* because they encourage isometric muscle contraction, which can aggravate skeletal muscle injury and promote lactic acidosis (19).

CYPROHEPTADINE: Cyproheptadine is a serotonin antagonist that can be given in severe cases of SS (20). This drug is available for oral administration only, but tablets can be broken up and administered through a nasogastric tube.

> Regimen: The initial dose is 12 mg, followed by 2 mg every 2 hrs for persistent symptoms. The maintenance dose is 8 mg every 6 hours.

Cyproheptadine can be sedating, but this should aid in the control of agitation in SS.

Neuromuscular paralysis may be required in severe cases of SS to control muscle rigidity and extreme elevations of body temperature (> 41°C). Nondepolarizing agents (e.g., vecuronium) should be used for muscle paralysis because succinylcholine can aggravate the hyperkalemia that accompanies rhabdomyolysis. Dantrolene does not reduce muscle rigidity or hyperthermia in SS (17).

HYPOTHERMIA

Hypothermia is defined as a decrease in body temperature below 35°C (95°F), and can be the result of environmental forces (accidental hypothermia), a metabolic disorder (secondary hypothermia), or a therapeutic intervention (induced hypothermia). This section will focus primarily on environmental (accidental) hypothermia.

Adaptation to Cold

Physiologically, the human body is better equipped to survive in hot rather than cold environments. The physiological response to cold includes cutaneous vasoconstriction (to reduce convective heat loss) and shivering (which can double metabolic heat production). These physiological adaptations are protective only in mild hypothermia (see later in the text); otherwise, protection from the cold is dependent on behavioral responses (e.g., wearing warm clothing and seeking shelter from the cold). Because of the importance of behavioral responses, hypothermia is particularly pronounced when these responses are impaired (e.g., in the intoxicated or confused patient).

Accidental Hypothermia

Environmental hypothermia is most likely to occur in the following situations: (a) prolonged submersion in cold water (the transfer of heat to cold water occurs much more readily than the transfer of heat to cold air), (b) exposure to cold wind (wind promotes heat loss by convection, as described earlier in the chapter), (c) when the physiological response to cold is impaired (e.g., the vasoconstrictive response to cold is impaired by alcohol consumption), and (d) when the behavioral responses to cold are impaired (as mentioned in the previous paragraph).

Temperature Recordings

Most standard thermometers measure temperatures down to 34°C (94°F). For more accurate recordings in hypothermia, electronic temperature probes are available that can record temperatures down to 25°C (77°F), and can be placed in the bladder, rectum, or esophagus.

Clinical Features

The consequences of progressive hypothermia are summarized in Table 42.5.

Table 42.5	Manifestations of Progressive Hypothermia	
Severity	**Body Temp**	**Clinical Manifestations**
Mild	32–35°C 90–95°F	Confusion, cold and pale skin, shivering, tachycardia
Moderate	28–31.9°C 82–89.9°F	Lethargy, reduced or absent shivering, bradycardia, bradypnea
Severe	<28°C <82°F	Obtundation or coma, no shivering, edema, dilated and fixed pupils, bradycardia, hypotension, oliguria
Fatal	<25°C <77°F	Apnea, asystole

MILD HYPOTHERMIA: In mild hypothermia (32–35°C or 90–95°F), patients are usually confused, and show signs of adaptation to cold; i.e., cold, pale skin from cutaneous vasoconstriction. There is brisk shivering, and a rapid heart rate.

MODERATE HYPOTHERMIA: In moderate hypothermia (28–31.8°C or 82–89°F), shivering may be absent, and patients are lethargic. Bradycardia and a decreased respiratory rate (bradypnea) become evident, and pupillary light reflexes can be absent.

SEVERE HYPOTHERMIA: In severe hypothermia (< 28°C or < 82°F), patients are usually obtunded or comatose with dilated, fixed pupils (which are not a sign of brain death in this situation). Additional findings include hypotension, severe bradycardia, oliguria, and generalized edema. Apnea and asystole are expected at body temperatures below 25°C (77°F).

Laboratory Evaluation

The laboratory tests of interest in hypothermia include arterial blood gases, serum electrolytes (particularly potassium), tests of coagulation, and tests of renal function. A generalized coagulopathy (with elevation of the INR and prolonged partial thromboplastin times) is common in hypothermia (21), but may not be evident if the coagulation profile is run at normal body temperatures. Arterial blood gases (which should be run at normal body temperatures) can reveal a respiratory acidosis or a metabolic acidosis (21). Serum electrolytes can reveal hyperkalemia, which is presumably due to potassium release by skeletal muscle from shivering or rhabdomyolysis. Serum creatinine levels can be elevated as a result of rhabdomyolysis, acute renal failure, or *cold diuresis* (caused by diminished renal tubular responsiveness to antidiuretic hormone).

Electrocardiogram

About 80% of patients with hypothermia will have prominent J waves at the QRS–ST junction on the electrocardiogram (see Figure 42.1). These waves, which are called *Osborn waves*, are not specific for hypothermia, and can occur with hypercalcemia, subarachnoid hemorrhage, cerebral injuries, and myocardial ischemia (22). Despite the attention these waves have received, they are merely a curiosity, and have little or no diagnostic or prognostic value in hypothermia (21–13).

ARRHYTHMIAS: A multitude of rhythm disturbances can occur in hypothermia, including first, second, and third-degree heart block, sinus and junctional bradycardia, idioventricular rhythm, premature atrial and ventricular beats, and atrial and ventricular fibrillation (22).

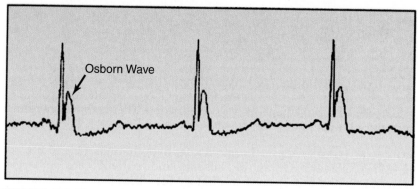

FIGURE 42.1 The (overhyped) Osborn wave.

Rewarming

EXTERNAL REWARMING: External rewarming (removing wet clothes, covering the patient in blankets, etc.) can increase body temperature at a rate of 1–2°C per hour (21), and is *adequate for most cases of hypothermia* (23). There is a risk of a further decrease in body temperature during external rewarming (called *afterdrop*), which can trigger ventricular fibrillation (24). This phenomenon is attributed to central displacement of cold blood in cutaneous blood vessels. Fortunately, serious cardiac arrhythmias are not common, and do not contribute to mortality during external rewarming for severe hypothermia (23,24).

INTERNAL REWARMING: There are several methods of internal rewarming, but they are invasive, time-consuming, and are needed only in the most severe cases of hypothermia. The easiest internal warming technique is to increase the temperature of inhaled gases to 40–45°C (104–113°F), which can raise the core temperature at a rate of 2.5°C per hour in intubated patients (21). Other internal warming techniques include peritoneal lavage with heated fluids (21), extracorporeal blood rewarming (25), and heated intravenous fluids (26). Warmed gastric lavage is ineffective (21).

REWARMING SHOCK: Rewarming from moderate or severe hypothermia is often accompanied by hypotension (*rewarming shock*). This is attributed to a combination of factors, including hypovolemia (from cold diuresis), myocardial depression, and vasodilation (23,24). Volume infusion will help to alleviate this problem, but the infusion of fluids at room temperature (21°C or 70°F) can aggravate the hypothermia, so the infused fluids should be heated. Vasoactive drugs are required in about half of patients with severe hypothermia, and this requirement indicates a poor prognosis (24).

Induced Hypothermia

Intentional cooling to a body temperature of 32–34°C (89.6–93.2°F) is now a popular treatment modality for patients who remain comatose after resuscitation from cardiac arrest. This topic is presented in Chapter 17 (see pages 336–339).

A FINAL WORD

The Adaptable Human

The number of deaths from heat exposure is estimated at only 400 per year in the United States (27), and in a 20-year survey of a large urban hospital in France, severe hypothermia accounted for only 0.4% of admissions to the ICU (24). These small numbers are a testament to the human ability to adapt (both physiologically and behaviorally) to environmental extremes.

REFERENCES

1. Keel CAm Neil E, Joels N. Regulation of body temperature in man. In: Samson Wright's Applied Physiology, 13th ed. New York: Oxford University Press, 1982:346.

2. Guyton AC, Hall JE. Body temperature, temperature regulation, and fever. In: Medical Physiology, 10th ed. Philadelphia, WB Saunders, 2000:822–833.

Heat-Related Illness

3. Khosla R, Guntupalli KK. Heat-related illnesses. Crit Care Clin 1999; 15:251–263.

4. Lugo-Amador NM, Rothenhaus T, Moyer P. Heat-related illness. Emerg Med Clin N Am 2004; 22:315–327.

5. Glazer JL. Management of heat stroke and heat exhaustion. Am Fam Physician 2005; 71:2133–2142.

6. Hadad E, Rav-Acha M, Heled Y, et al. Heat stroke: a review of cooling methods. Sports Med 2004; 34:501–511.

7. Ward MM. Factors predictive of acute renal failure in rhabdomyolysis. Arch Intern Med 1988; 148:1553–1557.

8. Sharp LS, Rozycki GS, Feliciano DV. Rhabdomyolysis and secondary renal failure in critically ill surgical patients. Am J Surg 2004; 188:801–806.

Malignant Hyperthermia

9. Rusyniakn DE, Sprague JE. Toxin-induced hyperthermic syndromes. Med Clin N Am 2005;89:1277–1296.

10. Litman RS, Rosenberg H. Malignant hyperthermia. J Am Med Assoc 2005; 293:2918–2924.

11. McEvoy GK, ed. AHFS Drug Information, 2001. Bethesda, MD: American Society of Health-System Pharmacists, 2001, pp. 1328–1331.

Neuroleptic Malignant Syndrome

12. Bhanushali NJ, Tuite PJ. The evaluation and management of patients with neuroleptic malignant syndrome. Neurol Clin N Am 2004; 22:389–411.

13. Khaldarov V. Benzodiazepines for treatment of neuroleptic malignant syndrome. Hosp Physician, 2003 (Sept):51–55.

14. Otani K, Horiuchi M, Kondo T, et al. Is the predisposition to neuroleptic malignant syndrome genetically transmitted? Br J Psychiatry 1991; 158:850–853.

15. Lev R, Clark RF. Neuroleptic malignant syndrome presenting without fever: case report and review of the literature. J Emerg Med 1996; 12:49–55.

16. Guze BH, Baxter LR. Neuroleptic malignant syndrome. N Engl J Med 1985; 313:163–166.

Serotonin Syndrome

17. Boyer EH, Shannon M. The serotonin syndrome. N Engl J Med 2005; 352:1112–1120.

18. Demirkiran M, Jankivic J, Dean JM. Ecstacy intoxication: an overlap between serotonin syndrome and neuroleptic malignant syndrome. Clin Neuropharmacol 1996; 19:157–164.

19. Hick JL, Smith SW, Lynch MT. Metabolic acidosis in restraint-associated cardiac arrest. Acad Emerg Med 1999; 6:239–245.

20. Graudins A, Stearman A, Chan B. Treatment of serotonin syndrome with cyproheptadine. J Emerg Med 1998; 16:615–619.

Hypothermia

21. Hanania NA, Zimmerman NA. Accidental hypothermia. Crit Care Clin 1999; 15:235–249.

22. Aslam AF, Aslam AK, Vasavada BC, Khan IA. Hypothermia: evaluation, electrocardiographic manifestations, and management. Am J Med 2006; 119:297–301.

23. Cornell HM. Hot topics in cold medicine: controversies in accidental hypothermia. Clin Ped Emerg Med 2001; 2:179–191.

24. Vassal T, Bernoit-Gonin B, Carrat F, et al. Severe accidental hypothermia treated in an ICU. Chest 2001; 120:1998–2003.

25. Ireland AJ, Pathi VL, Crawford R, et al. Back from the dead: Extracorporeal rewarming of severe accidental hypothermia victims in accidental emergency. J Accid Emerg Med 1997; 14:255–303.

26. Handrigen MT, Wright RO, Becker BM, et al. Factors and methodology in achieving ideal delivery temperatures for intravenous and lavage fluid in hypothermia. Am J Emerg Med 1997; 15:350–359.

A Final Word

27. Morbidity and Mortality Weekly Report, 2002; 51:567–570.

Chapter 43

FEVER IN THE ICU

Give me the power to produce fever,
and I will cure all diseases.

Parmenides
ca 500 B.C

The appearance of a new fever is always a matter of concern in a hospitalized patient. This chapter presents a practical approach to the ICU patient with a new-onset fever, and includes: (a) the definition of fever in ICU patients, (b) the appropriate sites for measuring body temperature, (c) the optimal method for obtaining blood cultures, and (d) the potential sources of fever in the ICU (1,2). The final section focuses on the practice of suppressing fever, and why Parmenides might disapprove of this practice.

BODY TEMPERATURE

Two scales (Celsius and Fahrenheit) are used to record body temperature, and the conversion from one scale to the other is shown in Table 43.1. Although readings on the Celsius scale are often called "degrees centigrade," this unit is intended for the degrees on a compass, not for temperatures (3). The appropriate term for temperatures on the Celsius scale is *degrees Celsius*.

Normal Body Temperature

The definition of a normal body temperature is not straightforward, as demonstrated by the following observations.

1. The traditional norm of 37°C (98.6°F) is a mean value derived from a study of axillary temperatures in 25,000 healthy adults, conducted in the late 19th century (4). However, axillary temperatures can vary by as much as 1.0°C (1.8°F) from core body temperatures (5), and axillary temperatures are not advised in ICU patients (1).

2. Core body temperature can be 0.5°C (0.9°F) higher than oral temperatures (6), and 0.2–0.3°C lower than rectal temperatures (1).

3. Elderly subjects have a mean body temperature about 0.5°C (0.9°F) lower than younger adults (4,7).

4. Body temperature has a diurnal variation, with the nadir in the early morning (between 4 and 8 a.m.) and the peak in the late afternoon (between 4 and 6 p.m.). The range of diurnal variation varies, but can be as high as 1.3°C (2.4°F) (8).

These observations indicate that the normal body temperature is influenced by age, measurement site, and time of day. As such, the best definition of a normal body temperature is the usual range of temperatures for an individual patient, measured at the same site, over a 24-hour period.

Table 43.1		Converting Celsius and Fahrenheit Temperatures
°C	°F	Conversion Formulas
100	212	Conversions are based on the corresponding
40	104	temperatures at the freezing point of water,
39	102.2	0°C = 32°F
38	100.4	and the corresponding temperature ranges from freezing point to boiling point of water,
37	98.6	Δ100°C = Δ180°F
36	95	which can be reduced to:
35	95	Δ5°C = Δ9°F
34	93.2	These relationships are then combined to derive the following formulas:
33	91.4	°F = (9/5 °C) + 32
0	32	°C = 5/9 (°F − 32)

Thermometry

The most recent guidelines on fever in the ICU (1) contain the following recommendations for measuring body temperature.

1. The most accurate measurements are obtained with thermistor-equipped catheters placed in the pulmonary artery, esophagus, or urinary bladder.

2. Less accurate measurements are obtained with rectal, oral, and tympanic membrane temperatures, in that order. Rectal temperatures are not advised in neutropenic patients (1), and oral temperatures should be measured with electronic probes (not mercury thermometers) placed in the right or left sublingual pockets.

3. The axillary and temporal artery sites are not recommended for temperature measurements in ICU patients.

Thermistor-equipped urinary bladder catheters seem ideal for patients who require a bladder drainage catheter (which includes most patients in an ICU). These devices not only provide accurate measurements of body temperature, they also permit continuous temperature monitoring, which allows you to identify the normal temperature range for each patient.

Definition of Fever

Fever is best defined as a temperature that exceeds the normal daily variation in temperature for each patient. However, this is not a practical definition because the normal temperature range for each patient cannot be determined with periodic measurements. The current recommendations for the definition of a fever in ICU patients are as follows (1):

1. A body temperature of 38.3°C (101°F) or higher represents a fever, and deserves further evaluation.

2. A lower threshold of 38.0°C (100.4°F) can be used for immunocompromised patients, particularly those with neutropenia.

The Febrile Response

Fever is the result of inflammatory cytokines (called endogenous pyrogens) that act on the hypothalamus to elevate the body temperature. Any condition that triggers a systemic inflammatory response will, therefore, produce a fever. Some implications of the febrile response are stated below.

1. Fever is a sign of inflammation, not infection, and about 50% of ICU patients who develop a fever have no apparent infection (9,10).

2. The severity of the fever does not correlate with the presence or severity of infection. High fevers can be the result of a noninfectious process such as a drug fever (see later), while fever can be absent in life-threatening infections (1).

The distinction between inflammation and infection is an important one, not only for the evaluation of fever, but also for curtailing the indiscriminate use of antibiotics.

Fever as an Adaptive Response

Unlike hyperthermia, which is the result of abnormal temperature regulation (see Chapter 42), fever is a condition where the thermoregulatory system is intact, but is operating at a higher set point (11). Elevated body temperatures serve to enhance immune function and inhibit bacterial and viral replication, indicating that fever can be viewed as an adaptive response that aids the host in defending against infection (12). The beneficial effects of fever are described in more detail later in the chapter.

Sources of Fever

Any condition capable of triggering an inflammatory response is capable of causing a fever. The notable sources of nosocomial fever in the ICU are shown in Figure 43.1.

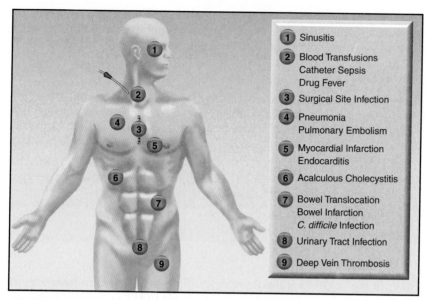

1. Sinusitis
2. Blood Transfusions
   Catheter Sepsis
   Drug Fever
3. Surgical Site Infection
4. Pneumonia
   Pulmonary Embolism
5. Myocardial Infarction
   Endocarditis
6. Acalculous Cholecystitis
7. Bowel Translocation
   Bowel Infarction
   C. difficile Infection
8. Urinary Tract Infection
9. Deep Vein Thrombosis

FIGURE 43.1 Potential sources of nosocomial fever in the ICU.

NONINFECTIOUS SOURCES

As mentioned earlier, infection is responsible for only half of ICU-acquired fevers (9,10). The conditions described in this section are responsible for most of the remaining 50% of ICU-acquired fevers. The ones that deserve mention are included in Table 43.2.

Table 43.2	Noninfectious Causes of ICU-Acquired Fever
More Common	**Less Common Causes**
SIRS	Drug Fever
Early Postop Fever	Adrenal Failure
Pulmonary Embolism	Acalculous Cholecystitis
Platelet Transfusions	Iatrogenic Fever

SIRS

The clinical entity known as the *systemic inflammatory response syndrome* (SIRS) is characterized by signs of systemic inflammation (see Table 14.2), and may not be associated with infection. Noninfectious sources of SIRS include tissue injury (e.g., from ischemia or major surgery), and translocation of endotoxin and inflammatory cytokines from the GI tract. SIRS can be accompanied by inflammatory injury in one or more vital organs (e.g., acute respiratory distress syndrome), and can have a fatal outcome. This condition is described in more detail in Chapter 14.

Early Postoperative Fever

Major surgery is itself a source of tissue injury. (In the words of Dr. John Millili, a surgeon and close friend, major surgery is like being hit with a baseball bat!) Because inflammation and fever are the normal response to tissue injury, it is no surprise that fever in the first postoperative day is reported in 15–40% of cases of major surgery (13–15) and, in most cases, there is no apparent infection (13,14). These fevers are short-lived, and usually resolve within 24–48 hours.

Atelectasis Does Not Cause Fever

There is a long-standing misconception that atelectasis is a common cause of fever in the early postoperative period. One possible source of this misconception is the high incidence of atelectasis in patients who develop a postoperative fever. This is demonstrated in Figure 43.2 (see the graph on the left), which is from a study involving patients who underwent open heart surgery (15). Close to 90% of the patients with a fever on the first postoperative day had radiographic evidence of atelectasis. This, however, is not evidence that the atelectasis is the source of fever. In fact, the graph on the right in Figure 43.2 shows that most (75%) of the patients with atelectasis did not have a fever. The inability of atelectasis to produce fever was demonstrated over 50 years ago in an animal study where lobar atelectasis produced by ligation of a mainstem bronchus was not accompanied by fever (16).

To summarize, atelectasis is a common complication of major surgery, and occurs in over 90% of cases of general anesthesia (17). However, it is not a common cause of postoperative fever. Most fevers that appear in the first 24 hours after surgery are the result of the tissue injury sustained during the procedure.

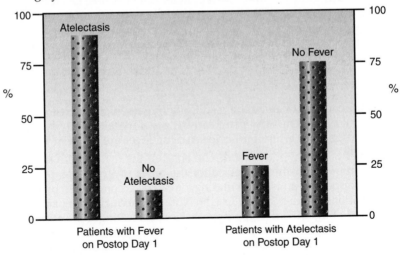

FIGURE 43.2 The relationships between fever and atelectasis in the first postoperative day in 100 consecutive patients who had open heart surgery. The graph on the left shows that most patients with fever had atelectasis, but the graph on the right shows that most patients with atelectasis did not have a fever. Data from Reference 15.

Malignant Hyperthermia

An uncommon but treatable cause of elevated body temperatures in the immediate postoperative period is *malignant hyperthermia,* an inherited disorder characterized by muscle rigidity, hyperpyrexia (temperature > 40°C or 104°F), and rhabdomyolysis in response to halogenated inhalational anesthetics. This disorder is described in Chapter 42.

Venous Thromboembolism

Several groups of patients are at risk for venous thromboembolism (see Table 6.1 and Figure 6.1), but the risk is highest in trauma victims and postoperative patients. Most cases of hospital-acquired deep vein thrombosis are asymptomatic, but acute pulmonary embolism can produce a fever that lasts up to 1 week (18). The diagnostic approach to acute pulmonary embolism is outlined in Figure 6.2.

Blood Transfusions

Erythrocyte Transfusions

Febrile non-hemolytic transfusion reactions occur in 0.5% of erythrocyte transfusions. These reactions are the result of antileukocyte antibodies in the recipient that react with donor leukocytes, and they are more likely to occur in patients who have received multiple transfusions. The fever usually appears during, or up to 6 hours after, the transfusion. For more information on these reactions, see pages 360–361.

Platelet Transfusions

Fever is much more common with platelet transfusions; i.e., the reported incidence is as high as 30% (see page 380). These reactions are also caused by antibodies to donor leukocytes, and the frequent appearance of these reactions with platelet transfusions is probably due to the multiple donors used for routine platelet transfusions.

Drug Fever

Drug-induced fever can be the result of a hypersensitivity reaction or an idiosyncratic reaction. Any drug can trigger a hypersensitivity reaction, but the drugs most often implicated in drug fever are listed in Table 43.3.

Drug fever is poorly understood. The onset of the fever varies from a few hours to more than three weeks after the onset of drug therapy (1). The fever can appear as an isolated finding, or can be accompanied by the other manifestations listed in Table 43.3 (19). Note that about half of patients have rigors, and about 20% develop hypotension, indicating that *patients with a drug fever can appear seriously ill.* Evidence of a hypersensitivity reaction (i.e., eosinophilia and rash) is absent in over 75% of cases of drug fever (19).

Suspicion of drug fever usually occurs when there are no other likely sources of fever. When suspected, possible offending drugs should be discontinued, if possible. The fever should disappear in 2–3 days, but it can persist for up to 7 days (20).

Table 43.3	Drug-Associated Fever in the ICU	
Common Offenders	**Occasional Offenders**	**Clinical Findings***
Amphotericin	Cimetidine	Rigors (53%)
Cephalosporins	Carbamazepine	Myalgias (25%)
Penicillins	Hydralazine	Leukocytosis (22%)
Phenytoin	Rifampin	Eosinophilia (22%)
Procainamide	Streptokinase	Rash (18%)
Quinidine	Vancomycin	Hypotension (18%)

From Reference 19.

Drug-Induced Hyperthermia Syndromes

The drug-induced hyperthermia syndromes include malignant hyperthermia (mentioned earlier), neuroleptic malignant syndrome, and serotonin syndrome. These disorders are characterized by muscle rigidity, hyperpyrexia (temperature > 40°C or 104°F), and rhabdomyolysis, and are described in detail in Chapter 42. The neuroleptic malignant syndrome is a particular concern in patients receiving haloperidol for sedation.

Other Sources

There are several other potential causes of noninfectious fever, and the most notable of these are included in the following text.

Acalculous Cholecystitis

Acalculous cholecystitis is an uncommon but serious disorder reported in 1.5% of critically ill patients (21). It is believed to be the result of ischemia and stasis within the gallbladder, resulting in edema of the cystic duct that blocks drainage of the gallbladder. The diagnosis and management of this condition is described in Chapter 40.

Endocrine Disorders

The endocrine disorders known to produce fever are thyrotoxicosis and adrenal crisis. Thyrotoxicosis is unlikely to appear *de novo* in the ICU, but adrenal crisis due to spontaneous adrenal hemorrhage is a recognized complication of anticoagulant therapy and disseminated intravascular coagulation (DIC). These endocrine disorders are described in Chapter 50.

Iatrogenic Fever

Faulty thermal regulators in water mattresses and aerosol humidifiers can cause fever by transference (22). It takes only a minute to check the temperature settings on heated mattresses and ventilators, but it can take far longer to explain why such a simple cause of fever was overlooked.

NOSOCOMIAL INFECTIONS

The incidence of ICU-acquired infections in medical and surgical ICU patients is shown in Table 43.4 (23). Four infections account for over three-quarters of ICU-acquired infections (pneumonia, urinary tract infections, bloodstream infections, and surgical site infections), and three of these infections involve indwelling plastic devices: i.e., 83% of the pneumonias occur in intubated patients, 97% of the urinary tract infections occur in catheterized patients, and 87% of bloodstream infections originate from intravascular catheters (23).

Table 43.4	Nosocomial Infections in Medical and Surgical ICU Patients	
Nosocomial Infection	**% Total Infections**	
	Medical Patients	**Surgical Patients**
Pneumonia	30% ⎫	33% ⎫
Urinary Tract Infection	30% ⎬ 76%	18% ⎬
Bloodstream Infection	16% ⎭	13% ⎬ 78%
Surgical Site Infection	——	14% ⎭
Cardiovascular Infection	5%	4%
GI Tract Infection	5%	4%
Ear, Nose & Throat Infection	4%	4%
Skin & Soft Tissue Infection	3%	3%
Others	7%	7%

From Reference 23.

Common Nosocomial Infections

The three most common ICU-acquired infections in Table 43.4 are described elsewhere in this book. The diagnosis and management of these conditions can be found in Chapter 3 (for vascular catheter-related infections), Chapter 29 (for ventilator-associated pneumonia), and Chapter 41 (for urinary tract infections). The following are some other nosocomial infections that should be considered in a patient with ICU-acquired fever.

Surgical Site Infections

Surgical site infections (SSIs) continue to be a considerable source of postoperative morbidity despite attention to preventive measures (24). These infections typically appear 5–7 days after surgery. Superficial infections are less likely to produce fever than infections with deep tissue involvement. Sternal wound infections following open heart surgery show a particular propensity for deep tissue involvement (i.e., mediastinitis) (25). For patients with fever following open heart surgery, sternal instability can be an early sign of sternal wound infection.

The pathogens involved in SSIs are determined by the surgical procedure. SSIs from clean surgical procedures (where the chest or abdomen has not been opened) usually involve *Staphylococcus aureus*, while SSIs from contaminated procedures (where the chest or abdomen has been opened) often involve organisms that are part of the indigenous flora of the organ that was surgically repaired (e.g., infections following bowel surgery typically involve Gram-negative aerobic bacilli and anaerobes) (1).

Management

Superficial infections can usually be managed with debridement only. The management of deep-seated infections is dependent on the character of the infection. Localized collections (abscesses) can often be managed with drainage only, while more diffuse involvement of deep tissues should prompt antimicrobial therapy.

Necrotizing Wound Infections

Necrotizing wound infections are produced by *Clostridium* species or β-hemolytic streptococci (1). Unlike other wound infections (which typically appear 5–7 days after surgery), necrotizing infections are evident in the first few postoperative days. There is often marked edema, and fluid-filled bullae, around the incision, and crepitance may be present. Spread to deeper structures is rapid, and progressive disease is often accompanied by rhabdomyolysis and myoglobinuric renal failure. Treatment involves extensive debridement and intravenous penicillin. The mortality rate is high (> 60%) when treatment is delayed.

Paranasal Sinusitis

Indwelling nasogastric and nasotracheal tubes can block the ostia that drain the paranasal sinuses, leading to accumulation of infected secretions in the sinuses. The maxillary sinuses are almost always involved, and the resulting acute sinusitis can be an occult source of fever. Paranasal sinusitis is reported in 15–20% of patients with indwelling nasal tubes (26,27), and can be a source of fever and bacteremia. However, the clinical significance of this condition, in many cases, is unclear (see later).

Microbiology

The pathogens involved in ICU-acquired sinusitis are the same ones that colonize the oropharynx in critically ill patients. The most frequent isolates are Gram-negative aerobic bacilli (in 60% of cases), followed by Gram-positive aerobic cocci (particularly *Staph. aureus* and coagulase-negative staphylococci) in 30% of cases, and yeasts (mostly *Candida albicans*) in 5–10% of cases (1).

Diagnosis

Purulent drainage from the nares is absent in about 75% of cases (1), and the diagnosis is suggested by radiographic features of sinusitis (i.e., opacification or air–fluid levels in the involved sinuses). Although CT scans are recommended for the diagnosis of nosocomial sinusitis (26,27), portable sinus films obtained at the bedside can also be revealing, as shown in Figure 43.3. The maxillary sinuses can be viewed with a single occipitomental view, also called a "Waters view," which can be obtained at the bedside (28). (Avoiding a CT scan also avoids the risks and man-power involved in transporting a patient out of the ICU.)

Radiographic or CT evidence of sinusitis is not sufficient for the diagno-sis of sinusitis because 30–40% of patients with evidence of sinusitis on imaging studies do not have an infection documented by aspiration of the involved sinus (26,27). The diagnosis requires aspiration of the involved sinus with a quantitative culture that grows $\geq 10^3$ colony form-ing units per mL (26,27).

Management

A trial of empiric antibiotic therapy is warranted when there is radi-ographic evidence of sinusitis in a febrile patient with no other apparent source of fever. The antibiotic regimen should provide coverage for Gram-negative aerobic bacilli and staphylococci. Single-agent therapy with imipenem or meropenem should be adequate if MRSA has not been isolated on routine nasal swabs. If MRSA has been isolated on a nasal swab, or MRSA is a frequent isolate in your ICU, then vancomycin should be added to the Gram-negative coverage. In addition, nasal tubes should be removed and replaced with oral tubes. If there is no improve-ment with empiric antibiotics, sinus puncture for Gram stain and quan-titative culture is warranted (1).

Clinical Significance

Despite the fact that nosocomial sinusitis is documented in 15–20% of patients with indwelling nasal tubes (26,27), sinusitis is often overlooked in the evaluation of ICU-acquired fever, without apparent harm. This cre-ates uncertainty about the clinical significance of ICU-acquired sinusitis.

Clostridium difficile **Infection**

ICU-acquired fever that is associated with new-onset diarrhea should always prompt suspicion of *Clostridium difficile* enterocolitis. The diagno-sis and management of this condition are described in Chapter 40 (see pages 738–742).

Patient-Specific Infections

Infections that should be considered in specific patient populations include: (a) abdominal abscesses in patients who have had a laparotomy or laparoscopy (see pages 744–745), (b) endocarditis in patients with prosthetic or damaged valves, (c) meningitis in neurosurgery patients, and (d) spontaneous bacterial peritonitis in patients with cirrhosis and ascites (see pages 725–726).

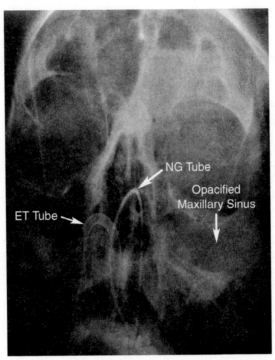

FIGURE 43.3 Portable sinus film (Waters view) showing opacification of the left maxillary and frontal sinuses in a patient with indwelling nasotracheal and nasogastric tubes. The diagnosis of paranasal sinusitis was subsequently confirmed by a maxillary sinus puncture at the bedside, with the aspirate growing *Staph. epidermidis* at 10^3 cfu/mL.

INITIAL APPROACH

The appearance of an ICU-acquired fever is not a license to perform an extensive evaluation and start empiric antimicrobial therapy. Instead, an evaluation should be made to determine the likelihood of a noninfectious or infectious source of fever. If a noninfectious source of fever is unlikely, the following measures are relevant.

Blood Cultures

Blood cultures are recommended for all cases of ICU-related fever where a noninfectious source is unlikely (1). The yield from blood cultures is dependent on the volume of blood withdrawn during a venipuncture, and the number of venipuncture sites.

Influence of Volume

The yield from blood cultures is optimal when 20–30 mL of blood is withdrawn from each venipuncture site (1). The standard practice is to withdraw 20 mL of blood from a venipuncture site: one-half (10 mL) is then injected into each of the two bottles of broth (one aerobic and one anaerobic) provided in a blood culture set. Increasing from 20 mL to 30 mL of blood increases the yield from blood cultures by about 10% (29). When using 30 mL per venipuncture, the extra 10 mL aliquot of blood should be injected into an aerobic broth bottle (29).

Number of Blood Cultures

In the terminology of blood cultures, one blood culture refers to a single venipuncture site. (For example, culture of blood specimens from each lumen of a multilumen catheter still represents one blood culture.) The relationship between the number of blood cultures and the detection of bacteremia is shown in Figure 43.4 (30). This is from a study of patients with bacteremia documented by four or more blood cultures drawn over a 24 hour period. The two curves in the graph represent patients with endocarditis and patients with other infections. The majority of the bacteremias (94%) were detected with two blood cultures in the patients with endocarditis, while three blood cultures were required to detect over 90% of the bacteremias in patients with other infections. The enhanced detection rate in endocarditis is due to the continuous bacteremia associated with endocarditis.

Based on the data in Figure 43.4, *three blood cultures drawn over a 24-hour period will detect a majority (> 90%) of bacteremias* (1). However, two blood cultures will detect a majority of bacteremias in patients with endocarditis.

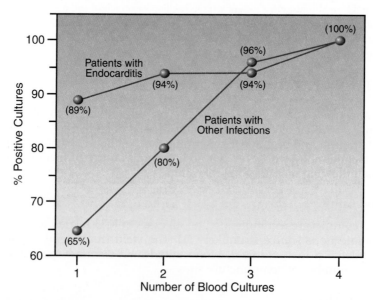

FIGURE 43.4 Relationship between the number of blood cultures drawn over a 24-hour period (20 mL per blood culture) and the detection rate for bacteremia. See text for explanation. Data from Reference 30.

Empiric Antimicrobial Therapy

Empiric antibiotic therapy is recommended when the likelihood of infection is high. Prompt initiation of antimicrobial therapy is considered essential, *particularly in patients with neutropenia* (absolute neutrophil count < 500), where delays of only a few hours can have a negative impact on outcomes (31).

1. Empiric coverage should always include an antibiotic that is active against Gram-negative aerobic bacilli, which are the most prevalent pathogens in ICU-acquired infections. Popular choices include the *carbapenems (imipenem or meropenem), piperacillin/tazobactam, or cefepime.*

2. Coverage for staphylococci (*S. aureus* and coagulase-negative staphylococci) should be included if vascular catheter-related septicemia is a possibility. *Vancomycin* is the antibiotic-of-choice for this purpose.

3. An antifungal agent should be considered when unexplained fever persists for longer than 3 days after the start of empiric antibiotics. This is most appropriate for patients who are at-risk for disseminated candidiasis (e.g., long hospital stay, recent antimicrobial therapy, immunosuppressed, *Candida* colonizing multiple sites). *Fluconazole* is adequate for most patients, while an alternative agent (e.g., caspofungin) is recommended for neutropenic patients.

See Chapter 52 for more information on the antimicrobial agents just mentioned, including dosing recommendations.

ANTIPYRETIC THERAPY

The popular perception of fever as a malady that must be corrected is rooted in hearsay. In fact, *fever is a normal adaptive response that enhances the ability to eradicate infection* (12). This section contains some observations about fever that are intended to make you think twice about starting antipyretic therapy in critically ill patients.

Fever as a Host Defense Mechanism

An increase in body temperature can enhance immune function by increasing the production of antibodies and cytokines, activating T-lymphocytes, facilitating neutrophil chemotaxis, and enhancing phagocytosis by neutrophils and macrophages (32,33). In addition, high temperatures inhibit bacterial and viral replication. The effect of body temperature on the growth of bacteria in blood is demonstrated in Figure 43.5 (34). Note that an increase in temperature of 4°C completely suppresses growth. Similar results have been demonstrated in an animal model of pneumococcal meningitis (35).

Clinical Studies

The benefits of fever as a host defense against infection is supported in

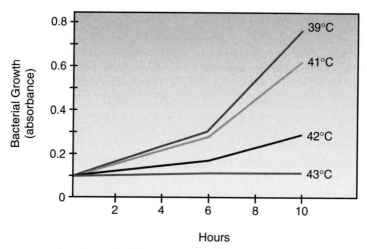

FIGURE 43.5 The influence of body temperature on the growth of *Pasteurella multocida* in the blood of infected laboratory animals. The range of temperatures in the figure is the usual range of febrile temperatures for the study animal (rabbits). Data from Reference 34.

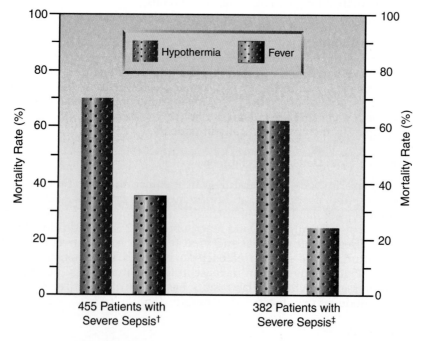

FIGURE 43.6 The relationship between body temperature and survival in two clinical studies of patients with severe sepsis. Data from References [†]36 and [‡]37.

clinical studies showing that septic patients who develop hypothermia have at least twice the mortality rate of septic patients who develop a fever (36,37). The results of these studies are shown in Figure 43.6. Although these studies cannot establish a causal relationship between body temperature and outcomes, they do show that higher body temperatures are associated with improved outcomes. A more recent observational study showed that antipyretic therapy was associated with higher mortality rates in septic patients (38).

Is Fever Harmful?

Tachycardia

One of the claims in support of suppressing fever is the assumed effect of fever in promoting tachycardia, which can be harmful in patients with heart disease. However, the association between fever and tachycardia was established in animal models of sepsis, and it is likely that the inflammatory response to sepsis is the source of tachycardia, and not an elevation in body temperature.

Neurologic Injury

There is convincing evidence that increased body temperatures aggravate ischemic brain injury following cardiac arrest (see Chapter 17) and ischemic stroke (see Chapter 46). However, the effects of increased body temperatures in the non-ischemic brain have not been adequately studied. The popular claim that hyperpyrexia (temperature $\geq 40°C$ or $\geq 104°F$) promotes injury in the non-ischemic brain can neither be supported nor refuted because hyperpyrexia is rarely left untreated in clinical practice.

Summary Statements

The available evidence at the present time indicates the following:

1. Fever is not a pathological condition, but is a normal adaptive response that serves an antimicrobial defense mechanism.
2. Except for the early period following cardiac arrest or ischemic stroke, fever provides a documented benefit in patients with infection.
3. The professed harm of hyperpyrexia ($\geq 40°C$ or $\geq 104°F$) in a nonischemic brain is more assumption than documented fact.

Antipyretic Drugs

Prostaglandin E mediates the febrile response to endogenous pyrogens, and drugs that interfere with prostaglandin E synthesis are effective in reducing fever (39). These drugs include aspirin, acetaminophen, and nonsteroidal anti-inflammatory agents (NSAIDS). Only the latter two are used for fever suppression in the ICU.

Acetaminophen

Acetaminophen is the favored drug for antipyresis, despite the fact that it is the leading cause of acute liver failure in the United States (see Chapter 54). Acetaminophen is contraindicated in patients with hepatic insufficiency.

DOSING REGIMENS: Acetaminophen is usually given orally or by rectal suppository in a dose of 650 mg every 4–6 hrs, with a maximum daily dose of 4 grams. An intravenous preparation is now available in the United States (OFIRMEV™), and the recommended dose for adults ≥ 50 kg is 650 mg every 4 hrs, or 1,000 mg every 6 hrs, with a maximum dose of 4 grams daily (40). This dosing regimen is equivalent to oral acetaminophen for suppressing fever in adults (41). Intravenous acetaminophen is costly, and is recommended only for patients who cannot tolerate oral or rectal drug administration.

NSAIDs

Ibuprofen is a popular over-the-counter NSAID that provides safe and effective antipyresis at an intravenous dose of 400–800 mg every six hours (42). *Ketorolac* is another intravenous NSAID that has been effective in suppressing fever (in a single dose of 0.5 mg/kg) (43). See Chapter 51 for more information on these drugs.

Cooling Blankets

Cooling blankets are inappropriate for the treatment of fever. The febrile response raises the body temperature by promoting cutaneous vasoconstriction and increasing skeletal muscle activity (via rigors and shivering). This is what the body normally does in response to a cold environment, so the febrile response mimics the physiological response to cold. Stated another way, *the febrile response makes the body behave like it is wrapped in a cooling blanket.* Adding a cooling blanket will only aggravate the cutaneous vasoconstriction and increased muscle activity involved in the febrile response. This explains why cooling blankets are notoriously ineffective in reducing fever.

Cooling blankets are more appropriate for hyperthermia syndromes, when normal thermoregulation is faulty (see Chapter 42).

A FINAL WORD

Right vs. Wrong

There's a wrong way and a right way to approach a new-onset fever in the ICU. The wrong way is to culture everything available, order a barrage of laboratory tests and imaging studies, and start antibiotics without hesitation. The right way is to make sure the fever is real (and not the result of an iatrogenic problem), and then evaluate the patient for the likelihood of an infectious or noninfectious source of the fever. Remember that there is a 50-50 chance of finding an underlying infection, so don't start antibiotics unless an infection is apparent or highly suspected, or the patient is immunocompromised. And finally, *please* think twice about suppressing fever, and stay away from cooling blankets.

REFERENCES

Reviews

1. O'Grady NP, Barie PS, Bartlett J, et al. Guidelines for the evaluation of new fever in critically ill adult patients: 2008 update from the American College of Critical Care Medicine and the Infectious Disease Society of America. Crit Care Med 2008; 36:1330–1349.

2. Laupland KB. Fever in the critically ill medical patient. Crit Care Med 2009; 37(Suppl):S273–S278.

Body Temperature

3. Stimson HF. Celsius versus centigrade: the nomenclature of the temperature scale of science. Science 1962; 136:254–255.

4. Wunderlich CA, Sequine E. Medical thermometry and human temperature. New York: William Wood, 1871.

5. Mellors JW, Horwitz RI, Harvey MR, et al. A simple index to identify occult bacterial infection in adults with acute unexplained fever. Arch Intern Med 1987; 147:666–671.

6. Tandberg D, Sklar D. Effect of tachypnea on the estimation of body temperature by an oral thermometer. N Engl J Med 1983; 308:945–946.

7. Marion GS, McGann KP, Camp DL. Core body temperature in the elderly and factors which influence its measurement. Gerontology 1991; 37:225–232.

8. Mackowiak PA, Wasserman SS, Levine MM. A critical appraisal of 98.6°F, the upper limit of the normal body temperature, and other legacies of Carl Reinhold August Wunderlich. JAMA 1992; 268:1578–1580.

9. Commichau C, Scarmeas N, Mayer SA. Risk factors for fever in the intensive care unit. Neurology 2003; 60:837–841.

10. Peres Bota D, Lopes Ferriera F, Melot C, et al. Body temperature alterations in the critically ill. Intensive Care Med 2004; 30:811–816.

11. Saper CB, Breder CB. The neurologic basis of fever. N Engl J Med 1994; 330:1880–1886.

12. Kluger MJ, Kozak W, Conn CA, et al. The adaptive value of fever. Infect Dis Clin North Am 1996; 10:1–20.

Noninfectious Sources of Fever

13. Fry DE. Postoperative fever. In: Mackowiak PA, ed. Fever: basic mechanisms and management. New York: Raven Press, 1991; 243–254.

14. Freischlag J, Busuttil RW. The value of postoperative fever evaluation. Surgery 1983; 94:358–363.

15. Engoren M. Lack of association between atelectasis and fever. Chest 1995; 107:81–84.

16. Shelds RT. Pathogenesis of postoperative pulmonary atelectasis: an experimental study. Arch Surg 1949; 48:489–503.

17. Warlitier DC. Pulmonary atelectasis. Anesthesiology 2005; 102:838–854.

18. Murray HW, Ellis GC, Blumenthal DS, et al. Fever and pulmonary thrombo-embolism. Am J Med 1979; 67:232–235.

19. Mackowiak PA, LeMaistre CF. Drug fever: a critical appraisal of conventional concepts. Ann Intern Med 1987; 106:728–733.

20. Cunha B. Drug fever: The importance of recognition. Postgrad Med 1986; 80:123–129.

21. Walden DT, Urrutia F, Soloway RD. Acute acalculous cholecystitis. J Intensive Care Med 1994; 9:235–243.

22. Gonzalez EB, Suarez L, Magee S. Nosocomial (water bed) fever. Arch Intern Med 1990; 150:687 (letter).

Nosocomial Infections

23. Richards MJ, Edwards JR, Culver DH, Gaynes RP. The National Nosocomial Infections Surveillance System. Nosocomial infections in combined medical-surgical intensive care units in the United States. Infect Control Hosp Epidemiol 2000; 21:510–515.

24. Alexander JW, Solomkin JS, Edwards MJ. Updated recommendations for control of surgical site infections. Ann Surg 2011; 253:1082–1093.

25. Loopp FD, Lytle BW, Cosgrove DM, et al. Sternal wound complications after isolated coronary artery bypass grafting: early and late mortality, morbidity, and cost of care. Ann Thorac Surg 1990; 49:179–187.

26. Holzapfel L, Chevret S, Madinier G, et al. Influence of long-term oro- or nasotracheal intubation on nosocomial maxillary sinusitis and pneumonia: results of a prospective, randomized, clinical trial. Crit Care Med 1993; 21:1132–1138.

27. Rouby J-J, Laurent P, Gosnach M, et al. Risk factors and clinical relevance of nosocomial maxillary sinusitis in the critically ill. Am Rev Respir Dis 1994; 150:776–783.

28. Diagnosing sinusitis by x-ray: is a single Waters view adequate? J Gen Intern Med 1992; 7:481–485.

Initial Approach

29. Patel R, Vetter EA, Harmsen WS, et al. Optimized pathogen detection with 30- compared to 20-milliliter blood culture draws. J Clin Microbiol 2011; 49:4047–4051.

30. Cockerill FR, Wilson JW, Vetter EA, et al. Optimal testing parameters for blood cultures. Clin Infect Dis 2004; 38:1724–1730.

31. Hughes WH, Armstrong D, Bodey GP, et al. 2002 guidelines for the use of antimicrobial agents in neutropenic patients with cancer. Clin Infect Dis 2002; 34(6):730–751.

Antipyretic Therapy

32. van Oss CJ, Absolom DR, Moore LL, et al. Effect of temperature on the chemotaxis, phagocytic engulfment, digestion, and O_2 consumption of human polymorphonuclear leukocytes. J Reticuloendothel Soc 1980; 27:561–565.

33. Azocar J, Yunis EJ, Essex M. Sensitivity of human natural killer cells to hyperthermia. Lancet 1982; 1:16–17.

34. Kluger M, Rothenburg BA. Fever and reduced iron: their interaction as a host defense response to bacterial infection. Science 1979; 203:374–376.

35. Small PM, Tauber MG, Hackbarth CJ, Sande MA. Influence of body temperature on bacterial growth rates in experimental pneumococcal meningitis in rabbits. Infect Immun 1986; 52:484–487.

36. Arons MM, Wheeler AP, Bernard GR, et al. Effects of ibuprofen on the physiology and survival of hypothermic sepsis. Critical Care Med 1999; 27:699–707.

37. Clemmer TP, Fisher CJ, Bone RC, et al. Hypothermia in the sepsis syndrome and clinical outcome. Crit Care Med 1990; 18:801–806.

38. Lee BH, Inui D, Sun GY, et al, for Fever and Antipyretic in Critically Ill patients Evaluation (FACE) Study Group. Association of body temperature and antipyretic treatments with mortality of critically ill patients with and without sepsis: multi-centered prospective observational study. Crit Care 2012; 16:R33.

39. Plaisance KI, Mackowiak PA. Antipyretic therapy. Physiologic rationale, diagnostic implications, and clinical consequences. Arch Intern Med 2000; 160:449–456.

40. Drug prescribing information on IV acetaminophen. Cadence Pharmaceuticals. Available at www.ofirmev.com (accessed 6/22/2013).

41. Peacock WF, Breitmeyer JB, Pan C, et al. A randomized study of the efficacy and safety of intravenous acetaminophen compared to oral acetaminophen for the treatment of fever. Acad Emerg Med 2011; 18:360–366.

42. Scott LJ. Intravenous ibuprofen. Drugs 2012; 72:1099–1109.

43. Gerhardt RT, Gerharst DM. Intravenous ketorolac in the treatment of fever. Am J Emerg Med 2000; 18:500–501 (Letter).

NERVOUS SYSTEM DISORDERS

There is no delusion more damaging than to get the idea in your head that you understand the functioning of your brain.

Lewis Thomas
1983

Chapter 44

DISORDERS OF CONSCIOUSNESS

I think, therefore I am.

René Descartes
1644

The ability to recognize and interact with the surroundings (i.e., consciousness) is the *sina qua non* of the life experience, and loss of this ability is one of the dominant (and most prevalent) signs of a life-threatening illness. This chapter describes the principal disorders of consciousness encountered in the ICU, including delirium, coma, and the ultimate disorder of consciousness, brain death.

ALTERED CONSCIOUSNESS

Consciousness has two components: *arousal* and *awareness*.

1. Arousal is the ability to experience your surroundings, and is also known as *wakefulness*.
2. Awareness is the ability to understand your relationship to your surroundings, and is also known as *responsiveness*.

These two components are used to identify the altered states of consciousness in Table 44.1.

Table 44.1	Altered States of Consciousness	
Aroused & Aware	**Aroused & Unaware**	**Unaroused & Unaware**
Anxiety	Delirium	Coma
Lethargy	Dementia	Brain Death
Locked-In State	Psychosis	
	Vegetative State	

Altered States of Consciousness

The principal states of altered consciousness are as follows:

1. *Anxiety* and *lethargy* are conditions where arousal and awareness are intact, but there is a change in *attentiveness* (i.e., the degree of awareness).

2. A *locked-in state* is a condition where arousal and awareness are intact, but there is almost total absence of motor responsiveness. This condition is caused by bilateral injury to the motor pathways in the ventral pons, which disrupts all voluntary movements except up-down ocular movements and eyelid blinking (1).

3. *Delirium* and *dementia* are conditions where arousal is intact, but awareness is altered. The change in awareness can be fluctuating (as in delirium) or permanent (as in dementia).

4. A *vegetative state* is a condition where there is some degree of arousal (eyes can open), but there is no awareness. Spontaneous movements and motor responses to deep pain can occur, but the movements are purposeless. After one month, this condition is called a *persistent vegetative state* (2).

5. *Coma* is characterized by the total absence of arousal and awareness (i.e., unarousable unawareness). Spontaneous movements and motor responses to deep pain can occur, but the movements are purposeless.

6. *Brain death* is similar to coma in that there is a total absence of arousal and awareness. However, brain death differs from coma in two ways: (a) it involves loss of all brainstem function, including cranial nerve activity and spontaneous respirations, and (b) it is always irreversible.

Sources of Altered Consciousness

The nontraumatic causes of altered consciousness are indicated in Figure 44.1. In a prospective survey of neurologic complications in a medical ICU (3), ischemic stroke was the most frequent cause of altered consciousness on admission to the ICU, and septic encephalopathy was the most common cause of altered consciousness that developed after admission to the ICU. Nonconvulsive status epilepticus should always be considered when the source of altered consciousness is not clear (see Chapter 45).

Septic Encephalopathy

Septic encephalopathy is a global brain disorder associated with infections that originate outside the central nervous system. This condition is reported in 50–70% of ICU patients with sepsis, and can be an early sign of infection, especially in elderly patients (3,4). Septic encephalopathy is similar to hepatic encephalopathy (described in Chapter 39) in that both conditions are characterized by cerebral edema, and involve the accumu-

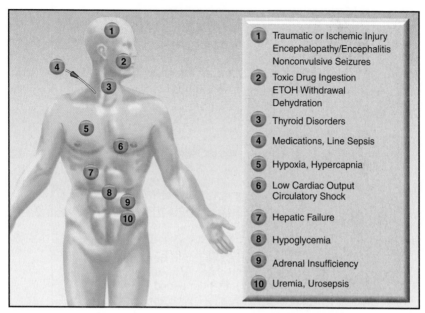

FIGURE 44.1 Sources of altered consciousness in ICU patients.

lation of ammonia and aromatic amino acids (e.g., tryptophan) in the central nervous system (4,5). The origins of septic encephalopathy may be the actions of inflammatory mediators to increase the permeability of the blood-brain barrier, which then allows ammonia and other toxic substances to gain entry into the central nervous system. This is similar to the capillary leak that promotes peripheral edema in septic and anaphylactic shock.

DELIRIUM

Delirium is reported in 16–89% of ICU patients (6), and is particularly prevalent in ventilator-dependent patients (7), and elderly postoperative patients (8). The delirium that accompanies alcohol withdrawal is a different entity than hospital-acquired delirium, and is described in a separate section.

Clinical Features

The clinical features of delirium are summarized in Figure 44.2 (9). Delirium is an acute confusional state with attention deficits, disordered thinking, and a fluctuating course (the fluctuations in behavior occur over a 24-hour period). Over 40% of hospitalized patients with delirium have psychotic symptoms (e.g., visual hallucinations) (10); as a result, delirium is often inappropriately referred to as "ICU psychosis" (11).

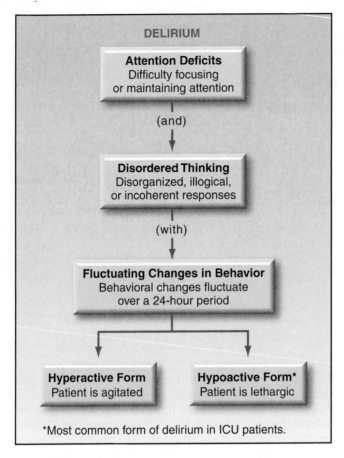

FIGURE 44.2 The clinical features of delirium

Subtypes

The following subtypes of delirium are recognized:

1. *Hyperactive delirium* is characterized by restless agitation. While this form of delirium is common in alcohol withdrawal, it *is rare in hospital-acquired delirium*, accounting for ≤2% of cases (6).

2. *Hypoactive delirium* is characterized by lethargy and somnolence. This *is the most common form of hospital-acquired delirium*, and is responsible for 45–64% of cases (6).

3. *Mixed delirium* is characterized by episodes of delirium that alternate between hyperactive and hypoactive forms of the illness. This type of delirium is reported in 6–55% of patients with hospital-acquired delirium (6).

As indicated, the popular perception of delirium as a state of agitated confusion does not apply to hospital-acquired delirium, where the most common presentation of delirium is lethargy and somnolence. Failure to recognize the hypoactive form of delirium may explain why the diagnosis of delirium is missed in as many as 75% of patients (12).

Delirium vs. Dementia

Delirium and dementia are distinct mental disorders that are often confused because they have overlapping clinical features (i.e., attention deficits and disordered thinking). Furthermore, as many as two-thirds of hospitalized patients with dementia can have a superimposed delirium (8,13), which further blurs the distinction between these two conditions. *The principal features of delirium that distinguish it from dementia are the acute onset and fluctuating course.*

Predisposing Conditions

Several conditions promote delirium in hospitalized patients, including (a) advanced age, (b) sleep deprivation, (c) unrelieved pain, (d) prolonged bed rest, (e) major surgery, (f) encephalopathy, (g) systemic inflammation, and (h) *deliriogenic* drugs (6,8,11).

Deliriogenic Drugs

Several types of drugs can promote delirium, including (a) anticholinergic drugs, (b) dopaminergic drugs, (c) seritonergic drugs, and (d) drugs that promote gamma-amino-butyric-acid (GABA)-mediated neurotransmission, such as benzodiazepines and propofol (6).

Diagnosis

Validated screening tools are recommended for the detection of delirium because (as mentioned earlier) the diagnosis of delirium is frequently missed (12). The *Confusion Assessment Method for the ICU* (CAM-ICU) is the most reliable tool for the detection of delirium (6,9), and it is available (along with an instructional video) at www.icudelirium.org.

Management

Preventive Measures

Recommended measures for reducing the risk of delirium in the ICU include (a) adequate treatment of pain, (b) maintaining regular sleep-wake cycles, (c) promoting out-of-bed time, (d) encouraging family visitation, and (e) limiting the use of deliriogenic drugs like midazolam and lorazepam, if possible (6,8).

DEXMEDETOMIDINE: Sedation with dexmedetomidine, an alpha-2-adrenergic receptor antagonist, is associated with fewer episodes of delirium than lorazepam or midazolam (14,15). This drug provides an alternative to benzodiazepines for sedation in ICU patients who are at risk for delirium (which includes most ICU patients). For more information on dexmedetomidine, see Chapter 51.

Drug Therapy

Drug therapy may be necessary for patients with agitated delirium and disruptive behavior. It is important to *avoid GABA-ergic drugs (e.g., benzodiazepines) for sedation in patients with hospital-acquired delirium* because these drugs promote delirium (6).

DEXMEDETOMIDINE: The most recent guidelines on sedation in the ICU recommend dexmedetomidine for sedation of patients with hospital-acquired delirium (16).

Dosage: Load with 1 µg/kg over 10 min, then infuse at 0.2–0.7 µg/kg/hr.

This drug can cause bradycardia and hypotension (see Chapter 51).

Alcohol Withdrawal Delirium

Alcohol withdrawal delirium, also known as *delirium tremens* or DTs, is characterized by increased motor activity and increased activity on the electroencephalogram (EEG). In contrast, hospital-acquired delirium is characterized by decreased motor activity and slowing of the EEG activity (6).

Pathogenesis

The central nervous system depressant effects of ethanol are the result of stimulation of GABA receptors (the major inhibitory pathway in the brain) and inhibition of N-methyl-D-aspartate (NMDA) receptors (the major excitatory pathway in the brain). When ethanol is withdrawn, the resulting effects on both receptors results in central nervous system excitation, which leads to the agitation, delirium, and seizures that are characteristic features of alcohol withdrawal.

Clinical Features

The clinical features of alcohol withdrawal are shown in Table 44.2. About 5% of patients who experience alcohol withdrawal symptoms will develop DTs (17). Risk factors include a prolonged drinking history, prior episodes of DTs, comorbid illness, and time since last drink. Signs of DTs usually appear 2–3 days after the last drink, and include agitated delirium, low-grade fever, tachycardia, hypertension, diaphoresis, nausea, and vomiting. Associated conditions include dehydration, hypo-kalemia, hypomagnesemia, and generalized seizures. The condition typically lasts for 3–5 days (17), but severe cases can last for up to 2 weeks (personal observation). The reported mortality is 5–15% (17).

WERNICKE'S ENCEPHALOPATHY: Alcoholic patients who are admitted with borderline thiamine stores and receive an intravenous glucose load can develop acute Wernicke's encephalopathy from thiamine deficiency (because thiamine is a cofactor for enzymes involved in glucose metabolism) (18). In this situation, the acute changes in mental status occur 2–3 days after admission, and can be confused with alcohol withdrawal delirium. The presence of nystagmus or oculomotor palsies (e.g., lateral gaze paralysis) will help to identify Wernicke's encephalopathy. (For more information on thiamine deficiency, see Chapter 47.)

Table 44.2	Clinical Features of Alcohol Withdrawal	
Features	**Onset after Last Drink**	**Duration**
Early Withdrawal Anxiety Tremulousness Nausea	6–8 hours	1–2 days
Generalized Seizures	6–48 hours	2–3 days
Hallucinations Visual Auditory Tactile	12–48 hours	1–2 days
Delirium Tremens Fever Tachycardia Hypertension Agitation Delirium	48–96 hours	1–5 days

Adapted from Reference 17.

Treatment

The drugs of choice for treating alcohol withdrawal delirium are the *benzodiazepines* (19), which mimic the CNS depressant effects of alcohol by stimulating GABA receptors in the brain. An added benefit of benzodiazepines is protection against generalized seizures.

ICU REGIMEN: For patients who require care in the ICU, *intravenous lorazepam* is an appropriate choice for the management of DTs (19). For initial control, give 2–4 mg IV every 5–10 minutes until the patient is calm. Thereafter, administer IV lorazepam every 1–2 hours in a dose that maintains calm (a dose of 2–4 mg should be sufficient in most cases). After at least 24 hours of calm, the dose can be tapered to determine if the delirium persists. It is important to taper benzodiazepines as soon as possible because they accumulate and can produce prolonged sedation and a prolonged ICU stay. An additional concern with prolonged administration of IV lorazepam is *propylene glycol toxicity* (see page 605). For more information on benzodiazepines, see Chapter 51.

THIAMINE: The clinical manifestations of DTs can mask an acute Wernicke's encephalopathy that is precipitated by glucose infusions in IV fluids, as described earlier. Therefore, thiamine supplementation is a standard practice during the treatment of DTs. The popular dose is 100 mg daily, which can be given intravenously without harm.

COMA

The patient who is comatose (i.e., unarousable and unaware) is one of the most challenging problems in critical care practice, and the management includes not only the patient, but the patient's family and other intimates as well.

Etiologies

Coma can be the result of any of the following conditions:

1. Diffuse, bilateral cerebral damage.
2. Unilateral cerebral damage causing midline shift with compression of the contralateral cerebral hemisphere.
3. Supratentorial mass lesion causing transtentorial herniation and brainstem compression.
4. Posterior fossa mass lesion causing direct brainstem compression.
5. Toxic or metabolic encephalopathies (including drug overdose).
6. Nonconvulsive status epilepticus.
7. Apparent coma (i.e., locked-in state, hysterical reaction).

The most common causes of coma in one study were cardiac arrest (31%), and either stroke or intracerebral hemorrhage (36%) (20).

Bedside Evaluation

The bedside evaluation of coma should include an evaluation of cranial nerve reflexes, spontaneous eye and body movements, and motor reflexes (20,21). The following elements of the evaluation deserve mention.

Motor Responses

Spontaneous myoclonus (irregular, jerking movements) can be a nonspecific sign of diffuse cerebral dysfunction, or can represent seizure activity (myoclonic seizures), while flaccid extremities can indicate diffuse brain injury or injury to the brainstem. Clonic movements elicited by flexion of the hands or feet (asterixis) is a sign of a diffuse metabolic encephalopathy (20). A focal motor defect in the extremities (e.g., hemiparesis or asymmetric reflexes) is a sign of a space-occupying lesion or spinal cord injury.

RESPONSE TO PAIN: Painful stimulation that elicits a purposeful response (i.e., localization to pain) is not a feature of the comatose state. The responses to pain in the comatose state are either purposeless or absent. With injury to the thalamus, painful stimuli provoke flexion of the upper extremity, which is called *decorticate posturing*. With injury to the midbrain and upper pons, the arms and legs extend and pronate in response to pain; this is called *decerebrate posturing*. Finally, with injury involving the lower brainstem, the extremities remain flaccid during painful stimulation.

Eye Opening

Spontaneous eye opening is an indication of arousal, and is not consistent with the diagnosis of coma. Spontaneous eye opening can be associated with awareness (i.e., locked-in state) or lack of awareness (i.e., vegetative state).

Examination of Pupils

The conditions that affect pupillary size and light reactivity are shown in Table 44.3 (21,22,24).

Table 44.3	Conditions That Affect Pupillary Size and Reactivity
Pupil Size & Reactivity	**Associated Conditions**
⬤ ⬤ (+) (+)	Atropine, anticholinergic toxicity, adrenergic agonists (e.g., dopamine), stimulant drugs (e.g., amphetamines), or nonconvulsive seizures
⬤ ⬤ (–) (–)	Diffuse brain injury, hypothermia (<28°C), or brainstem compression from an expanding intracranial mass or intracranial hypertension
⬤ ⬤ (–) (+)	Expanding intracranial mass (e.g., uncal herniation), ocular trauma or surgery, or focal seizure
⬤ ⬤ (+) (+)	Toxic/metabolic encephalopathy, sedative overdose, or neuromuscular blockade
⬤ ⬤ (–) (–)	Acute liver failure, postanoxic encephalopathy, or brain death
⬤ ● (+) (+)	Horner's Syndrome
● ● (+/–) (+/–)	Opiate overdose, toxic/metabolic encephalopathy, hypercapnia or pontine injury

(+) and (–) indicate a reactive and nonreactive pupil, respectively. From References 21, 22, and 24.

Pupillary findings can be summarized as follows:

1. Dilated, reactive pupils can be the result of drugs (anticholinergics, CNS stimulants, or adrenergic agonists) or nonconvulsive seizures, while dilated, unreactive pupils are a sign of diffuse brain injury or brainstem compression (e.g., from an expanding intracranial mass).

2. A unilateral, dilated and fixed pupil can be the result of ocular trauma or recent ocular surgery, or can be evidence of third cranial nerve dysfunction from an expanding intracranial mass.

3. Midposition, reactive pupils can be the result of a metabolic encephalopathy, a sedative overdose, or neuromuscular blocking drugs, while midposition, unreactive pupils can be seen with acute liver failure, postanoxic encephalopathy, or brain death.

4. Small, reactive pupils can be the result of a metabolic encephalopathy, while pinpoint pupils can be the result of opiate overdose (pupils reactive) or pontine injury (pupils unreactive).

Ocular Motility

Spontaneous eye movements (conjugate or dysconjugate) are a nonspecific sign of toxic or metabolic encephalopathies (22). However, a fixed gaze preference involving one or both eyes is highly suggestive of a mass lesion or seizure activity.

Ocular Reflexes

The ocular reflexes are used to evaluate the functional integrity of the lower brainstem (22). These reflexes are illustrated in Figure 44.3.

OCULOCEPHALIC REFLEX: The oculocephalic reflex is assessed by briskly rotating the head from side-to-side. When the cerebral hemispheres are impaired but the lower brainstem is intact, the eyes will deviate away from the direction of rotation and maintain a forward field of view. When the lower brainstem is damaged (or the patient is awake), the eyes will follow the direction of head rotation. The oculocephalic reflex should *not* be attempted in patients with an unstable cervical spine.

OCULOVESTIBULAR REFLEX: The oculovestibular reflex is performed by injecting 50 mL of cold saline in the external auditory canal of each ear (using a 50 mL syringe and a 2-inch soft plastic angiocatheter). Before the test is performed, check to make sure that the tympanic membrane is intact and that nothing is obstructing the ear canal. When brainstem function is intact, both eyes will deviate slowly toward the irrigated ear. This conjugate eye movement is lost when the lower brainstem is damaged. After the test is performed on one side, wait for 5 minutes before testing the opposite side.

The Glasgow Coma Score

The Glasgow Coma Scale, which is shown in Table 44.4, was introduced to evaluate the severity of traumatic brain injuries (25,26), but has been adopted for use in patients with nontraumatic brain injuries. The Scale consists of three components: 1) eye opening, 2) verbal communication, and 3) motor response to verbal or noxious stimulation. The *Glasgow Coma Score* (GCS) is the sum of the three components. A minimum score of 3 indicates total absence of awareness and responsiveness, while a maximum score of 15 is normal.

Interpretations

The GCS is not reliable in patients who are paralyzed, heavily sedated, or hypotensive. Otherwise, the GCS (best score) can be used as follows:

1. To define coma (GCS ≤ 8).

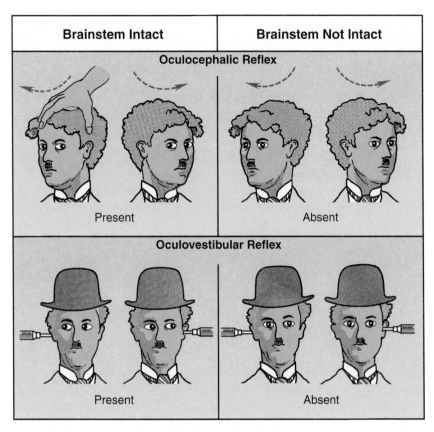

Brainstem Intact	Brainstem Not Intact
Oculocephalic Reflex	
Present	Absent
Oculovestibular Reflex	
Present	Absent

FIGURE 44.3 The ocular reflexes in the evaluation of coma.

2. To stratify the severity of head injury (mild: GCS = 13–15, moderate: GCS = 9–12, severe: GCS ≤ 8) (25,26).

3. To identify candidates for intubation; i.e., airway protective reflexes are typically defective at a GCS ≤ 8, which is used as an indication for endotracheal intubation.

4. As a prognostic marker; e.g., in the initial evaluation of nontraumatic coma, patients with a GCS ≥ 6 are seven-times more likely to awaken within two weeks than patients with a GCS ≤ 5 (27).

5. The influence of induced hypothermia on the prognostic value of the GCS is described in Chapter 17 (see Table 17.5).

INTUBATED PATIENTS: One of the major shortcomings of the Glasgow Coma Scale is the inability to evaluate verbal responses in intubated patients. These patients are assigned a verbal pseudoscore of 1 (for a maximum GCS of 11).

Table 44.4	The Glasgow Coma Scale and Score	
	Points	
Eye Opening:		
Spontaneous	4	
To speech	3	
To pain	2	
None	1	☐ Points
Verbal Communication:		
Oriented	5	
Confused conversation	4	
Inappropriate but recognizable words	3	
Incomprehensible sounds	2	
None	1	☐ Points
Motor Response:		
Obeys commands	6	
Localizes to pain	5	
Withdraws to pain	4	
Abnormal flexion (decorticate response)	3	
Abnormal extension (decerebrate response)	2	
No movement	1	☐ Points
Glasgow Coma Score (Total of 3 scales)*		☐ Points

*Worst score is 3 points, and best score is 15 points. With endotracheal intubation, the highest score is 11.

BRAIN DEATH

The Uniform Determination of Death Act states the following: "An individual who has sustained either 1) irreversible cessation of circulatory and respiratory functions, or 2) irreversible cessation of all functions of the entire brain, including the brainstem, is dead." (28). The second requirement in this statement is the purpose of the brain death determination described here.

Brain death is not a common consequence of the conditions listed in Figure 44.1, and is most often the result of traumatic brain injury and intracerebral hemorrhage, where increased intracranial pressure results in cessation of blood flow to all areas of the brain (29).

Diagnosis

A checklist for the diagnosis of brain death in adults is shown in Table 44.5 (30–32). There is a lack of consensus about minor aspects of the brain

Table 44.5	Checklist for Brain Death Determination in Adults

Instructions:

The patient can be declared legally dead if Steps 1–4 are confirmed, or there is a positive confirmatory test.

Check (✔) Item if Confirmed

Step 1: Prerequisite to Exam:

All of the following conditions should be corrected before beginning the brain death evaluation.   ❑

- Hypotension (mean arterial pressure <65 mm Hg)
- Hypothermia (core temp <32°C or <90°F)
- Hypothyroidism
- Hypoglycemia
- Effects of CNS depressant drugs

Step 2: Establish the Cause of Coma:

The cause of coma is known, and is sufficient to account for irreversible brain death.   ❑

Step 3: Absence of Brain and Brainstem Function:

This step involves two sequential exams. There is no agreement about the length of time required between exams, but 6 hours is a popular choice.

	First Exam	Second Exam
A. The patient is comatose (unaware and unresponsive).	❑	❑
B. The following brainstem reflexes are absent:	❑	❑

- Absent pupillary response to bright light
- Absent corneal reflex
- Absent gag and cough reflexes
- Absent oculocephalic reflex
- Absent deviation of eyes with cold water stimulation of the tympanic membrane

Step 4: Absence of Spontaneous Breathing Efforts:

There are no spontaneous breathing efforts when the arterial PCO_2 is 20 mm Hg above the patient's baseline level (positive apnea test).   ❑

Step 5: Consider Confirmatory Tests:[†]

Confirmatory tests may be necessary when Steps 1–4 cannot be completed or unequivocally interpreted.

[†]Confirmatory testing can include: electroencephalography, transcranial Doppler flow study, somatosensory evoked potentials, brain scan with technetium-99m, or cerebral angiography.

From References 30–32.

death determination, but the consensus goal is to establish: (a) irreversible coma, (b) the absence of brainstem reflexes, and (c) the absence of spontaneous respirations. Prior to performing a brain death examination, other confounding conditions (e.g., hypothermia) should be corrected. If the etiology of the coma is unclear, an electroencephalogram should be performed to search for nonconvulsive status epilepticus. If the clinical evaluation for brain death is equivocal, then confirmatory testing may be required. (See the bottom of Table 44.5 for a list of the accepted confirmatory tests).

The Apnea Test

The most convincing evidence of brain death is the absence of spontaneous respiratory efforts in the face of an acute increase in arterial PCO_2 (which is normally a potent respiratory stimulus). This is evaluated with the apnea test, which involves removing the patient from ventilatory support and observing for spontaneous breathing efforts as the arterial PCO_2 rises. Because the apnea test can cause hypotension, hypoxemia and cardiac arrhythmias, it is typically the last test performed in the brain death determination. The following steps are involved in the apnea test:

1. Prior to the test, the patient is preoxygenated with 100% O_2, and an arterial blood gas is obtained to establish the baseline arterial PCO_2 ($PaCO_2$).

2. The patient is then separated from the ventilator and oxygen is insufflated into the endotracheal tube (apneic oxygenation) to help prevent O_2 desaturation during the apneic period. (A pulse oximeter should be used to monitor the arterial O_2 saturation.)

3. The goal of the apnea test is to allow the $PaCO_2$ to rise 20 mm Hg above baseline. The $PaCO_2$ rises about 3 mm Hg per minute during apnea at normal body temperatures (33), so an apnea period of 6–7 minutes should be sufficient for achieving the target $PaCO_2$. A repeat arterial blood gas is obtained at the end of the apnea period, and the patient is placed back on the ventilator.

4. If apnea persists despite a rise in $PaCO_2 \geq 20$ mm Hg, the test confirms the diagnosis of brain death.

5. The apnea test is risky, and often cannot be completed because of severe O_2 desaturation, hypotension, or serious cardiac arrhythmias (34). If the apnea test cannot be completed, confirmatory testing may be required to establish the diagnosis of brain death.

Lazarus' Sign

Brain-dead patients can exhibit brief, spontaneous movements of the head, torso, or upper extremities (*Lazarus' Sign*), especially after they are removed from the ventilator (35). These movements are the result of neuronal discharges in the cervical spinal cord, possibly in response to hypoxemia, and they can be a source of angst when they appear after the patient has been pronounced brain dead and is removed from the ventilator.

The Potential Organ Donor

For the potential organ donor, the following measures can be used to enhance organ viability (36).

Hemodynamics

Potential organ donors should have a mean arterial pressure ≥ 65 mm Hg and a urine output ≥ 1 mL/kg per hour, and fluids and vasopressors should be used, if necessary, to achieve these goals. Circulatory support for the potential organ donor should follow the same principles of circulatory support used for other critically ill patients (see pages 270–272).

Pituitary Failure

More than half of patients with brain death will develop pituitary failure with *diabetes insipidus and secondary adrenal insufficiency* (37). Both conditions can lead to profound hypovolemia (with reduced organ perfusion) and hypertonic hypernatremia (with cell dehydration). If there is evidence of central diabetes insipidus (i.e., spontaneous diuresis with a urine osmolality below 200 mOsm/L), treatment with *desmopressin*, a vasopressin analog that does not cause vasoconstriction, is advised (38). The usual dose of desmopressin is 0.5–2.0 µg IV every 2–3 hours, with dose titration to maintain a urine output of 100–200 mL/hr.

A FINAL WORD

Family Care

In the care of the patient with persistent coma or a persistent vegetative state, spending time with the patient's family (or other intimates) is as important as patient care. These people will look to you for guidance, and avoiding the *conspiracy of silence* (39) is one of the greatest services you can perform as a physician.

REFERENCES

Altered Consciousness

1. León-Carrión J, van Eeckhout P, Dominguez-Morales Mdel R. The locked-in syndrome: a syndrome looking for a therapy. Brain Inj 2002; 16:555–569.

2. The Multi-Society Task Force on PVS. Medical aspects of the persistent vegetative state (Part 1). N Engl J Med 1994; 330:1499–1508.

3. Bleck TP, Smith MC, Pierre-Louis SJ, et al. Neurologic complications of critical medical illnesses. Crit Care Med 1993; 21:98–103.

4. Papadopoulos M, Davies D, Moss R, et al. Pathophysiology of septic encephalopathy: a review. Crit Care Med 2000; 28:3019–3024.

5. Sprung CL, Cerra FB, Freund HR, et al. Amino acid alterations and encephalopathy in the sepsis syndrome. Crit Care Med 1991; 19:753–757.

Delirium

6. Zaal IJ, Slooter AJC. Delirium in critically ill patients: epidemiology, pathophysiology, diagnosis and management. Drugs, 2012; 72:1457–1471.

7. Ely EW, Shintani A, Truman B, et al. Delirium as a predictor of mortality in mechanically ventilated patients in the intensive care unit. JAMA 2004; 291:1753–1762.

8. Inouye SK. Delirium in older persons. N Engl J Med 2006; 354:1157–1165.

9. Ely EW, Margolin R, Francis J, et al. Evaluation of delirium in critically ill patients: validation of the Confusion Assessment Method for the Intensive Care Unit (CAM-ICU). Crit Care Med 2001; 29:1370–1379.

10. Webster R, Holroyd S. Prevalence of psychotic symptoms in delirium. Psychosomatics 2000; 41:519–522.

11. McGuire BE, Basten CJ, Ryan CJ, et al. Intensive care unit syndrome: a dangerous misnomer. Arch Intern Med 2000; 160:906–909.

12. Inouye SK. The dilemma of delirium: clinical and research controversies regarding diagnosis and evaluation of delirium in hospitalized elderly medical patients. Am J Med 1994; 97:278–288.

13. Fick DM, Agostini JV, Inouye SK. Delirium superimposed on dementia: a systematic review. J Am Geriatr Soc 2002; 50:1723–1732.

14. Pandharipande PP, Pun BT, Herr DL, et al. Effect of sedation with dexmedetomidine vs. lorazepam on acute brain dysfunction on mechanically ventilated patients: the MENDS randomized controlled trial. JAMA 2007; 298:2644–2653.

15. Riker RR, Shehabi Y, Bokesch PM, et al. Dexmedetomidine vs. midazolam for sedation of critically ill patients: a randomized trial. JAMA 2009; 301:489–499.

16. Barr J, Fraser G, Puntillo K, et al. Clinical practice guidelines for the management of pain, agitation, and delirium in adult patients in the intensive care unit. Crit Care Med 2013; 41:263–306.

Delirium Tremens

17. Tetrault JM, O'Connor PG. Substance abuse and withdrawal in the critical care setting. Crit Care Clin 2008; 24:767–788.

18. Attard O, Dietermann JL, Diemunsch P, et al. Wernicke encephalopathy: a complication of parenteral nutrition diagnosed by magnetic resonance imaging. Anesthesiology 2006; 105:847–848.

19. Mayo-Smith MF, Beecher LH, Fischer TL, et al. Management of alcohol withdrawal delirium: an evidence-based practice guideline. Arch Intern Med 2004; 164:1405–1412.

Coma

20. Hamel MB, Goldman L, Teno J, et al. Identification of comatose patients at high risk for death or severe disability. JAMA 1995; 273:1842–1848.

21. Stevens RD, Bhardwaj A. Approach to the comatose patient. Crit Care Med 2006; 34:31–41.

22. Bateman DE. Neurological assessment of coma. J Neurol Neurosurg Psychiatry 2001; 71:i13–i17.

23. Kunze K. Metabolic encephalopathies. J Neurol 2002; 249:1150–1159.

24. Wijdicks EFM. Neurologic manifestations of pharmacologic agents commonly used in the intensive care unit. In: Neurology of critical illness. Philadelphia: F.A. Davis, Co., 1995:3–17.

25. Teasdale G, Jennett B. Assessment of coma and impaired consciousness. A practical scale. Lancet 1974; 2:81–84.

26. Teasdale G, Jennett B. Assessment and prognosis of coma after head injury. Acta Neurochir (Wien) 1976; 34:45–55.

27. Sacco RL, VanGool R, Mohr JP, et al. Nontraumatic coma. Glasgow coma score and coma etiology as predictors of 2-week outcome. Arch Neurol 1990; 47:1181–1184.

Brain Death

28. Uniform Determination of Death Act, 12 uniform laws annotated 589 (West 1993 and West suppl 1997).

29. Smith AJ, Walker AE. Cerebral blood flow and brain metabolism as indicators of cerebral death. A review. Johns Hopkins Med J 1973; 133:107–119.

30. The Quality Standards Subcommittee of the American Academy of Neurology. Practice parameters for determining brain death in adults (summary statement). Neurology 1995; 45:1012–1014.

31. Wijdicks EFM, Varelas PNV, Gronseth GS, Greer DM. Evidence-based guideline update: determining brain-death in adults. Report of the Quality Standards Subcommittee of the American Academy of Neurology. Neurology 2010; 74:1911–1918.

32. Wijdicks EF. The diagnosis of brain death. N Engl J Med 2001; 344:1215–1221.

33. Dominguez-Roldan JM, Barrera-Chacon JM, Murillo-Cabezas F, et al. Clinical factors influencing the increment of blood carbon dioxide during the apnea test for the diagnosis of brain death. Transplant Proc 1999; 31:2599–2600.

34. Goudreau JL, Wijdicks EF, Emery SF. Complications during apnea testing in the determination of brain death: predisposing factors. Neurology 2000; 55:1045–1048.

35. Ropper AH. Unusual spontaneous movements in brain-dead patients. Neurology 1984; 34:1089–1092.

The Potential Organ Donor

36. Wood KE, Becker BN, McCartney JG, et al. Care of the potential organ donor. N Engl J Med 2004; 351:2730–2739.

37. Detterbeck FC, Mill MR. Organ donation and the management of the multiple organ donor. Contemp Surg 1993; 42:281–285.

38. Guesde R, Barrou B, Leblanc I, et al. Administration of desmopressin in brain-dead donors and renal function in kidney recipients. Lancet 1998; 352:1178–1181.

A Final Word

39. Fallowfield LJ, Jenkins VA, Beveridge HA. Truth may hurt but deceit hurts more: communication in palliative care. Palliative Med 2002; 16:297–303.

Chapter 45

DISORDERS OF MOVEMENT

When we contemplate this life, we see motion as its principal characteristic,
and when we take a farther view, we see that this motion must necessarily
waste the machine in which it resides.

John Young
Senior Dissertation
Univ. PA School of Medicine
1803

This chapter describes three types of movement disorder that you are likely to encounter in the ICU: (a) involuntary movements (i.e., seizures), (b) weak or ineffective movements (i.e., neuromuscular weakness), and (c) no movements (i.e., drug-induced paralysis). These disorders share one common trait, which is the ability to "waste" the human machine.

SEIZURES

Seizures are second only to metabolic encephalopathy as the most common neurological complication in critically ill patients (1). The incidence of new-onset seizures in ICU patients is 0.8–3.5% (1,2).

Types Of Seizures

Seizures are classified by the extent of brain involvement (generalized vs. focal seizures), the presence or absence of abnormal movements (convulsive vs. nonconvulsive seizures), and the type of movement abnormality (e.g., tonic-clonic, myoclonic movements).

Abnormal Movements

The movements associated with seizures can be *tonic* (caused by sustained muscle contraction), *clonic* (rhythmic movements with a regular amplitude and frequency), or *myoclonic* (irregular movements that vary

817

in amplitude and frequency) (3). Some movements are familiar (e.g., chewing) but repetitive; these are called *automatisms*.

Generalized Seizures

Generalized seizures arise from synchronous, rhythmic electrical discharges that involve most of the cerebral cortex, and they are always associated with loss of consciousness (3). These seizures typically produce tonic-clonic movements of the extremities, but they can also occur without abnormal movements (generalized nonconvulsive seizures) (4).

Partial Seizures

Partial seizures can arise from diffuse or localized rhythmic discharges in the brain, and the clinical manifestations can vary widely, as demonstrated by the following two examples of partial seizures.

1. *Partial complex seizures* are nonconvulsive seizures that produce behavioral changes. The typical manifestation is a patient who is awake but not aware of the surroundings (similar to absence seizures). They are often preceded by an aura (e.g., a particular smell), and can be accompanied by repetitive chewing motions or lip smacking (automatisms).

2. *Epilepsia partialis continua* is a convulsive seizure that is characterized by persistent tonic-clonic movements of the facial and limb muscles on one side of the body.

Myoclonus

Myoclonus is characterized by irregular jerking movements of the extremities, which can occur spontaneously, or in response to painful stimuli or loud noises (*startle myoclonus*). These movements can be seen in any type of encephalopathy (metabolic, ischemic). In patients who do not awaken in the hours following a cardiac arrest, the presence of myoclonus that lasts longer than 24 hours carries a poor prognosis for neurologic recovery (5). Myoclonus is not universally regarded as a seizure, because it is not associated with rhythmic discharges on the EEG (6).

Status Epilepticus

Status epilepticus is traditionally defined as more than 30 minutes of either continuous seizure activity, or recurrent seizure activity without a period of recovery (6). Since generalized convulsive seizures are unlikely to stop after 5 minutes, a recently proposed definition of *status epilepticus is 5 minutes of continuous seizure activity, or two seizures without an intervening period of consciousness* (7). Status epilepticus can involve any type of seizure, and can be "convulsive" (i.e., associated with abnormal body movements) or "nonconvulsive" (i.e., not associated with abnormal body movements).

NONCONVULSIVE STATUS EPILEPTICUS: Most cases of nonconvulsive status epilepticus involve partial complex seizures (which are not common in ICU patients), but as many as 25% of generalized seizures can be nonconvulsive (8). Generalized nonconvulsive status epilepticus is also known as *subtle status epilepticus*, and typically occurs when generalized convulsive seizures have not been adequately treated (4). These seizures are associated with loss of consciousness, and they are a source of unexplained coma in the ICU. In one study, generalized nonconvulsive seizures were responsible for 8% of cases of coma in ICU patients (9). The diagnosis requires evidence of epileptiform discharges on the EEG.

Predisposing Conditions

A variety of conditions can produce seizures in critically ill patients, as indicated in Table 45.1. In one survey of new-onset seizures in ICUs, the most common predisposing conditions were drug intoxication, drug withdrawal, and metabolic abnormalities (e.g., hypoglycemia) (2).

Table 45.1	Conditions That Promote Seizures in the ICU
Most Common†	**Less Common**
Drug Toxicity	**Ischemic**
Amphetamines	Stroke
Cocaine	Cardiac arrest
Tricyclics	
	Traumatic
Drug Withdrawal	Intracranial hemorrhage
Barbiturates	Intracranial hypertension
Benzodiazepines	
Ethanol	**Infectious**
Opiates	Abscess
	Meningoencephalitis
Metabolic	Septic Emboli
Hypoglycemia	
Hypoxia	**Hematologic**
Uremia	DIC
Liver failure	TTP

†From Reference 2. DIC = disseminated intravascular coagulopathy, TTP = thrombotic thrombocytopenia purpura.

Acute Management

The acute management described here pertains to generalized status epilepticus (GSE), both convulsive and nonconvulsive. The approach is divided into three stages, and the recommended drug dosing regimens for each stage are shown in Tables 45.2 and 45.3 (6,7).

Stage 1 Drugs

The most effective drugs for rapid termination of generalized seizures are the benzodiazepines, which terminate 65–80% of convulsive seizures within 2–3 minutes (10,11).

LORAZEPAM: Intravenous lorazepam (4 mg IV over 2 minutes) is the drug regimen of choice for terminating GSE. The onset of action is less than two minutes, and the effect lasts for 12–24 hours (11,12).

MIDAZOLAM: The benefit of midazolam is rapid uptake when given by intramuscular (IM) injection. When intravenous access is not available or difficult to establish, midazolam can be given IM in a dose of 10 mg, and the efficacy in terminating GSE is equivalent to IV lorazepam (13). If the time to establish intravenous access is considered, IM midazolam produces more rapid suppression of seizures (3–4 minutes) than IV lorazepam (13). This approach is well suited for prehospital control of GSE.

Stage 2 Drugs

Stage 2 drugs are used for seizures that are refractory to benzodiazepines, or are likely to recur within 24 hours. The drug-of-choice for this purpose is phenytoin.

PHENYTOIN: The initial IV dose of phenytoin is 20 mg/kg, with a second dose of 10 mg/kg, if necessary. The goal is a serum phenytoin level of 10–20 µg/mL. Phenytoin cannot be infused at a rate above 50 mg/min because of the risk of cardiac depression and hypotension. This means that, for a 70 kg adult, the initial dose of phenytoin (20 mg/kg) will require 30 minutes to complete, and this is a disadvantage when GSE has not resolved (i.e., is refractory to benzodiazepines). The cardiac depression is attributed propylene glycol, which is used as a solvent in IV phenytoin preparations.

FOSPHENYTOIN: Fosphenytoin is a water-soluble phenytoin analogue that produces less cardiac depression than phenytoin because it does not contain propylene glycol. As a result, fosphenytoin can be infused three times faster than phenytoin (150 mg/min vs. 50 mg/min) (14). Fosphenytoin is a prodrug (must be converted to phenytoin), and is given in the same doses as phenytoin.

ALTERNATIVE DRUGS: Intravenous *valproic acid* (20–40 mg/kg) is as effective as phenytoin in terminating GSE (15), but is recommended only when phenytoin cannot be given (e.g., because of a drug allergy) (6,7). Another alternative to phenytoin is *levetiracetam* (1,000–3,000 mg IV), which has a better safety profile than valproic acid, but has not been evaluated as extensively.

Stage 3: Refractory Status Epilepticus

Ten percent of patients with GSE are refractory to stage 1 and 2 drugs (8). The recommended treatment at this point is anesthetic doses of one of the drugs in Table 45.3. Pentobarbital may be the favored drug in this situation (16). At this stage, a neurology consult is the best option.

Table 45.2	Drug Regimens for Generalized Status Epilepticus
Drug	**Dosing Regimens and Comments**
Stage 1 Drugs	
Lorazepam	Dosing: 4 mg IV over 2 min. Repeat in 5 min, if necessary.
	Comment: The drug regimen of choice for terminating generalized seizure. The effect lasts 12–24 hrs.
Midazolam	Dosing: 10 mg by intramuscular (IM) injection.
	Comment: IM midazolam can be used when IV access is not available (e.g., in the field). As effective as IV lorazepam.
Stage 2 Drugs	
Phenytoin	Dosing: 20 mg/kg IV at ≤50 mg/min. Another 10 mg/kg can be given 10 min. after the initial dose, if necessary.
	Comment: IV preparation has propylene glycol as solvent, which promotes hypotension when injected rapidly.
Fosphenytoin	Dosing: 20 mg/kg IV at ≤150 mg/min. Another 10 mg/kg can be given 10 min. after the initial dose, if necessary.
	Comment: Can be given 3 times faster than phenytoin because it is water soluble, and has no propylene glycol.
Alternate Stage 2 Drugs	
Valproic Acid	Dosing: 20–40 mg/kg IV at 3–6 mg/kg/min. Can give another 20 mg/kg IV at 10 min after the initial dose, if necessary.
	Comment: May be as effective as phenytoin, but is recommended only when phenytoin cannot be used (e.g., drug allergy).
Levetiracetam	Dosing: 1,000–3,000 mg IV over 5–10 min.
	Comment: This drug has a better safety profile than valproic acid, but the clinical experience in status epilepticus is limited.

Dosing regimens from References 6 and 7.

Outcomes

The in-hospital mortality rates are as high as 21% for convulsive GSE, as high as 52% for nonconvulsive GSE, and as high as 61% for refractory GSE (7).

Table 45.3	Drug Regimens for Refractory Status Epilepticus
Drug	**Dosing Regimens**
Pentobarbital	Load with 5–15 mg/kg IV over one hr, then infuse at 0.5–1 mg/kg/hr. If necessary, increase infusion rate up to 3 mg/kg/hr (maximum rate).
Thiopental	Start with an IV bolus of 3–5 mg/kg, and follow with 1–2 mg/kg every 2–3 min until seizures subside. Then infuse 3–7 mg/kg/hr for the next 24 hrs.
Midazolam	Load with 0.2 mg/kg IV, then infuse at 4–10 mg/kg/hr.
Propofol	Start with IV bolus of 2–3 mg/kg, and use further boluses of 1–2 mg/kg, if needed, until seizure activity subsides. Then infuse at 4–10 mg/kg/hr for 24 hrs.

Dosing regimens from Reference 6.

NEUROMUSCULAR WEAKNESS SYNDROMES

The following is a description of the acute neuromuscular weakness syndromes that you may encounter in an ICU.

Myasthenia Gravis

Myasthenia gravis (MG) is an autoimmune disease produced by antibody-mediated destruction of acetylcholine receptors on the postsynaptic side of neuromuscular junctions (17).

Predisposing Conditions

MG can be triggered by major surgery or a concurrent illness. Thymic tumors are responsible for up to 20% of cases, and hyperthyroidism is the culprit in 5% of cases. Several drugs can precipitate or aggravate MG (17). The principal offenders are antibiotics (e.g., aminoglycosides, ciprofloxacin) and cardiac drugs (e.g., beta-adrenergic blockers, lidocaine, procainamide, quinidine).

Clinical Features

The muscle weakness in MG has the following features:

1. The weakness worsens with activity and improves with rest.
2. Weakness is first apparent in the eyelids and extraocular muscles, and limb weakness follows in 85% of cases (19).
3. Progressive weakness often involves the chest wall and diaphragm, and rapid progression to respiratory failure, called *myasthenic crisis,* occurs in 15–20% of patients (18).
4. The deficit is purely motor, and deep tendon reflexes are preserved (see Table 45.4).

Diagnosis

The diagnosis of MG is suggested by weakness in the eyelids or extraocular muscles that worsens with repeated use. The diagnosis is confirmed by: (a) increased muscle strength after the administration of edrophonium (Tensilon), an acetylcholinesterase inhibitor, and (b) a positive assay for acetylcholine receptor antibodies in the blood, which are present in 85% of patients of MG (17).

Treatment

The first line of therapy is an acetylcholinesterase inhibitor, *pyridostigmine* (Mestinon), which is started at an oral dose of 60 mg every 6 hours, and can be increased to 120 mg every 6 hours if necessary (20,21). Pyridostigmine can be given intravenously to treat myasthenic crisis: the IV dose is 1/30th of the oral dose (19,20).

Immunotherapy is added, if needed, using either *prednisone* (1–1.5 mg/kg/day), *azathioprine* (1–3 mg/kg/day), *or cyclosporine* (2.5 mg/kg twice daily) (21). To reduce the need for long-term immunosuppressive therapy, surgical thymectomy is often advised in patients under 60 years of age (21).

ADVANCED CASES: In advanced cases requiring mechanical ventilation, there are two treatment options: (a) plasmapharesis to clear pathological antibodies from the bloodstream, or (b) administration of immunoglobulin G (0.4 or 2 gm/kg/day IV for 2–5 days) to neutralize the pathologic antibodies. Both approaches are equally effective (19,21), but plasmapharesis produces a more rapid response (21).

Table 45.4	Comparative Features of Myasthenia Gravis and Guillain-Barré Syndrome	
Features	Myasthenia Gravis	Guillain-Barré Syndrome
Ocular weakness	Yes	No
Fluctuating weakness	Yes	No
Bulbar weakness	Yes	No
Deep tendon reflexes	Intact	Depressed
Autonomic instability	No	Yes
Nerve conduction	Normal	Slowed

Guillain-Barré Syndrome

The Guillain-Barré syndrome is a *subacute inflammatory demyelinating polyneuropathy* that often follows an acute infectious illness (by 1–3 weeks) (22,23). An immune etiology is suspected.

Clinical Features

The presenting features of the Guillain-Barré syndrome include paresthesias and symmetric limb weakness that evolves over a period of a few days to a few weeks. Progression to respiratory failure occurs in 25% of cases (22), and autonomic instability can be a feature in advanced cases (24). The condition resolves spontaneously in about 80% of cases, but residual neurological deficits are common (22).

Diagnosis

The diagnosis of Guillain-Barré syndrome is based on the clinical presentation (paresthesias and symmetric limb weakness), nerve conduction studies (slowed conduction), and cerebrospinal fluid analysis (elevated protein in 80% of cases) (22). The features that distinguish the Guillain-Barré syndrome from myasthenia gravis are shown in Table 45.4.

Treatment

Treatment is mostly supportive, but in advanced cases with respiratory failure, *plasmapharesis or intravenous immunoglobulin G* (0.4 g/kg/day for 5 days) are equally effective in producing short-term improvement (23). Immunoglobulin G is often preferred because it is easier to carry out.

Critical Illness Neuromyopathy

The disorders known as *critical illness polyneuropathy* (CIP) and *critical illness myopathy* (CIM) are secondary disorders, and typically accompany severe sepsis and other conditions associated with progressive systemic inflammation (25). These disorders often co-exist in the same patient, and become apparent when patients fail to wean from mechanical ventilation.

Pathogenesis

CIP is a diffuse sensory and motor axonal neuropathy that is discovered in at least 50% of patients with severe sepsis and septic shock (25–27). The onset is variable, occurring from 2 days to a few weeks after the onset of the septic episode. CIP is considered the most common peripheral neuropathy in critically ill patients (28)

CIM is a diffuse inflammatory myopathy that involves both limb and truncal muscles (29). Predisposing conditions include severe sepsis and septic shock, and prolonged periods of drug-induced neuromuscular paralysis, particularly when combined with high-dose corticosteroid therapy (25,26,29). CIM has also been reported in one-third of patients with status asthmaticus who are treated with high-dose corticosteroids (29).

Clinical Features

As just mentioned, CIP and CIM often go undetected until there is an unexplained failure to remove a patient from mechanical ventilation. Physical examination will then reveal a flaccid quadriparesis with hyporeflexia or areflexia. The diagnosis of CIP can be confirmed by nerve conduction studies (which show slowed conduction in sensory and motor fibers) (27), and the diagnosis of CIM can be confirmed by electromyography (which shows myopathic changes) and by muscle biopsy (which shows atrophy, loss of myosin filaments, and inflammatory infiltration) (29).

There is no treatment for CIP or CIM. Complete recovery is expected in about half the patients (27), but it can takes months to recover.

DRUG-INDUCED PARALYSIS

Drug-induced paralysis is used in the following situations: (a) to facilitate endotracheal intubation, (b) to prevent shivering during induced hypothermia (in comatose survivors of cardiac arrest), and (c) to facilitate mechanical ventilation in severely agitated patients (30). The latter practice is frowned upon for reasons stated later.

Neuromuscular blocking agents act by binding to acetylcholine receptors on the postsynaptic side of the neuromuscular junction. Once bound, there are two different modes of action: (a) *depolarizing agents* act like acetylcholine and produce a sustained depolarization of the post-synaptic membrane, and (b) *non-depolarizing agents* act by inhibiting depolarization of the post-synaptic membrane.

Commonly Used Agents

The comparative features of three commonly used neuromuscular blocking agents are shown in Table 45.5 (31).

Table 45.5	Features of Commonly Used Neuromuscular Blocking Agents		
	Succinylcholine	**Rocuronium**	**Cisatracurium**
IV Bolus Dose	1 mg/kg	0.6 mg/kg	0.1 mg/kg
Onset Time	1–1.5 min	1.5–3 min	5–7 min
Recovery Time	10–12 min	30–40 min	40–50 min
Infusion Rate	—	5–10 µg/kg/min	2–5 µg/kg/min
Cardiovascular Effects	Bradycardia	None	None
Effects of Renal or Liver Failure	None	Prolonged effect in liver failure	None

From Reference 2.

Succinylcholine

Succinylcholine is a depolarizing agent with a rapid onset of action (60–90 seconds) and a rapid recovery time (10–12 minutes). Because of these features, succinylcholine is used to facilitate endotracheal intubation.

SIDE EFFECTS: Succinylcholine-induced depolarization of skeletal muscle promotes the efflux of potassium from muscle cells. This can be associated with a 0.5 mEq/L rise in the serum potassium (32), but this effect is transient and without consequence. However, life-threatening hyperkalemia can occur when succinylcholine is given to patients with skeletal muscle "denervation injury" (e.g., from head or spinal cord injury), or patients with rhabdomyolysis, burns, or chronic immobility. As a result, succinylcholine is not advised for patients with these conditions.

Rocuronium

Rocuronium is a non-depolarizing neuromuscular blocker with a rapid onset of action (1.5–3 minutes) and an "intermediate" recovery time (30–40 min). Because of the rapid onset of action, rocuronium can be used for endotracheal intubation when succinylcholine is not advised. However, larger doses (1 mg/kg) are required for intubation, and this will prolong the recovery time (31). Rocuronium can be infused at a rate of 5–10 µg/kg/min for prolonged neuromuscular paralysis. The drug is well tolerated, and has no cardiovascular side effects. Rocuronium has gradually replaced a related neuromuscular blocker, vecuronium, because of its rapid onset of action.

Cisatracurium

Cisatracurium is a non-depolarizing agent with a prolonged onset of action (5–7 min) and an "intermediate" recovery time. It is an isomer of atracurium (another neuromuscular blocker), and was developed to eliminate the histamine release associated with atracurium. Cisatracurium can be infused at a rate of 2–5 µg/kg/min for prolonged neuromuscular paralysis, and the drug is well suited for ICU patients because blood levels are not influenced by renal or liver dysfunction (31).

Monitoring

The standard method of monitoring drug-induced paralysis is to apply a series of four low-frequency (2 Hz) electrical pulses to the ulnar nerve at the forearm, and observe for adduction of the thumb. Total absence of thumb adduction is evidence of excessive block. The desired goal is 1 or 2 perceptible twitches, and the drug infusion is adjusted to achieve that end-point (30).

Avoiding Drug-Induced Paralysis

The experience of being awake while paralyzed is both horrifying and painful (33), and it is imperative to keep patients heavily sedated while they are paralyzed. However, it is not possible to evaluate the adequacy of sedation or pain control while a patient is paralyzed. The inability to insure adequate sedation and pain control is the major reason to avoid drug-induced paralysis whenever possible. Avoiding prolonged periods of neuromuscular paralysis will also reduce the risk of the following complications:

1. Critical illness myopathy (explained earlier).
2. "Hypostatic" pneumonia (from pooling of respiratory secretions in dependent lung regions).
3. Venous thromboembolism (from prolonged immobilization).
4. Pressure ulcers on the skin (also from prolonged immobilization).

A FINAL WORD

Inflammation Strikes Again

One of the central themes in this book is the widespread harm inflicted by progressive systemic inflammation in critically ill patients. Inflammatory injury is responsible for the acute respiratory distress syndrome (see Chapter 23) and acute kidney injury (see Chapter 34), as well as the multiorgan failure associated with septic shock (see Chapter 14). In this chapter, we learn that inflammation can also damage peripheral nerves (i.e., critical illness polyneuropathy) and skeletal muscle (i.e., critical illness myopathy). These injuries support the notion that inflammation is the most lethal force that you will face in the ICU.

REFERENCES

Seizures

1. Bleck TP, Smith MC, Pierre-Louis SJ, et al. Neurologic complications of critical medical illnesses. Crit Care Med 1993; 21:98–103.
2. Wijdicks EF, Sharbrough FW. New-onset seizures in critically ill patients. Neurology 1993; 43:1042–1044.
3. Chabolla DR. Characteristics of the epilepsies. Mayo Clin Proc 2002; 77:981–990.
4. Holtkamp M, Meierkord H. Nonconvulsive status epilepticus: a diagnostic and therapeutic challenge in the intensive care setting. Ther Adv Neurol Disorders 2011; 4:169–181.
5. Wijdicks EF, Parisi JE, Sharbrough FW. Prognostic value of myoclonus status in comatose survivors of cardiac arrest. Ann Neurol 1994; 35:239–243.
6. Meierkord H, Boon P, Engelsen B, et al. EFNS guideline on the management of status epilepticus in adults. Eur J Neurol 2010; 17:348–355.
7. Brophy GM, Bell R, Claassen J, et al. Guidelines for the evaluation and management of status epilepticus. Neurocrit Care 2012; 17:3–23.
8. Marik PE, Varon J. The management of status epilepticus. Chest 2004; 126:582–591.
9. Towne AR, Waterhouse EJ, Boggs JG, et al. Prevalence of nonconvulsive status epilepticus in comatose patients. Neurology 2000; 54:340–345.

10. Treiman DM, Meyers PD, Walton NY, et al. A comparison of four treatments for generalized convulsive status epilepticus. N Engl J Med 1998; 339:792–798.

11. Lowenstein DH, Alldredge BK. Status epilepticus. N Engl J Med 1998; 338:970–976.

12. Manno EM. New management strategies in the treatment of status epilepticus. Mayo Clin Proc 2003 ;78:508–518.

13. Silbergleit R, Durkalsi V, Lowenstein D, et al. Intramuscular versus intravenous therapy for prehospital status epilepticus. N Engl J Med 2012; 366:591–600.

14. Fischer JH, Patel TV, Fischer PA. Fosphenytoin: clinical pharmacokinetics and comparative advantages in the acute treatment of seizures. Clin Pharmacokinet 2003; 42:33–58.

15. Misra UK, Kalita J, Patel R. Sodium valproate vs. phenytoin in status epilepticus: a pilot study. Neurology 2006; 67:340–342.

16. Claassen J, Hirsch LJ, Emerson RG, et al. Treatment of refractory status epilepticus with pentobarbital, propofol, or midazolam: a systematic review. Epilepsia 2002; 43:146–153.

Myasthenia Gravis

17. Vincent A, Palace J, Hilton-Jones D. Myasthenia gravis. Lancet 2001; 357:2122–2128.

18. Wittbrodt ET. Drugs and myasthenia gravis. An update. Arch Intern Med 1997; 157:399–408.

19. Drachman DB. Myasthenia gravis. N Engl J Med 1994; 330:1797–1810.

20. Berrouschot J, Baumann I, Kalischewski P, et al. Therapy of myasthenic crisis. Crit Care Med 1997; 25:1228–1235.

21. Saperstein DS, Barohn RJ. Management of myasthenia gravis. Semin Neurol 2004; 24:41–48.

Guillain-Barré Syndrome

22. Hughes RA, Cornblath DR. Guillain-Barré syndrome. Lancet 2005; 366:1653–1666.

23. Hund EF, Borel CO, Cornblath DR, et al. Intensive management and treatment of severe Guillain-Barré syndrome. Crit Care Med 1993; 21:433–446.

24. Pfeiffer G, Schiller B, Kruse J, et al. Indicators of dysautonomia in severe Guillain-Barré syndrome. J Neurol 1999; 246:1015–1022.

Critical Illness Neuromyopathy

25. Hund E. Neurological complications of sepsis: critical illness polyneuropathy and myopathy. J Neurol 2001; 248:929–934.

26. Bolton CF. Neuromuscular manifestations of critical illness. Muscle & Nerve 2005; 32:140–163.

27. van Mook WN, Hulsewe-Evers RP. Critical illness polyneuropathy. Curr Opin Crit Care 2002; 8:302–310.

28. Maramatton BV, Wijdicks EFM. Acute neuromuscular weakness in the intensive care unit. Crit Care Med 2006; 34:2835–2841.

29. Lacomis D. Critical illness myopathy. Curr Rheumatol Rep 2002; 4:403–408.

Drug-Induced Paralysis

30. Murray MJ, Cowen J, DeBlock H, et al. Clinical practice guidelines for sustained neuromuscular blockade in the adult critically ill patient. Crit Care Med 2002; 30:142–156.

31. Donati F, Bevan DR. Neuromuscular blocking agents. In: Barash PG, Cullen BF, Stoelting RK, et al, eds. Clinical Anesthesia. 6th ed. Philadelphia: Lippincott Williams & Wilkins, 2009:498–530.

32. Koide M, Waud BE. Serum potassium concentrations after succinylcholine in patients with renal failure. Anesthesiology 1972; 36:142–145.

33. Parker MM, Schubert W, Shelhamer JH, et al. Perceptions of a critically ill patient experiencing therapeutic paralysis in an ICU. Crit Care Med 1984; 12:69–71.

Chapter 46

ACUTE STROKE

Disease makes men more physical,
it leaves them nothing but body.

Thomas Mann

The focus of this chapter is a cerebrovascular disorder that was first described over 2,400 years ago, and since then has suffered through a variety of inappropriate names like *apoplexy, cerebrovascular accident* (what accident?), *stroke,* and the most recent embarrassment, *brain attack.* Considering that this disorder is responsible for one death every 4 seconds in the United States (1), it deserves a better name.

This chapter describes the initial evaluation and management of acute stroke, with an emphasis on the recommendations for thrombolytic therapy in acute stroke from the American Heart Association (2).

DEFINITIONS

Stroke

Stroke is defined as "an acute brain disorder of vascular origin accompanied by neurological dysfunction that persists for longer than 24 hours" (3). The neurological dysfunction is usually localized or focal (which is typical of vascular occlusion); however, global dysfunction can occur when vascular rupture leads to hemorrhage and mass effect.

Classification

Stroke is classified according to the responsible mechanism.

1. *Ischemic stroke* accounts for 87% of all strokes (1): 80% of ischemic strokes are *thrombotic strokes,* and 20% are *embolic strokes.* Most emboli originate from thrombi in the left atrium (from atrial fibrillation) or left ventricle (from acute MI), but some originate from venous thrombi in the legs that reach the brain through a patent foramen ovale (4).

2. *Hemorrhagic stroke* accounts for 13% of all strokes: 97% of hemor-

rhagic strokes involve intracerebral hemorrhage, and 3% are the result of subarachnoid hemorrhage (1).

Transient Ischemic Attack

A transient ischemic attack (TIA) is an acute episode of ischemia with focal loss of brain function that lasts less than 24 hours (3). The feature that distinguishes TIA from stroke is the *reversibility of clinical symptoms* in TIAs. This does not apply to reversibility of cerebral injury, because *one-third of TIAs are associated with cerebral infarction* (5,6).

INITIAL EVALUATION

The evaluation of a patient with suspected acute stroke must proceed quickly. *Each minute of cerebral infarction results in the destruction of 1.9 million neurons and 7.5 miles of myelinated nerves* (7), and continued tissue destruction eventually leads to a point where reperfusion of occluded arteries with thrombolytic therapy will not promote neurological recovery. This point occurs 4–5 hours after stroke onset, where the benefit from thrombolytic therapy is lost.

Bedside Evaluation

Stroke has traditionally been a clinical diagnosis (although diffusion-weighted MRI will change this, as described later), and the area of brain that is injured determines the clinical presentation. Figure 46.1 shows the clinical features of stroke in relation to the area of brain that is damaged. Some of the notable manifestations of acute stroke are described next.

Mental Status

Most cerebral infarctions are unilateral, and do not result in loss of consciousness (8). When focal neurological deficits are accompanied by coma, the most likely conditions are intracerebral hemorrhage, brainstem infarction, or nonconvulsive seizures.

APHASIA: Injury in the left cerebral hemisphere (which is the dominant hemisphere for speech in 90% of patients) produces *aphasia*, which is a disturbance in the comprehension and/or formulation of language. Patients with aphasia can have difficulty with verbal comprehension (*receptive aphasia*), or difficulty with verbal expression (*expressive aphasia*), or both (*global aphasia*).

Sensorimotor Loss

The hallmark of injury involving one cerebral hemisphere is weakness on the opposite or contralateral side of the face and body (i.e., hemiparesis). The presence of hemiparesis or isolated limb weakness creates a high index of suspicion for stroke (or TIA), but focal limb weakness can be the result of nonconvulsive status epilepticus, and hemiparesis has been reported in patients with hepatic and septic encephalopathy (9,10).

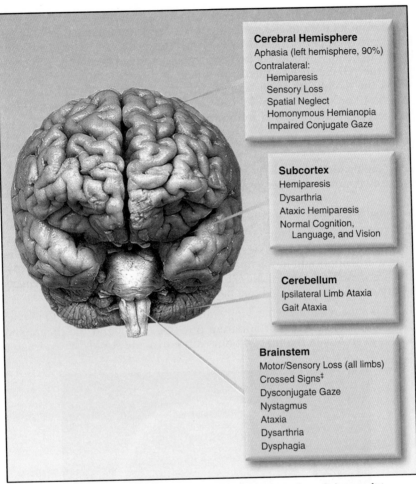

Cerebral Hemisphere
Aphasia (left hemisphere, 90%)
Contralateral:
  Hemiparesis
  Sensory Loss
  Spatial Neglect
  Homonymous Hemianopia
  Impaired Conjugate Gaze

Subcortex
Hemiparesis
Dysarthria
Ataxic Hemiparesis
Normal Cognition,
  Language, and Vision

Cerebellum
Ipsilateral Limb Ataxia
Gait Ataxia

Brainstem
Motor/Sensory Loss (all limbs)
Crossed Signs[‡]
Dysconjugate Gaze
Nystagmus
Ataxia
Dysarthria
Dysphagia

FIGURE 46.1 Areas of brain injury and corresponding neurological abnormalities.
‡Indicates deficits involving the same side of the face and the opposite side of the body.

Stroke Mimics

For patients admitted to the hospital with a suspected stroke based on clinical findings, as many as 30% of the patients will have another condition that mimics an acute stroke (11). The most common stroke mimics are seizures, sepsis, metabolic encephalopathies, and space-occupying lesions (in that order) (11). Since stroke is primarily a clinical diagnosis, at least in the first 24–48 hours, stroke mimics are a source of excessive hospital admissions (and thrombolytic therapy) for suspected stroke.

NIH Stroke Scale

The use of a clinical scoring system is recommended to standardize the evaluation of acute stroke (2), and the most validated scoring system is the NIH Stroke Scale (NIHSS). The NIHSS evaluates 11 different aspects of performance, and rates each performance with a number from zero to 3 or 4. The total score is a measure of the severity of illness, and ranges from zero (best performance) to 41 (worst performance). A score of 22 or higher generally indicates a poor prognosis. Trained personnel can complete the NIHSS in less than 5 minutes, and the score can be used to assess the likelihood of an acute stroke (i.e., a stroke is unlikely if the score is 10 or lower) and to follow the clinical course of the illness. (The NIHSS can be downloaded from http://stroke.nih.gov/documents.)

Diagnostic Imaging

The imaging techniques described next have become an integral part of the stroke evaluation, and each technique has a specific role in the evaluation.

Computed Tomography

Noncontrast computed tomography (NCCT) is a reliable method for visualizing intracranial hemorrhage, as shown in Figure 46.2. This reliability is particularly important in the decision to administer thrombolytic therapy, which is contraindicated if NCCT reveals intracranial bleeding. The sensitivity of NCCT for intracranial hemorrhage is close to 100% (5).

NCCT is *not* a reliable method for visualizing ischemic changes. One-half of ischemic strokes are not apparent on NCCT (12), and the diagnostic yield is even less in the first 24 hours after an acute stroke (when infarct

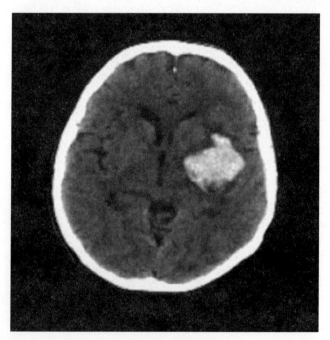

FIGURE 46.2 Noncontrast CT scan showing a high-density mass with adjacent low-density areas in the left hemisphere representing hematoma with adjacent areas of edema. CT is a reliable method for visualizing intracranial hemorrhage.

size is the smallest) (13). The nonvalue of CT imaging in the early post-infarct period is demonstrated in Figure 46.3 (13). The CT image on day 3 shows a large area of infarction with mass effect, which is not apparent in the CT image on day 1 (the day of the stroke). These images demonstrate why, *in the initial evaluation of suspected stroke, a negative CT scan does not eliminate the possibility of an ischemic stroke.*

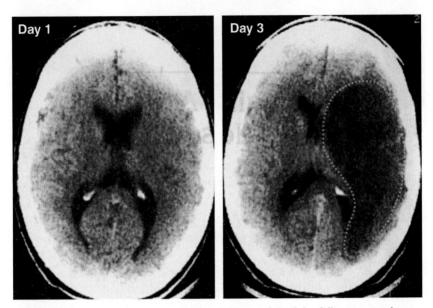

FIGURE 46.3 Noncontrast CT scans from the first and third day following an ischemic stroke. The CT scan on day 1 is unrevealing, while the CT scan on day 3 shows a large hypodense area (outlined by the dotted line) with mass effect, representing extensive tissue destruction with intracerebal edema. Images from Reference 13.

Magnetic Resonance Imaging

MRI with diffusion-weighted imaging (DWI) is the most sensitive and specific technique for the detection of ischemic stroke (2). This technique, which is based on water movement through tissues, can detect ischemic changes within 5–10 minutes after onset (14), and it has a sensitivity of 90% for the detection of ischemic stroke in the early period after stroke onset (5). The appearance of diffusion-weighted MRI in ischemic stroke is shown in Figure 46.4 (15). The image on the left shows a large, hyperdense area representing ischemic changes. (This differs from CT scans, which show ischemic changes as hyopodense areas.) The image on the right is a time-delay technique that detects regions of hypoperfusion using the adjacent color palette. If the ischemic areas on the DWI image are digitally subtracted from the areas of hypoperfusion in the time-delay image, the remaining colored areas on the time-delay map would represent areas of threatened infarction. This digital subtraction technique allows an assessment of continued risk in patients with acute ischemic stroke.

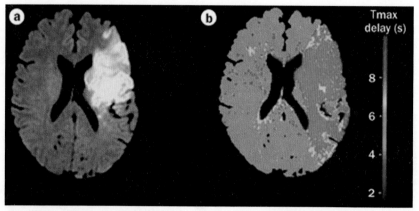

FIGURE 46.4 Diffusion-weighted MRI showing a large area of ischemic change (image on the left). The colored image on the right is a time-delay map, which shows areas of hypoperfusion in red and yellow. Digital subtraction of the ischemic area (image on the left) from the area of hypoperfusion (image on the right) would reveal the areas of threatened infarction. Images from Reference 15.

Echocardiography

The principal role of echocardiography in acute stroke includes the following:

1. Identify a source of cerebral emboli when ischemic stroke is associated with atrial fibrillation, acute MI, or left-sided endocarditis.

2. Identify a patent foramen ovale in patients with ischemic stroke and recent or prior thromboembolism.

THROMBOLYTIC THERAPY

When the initial evaluation identifies a patient with suspected acute stroke, the next step is to determine if the patient is a candidate for thrombolytic therapy.

Selection Criteria

The selection criteria for thrombolytic therapy in ischemic stroke are presented as a checklist in Table 46.1. Some comments about the criteria are presented next.

Time Restriction

The use of thrombolytic therapy in ischemic stroke was prompted by a single study (16), which showed that a 60-minute infusion of recombinant tissue plasminogen activator (tPA) was associated with improved neurologic recovery (not survival), but only when the drug infusion started within 3 hours after the onset of symptoms. The FDA subsequently approved the use of tPA in ischemic stroke (in 1996), but with the restriction that drug administration must be started within 3 hours of symptom onset. This 3-hour time restriction has limited the use of thrombolytic therapy in ischemic stroke; i.e., surveys indicate that *only 2% of patients with ischemic stroke receive thrombolytic therapy (17).*

Table 46.1	**Checklist for Thrombolytic Therapy in Ischemic Stroke**

Step 1: Inclusion Criteria

☑ Time of symptom onset can be identified accurately.

☑ Thrombolytic therapy can be started within 4.5 hrs of symptom onset.

If both boxes are checked, proceed to Step 2.

Step 2: Exclusion Criteria

☐ Evidence of active bleeding

☐ Systolic pressure ≥185 mm Hg or diastolic pressure ≥110 mm Hg

☐ History of previous intracranial hemorrhage

☐ Intracranial neoplasm, aneurysm, or AV malformation

☐ Intracranial/intraspinal surgery, serious head trauma, or stroke in past 3 months

☐ Thrombin inhibitor or factor Xa inhibitor in past 2 days

☐ Laboratory evidence of a coagulopathy (e.g., platelets <100,000/µL)

☐ Blood glucose <50 mg/dL (2.7 mmol/L)

☐ CT scan shows multilobar infarction (hypodense area >1/3 cerebral hemispheres)

If no boxes are checked, proceed to Step 3.

Step 3: Relative Exclusion Criteria

☐ Major surgery or serious trauma in past 14 days

☐ GI or urinary tract bleeding within past 21 days

☐ Acute MI within past 3 months

☐ Seizure since onset with continued postictal state

Additional criteria for thrombolytic therapy at 3–4.5 hrs after symptom onset:

☐ Age >80 years   ☐ Oral anticoagulant therapy, regardless of INR

☐ Severe stroke   ☐ Diabetes plus a previous stroke
(NIHSS >25)

Proceed to Step 4 when no boxes are checked, or when 1 or more boxes are checked, but a risk-benefit analysis favors thrombolytic therapy.

Step 4: Thrombolytic Therapy (begin immediately)

From Reference 2.

EXPANDED TIME LIMIT: A more recent clinical study has shown that thrombolytic therapy started between 3 and 4.5 hours after the onset of ischemic stroke also improves neurologic recovery (18). Based on these results, *the time for initiating thrombolytic therapy has recently been expanded to 4.5 hours after the onset of ischemic stroke* (2). There are additional exclusion criteria for the expanded time limit, and these are included in Table 46.1.

Why adhere to these time restrictions? Because about 6% of patients who receive thrombolytic therapy for ischemic stroke will suffer from an intracerebral hemorrhage, so evidence of benefit is necessary to justify this therapy.

Time of Stroke Onset

The time restriction for thrombolytic therapy makes it imperative to pinpoint the time when the stroke began (i.e., became symptomatic). This can be difficult, because patients are unable to provide a reliable history and, in many cases, the onset of symptoms is not witnessed (or occurs during sleep).

Hypertension

One of the exclusion criteria for thrombolytic therapy is an elevated blood pressure; i.e., a systolic pressure ≥ 185 mm Hg, or a diastolic pressure ≥ 110 mm Hg (see Table 46.1). If the patient is otherwise a candidate for thrombolytic therapy, the blood pressure can be lowered to qualify for thrombolytic therapy using the drug regimens shown in Table 46.2 (1). The methods and concerns with blood pressure reduction in acute stroke are described in the last section of the chapter. If the blood pressure reduction is successful and the patient receives thrombolytic therapy, the blood pressure should be maintained at < 180/105 for the next few days to limit the risk of intracranial hemorrhage.

Table 46.2	Blood Pressure Control in Acute Stroke
Trigger	**Drugs & Dosing Regimens**
†SBP >185 mm Hg or DBP >110 mm Hg	Labetalol: 10–20 mg IV over 1–2 min. Can repeat once after 10 min.
	Nicardipine: Infuse at 5 mg/hr, and increase by 2.5 mg/hr every 5–15 min, if necessary, up to 15 mg/hr.
SBP >220 mm Hg or DBP >120 mm Hg	Labetalol: 10 mg IV bolus, then infuse at 2–8 mg/min.
	Nicardipine: Infuse at 5 mg/hr, and increase by 2.5 mg/hr every 5–15 min, if necessary, up to 15 mg/hr.
DBP >140 mm Hg	Nitroprusside: Infuse at 0.2 µg/kg/min and titrate to desired effect.

†Blood pressure reduction to allow thrombolytic therapy.
Adapted from Reference 2.

Thrombolytic Regimen

Thrombolytic therapy should be initiated as soon as possible, because earlier initiation is associated with better outcomes (2). Recombinant tissue plasminogen activator (tPA) is the only thrombolytic agent approved for use in acute stroke.

Dosing Regimen: The dose of tPA is 0.9 mg/kg, up to a maximum dose of 90 mg. Ten percent of the dose is given IV over 1–2 minutes, and the remainder is infused over 60 minutes (2).

The infusion should be stopped for any signs of possible intracerebral hemorrhage, such as a deteriorating neurological status, a sudden rise in blood pressure, or a complaint of headache. After the infusion is stopped, an emergent CT scan (without contrast) should be obtained. Following successful completion of the thrombolytic regimen, patients are typically admitted to an ICU for 24 hours. *The administration of any anticoagulant or antiplatelet agent is contraindicated for the first 24 hours after thrombolytic therapy.*

Antithrombotic Therapy

Heparin

Several studies have failed to show a beneficial effect of heparin anticoagulation in ischemic stroke (2). This lack of benefit, combined with the risks associated with heparin (i.e., bleeding and thrombocytopenia) is the reason that heparin anticoagulation is not recommended in ischemic stroke (2). The only recommended use of heparin in acute stroke is for prevention of thromboembolism (2).

Aspirin

Despite the apparent lack of benefit, aspirin therapy is recommended as a routine measure in ischemic stroke (2). The initial dose is 325 mg (oral), which is given 24–48 hours after stroke onset (or after thrombolytic therapy), and the daily maintenance dose is 75–150 mg (2). Additional antiplatelet agents are not recommended.

PROTECTIVE MEASURES

The measures described in this section are designed to protect the brain from further injury following an acute stroke.

Oxygen Therapy

Oxygen inhalation has been a routine practice in patients with ischemic stroke, even when arterial oxygenation is adequate. This practice has no proven benefit (19), and it neglects the toxic effects of oxygen metabolites (especially the participation of superoxide radicals in reperfusion injury), and the fact that *oxygen promotes cerebral vasoconstriction* (20).

The latest guidelines on stroke management acknowledge the lack of evidence that oxygen breathing is beneficial in patients with ischemic stroke, and recommend supplemental oxygen only when the arterial O_2 saturation falls below 94% (2). This parallels the latest recommendations for oxygen therapy in acute coronary syndromes (see page 306). Although the threshold for oxygen breathing could be lowered to 90%, the new recommendations are a step in the right direction.

Hypertension

Hypertension is reported in 60–65% of patients with acute stroke (21), and is attributed to several factors, including activation of the sympathetic nervous system, cerebral edema, and a prior history of hypertension. Blood pressures usually return to baseline levels in 2–3 days. Patients with stroke-associated hypertension have more extensive neurologic deficits, but blood pressure reduction is not routinely recommended (2). The indications for blood pressure reduction include a systolic pressure > 220 mm Hg, a diastolic blood pressure > 120 mm Hg, or a complication of hypertension (e.g., acute MI).

Treatment Regimens

Table 46.2 shows the recommended drugs and dosing regimens for blood pressure reduction in patients with acute stroke. *Labetalol* (a combined α, β-adrenergic receptor antagonist) and *nicardipine* (a calcium channel blocker) share the ability to decrease blood pressure while preserving cardiac output (and cerebral blood flow). Labetalol is probably the preferred drug because it does not cause tachycardia, but there are no studies comparing these drugs for blood pressure control in acute stroke. *Sodium nitroprusside* is recommended for severe hypertension (diastolic BP > 140 mm Hg) (2), but nitroprusside infusions are accompanied by an increase in intracranial pressure (22), which is not a desirable condition in the patient with ischemic brain injury.

Fever

Fever develops within 48 hours in 30% of patients with acute stroke (2), and the presence of fever is associated with worse clinical outcomes (23).

Source of Fever

Fever typically appears within 48 hours after stroke onset (24), which suggests a noninfectious origin (e.g., from tissue necrosis or intracerebral blood). However, some studies have found infections in a majority of patients with stroke-related fever (25). Therefore, stroke-related fever should be evaluated as potentially infectious in origin.

Antipyresis

There is convincing evidence from animal studies that fever is harmful for ischemic brain tissue (27), and thus antipyretic therapy is justified for stroke-related fever. Antipyretic therapy is described in Chapter 43.

A FINAL WORD

Where's the Beef?

The success of thrombolytic therapy in coronary occlusive syndromes created high expectations for thrombolytic therapy in acute, ischemic stroke, and these expectations prompted a massive effort to create "stroke centers" in major hospitals, each with a "stroke team" to direct the management of acute stroke. The following is an accounting of what this effort has accomplished.

Number of strokes each year in the United States	700,000
Number of ischemic strokes (88%)	616,000
Number of stroke patients who receive lytic therapy (2%)	12,320
Number of patients who benefit from lytic therapy (1 in 9)	1,369
Percent of strokes that benefit from lytic therapy (1369/700,000)	0.2%

Enough said.

REFERENCES

1. Go AS, Mozaffarian D, Roger VL, et al. Heart disease and stroke statistics – 2013 update: A report from the American Heart Association. Circulation 2013; 127:e6–e245.

Clinical Practice Guideline

2. Jauch EC, Saver JL, Adams HP, et al. Guidelines for the early management of patients with acute ischemic stroke. A guideline for healthcare professionals from The American Heart Association/American Stroke Association. Stroke 2013; 44:1–78.

Definitions

3. Special report from the National Institute of Neurological Disorders and Stroke. Classification of cerebrovascular diseases III. Stroke 1990; 21:637–676.

4. Kizer JR, Devereux RB. Clinical practice. Patent foramen ovale in young adults with unexplained stroke. N Engl J Med 2005; 353:2361–2372.

5. Culebras A, Kase CS, Masdeu JC, et al. Practice guidelines for the use of imaging in transient ischemic attacks and acute stroke. A report of the Stroke Council, American Heart Association. Stroke 1997; 28:1480–1497.

6. Ovbiagele B, Kidwell CS, Saver JL. Epidemiological impact in the United States of a tissue-based definition of transient ischemic attack. Stroke 2003; 34:919–924.

Initial Evaluation

7. Saver JL. Time is brain—quantified. Stroke 2006; 37:263–266.

8. Bamford J. Clinical examination in diagnosis and subclassification of stroke. Lancet 1992; 339:400–402.

9. Atchison JW, Pellegrino M, Herbers P, et al. Hepatic encephalopathy mimicking stroke. A case report. Am J Phys Med Rehabil 1992; 71:114–118.

10. Maher J, Young GB. Septic encephalopathy. Intensive Care Med 1993; 8:177–187.

11. Hand PJ, Kwan J, Lindley RI, et al. Distinguishing between stroke and mimic at the bedside: the brain attack study. Stroke 2006; 37:769–775.

12. Warlow C, Sudlow C, Dennis M, et al. Stroke. Lancet 2003; 362:1211–1224.

13. Graves VB, Partington VB. Imaging evaluation of acute neurologic disease. In: Goodman LR Putman CE, eds. Critical care imaging. 3rd ed. Philadelphia: W.B. Saunders, Co., 1993; 391–409.

14. Moseley ME, Cohen Y, Mintorovich J, et al. Early detection of regional cerebral ischemia in cats: comparison of diffusion- and T2-weighted MRI and spectroscopy. Magn Reson Med 1990; 14:330–346.

15. Asdaghi N, Coutts SB. Neuroimaging in acute stroke – where does MRI fit in? Nature Rev Neurol 2011; 7:6–7.

Thrombolytic Therapy

16. Tissue plasminogen activator for acute ischemic stroke. The National Institute of Neurological Disorders and Stroke rt-PA Stroke Study Group. N Engl J Med 1995; 333:1581–1587.

17. Caplan LR. Thrombolysis 2004: the good, the bad, and the ugly. Rev Neurol Dis 2004; 1:16–26.

18. Hacke W, Kaste M, Bluhmki E, et al. Thrombolysis with alteplase 3 to 4.5 hours after acute ischemic stroke. N Engl J Med 2008; 359:1317–1329.

Protective Measures

19. Ronning OM, Guldvog B. Should stroke victims routinely receive supplemental oxygen. A quasi-randomized controlled trial. Stroke 1999; 30:2033–2037.

20. Kety SS, Schmidt CF. The effects of altered tensions of carbon dioxide and oxygen on cerebral blood flow and cerebral oxygen consumption of normal young men. J Clin Invest 1984; 27:484–492.

21. Qureshi AI, Ezzeddine MA, Nasar A, et al. Prevalence of elevated blood pressure in 563,704 adult patients with stroke presenting to the ED in the United States. Am J Emerg Med 2007; 25:32–38.

22. Candia GJ, Heros RC, Lavyne MH, et al. Effect of intravenous sodium nitroprusside on cerebral blood flow and intracranial pressure. Neurosurgery 1978; 3:50–53.

23. Reith J, Jorgensen HS, Pedersen PM, et al. Body temperature in acute stroke: relation to stroke severity, infarct size, mortality, and outcome. Lancet 1996; 347:422–425.

24. Wrotek SE, Kozak WE, Hess DC, Fagan SC. Treatment of fever after stroke: conflicting evidence. Pharmacotherapy 2011; 31:1085–1091.

25. Grau AJ, Buggle F, Schnitzler P, et al. Fever and infection early after ischemic stroke. J Neurol Sci 1999; 171:115–120.

26. Baena RC, Busto R, Dietrich WD, et al. Hyperthermia delayed by 24 hours aggravates neuronal damage in rat hippocampus following global ischemia. Neurology 1997; 48:768–773.

27. Sulter G, Elting JW, Mauritis N, et al. Acetylsalicylic acid and acetaminophen to combat elevated temperature in acute ischemic stroke. Cerebrovasc Dis 2004; 17:118–122.

NUTRITION & METABOLISM

The more impure bodies are fed, the more diseased they will become.

Hippocrates
Aphorisms

Chapter 47

NUTRITIONAL REQUIREMENTS

What is food to one man, may be fierce poison to others.

Lucretius
(99–55 BC)

The fundamental goal of nutritional support is to provide the daily nutrient and energy needs of each patient. This chapter will describe how to evaluate those needs in critically ill patients (1), and will try to do so without pretending that anyone knows how to support metabolism in patients who are critically ill.

DAILY ENERGY EXPENDITURE

Oxidation of Nutrient Fuels

Oxidative metabolism captures the energy stored in nutrient fuels (carbohydrates, lipids, and proteins) and uses this energy to sustain life. This process consumes oxygen, and generates carbon dioxide, water, and heat. The quantities involved in the oxidation of each type of nutrient fuel are shown in Table 47.1. The following points deserve mention.

1. The heat generated by the complete oxidation of a nutrient fuel is equivalent to the energy yield (in kcal/g) of that fuel.
2. Lipids have the highest energy yield (9.1 kcal/gram), while glucose has the lowest energy yield (3.7 kcal/gram).

The summed metabolism of all three nutrient fuels determines the whole-body O_2 consumption (VO_2), CO_2 production (VCO_2), and heat production for any given time period. The 24-hour heat production is equivalent to the daily energy expenditure (in kcal) for each patient. *The daily energy expenditure determines how many calories to provide each day in nutritional support,* and it can be calculated or measured.

Table 47.1	Oxidative Metabolism of Nutrient Fuels		
Fuel	O_2 Consumption	CO_2 Production	Heat Production[†]
Glucose	0.74 L/g	0.74 L/g	3.7 kcal/g
Lipid	2.00 L/g	1.40 L/g	9.1 kcal/g
Protein	0.96 L/g	0.78 L/g	4.0 kcal/g

[†]The energy yield from each nutrient fuel.

Indirect Calorimetry

It is not possible to measure metabolic heat production in hospitalized patients, but if the whole-body O_2 consumption (VO_2) and CO_2 production (VCO_2) are known, the relationships in Table 47.1 can be used to determine the metabolic heat production. This is the principle of *indirect calorimetry*, which measures the *resting energy expenditure* (REE) using the following relationships (2):

$$REE\ (kcal/min) = (3.6 \times VO_2) + (1.1 \times VCO_2) - 61 \qquad (47.1)$$

Methodology

Indirect calorimetry is performed with "metabolic carts" that measure whole-body VO_2 and VCO_2 at the bedside by measuring the concentrations of O_2 and CO_2 in inhaled and exhaled gas (usually in intubated patients). Steady-state measurements are obtained for 15–30 minutes to determine the REE (kcal/min), which is then multiplied by 1,440 (the number of minutes in 24 hours) to derive the daily energy expenditure (kcal/24 hr) (3). Clinical studies have shown that REE measurements obtained over 30 minutes and extrapolated to 24 hours are equivalent to REE measurements performed for 24 hours (4). The oxygen sensor in metabolic carts is not reliable at O_2 concentrations above 60% (3), so indirect calorimetry can be unreliable when inhaled O_2 concentrations are ≥60%.

Although indirect calorimetry is the most accurate method for determining daily energy requirements, it requires expensive equipment along with trained personnel, and is not universally available. As a result, daily energy requirements are usually estimated, as described next.

The Simple Way

There are more than 200 cumbersome equations available for estimating daily energy requirements (1), but none is considered more predictive than the following relationship:

$$REE\ (kcal/day) = 25 \times body\ weight\ (kg) \qquad (47.2)$$

This simple predictive relationship is remarkably accurate in most ICU patients (5) and is considered suitable for estimating daily energy requirements in the ICU (1). Actual body weight is used unless it is 25% higher than ideal body weight. When actual weight is more than 125% of ideal weight, the adjusted weight (wt) can be used, as determined by the following equation (6):

$$\text{Adjusted wt (kg)} = [(\text{actual} - \text{ideal}) \text{ wt} \times 0.25] + \text{ideal wt} \qquad (47.3)$$

SUBSTRATE REQUIREMENTS

Nonprotein Calories

The daily energy requirement is provided by nonprotein calories from carbohydrates and lipids, while protein intake is used to maintain essential enzymatic and structural proteins.

Carbohydrates

Standard nutrition regimens use carbohydrates to provide about 70% of the nonprotein calories. The human body has limited carbohydrate stores (Table 47.2), and daily intake of carbohydrates is necessary to ensure proper functioning of the central nervous system, which relies heavily on glucose as a nutritive fuel. However, excessive carbohydrate intake promotes hyperglycemia, which has several deleterious effects, including impaired immune responsiveness in leukocytes (7).

Table 47.2	Endogenous Fuel Stores in Healthy Adults	
Fuel Source	**Amount (kg)**	**Energy Yield (kcal)**
Adipose Tissue Fat	15.0	141,000
Muscle Protein	6.0	24,000
Total Glycogen	0.09	900
		Total: 165,900

Data from Cahill GF. Jr. N Eng J Med 1970; 282:668–675.

Lipids

Standard nutrition regimens use lipids to provide approximately 30% of the daily energy needs. Dietary lipids have the highest energy yield of the three nutrient fuels (Table 47.1), and lipid stores in adipose tissues represent the major endogenous fuel source in healthy adults (Table 47.2).

Linoleic Acid

Dietary lipids are triglycerides, which are composed of a glycerol molecule linked to three fatty acids. The only dietary fatty acid that is considered essential (i.e., must be provided in the diet) is *linoleic acid*, a long chain, polyunsaturated fatty acid with 18 carbon atoms (8). A deficient intake of this essential fatty acid produces a clinical disorder characterized by a scaly dermopathy, cardiac dysfunction, and increased susceptibility to infections (8). This disorder is prevented by providing 0.5% of the dietary fatty acids as linoleic acid. Safflower oil is used as the source of linoleic acid in most nutritional support regimens.

Propofol

Propofol, an intravenous anesthetic agent that is popular for short-term sedation in the ICU, is mixed in a 10% lipid emulsion very similar to 10% Intralipid (Baxter Healthcare) that provides 1.1 kcal/mL. As a result, the calories provided by propofol infusions must be considered when calculating the nonprotein calories in a nutrition support regimen (1).

Protein Requirements

The daily protein requirement is dependent on the rate of protein catabolism. The normal daily protein intake is 0.8–1 grams/kg, but in ICU patients, the daily protein intake is higher at 1.2–1.6 grams/kg because of hypercatabolism (9).

Nitrogen Balance

The adequacy of protein intake can be evaluated with the nitrogen balance; i.e., the difference between intake and excretion of protein-derived nitrogen.

1. *Nitrogen Excretion:* Two-thirds of the nitrogen derived from protein breakdown is excreted in the urine (8), and about 85% of this nitrogen is contained in urea (the remainder is in ammonia and creatinine). Thus, the *urinary urea nitrogen* (UUN), measured in grams excreted in 24 hours, represents the bulk of nitrogen derived from protein breakdown. The remainder of the protein-derived nitrogen (usually about 4–6 grams/day) is excreted in the stool. Therefore, protein-derived nitrogen excretion can be expressed as follows:

$$\text{Nitrogen Excretion (g/24h)} = \text{UUN} + (4-6) \qquad (47.4)$$

If the UUN is greater than 30 g/24 h, 6 grams is more appropriate for the estimated non-urinary nitrogen losses (10). In the presence of diarrhea, non-urinary nitrogen losses cannot be estimated accurately, and nitrogen balance determinations are unreliable.

2. *Nitrogen Intake:* Protein is 16% nitrogen, so each gram of protein contains 1/6.25 grams of nitrogen. Therefore, protein-derived nitrogen intake is derived as follows:

$$\text{Nitrogen Intake (g/24 h)} = \text{Protein Intake (g/24h)} / 6.25 \qquad (47.5)$$

3. *Nitrogen Balance:* The equations for nitrogen intake and nitrogen excretion are combined to determine the daily nitrogen balance.

$$\text{Nitrogen Balance (g/24h)} = \text{Protein Intake}/6.25 - [\text{UUN} + (4-6)] \qquad (47.6)$$

The goal of nutritional support is a positive nitrogen balance of 4–6 grams.

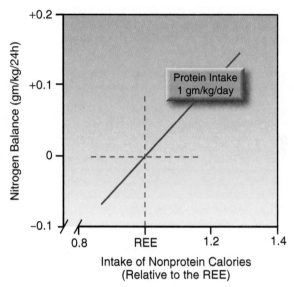

FIGURE 47.1 Relationship between nitrogen balance and the daily intake of nonprotein calories relative to daily calorie requirements. Protein intake is constant. REE = resting energy expenditure.

Nitrogen Balance & Nonprotein Calories

The first step in achieving a positive nitrogen balance is to provide enough nonprotein calories to spare proteins from being degraded to provide energy. This is demonstrated in Figure 47.1. When the daily protein intake is constant, the nitrogen balance becomes positive only when the intake of nonprotein calories is sufficient to meet the daily energy needs (i.e., the REE). *Therefore, increasing protein intake will not achieve a positive nitrogen balance unless the intake of nonprotein calories is adequate.*

VITAMIN REQUIREMENTS

Thirteen vitamins are considered an essential part of the daily diet, and Table 47.3 shows the recommended daily dose and the maximum tolerable daily dose of these vitamins. The daily vitamin requirements have not been identified in critically ill patients (and probably vary with each patient) but they are likely to be higher than the recommended daily doses in Table 47.3. This is supported by reports of vitamin deficiencies in hospitalized patients who were receiving daily vitamin supplementation (11,12). Two vitamin deficiencies that deserve mention are described next.

Thiamine Deficiency

Thiamine (vitamin B_1) plays an essential role in carbohydrate metabolism, where it serves as a coenzyme (thiamine pyrophosphate) for pyruvate dehydrogenase, the enzyme that allows pyruvate to enter mitochondria and undergo oxidative metabolism to generate high-energy ATP molecules (13). Thiamine deficiency can thus have an adverse effect on cellular energy production, particularly in the brain, which relies heavily on glucose metabolism.

Table 47.3	Dietary Allowances for Vitamins	
Vitamin	Recommended Daily Intake	Maximum Daily Intake
Vitamin A	900 μg	3,000 μg
Vitamin B_{12}	2 μg	5 μg
Vitamin C	90 mg	2,000 mg
Vitamin D	15 μg	100 μg
Vitamin E	15 mg	1,000 mg
Vitamin K	120 μg	ND
Thiamine (B_1)	1 mg	ND
Riboflavin (B_2)	1 mg	ND
Niacin (B_3)	16 mg	35 mg
Pyridoxine (B_6)	2 mg	100 mg
Pantothenic acid (B_1)	5 mg	ND
Biotin	30 μg	ND
Folate	400 μg	1,000 μg

Intakes for adult males, age 51–70 yrs. From the Food & Nutrition Board, Institute of Medicine. Available at the Food & Nutrition Information Center (http://fnic.nal.usda.gov). Accessed July 2013. Doses rounded off to the nearest whole number. ND = not determined.

Predisposing Factors

The prevalence of thiamine deficiency in ICU patients is not known, but the are several conditions in ICU patients that promote thiamine deficiency, including alcoholism, hypermetabolic states like trauma (14), increased urinary thiamine excretion by furosemide (15), and magnesium depletion (16). Furthermore, thiamine is degraded by sulfites (used as preservatives) in parenteral nutrition solutions (17), so thiamine-containing multivitamin preparations should not be mixed with parenteral nutrition solutions.

Clinical Manifestations

The consequences of thiamine deficiency include cardiomyopathy (wet beriberi), Wernicke's encephalopathy (18), lactic acidosis (19), and a peripheral neuropathy (dry beriberi). Cardiomyopathies, encephalopathies, and lactic acidosis are common in ICU patients, and the possible contribution of thiamine deficiency to these conditions should not be overlooked.

Diagnosis

The laboratory evaluation of thiamine status is shown in Table 47.4. Plasma levels of thiamine can be useful in detecting thiamine depletion, but the most reliable measure of functional thiamine stores is the *erythrocyte transketolase assay* (21). This assay measures the activity of a thiamine pyrophosphate-dependent (transketolase) enzyme in the patient's red blood cells in response to the addition of thiamine pyrophosphate (TPP). An increase in enzyme activity of greater than 25% after the addition of TPP indicates functional thiamine deficiency.

Table 47.4	Laboratory Evaluation of Thiamine Status

Plasma Thiamine

Thiamine Fraction	Normal Range
Total	3.4–4.8 µg/dL
Free	0.8–1.1 µg/dL
Phosphorylated	2.6–3.7 µg/dL

Erythrocyte Transketolase Activity†

Enzyme activity measured in response to thiamine pyrophosphate (TPP)

1. <20% increase in activity after TPP indicates normal thiamine levels.
2. >25% increase in activity after TPP indicates thiamine deficiency.

†From Reference 21.

Vitamin E Deficiency

Vitamin E is the major lipid-soluble antioxidant in the body, and plays a major role in preventing damage from lipid peroxidation in cell membranes (22). The incidence of vitamin E deficiency in ICU patients is not known, but vitamin E deficiency is common during parenteral nutrition (23). The reperfusion injury that follows aortic cross-clamping is associated with reduced blood levels of vitamin E, and pre-treatment with vitamin E ameliorates this reperfusion injury (24). Considering that oxidant stress plays an important role in the pathogenesis of inflammatory-mediated organ injury (25), attention to the status of vitamin E in critically ill patients seems warranted. The normal plasma concentration of vitamin E is 11.6–30.8 µmol/L (0.5–1.6 mg/dL) (26).

ESSENTIAL TRACE ELEMENTS

Daily Requirements

A trace element is a substance that is present in the body in amounts less than 50 µg per gram of body tissue (27). Seven trace elements are considered essential in humans (i.e., are associated with deficiency syndromes), and these are listed in Table 47.5, along with the recommended and maximum daily intake for each element. As mentioned for vitamins, the essential trace element requirements are not known in critically ill patients, and are probably higher than normal. The following trace elements deserve mention because of their relevance to oxidant cell injury.

Table 47.5	Dietary Allowances for Essential Trace Elements	
Trace Element	Recommended Daily Intake	Maximum Daily Intake
Chromium	30 µg	ND
Copper	900 µg	10,000 µg
Iodine	150 µg	1,100 µg
Iron	8 mg	45 mg
Manganese	2.3 mg	11 mg
Selenium	55 µg	400 µg
Zinc	11 mg	40 mg

Intakes for adult males, 51–70 yrs. From the Food & Nutrition Board, Institute of Medicine. Available at the Food & Nutrition Information Center (http://fnic.nal.usda.gov). Accessed July 2013. ND = not determined.

Iron

One of the interesting features of iron in the human body is how little is allowed to remain as free, unbound iron. The normal adult has approximately 4.5 grams of iron, yet there is virtually no free iron in plasma (28). Most of the iron is bound to hemoglobin, and the remainder is bound to ferritin in tissues and transferrin in plasma. Furthermore, the transferrin in plasma is only approximately 30% saturated with iron, so any increase in plasma iron will be quickly bound by transferrin, thus preventing any rise in plasma free iron.

Iron and Oxidant Injury

One reason for the paucity of free iron is the ability of free iron to promote oxidant-induced cell injury (28,29). Iron in the reduced state (Fe-II) promotes the formation of hydroxyl radicals (see Figure 22.6), and hydroxyl radicals are considered the most reactive oxidants known in biochemistry. In this context, the ability to bind and sequester iron has been called the major antioxidant function of blood (29). This might explain why hypoferremia is a common occurrence in patients who have conditions associated with hypermetabolism (30) (because this would limit the destructive effects of hypermetabolism).

In light of this description of iron, *a reduced serum iron level in a critically ill patient should not prompt iron replacement therapy* unless there is evidence of total-body iron deficiency. This latter condition can be detected with a plasma ferritin level; i.e., iron deficiency is likely if the plasma ferritin is below 18 µg/L, and is unlikely if the plasma ferritin is above 100 µg/L (31).

Selenium

Selenium is an endogenous antioxidant by virtue of its role as a co-factor for glutathione peroxidase (see Figure 22.7). The recommended daily requirement for selenium is 55 µg in healthy adults (32), but selenium utilization is increased in acute illness (33), so daily requirements are likely to be higher in critically ill patients. A recent review of studies evaluating selenium in patients with severe sepsis has shown that low plasma levels of selenium are common in severe sepsis, and selenium supplementation in severe sepsis is associated with a lower mortality rate (34). In light of this study, attention to monitoring serum selenium levels in severe sepsis, as well as other conditions associated with systemic inflammation, seems warranted. The normal plasma selenium concentration is 89–113 µg/L (35).

A FINAL WORD

The Problem with Nutrition Support in Critically Ill Patients

Before leaving this chapter, it is important to point out a fundamental problem with promoting nutrient intake in critically ill patients (36). The problem is the difference in mechanisms for the malnutrition associated with critical illness and the malnutrition associated with starvation; i.e.,

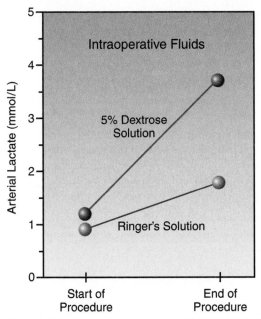

FIGURE 47.2 Influence of dextrose infusion on arterial lactate levels during abdominal aortic surgery. Each point represents the mean lactate level for 10 patients receiving Ringer's solution (closed squares) and 10 patients receiving 5% dextrose solution (open squares). Total volume infused is equivalent with both fluids. Data from Reference 38.

the malnutrition from starvation is due to depletion of essential nutrients, while *the malnutrition associated with critical illnesses is the result of abnormal nutrient processing*. Because malnutrition in critically ill patients is caused by metabolic derangements, providing nutrients will not correct the malnutrition until the metabolic derangements resolve.

An example of abnormal nutrient processing in acute illness is illustrated by the fate of a glucose load; i.e., less than 5% of glucose is metabolized to lactate in healthy subjects, while as much as 85% of a glucose load can be recovered as lactate in acutely ill patients (37). This is demonstrated in Figure 47.2 (38). In this case, patients undergoing abdominal aneurysm surgery were given intraoperative fluid therapy with either Ringer's solutions or 5% dextrose solutions. In the patients who received dextrose (an average of 200 grams), the blood lactate level increased by more than 3 mmol/L, whereas the blood lactate level increased < 1 mmol/L in the patients who received dextrose-free fluids. This demonstrates that nutrient intake can have very different consequences in critically ill patients, and the consequences can be toxic (e.g., the accumulation of an organic acid). It seems Lucretius had the right idea, over 2,000 years ago.

REFERENCES

Clinical Practice Guideline

1. McClave SA, Martindale RG, Vanek VW, et al. Guidelines for the provision and assessment of nutrition support therapy in the adult critically ill patient: Society of Critical Care Medicine and American Society for Parenteral and Enteral Nutrition. J Parent Ent Nutr 2009; 33:277–316.

Daily Energy Expenditure

2. Bursztein S, Saphar P, Singer P, et al. A mathematical analysis of indirect calorimetry measurements in acutely ill patients. Am J Clin Nutr 1989; 50:227–230.

3. Lev S, Cohen J, Singer P. Indirect calorimetry measurements in the ventilated critically ill patient: facts and controversies – the heat is on. Crit Care Clin 2010; 26:e1–e9.

4. Smyrnios NA, Curley FJ, Shaker KG. Accuracy of 30-minute indirect calorimetry studies in predicting 24-hour energy expenditure in mechanically ventilated critically ill patients. J Parenter Enteral Nutr 1997; 21:168–174.

5. Paauw JD, McCamish MA, Dean RE, et al. Assessment of caloric needs in stressed patients. J Am Coll Nutr 1984; 3:51–59.

6. Krenitsky J. Adjusted body weight, pro: Evidence to support the use of adjusted body weight in calculating calorie requirements. Nutr Clin Pract 2005; 20:468–473.

Substrate Requirements

7. Marik PE, Preiser J-C. Toward understanding tight glycemic control in the ICU. Chest 2010; 137:544–551.

8. Jones PJH, Kubow S. Lipids, Sterols, and Their Metabolites. In: Shils ME, et al., eds. Modern nutrition in health and disease. 10th ed. Philadelphia, PA: Lippincott, Williams & Wilkins, 2006; 92–121.

9. Matthews DE. Proteins and Amino Acids. In: Shils ME, et al., eds. Modern nutrition in health and disease. 10th ed. Philadelphia, PA: Lippincott, Williams & Wilkins, 2006; 23–61.

10. Velasco N, Long CL, Otto DA, et al. Comparison of three methods for the estimation of total nitrogen losses in hospitalized patients. J Parenter Enteral Nutr 1990; 14:517–522.

Vitamin Requirements

11. Dempsey DT, Mullen JL, Rombeau JL, et al. Treatment effects of parenteral vitamins in total parenteral nutrition patients. J Parenter Enteral Nutr 1987; 11:229–237.

12. Beard ME, Hatipov CS, Hamer JW. Acute onset of folate deficiency in patients under intensive care. Crit Care Med 1980; 8:500–503.

13. Butterworth RF. Thiamine. In: Shils ME, et al., eds. Modern nutrition in health and disease. 10th ed. Philadelphia, PA: Lippincott, Williams & Wilkins, 2006; 426–433.

14. McConachie I, Haskew A. Thiamine status after major trauma. Intensive Care Med 1988; 14:628–631.

15. Seligmann H, Halkin H, Rauchfleisch S, et al. Thiamine deficiency in patients with congestive heart failure receiving long-term furosemide therapy: a pilot study. Am J Med 1991; 91:151–155.

16. Dyckner T, Ek B, Nyhlin H, et al. Aggravation of thiamine deficiency by magnesium depletion. A case report. Acta Med Scand 1985; 218:129–131.

17. Scheiner JM, Araujo MM, DeRitter E. Thiamine destruction by sodium bisulfite in infusion solutions. Am J Hosp Pharm 1981; 38:1911–1916.

18. Tan GH, Farnell GF, Hensrud DD, et al. Acute Wernicke's encephalopathy attributable to pure dietary thiamine deficiency. Mayo Clin Proc 1994; 69:849–850.

19. Oriot D, Wood C, Gottesman R, et al. Severe lactic acidosis related to acute thiamine deficiency. J Parenter Enteral Nutr 1991; 15:105–109.

20. Koike H, Misu K, Hattori N, et al. Postgastrectomy polyneuropathy with thiamine deficiency. J Neurol Neurosurg Psychiatry 2001; 71:357–362.

21. Boni L, Kieckens L, Hendrikx A. An evaluation of a modified erythrocyte transketolase assay for assessing thiamine nutritional adequacy. J Nutr Sci Vitaminol (Tokyo) 1980; 26:507–514.

22. Burton GW, Ingold KU. Vitamin E as an in vitro and in vivo antioxidant. Ann NY Acad Sci 1989; 570:7–22.

23. Vandewoude MG, Vandewoude MFJ, De Leeuw IH. Vitamin E status in patients on parenteral nutrition receiving intralipid. J Parenter Enter Nutr 1986; 10:303–305.

24. Novelli GP, Adembri C, Gandini E, et al. Vitamin E protects human skeletal muscle from damage during surgical ischemia-reperfusion injury. Am J Surg 1996; 172:206–209.

25. Anderson BO, Brown JM, Harken AH. Mechanisms of neutrophil-mediated tissue injury. J Surg Res 1991; 51:170–179.

26. Meydani M. Vitamin E. Lancet 1995; 345:170–175.

Essential Trace Elements

27. Fleming CR. Trace element metabolism in adult patients requiring total parenteral nutrition. Am J Clin Nutr 1989; 49:573–579.

28. Halliwell B, Gutteridge JM. Role of free radicals and catalytic metal ions in human disease: an overview. Methods Enzymol 1990; 186:1–85.

29. Herbert V, Shaw S, Jayatilleke E, et al. Most free-radical injury is iron-related: it is promoted by iron, hemin, holoferritin and vitamin C, and inhibited by desferoxamine and apoferritin. Stem Cells 1994; 12:289–303.

30. Shanbhogue LK, Paterson N. Effect of sepsis and surgery on trace minerals. J Parenter Enteral Nutr 1990; 14:287–289.

31. Guyatt GH, Patterson C, Ali M, et al. Diagnosis of iron-deficiency anemia in the elderly. Am J Med 1990; 88:205–209.

32. Food and Nutrition Board, Institute of Medicine. Recommended dietary allowances and adequate intakes of trace elements. Available at the Food and Nutrition website (http://fnic.nal.usda.gov), accessed July, 2013.

33. Hawker FH, Stewart PM, Snitch PJ. Effects of acute illness on selenium homeostasis. Crit Care Med 1990; 18:442–446.

34. Alhazzani W, Jacobi J, Sindi A, et al. The effect of selenium therapy on mortality in patients with sepsis syndrome. Crit Care Med 2013; 41:1555–1564.

35. Geoghegan M, McAuley D, Eaton S, et al. Selenium in critical illness. Curr Opin Crit Care 2006; 12:136–141.

A Final Word

36. Marino PL, Finnegan MJ. Nutrition support is not beneficial and can be harmful in critically ill patients. Crit Care Clin 1996; 12:667–676.

37. Gunther B, Jauch KW, Hartl W, et al. Low-dose glucose infusion in patients who have undergone surgery. Possible cause of a muscular energy deficit. Arch Surg 1987; 122:765–771.

38. Degoute CS, Ray MJ, Manchon M, et al. Intraoperative glucose infusion and blood lactate: endocrine and metabolic relationships during abdominal aortic surgery. Anesthesiology 1989; 71:355–361.

Chapter 48

ENTERAL TUBE FEEDING

*Forced feeding . . . goes on because the
world still believes it can eat itself well.*

Herbert Shelton
1978

For patients who are unable to eat, the preferred method of nutrition support is the infusion of liquid feeding formulas into the stomach or small
bowel (1,2). This mimics the normal process of nutrition support, and
also serves as an infection control measure, as will be described.

This chapter presents the fundamentals of nutrition support with enteral
tube feedings, and will show you how to create a tube feeding regimen
for each patient in the ICU.

GENERAL CONSIDERATIONS

Infectious Risk

The preference for enteral over parenteral nutrition is based on numerous
studies showing that enteral nutrition is associated with fewer infections
(1–4), particularly pneumonias. This is attributed to the trophic effects of
nutritional bulk that maintain the barrier and immunological functions of
the bowel, as described next.

Mechanisms

The role of enteral tube feedings in protecting against infections is summarized in the following statements.

1. The presence of food or tube feedings in the lumen of the bowel has
   a trophic influence on the bowel mucosa that preserves the structural integrity of the mucosa (5,6). This maintains the barrier function
   of the bowel mucosa, which protects against invasion from enteric
   pathogens, a phenomenon known as *translocation* (7).

2. The trophic influence of luminal nutrition also extends to the immune defenses in the bowel, such as the production of immunoglobulin A (IgA) by monocytes in the bowel wall, which blocks the attachment of pathogens to the bowel mucosa (8).

3. These effects are triggered by the presence of nutritional bulk in the lumen of the bowel (9), and are mediated, in part, by the release of gastrin and cholecystokinin in response to gastric distension (1). Specific nutrients in the bowel lumen also participate in these effects. One of these nutrients is glutamine, which is a principal fuel for enterocytes in the bowel mucosa (10).

4. The trophic effects of nutritional bulk are lost during periods of bowel rest, and this results in progressive atrophy of the bowel mucosa (6), and can lead to translocation and the systemic spread of enteric pathogens (11). Parenteral nutrition does not prevent the deleterious effects of prolonged bowel rest (1,11).

The sum of these observations indicates that the normal antimicrobial defenses in the bowel are sustained by the presence of nutritional bulk in the bowel lumen. This is how nutrition support with enteral tube feedings serves as an infection control measure, as stated in the introduction to the chapter.

Who and When

Patients who are unable to eat and do not have the absolute contraindications described next are candidates for enteral tube feeding. *The presence of bowel sounds is not required to initiate enteral tube feedings* (1). Tube feedings should be started within 24–48 hours of admission to the ICU (1) to take advantage of the protective effects of tube feedings. There is evidence that early institution of enteral nutrition is associated with fewer septic complications and a shorter hospital stay (12).

Contraindications

Absolute contraindications to enteral tube feedings include complete bowel obstruction, bowel ischemia, ileus, and circulatory shock with high-dose vasopressor requirements (1,2). Gastric feedings can be attempted in stable patients on low doses of vasopressors (1), but any signs of intolerance should prompt immediate cessation of feedings.

FEEDING FORMULAS

There are at least 200 enteral feeding formulas that are commercially available, and many of the formulas used at individual hospitals are from the same manufacturer (because of contractual obligations). The following is a brief description of some characteristic features of feeding formulas. Examples are provided in Tables 48.1 and 48.2

Caloric Density

Feeding formulas are available with caloric densities of 1 kcal/mL, 1.5

kcal/mL, and 2 kcal/mL. Most tube feeding regimens use formulas with 1 kcal/mL. The high-calorie formulas (2 kcal/mL) are intended for patients with severe physiological stress (e.g., multisystem trauma and burns), but they are frequently used when volume restriction is a priority.

Table 48.1	Standard Formulas for Enteral Nutrition			
Feeding Formula	Caloric Density (kcal/mL)	Nonprotein Calories (%)	Protein (g/L)	Osmolality (mosm/kg H_2O)
Osmolite	1	86	37	300
Osmolite HN	1	83	44	300
Isocal	1	87	34	300
Isocal HN	1	83	44	300
Isocal HCN	2	85	75	690
Twocal HN	2	83	84	690

Nonprotein Calories

The caloric density of feeding formulas includes both protein and nonprotein calories, but daily caloric requirements should be provided by nonprotein calories (as mentioned in Chapter 47). In standard feeding formulas, nonprotein calories account for about 85% of the total calories (see Table 48.1).

Osmolality

The osmolality of feeding formulas is determined primarily by the caloric density. Feeding formulas with 1 kcal/mL have an osmolality similar to plasma (280–300 mosm/kg H_2O), and feeding formulas with 2 kcal/mL have an osmolality about twice that of plasma. Hypertonic feedings create little risk of diarrhea when they are delivered into the stomach, where the large volume of gastric secretions attenuates the osmolality.

Protein Content

Standard feeding formulas provide 35–40 grams of protein per liter. High-protein formulas, often designated by the suffix HN (for "high nitrogen"), provide about 20% more protein than the standard formulas (compare Isocal and Isocal HN in Table 48.1).

Most enteral formulas contain intact proteins that are broken down into amino acids in the upper GI tract. These are called *polymeric* formulas. Feeding formulas are also available that contain small peptides (called *semi-elemental* formulas) and individual amino acids (called *elemental* formulas) that are absorbed more readily than intact protein. Semi-elemental and elemental formulas promote water reabsorption from the bowel, and could benefit patients with troublesome diarrhea. However, the clinical benefit of these formulas is unproven (14). Examples of semi-elemental and elemental formulas include *Optimental, Peptamen, Perative, Vital HN,* and *Vivonex T.E.N.*

Carbohydrate Content

Carbohydrates (usually polysaccharides) are the major source of calories in feeding formulas, and provide 40–70% of the total calories. Low-carbohydrate formulas, in which carbohydrates provide 30–40% of the calories, are available for diabetics. One example of a low-carbohydrate formula is *Glucerna.*

Fiber

The term "fiber" refers to polysaccharides from plants that are not digested by humans. Fiber is fermented by bacteria in the colon, and is broken down into short-chain fatty acids, which are an important energy source for the mucosal cells in the large bowel (13). The uptake of these fatty acids into the bowel mucosa also promotes sodium and water absorption. This "fermentable" fiber promotes the growth and viability of the surface mucosa in the large bowel, and can also reduce the water content of stool. There is also "nonfermentable" fiber that is not broken down by gut bacteria. This type of fiber draws water into the bowel and increases the water content of stool.

Fiber is added to some feeding formulas to promote the viability of the mucosa in the large bowel, and some examples of fiber-containing formulas are shown in Table 48.2. The fiber in most feeding formulas is a mixture of fermentable and nonfermentable varieties.

Table 48.2	Feeding Formulas Enriched With Fiber			
Feeding Formula	Calories (kcal/mL)	Protein (g/L)	Fiber (g/L)	Osmolality (mosm/kg H_2O)
Jevity - 1 Cal	1	44	14	300
Jevity - 1.5 Cal	1.5	64	22	525
Promote with Fiber	1	63	14	380

Lipid Content

Standard feeding formulas contain polyunsaturated fatty acids from vegetable oils. The lipid content is adjusted to provide about 30% of the caloric density of the formula.

Omega-3 Fatty Acids

Polyunsaturated fatty acids from vegetable oils (which make up the lipid content of standard feeding formulas) can serve as precursors for inflam-

matory mediators (eicosanoids) that are capable of promoting inflammatory cell injury. This concern has prompted the introduction of feeding
solutions that contain polyunsaturated fatty acids from fish oils (omega-
3 fatty acids), which do not promote the production of inflammatory
mediators. Some of these feeding formulas are shown in Table 48.3. The
use of feeding formulas that influence the inflammatory response is
known as *immunonutrition* (14).

Table 48.3	Immune-Modulating Feeding Formulas			
Feeding Formula	Calories (kcal/mL)	Ω-3 FAs (g/L)	Arginine (g/L)	Antioxidants
Impact	1	1.7	13	Selenium, β-carotene
Impact 1.5	1.5	2.6	19	Selenium, β-carotene
Optimental	1	2.3	6	Vitamins C & E, β-carotene
Oxepa	1.5	4.6	0	Vitamins C & E, β-carotene

Ω-3 FAs = omega-3 fatty acids.

Clinical studies have shown that patients with acute respiratory distress
syndrome (ARDS) derive some benefit (fewer days on the ventilator)
from feeding formulas enriched with omega-3 fatty acids and antioxidants (15). However, the benefits are marginal, and there is a general
reluctance to adopt these feeding formulas for patients with ARDS.

Conditionally Essential Nutrients

Non-essential nutrients can become essential (i.e., require exogenous
support) in conditions of increased utilization. Two of these *conditionally
essential nutrients* deserve mention.

Arginine

Arginine is a preferred metabolic substrate for injured muscle, and can
become depleted in conditions like multisystem trauma. Arginine also
promotes wound healing, and is a precursor of nitric oxide (16). At
least 8 enteral feeding formulas contain arginine in concentrations of
8–19 g/L, but the optimal intake of arginine is not known because
there is no daily requirement for this amino acid.

POTENTIAL HARM: Arginine is a common additive in immune-modulating
feeding formulas, and postoperative patients seem to benefit most from
arginine-enriched feeding formulas (14). However, there are reports of
increased mortality associated with arginine-enriched feeding formulas

in patients with severe sepsis (1,17). The presumed mechanism is arginine-induced formation of nitric oxide, with subsequent vasodilation and hypotension. At the present time, arginine-containing feeding formulas are not advised for patients with severe sepsis (1).

Carnitine

Carnitine is necessary for the transport of fatty acids into mitochondria for fatty acid oxidation. Hypercatabolic conditions can promote carnitine deficiency (18), which is characterized by a myopathy involving the heart and skeletal muscle. A deficiency state is suggested by plasma carnitine concentration < 20 mmol/L.

The recommended daily intake of carnitine is 20–30 mg/kg in adults (19). Feeding formulas that provide supplemental carnitine include *Glucerna*, *Isocal HN*, *Jevity*, and *Peptamen*.

One Feeding Formula for All?

Despite the confusing array of liquid feeding formulas, including the "designer formulas," there is very little consistent or convincing evidence that one feeding formula, or one type of formula, is superior to the others. In other words *a single feeding formula could be used for all ICU patients (with an occasional exception), as long as it is used appropriately.*

CREATING A FEEDING REGIMEN

This section describes a simple four-step method for creating an enteral feeding regimen. This method is summarized in Table 48.4.

Step 1. Estimate daily energy and protein requirements.

The very first consideration is the patient's daily requirement for calories and protein, and both requirements can be estimated with the simple predictive formulas in Table 48.2. (See Chapter 47 for more information on these formulas.) You can use actual body weight in the formulas as long as actual body weight is not above 125% of the ideal weight. If actual body weight exceeds 125% of ideal body weight, you should use an adjusted body weight, which is derived in Equation 47.3. If available, indirect calorimetry should be used to measure the resting energy expenditure (see Chapter 47).

Step 2. Select a feeding formula.

A standard formula, with 1–1.5 kcal/mL, should be sufficient for most patients. Use formulas with higher caloric densities if volume restriction is a priority.

Step 3. Calculate the desired infusion rate.

To determine the desired infusion rate for feeding, first calculate the volume of the feeding formula that must be infused to meet the daily requirement for calories (i.e., the daily caloric requirement in kcal/day divided by the caloric density of the feeding formula in kcal/mL). Next, divide the feeding volume (L/hr) by the number of hours each day that the feeding formula will be infused.

There are two considerations at this stage:

a. If propofol is being infused, subtract the calories provided by propofol (1 kcal/mL) from the daily caloric requirement. Propofol is infused in a 10% lipid emulsion, which has a caloric density of 1 kcal/mL. Therefore, the hourly infusion rate of propofol (mL/hr) is equivalent to the hourly yield of calories from propofol (kcal/hr).

b. Use nonprotein calories to provide the daily caloric requirement (so protein can be used for muscle strength, etc). This requires an adjustment of the calories provided by the feeding formula. (In standard feeding formulas, nonprotein calories account for about 85% of the total calories.)

Step 4. Adjust the protein intake, if necessary.

The final step in the process is to determine if the feeding regimen will provide enough protein to satisfy the daily protein requirement (from step 1). The projected protein intake is simply the daily feeding volume multiplied by the protein concentration in the feeding formula. If the projected protein intake is less than the desired protein intake, powdered protein is added to the tube feedings to correct the discrepancy.

Table 48.4	Creating an Enteral Feeding Regimen

Step 1: Estimate daily calorie and protein requirements.

$$\text{Calories (kcal/day)} = 25 \times \text{wt (kg)}$$
$$\text{Protein (g/day)} = (1.2 - 1.6) \times \text{wt (kg)}$$

Step 2: Select feeding formula.

Step 3: Calculate desired infusion rate.

$$\text{Feeding volume (mL)} = \frac{\text{kcal/day required}}{\text{kcal/mL in feeding formula}}$$

$$\text{Infusion rate (mL/hr)} = \frac{\text{Feeding volume (mL)}}{\text{Feeding time (hrs)}}$$

Step 4: Adjust protein intake, if necessary.

a. Calculate the projected protein intake (g/day) as:

Feeding volume (L/day) × protein (g/L) in feedings

b. If the projected intake is less than desired intake, add protein to the feeding regimen to correct the discrepancy.

INITIATING TUBE FEEDINGS

Placement of Feeding Tubes

Feeding tubes are inserted through the nares and advanced blindly into the stomach or duodenum. The distance required to reach the stomach can be estimated by measuring the distance from the tip of the nose to the earlobe and then to the xiphoid process (typically 50–60 cm) (20). Once the tube is advanced the desired length, *a portable chest x-ray is required to verify proper tube position* before the feeding formula is infused. The common practice of *evaluating tube placement by pushing air through the tube and listening for bowel sounds is not reliable,* because sounds emanating from a misplaced tube in the distal airways or pleural space can be transmitted into the upper abdomen (21,22).

Tube Misplacement

Feeding tubes end up in the trachea during 1% of insertions (23). Intubated patients often do not cough when feeding tubes enter the trachea (unlike healthy subjects); as a result, feeding tubes can be advanced deep into the lungs without any warning signs, and can puncture the visceral pleura and create a pneumothorax (21,22). The portable chest x-ray in Figure 48.1 shows a feeding tube that has been advanced almost to the edge of the right lung in a patient with a tracheostomy. This was a routine post-insertion chest x-ray, and there was no evidence that the tube was in the airways other than the chest x-ray. This illustrates the value of a portable chest x-ray immediately after a feeding tube is inserted, and before the feeding formula is infused. (The pleural effusion on the right in Figure 48.1 was present prior to insertion of the feeding tube.)

Gastric vs. Duodenal Placement

Advancing the tip of the feeding tube into the duodenum, to reduce the risk of aspiration, is not necessary (1) because most studies show that *there is no difference in the risk of aspiration with gastric versus duodenal feedings* (24,25). However, duodenal placement may be necessary in patients who regurgitate intragastric feedings.

Starter Regimens

The traditional practice is to begin tube feedings at a low infusion rate (10–20 ml/hr), and then gradually advance to the target infusion rate over the next 6–8 hours. However, gastric feedings can begin at the desired (target) rate in most patients without the risk of vomiting or aspiration (26,27). Starter regimens are more appropriate for small bowel feedings (particularly in the jejunum) because of the limited reservoir capacity of the small bowel.

COMPLICATIONS

The complications associated with enteral tube feedings include occlu-

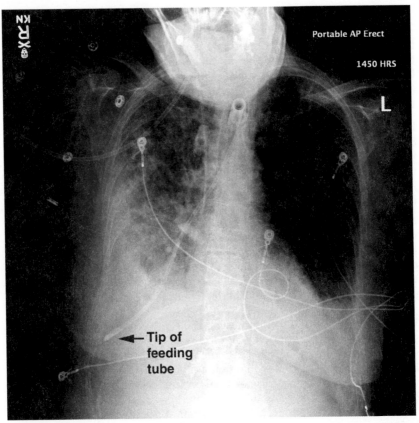

Tip of feeding tube

FIGURE 48.1 Routine chest x-ray following the insertion of a feeding tube. See text for explanation. Image digitally enhanced.

sion of the feeding tube, regurgitation of the feeding formula into the mouth and airways, and diarrhea.

Tube Occlusion

Narrow-bore feeding tubes can become occluded by protein precipitates that form when acidic gastric secretions reflux into the feeding tubes (28). Standard preventive measures include flushing the feeding tubes with 30 mL of water every 4 hours, and using a 10-mL water flush after medications are instilled.

Restoring Patency

If flow through the feeding tube is sluggish, flushing the tube with warm water can restore flow in 30% of cases (29). If this is ineffective, *pancreatic enzyme* (Viokase) can be used as follows (29):

Regimen: Dissolve 1 tablet of Viokase and 1 tablet of sodium carbonate (324 mg) in 5 mL of water. Inject this mixture into the feeding tube and clamp for 5 minutes.

Follow with a warm water flush. This should relieve the obstruction in about 75% of cases (17).

If the tube is completely occluded, advance a flexible wire or a drum cartridge catheter through the feeding tube in an attempt to clear the obstruction. If this is unsuccessful, replace the feeding tube without delay.

Regurgitation/Aspiration

Retrograde regurgitation of feeding formula is reported in as many as 80% of patients receiving gastric or duodenal feedings (18). The following measures are available for reducing the risk of regurgitation and aspiration pneumonia.

Gastric Residual Volume

A standard practice during enteral tube feeding is to measure the gastric residual volume periodically, and discontinue the feeding temporarily if the residual volume exceeds a preselected threshold. This results in frequent interruptions in feeding, and is a common cause of inadequate nutrition support. However, this practice is flawed, because there is no agreement on the residual volume that causes regurgitation.

WHAT VOLUME? Residual volumes of 150–250 mL are typically used to stop enteral feedings, but clinical studies have shown that residual volumes up to 500 mL do not increase the risk of aspiration pneumonia (31). In fact, a recent study shows that managing ventilator-dependent patients without monitoring gastric residual volumes has no adverse consequences on the risk of ventilator-associated pneumonia, or on clinical outcomes (32). This observation creates doubt about the benefits of monitoring gastric residual volumes routinely in the ICU.

RECOMMENDATIONS The most recent guidelines on nutrition support in the ICU recommends that gastric residual volumes of 200–500 mL should raise concern about the risk of aspiration, but tube feedings should not be stopped when the residual volumes are < 500 mL unless there are other signs of intolerance to feedings (e.g., vomiting) (1).

When regurgitation of enteral feedings is evident, the head of the bed should be elevated to 45° above horizontal, and the feeding tube should be advanced into the small bowel (if it's not already there). Prokinetic therapy is an additional option, but the benefits are questionable.

Prokinetic Therapy

The prokinetic agents and recommended dosing regimens are shown in Table 48.5. Prokinetic therapy can produce short-term improvement in indices of gastric motility, but the clinical significance of these effects have been difficult to demonstrate (33).

ERYTHROMYCIN: The macrolide antibiotic, erythromycin, promotes gastric emptying by stimulating motilin receptors in the GI tract (34). At a dose of 200 mg IV every 12 hours, erythromycin can decrease gastric residual volumes by 60% after 24 hours, but this effect diminishes rapidly over a few days (35). Erythromycin may be more effective than metoclopramide, but it is usually not favored because of concerns about antimicrobial resistance. Erythromycin is more effective when used in combination with metoclopramide (36).

Table 48.5	Prokinetic Therapy
Drug	**Dosing Regimens and Comments**
Metoclopramide	Dosing: 10 mg every 6 hrs. Comment: A dopamine antagonist in the GI tract. Can decrease gastric residual volume by 30%, but efficacy diminishes over a few days. IV may be more effective than PO therapy.
Erythromycin	Dosing: 200 mg IV every 12 hrs. Comment: Stimulates motilin receptors in the GI tract. May be more effective than metoclopramide, but efficacy wanes over a few days.
Enteral Naloxone	Dosing: 8 mg via nasogastric tube every 6 hrs. Comment: Blocks opiate receptors in the bowel without antagonizing the analgesic effects of opiates. Used only for gastric dysmotility associated with opiates.

From References 34–37.

METOCLOPRAMIDE: Metoclopramide promotes gastric emptying by antagonizing the actions of dopamine in the GI tract. At a dose of 10 mg IV every 6 hours, metoclopramide can decrease gastric residual volumes by 30% after 24 hours, but the effect wanes rapidly (35). Metoclopramide is more effective when given in combination with erythromycin (36).

ENTERAL NALOXONE: In critically patients who have gastric dysmotility associated with opiates, direct intragastric administration of the opioid antagonist naloxone (8 mg via nasogastric tube every 6 hours) can selectively block opioid receptors in the bowel and promote gastric emptying without antagonizing the analgesic effects of the opiate (37). The opiate antagonist methylnaltrexone, has also been shown to promote postoperative recovery of bowel function in opiate users (38).

RECOMMENDATION: For a trial of prokinetic therapy, either start with erythromycin, and add metoclopramide after 24 hours if needed, or start with both drugs. And don't expect much.

The Intolerant Patient

For patients who continue to be intolerant of tube feedings (e.g., repeatedly regurgitate feedings or develop abdominal distention), a switch to parenteral nutrition may be necessary. However, the infusion of tube feedings should be continued at a lower, tolerable rate, whenever possible, to provide some support for the antimicrobial defenses in the bowel.

Diarrhea

Diarrhea occurs in approximately 30% of patients receiving enteral tube feedings (26). The feeding formulas were originally implicated, but the consensus opinion now is that other factors are involved (39). The principal offender in tube-feeding diarrhea may be liquid drug preparations.

Liquid Drug Preparations

Liquid preparations are favored for drug delivery through narrow-bore feeding tubes because there is less risk of obstruction. However, liquid preparations have two features that create a risk for diarrhea: (a) they can be extremely hyperosmolar ($\geq 3,000$ mosm/kg H_2O), and (b) they can contain sorbitol (to improve palatability), a well-known laxative that draws water into the bowel lumen (40). Table 48.6 includes a list of diarrhea-prone liquid preparations that might be used in ICU patients. These preparations should be discontinued, if possible, in any patient who develops diarrhea of uncertain etiology during enteral nutrition.

Table 48.6	Liquid Drug Preparations That Promote Diarrhea
$\geq 3,000$ mosm/kg H_2O	**Contain Sorbitol**
Acetaminophen elixir	Acetaminophen liquid
Dexamethasone solution	Cimetidine solution
Ferrous sulfate liquid	Isoniazid syrup
Hydroxyzine syrup	Iatrogenic Fever
Metoclopramide syrup	Lithium syrup
Multivitamin liquid	Metoclopramide syrup
Potassium chloride liquid	Theophylline solution
Promethazine syrup	Tetracycline suspension
Sodium phosphate liquid	

From Reference 40.

A FINAL WORD

Eating as a Physical Defense Mechanism

The mucosal surface of the bowel is constantly changing, with new cells to replace the old ones every few days, and the force behind this dynamic process is the presence of food in the lumen of the bowel. Removing the nutritional bulk from the bowel lumen disrupts the normal process of renewal in the bowel mucosa, and makes us vulnerable to invasion by the hordes of enteric pathogens that inhabit the bowel. This is one of the major advantages of enteral tube feedings over total parenteral nutrition, and it also means that *eating is a defense against infection.*

REFERENCES

Clinical Practice Guidelines

1. McClave SA, Martindale RG, Vanek VW, et al. Guidelines for the provision and assessment of nutrition support therapy in the adult critically ill patient: Society of Critical Care Medicine and American Society for Parenteral and Enteral Nutrition. J Parent Ent Nutr 2009; 33:277–316.

2. Kreymann KG, Berger MM, Deutz NEP, et al. ESPEN guidelines on enteral nutrition: intensive care. Clin Nutr 2006; 25:210–223.

General Considerations

3. Simpson F, Doig GS. Parenteral vs enteral nutrition in the critically ill patient: a meta-analysis of trials using the intention to treat principle. Intensive Care Med 2005; 31:12–23.

4. Moore FA, Feliciano DV, Andrassay RJ, et al. Early enteral feeding, compared with parenteral, reduces postoperative septic complications: the results of a meta-analysis. Ann Surg 1992; 216:172–183.

5. Levine GM, Derin JJ, Steiger E, et al. Role of oral intake in maintenance of gut mass and disaccharide activity. Gastroenterology 1974; 67:975–982.

6. Alpers DH. Enteral feeding and gut atrophy. Curr Opin Clin Nutr Metab Care 2002; 5:679–683.

7. Wiest R, Rath HC. Gastrointestinal disorders of the critically ill. Bacterial translocation in the gut. Best Pract Res Clin Gastroenterol 2003; 17:397–425.

8. Ohta K, Omura K, Hirano K, et al. The effect of an additive small amount of a low residue diet against total parenteral nutrition-induced gut mucosal barrier. Am J Surg 2003; 185:79–85.

9. Spaeth G, Specian RD, Berg R, Deitch EA. Bulk prevents bacterial translocation induced by the oral administration of total parenteral nutrition solution. J Parenter Ent Nutrit 1990; 14:442–447.

10. Herskowitz K, Souba WW. Intestinal glutamine metabolism during critical illness: a surgical perspective. Nutrition 1990; 6:199–206.

11. Alverdy JC, Moss GS. Total parenteral nutrition promotes bacterial translocation from the gut. Surgery 1988; 104:185–190.

12. Marik PE, Zaloga GP. Early enteral nutrition in acutely ill patients: a systematic review. Crit Care Med 2001; 29:2264–2270.

Enteral Feeding Formulas

13. Lefton J, Esper DH, Kochevar M. Enteral formulations. In: The A.S.P.E.N Nutrition Support Core Curriculum. Silver Spring, MD: American Society for Parenteral and Enteral Nutrition, 2007: 209–232.

14. Heyland DK, Novak F, Drover JW. et al. Should immunonutrition become routine in critically ill patients? JAMA 2007; 286:944–953.

15. SingerP, Theilla M, Fisher H, et al. Benefit of an enteral diet enriched with eicosapentanoic acid and gamma-linolenic acid in ventilated patients with acute lung injury. Crit Care Med 2006; 34:1033–1038.

16. Kirk SJ, Barbul A. Role of arginine in trauma, sepsis, and immunity. J Parenter Ent Nutr 1990; 14(Suppl):226S–228S.

17. Bertolini G, Iapichino G, Radrizzani D, et al. Early enteral immunonutrition in patients with severe sepsis: results of an interim analysis of a randomized multicentre clinical trial. Intensive Care Med 2003; 29:834–840.

18. Rebouche CJ. Carnitine. In: Shils ME, et al., eds. Modern nutrition in health and disease. 10th ed. Philadelphia, PA: Lippincott, Williams & Wilkins, 2006; 537–544.

19. Karlic H, Lohninger A. Supplementation of L-carnitine in athletes: does it make sense? Nutrition (Burbank, CA) 2004; 20:709–715.

Initiating Tube Feedings

20. Stroud M, Duncan H, Nightingale J. Guidelines for enteral feeding in adult hospital patients. Gut 2003; 52 Suppl 7:vii1–vii2.

21. Kolbitsch C, Pomaroli A, Lorenz I, et al. Pneumothorax following nasogastric feeding tube insertion in a tracheostomized patient after bilateral lung transplantation. Intensive Care Med 1997; 23:440–442.

22. Fisman DN, Ward ME. Intrapleural placement of a nasogastric tube: an unusual complication of nasotracheal intubation. Can J Anaesth 1996; 43:1252–1256.

23. Baskin WN. Acute complications associated with bedside placement of feeding tubes. Nutr Clin Pract 2006; 21:40–55.

24. Neumann DA, DeLegge MH. Gastric vsersus small bowel tube feeding in the intensive care unit: a prospective comparison of efficacy. Crit Care Med 2002; 30:1436–1438.

25. Marik PE, Zaloga GP. Gastric versus post-pyloric feeding: a systematic review. Crit Care 2003; 7:R46–R51.

26. Rees RG, Keohane PP, Grimble GK, et al. Elemental diet administered nasogastrically without starter regimens to patients with inflammatory bowel disease. J Parenter Enteral Nutr 1986; 10:258–262.

27. Mizock BA. Avoiding common errors in nutritional management. J Crit Illness 1993; 10:1116–1127.

Complipations

28. Marcuard SP, Perkins AM. Clogging of feeding tubes. J Parenter Enteral Nutr 1988; 12:403–405.

29. Marcuard SP, Stegall KS. Unclogging feeding tubes with pancreatic enzyme. J Parenter Enteral Nutr 1990; 14:198–200.

30. Metheny N. Minimizing respiratory complications of nasoenteric tube feedings: state of the science. Heart Lung 1993; 22:213–223.

31. Montejo JC, Minambres E, Bordejé L, et al. Gastric residual volume during enteral nutrition in ICU patients: the REGANE study. Intensive Care Med 2010; 36:1386–1393.

32. Reignier K, Mercier E, Le Gouge A, et al. Effect of not monitoring residual gastric volume on risk of ventilator-associated pneumonia in adults receiving mechanical ventilation and early enteral feeding. JAMA 20113: 309:249–256.

33. Booth CM, Heyland DK, Paterson WG. Gastrointestinal promotility drugs in the critical care setting: a systematic review of the evidence. Crit Care Med 2002; 30:1429–1435.

34. Hawkyard CV, Koerner RJ. The use of erythromycin as a gastrointestinal prokinetic agent in adult critical care: benefits and risks. J Antimicrob Chemother 2007; 59:347–358.

35. Nguyen NO, Chapman MJ, Fraser RJ, et al. Erythromycin is more effective than metoclopramide in the treatment of feed intolerance in critical illness. Crit Care Med 2007; 35:483–489.

36. Nguyen NO, Chapman M, Fraser RJ, et al. Prokinetic therapy for feed intolerance in critical illness: one drug or two? Crit Care Med 2007; 35:2561–2567.

37. Meissner W, Dohrn B, Reinhart K. Enteral naloxone reduces gastric tube reflux and frequency of pneumonia in critical care patients during opioid analgesia. Crit Care Med 2003; 31:776–780.

38. Ladanyi A, Temkin SM, Moss J. Subcutaneous methylnaltrexone to restore postoperative bowel function in a long-term opiate user. Int J Gynecol Cancer 2010; 20:308–310 (abstract).

39. Edes TE, Walk BE, Austin JL. Diarrhea in tube-fed patients: feeding formula not necessarily the cause. Am J Med 1990; 88:91–93.

40. Williams NT. Medication administration through enteral feeding tubes. Am J Heath-Sys Pharm 2008; 65:2347–2357.

Chapter 49

PARENTERAL NUTRITION

To lengthen thy life, lessen thy meals.

Benjamin Franklin

When full nutritional support is not possible in the alimentary canal, the intravenous route is available for nutrient delivery. This chapter describes the basic features of intravenous nutritional support, and demonstrates how to create a parenteral nutrition regimen to meet the needs of individual patients.

SUBSTRATE SOLUTIONS

Dextrose Solutions

Standard nutrition support regimens use carbohydrates to supply approximately 70% of the daily (nonprotein) caloric requirements. The carbohydrate source for total parenteral nutrition (TPN) is dextrose (glucose), which is available in the solutions shown in Table 49.1. Because the energy yield from dextrose is relatively low (see Table 47.1), the dextrose solutions must be concentrated to provide enough calories to satisfy daily requirements. (The standard solution is 50% dextrose, or D_{50}.) These solutions are hyperosmolar, and must be infused through large central veins.

Table 49.1	Intravenous Dextrose Solutions		
Strength	**Concentration (g/L)**	**Energy Yield* (g/L)***	**Osmolarity (mosm/L)**
5%	50	170	253
10%	100	340	505
20%	200	680	1,080
50%	500	1,700	2,525
70%	700	2,380	3,530

*Based on an oxidative energy yield of 3.4 kcal/g for dextrose.

Amino Acid Solutions

Protein is provided as amino acid solutions that contain varying mixtures of essential (N = 9), semi-essential (N = 4), and nonessential (N = 10) amino acids. These solutions are mixed with dextrose solutions in a 1:1 volume ratio. Examples of standard and "specialty" amino acid solutions are shown in Table 49.2.

Table 49.2	Standard and Specialty Amino Acid Solutions		
	Aminosyn	**Aminosyn-HBC**	**Aminosyn RF**
Strengths	3.5%, 5%, 7%, 8.5%, 10%	7%	5.2%
Indications	Standard TPN	Hypercatabolism	Renal Failure
% EAA	50%	63%	89%
% BCAA	25%	46%	33%

EAA = essential amino acids; BCAA = branched chain amino acids.

Standard Solutions

Standard amino acid solutions (e.g., Aminosyn in Table 49.2) are balanced mixtures of 50% essential amino acids and 50% nonessential and semi-essential amino acids. Available concentrations range from 3.5 % up to 10%, but 7% solutions (70 g/L) are used most often.

Specialty Solutions

Specially designed amino acid solutions are available for patients with severe metabolic stress (e.g., from multisystem trauma or burns), and for patients with renal or liver failure.

1. Solutions designed for metabolic stress (e.g., Aminosyn-HBC in Table 49.2) are enriched with branched chain amino acids (isoleucine, leucine, and valine), which are preferred fuels in skeletal muscle when metabolic demands are high.

2. Renal failure solutions (e.g., Aminosyn RF in Table 49.2) are rich in essential amino acids, because the nitrogen in essential amino acids is partially recycled to produce nonessential amino acids, which results in smaller increments in blood urea nitrogen (BUN) when compared with breakdown of nonessential amino acids.

3. Solutions designed for hepatic failure (e.g., HepaticAid) are enriched with branched chain amino acids, which block the transport of aromatic amino acids across the blood-brain barrier (which is implicated in hepatic encephalopathy).

It is important to emphasize that none of these specialized formulas have improved the outcomes in the disorders for which they are designed (3).

Glutamine

Glutamine is the principal metabolic fuel for rapidly dividing cells like intestinal epithelial cells and vascular endothelial cells (4). Because of studies showing that glutamine is important for maintaining the integrity of the bowel mucosa (5), and studies showing a glutamine-associated decrease in infectious complications in ICU patients (6,7), glutamine has been recommended as a daily nutrional supplement in ICU patients (0.2–0.4 g/kg/day) (1). However, a recent multicenter study has shown a glutamine-associated increase in mortality rate in ICU patients with multiorgan failure (8), and until this issue is resolved, the recommendation for daily glutamine administration in ICU patients must be re-evaluated. (*Note:* Glutamine is not included in any of the commercially available amino acid solutions, so it must be added to the solutions by the pharmacy. This alone will limit the popularity of daily glutamine supplementation.)

Table 49.3	Intravenous Lipid Emulsions for Clinical Use			
Feature	**Intralipid**		**Liposyn II**	
	10%	**20%**	**10%**	**20%**
Calories (kcal/mL)	1.1	2	1.1	2
% calories as EFA (Linoleic acid)	50%	50%	66%	66%
Cholesterol (mg/dL)	250–300	250–300	13–22	13–22
Osmolarity (mosm/L)	260	260	276	258
Unit Volumes (mL)	50 100 250 500	50 100 250 500	100 200 500	200 500

EFA = essential fatty acid.

Lipid Emulsions

Lipids are provided as emulsions composed of submicron droplets of cholesterol, phospholipids, and triglycerides (9). The triglycerides are derived from vegetable oils (safflower or soybean oils) and are rich in linoleic acid, an essential fatty acid (10). Lipids are used to provide 30% of daily caloric requirements, and 4% of the daily calories should be provided as linoleic acid to prevent essential fatty acid deficiency (11).

As shown in Table 49.3, lipid emulsions are available in 10% and 20% strengths (the percentage refers to grams of triglyceride per 100 mL of solution). The 10% emulsions provide approximately 1 kcal/mL, and the 20% emulsions provide 2 kcal/mL. Unlike the hypertonic dextrose solutions, lipid emulsions are roughly isotonic to plasma and *can be infused through peripheral veins.* The lipid emulsions are available in unit volumes of 50 to 500 mL, and can be infused separately (at a maximum rate of 50 mL/hour) or added to the dextrose–amino acid mixtures. The triglycerides introduced into the bloodstream are not cleared for 8 to 10 hours, and lipid infusions often produce a transient, lipemic-appearing plasma.

ADDITIVES

Commercially available mixtures of electrolytes, vitamins, and trace elements are added directly to the dextrose–amino acid mixtures.

Electrolytes

There are more than 15 electrolyte mixtures available. Most have a volume of 20 mL, and contain sodium, chloride, potassium, and magnesium. You must check the mixture used at your hospital to determine if additional electrolytes must be added. Additional requirements for potassium or other electrolytes can be specified in the TPN orders.

Vitamins

Aqueous multivitamin preparations are added to the dextrose–amino acid mixtures. One unit vial of a standard multivitamin preparation will provide the normal daily requirements for most vitamins (see Table 47.3) (16). The daily vitamin requirements in ICU patients are not known (and probably varies with each patient). However, vitamin deficiencies are rcommon in ICU patients despite the provision of normal daily requirements, suggesting that critically ill patients have increased daily vitamin requirements.

Trace Elements

A variety of trace element additives are available, and one of the commercial preparations is shown in Table 49.4, along with the recommended daily requirement for trace elements. Note the poor correlation between the daily requirements and the trace element content of the commercial mixture. Trace element mixtures don't contain iron and iodine, and some don't contain selenium. Iron is not advised in critically ill patients because of its pro-oxidant effects (see Chapter 47 for more information on iron and oxidant injury). However, selenium should be given daily to ICU patients, particularly those with severe sepsis.

Selenium

The most important consideration regarding trace elements is selenium, which is a co-factor for glutathione peroxidase, an enzyme that participates in endogenous antioxidant protection (see Figure 22.7). Plasma levels of selenium are reduced in severe sepsis, and selenium replacement is associated with improved survival (12). The proposed daily requirement for selenium is 55 µg, but this is probably inadequate for critically ill patients. A daily dose of 200 µg is used in many studies, and doses of 400 µg daily are considered safe (see Table 47.3).

Table 49.4	Dietary Allowances for Essential Trace Elements	
Trace Element	**Daily Requirement†**	**Multitrace-5 Concentrated§**
Chromium	30 µg	10 µg
Copper	900 µg	1 mg
Iodine	150 µg	—
Iron	8 mg	—
Manganese	2.3 mg	0.5 mg
Selenium	55 µg	60 µg
Zinc	11 mg	5 mg

†From the Food and Nutrition Information Center (http://fnic.nal.usda.gov). Accessed July, 2013.
§Product description, America Reagent, Inc.

CREATING A TPN REGIMEN

The following is a stepwise approach to creating a standard TPN regimen for an individual patient. The patient in this example will be a 70-kg adult who is not malnourished and has no volume restrictions.

Step 1

The first step is to determine the daily requirement for calories and protein. There are two very simple approximations that can be used: i.e., the daily requirement for calories is 25 kcal/kg, and the daily protein requirement is 1.2–1.6 g/kg. (See Chapter 47 for more information on these estimates.) You can use actual body weight in these estimates as long as actual body weight is within 125% of the ideal weight. If actual body weight exceeds 125% of ideal body weight, you can use an adjusted body weight (see equation 47.3). If available, indirect calorimetry should be used to measure the resting energy expenditure (see Chapter 47).

For the 70 kg patient, we'll use actual body weight, and a daily protein requirement of 1.4 g/kg. Therefore, the daily requirement for calories and protein will be:

$$\text{Calories: } 25 \times 70 = 1{,}750 \text{ kcal/day}$$

$$\text{Protein: } 1.4 \times 70 = 98 \text{ grams/day} \tag{49.1}$$

Note: If propofol is being infused, you should determine the calories provided by propofol and subtract those calories from the daily caloric requirement. Propofol is infused in a 10% lipid emulsion, which has a caloric density equivalent to 10% Intralipid (1 kcal/mL). Therefore, the hourly infusion rate of propofol (mL/hr) is equivalent to the hourly yield of calories (kcal/hr).

Step 2

The next step is to take a standard mixture of 10% amino acids (500 mL) and 50% dextrose (500 mL) and determine the volume of this mixture that is needed to deliver the estimated daily protein requirement. Although the dextrose–amino acid mixture is referred to as A_{10}-D_{50}, the final mixture actually represents 5% amino acids (50 grams of protein per liter) and 25% dextrose (250 grams of dextrose per liter). The volume of the A_{10}-D_{50} mixture that will provide the daily protein requirement is equivalent to the daily protein requirement (98 g/day), divided by the protein concentration in the amino acid mixture (50 g/L); i.e.,

$$\text{Volume of } A_{10}D_{50} = 98 / 50 = 1.9 \text{ Liters} \tag{49.2}$$

If this mixture is infused over 24 hours, the infusion rate will be:

$$\text{Infusion rate} = 1{,}900 \text{ mL}/24 \text{ hr} = 81 \text{ mL/hr} \tag{49.3}$$

Step 3

Now, determine how many nonprotein calories will be provided by 1.9 liters of A_{10}-D_{50}. (Only nonprotein calories are used to provide the daily energy needs.) First, determine how much dextrose is in 1.9 liters of A_{10}-D_{50}:

$$250 \text{ g/L} \times 1.9 \text{ L} = 475 \text{ grams of dextrose} \tag{49.4}$$

Now, using an energy yield of 3.4 kcal/g for dextrose, calculate the calories provided by 475 grams of dextrose:

$$\text{Dextrose calories} = 475 \times 3.4 = 1{,}615 \text{ kcal/day} \tag{49.5}$$

Step 4

The next step is to use lipid calories to make up the difference between the calories supplied by dextrose and the daily requirement for calories, as shown below:

$$\text{Daily Requirement: } 1{,}750 \text{ kcal} \tag{49.6}$$

$$\text{Daily Dextrose Calories: } 1{,}615 \text{ kcal}$$

$$\text{Deficit: } 135 \text{ kcal}$$

The remaining 135 calories will be provided by lipids. If a 10% lipid emulsion (1 kcal/mL) is used, the volume will be 135 mL/day. (Lipid emulsions are available in unit volumes of 50 mL, so the volume can be adjusted to 150 mL to avoid wastage). The maximum infusion rate is 50 mL/hr.

Step 5

The TPN orders for this example can be written as follows:

1. A_{10}-D_{50} to run at 80 mL/hour.

2. 10% Intralipid, 150 mL, to infuse over 3 hours.

3. Add standard electrolytes, multivitamins, and trace elements.

TPN orders are rewritten each day. Specific electrolytes, vitamins, and trace elements are added to the daily orders when needed.

COMPLICATIONS

Catheter-Related Complications

As mentioned earlier, the hyperosmolarity of the dextrose and amino acid solutions requires infusion through large veins, so central venous cannulation, or a peripherally inserted central catheter (PICC), is required. The complications associated with these catheters are described in Chapters 2 and 3.

Misdirected Catheter

Insertion of subclavian vein catheters and peripherally inserted central catheters (PICCs) can occasionally result in advancement of a catheter into the internal jugular vein, like the one shown in Figure 49.1. In one survey (13), 10% of subclavian vein cannulations (mostly on the right) resulted in misplacement of the catheter in the internal jugular vein. The standard recommendation is to reposition such catheters because of the risk of thrombosis (13), but *there is no evidence to support this claim.*

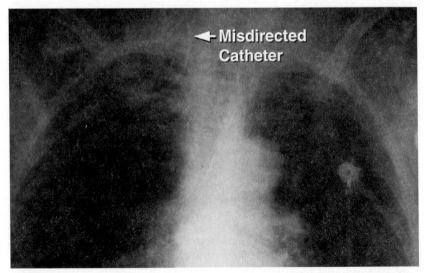

FIGURE 49.1 X-ray showing a central venous catheter misdirected into the neck.

Carbohydrate Complications

Hyperglycemia

Hyperglycemia is common during TPN; e.g., in one study, blood glucose levels above 300 mg/dL were recorded in 20% of postoperative patients receiving TPN (vs. 1.5% of control patients) (14). This is attributed to the glucose load in TPN. (A standard TPN regimen with 1,800 nonprotein calories has about 350 grams of glucose, compared to 230 grams in a standard tube feeding regimen.) Tight glycemic control is not recommended in critically ill patients because of the risk of hypoglycemia, which has more serious consequences than hyperglycemia (15). The current recommendation for hospitalized patients is *a target range of 140 – 180 mg/dL for blood glucose* (1,16).

INSULIN If insulin therapy is required, a variety of biosynthetic insulins are available, and the ones used most frequently are shown in Table 49.5 (17). A continuous infusion of regular insulin is preferred for critically ill patients who are unstable or have type 1 diabetes (2), to prevent wide swings in glucose levels. This can be accomplished by adding insulin to the TPN solutions. One shortcoming of intravenous insulin infusions is the propensity for insulin to adsorb to the plastic tubing in IV infusion sets. This has a variable effect on the bioavailability of insulin, but this variability can be reduced by priming the IV infusion set with an insulin solution (e.g., 20 mL of a saline containing 1 unit/mL of regular insulin). This stabilizes the bioavailability of infused insulin (at about 30–40%) for several days, but the priming procedure must be repeated each time the IV infusion set is changed (2).

Table 49.5	Insulin Preparations			
Type	**Name**	**Onset**	**Peak**	**Duration**
Rapid-Acting	Aspart	10–20 min	1–3 hr	3–5 hr
Rapid-Acting	Glulisine	25 min	45–50 min	4–5 hr
Rapid-Acting	Lispro	15–30 min	0.5–2.5 hr	3–6 hr
Short-Acting	Regular	30–60 min	1–5 hr	6–10 hr
Intermediate	NPH	1–2 hr	6–14 hr	16–24 hr
Long-Acting	Glargine	1 hr	2–20 hr	24 hr

From Reference 17.

Subcutaneous insulin can be used for patients who are stable. Regimens will vary in each patient, but the combination of an intermediate or long-acting insulin with a rapid-acting insulin, when needed, is a popular for hospitalized patients.

Hypophosphatemia

The movement of glucose into cells is associated with a similar movement of phosphate into cells, and this provides phosphate for co-factors (e.g., thiamine pyrophosphate) that participate in glucose metabolism. This intracellular shift of phosphate can result in hypophosphatemia if extracellular phosphate levels are marginal. This is the most common cause of hypophosphatemia in hospitalized patients (18), and plasma phosphate levels typically show a steady decline after TPN is initiated (see Table 38.2).

Hypokalemia

Glucose movement into cells is also accompanied by an intracellular shift of potassium (which is the basis for the use of glucose and insulin to treat severe hyperkalemia). This effect is usually transient, but continued glucose loading during TPN can lead to persistent hypokalemia.

Hypercapnia

Excess carbohydrate intake promotes CO_2 retention in patients with respiratory insufficiency. This was originally attributed to the high respiratory quotient (VCO_2/VO_2) associated with carbohydrate metabolism. However, CO_2 retention is a consequence of overfeeding, and not overfeeding with carbohydrates (19).

Lipid Complications

Overfeeding with lipids may contribute to hepatic steatosis. However, a more serious concern with lipid infusions is the potential to *promote inflammation*. The lipid emulsions used in TPN regimens are rich in oxidizable lipids (20), and the oxidation of infused lipids will trigger an inflammatory response. In fact, infusions of oleic acid, one of the lipids in TPN, is a standard method for producing the acute respiratory distress syndrome (ARDS) in animals (21), and this might explain why lipid infusions are associated with impaired oxygenation (22,23). The possible role of lipid infusions in promoting oxidant-induced injury deserves more attention.

Hepatobiliary Complications

Hepatic Steatosis

Fat accumulation in the liver (hepatic steatosis) is common in patients receiving long-term TPN, and is believed to be the result of chronic overfeeding with carbohydrates and lipids. Although this condition is associated with elevated liver enzymes in blood (24), it may not be a pathological entity.

Cholestasis

The absence of lipids in the proximal small bowel prevents cholecystokinin-mediated contraction of the gallbladder. This results in bile stasis and the accumulation of sludge in the gallbladder, and can lead to *acalculous cholecystitis* (25), which is described in Chapter 40.

Bowel Sepsis

The absence of nutritional bulk in the GI tract leads to atrophic changes in the bowel mucosa, and impairs bowel-associated immunity, and these changes can lead to the systemic spread of enteric pathogens. This topic is described in Chapter 48.

PERIPHERAL PARENTERAL NUTRITION

Peripheral parenteral nutrition (PPN) is a truncated form of TPN that can be used to provide nonprotein calories in amounts that will spare the breakdown of proteins to provide energy (i.e., *protein-sparing* nutrition support). PPN can be used as a supplement to enteral feeding, or as a source of calories during brief periods of inadequate nutrition. It is not intended for hypercatabolic or malnourished patients, who need full nutritional support,

The osmolarity of peripheral vein infusates should be kept below 900 mosm/L, with a pH between 7.2 and 7.4, to slow the rate of osmotic damage to vessels (26,27). This requires dilute amino acid and dextrose solutions, which limits nutrient intake. However, lipid emulsions are isotonic to plasma, and lipids can be used to provide a considerable portion of the nonprotein calories in PPN.

Method

A popular solution in PPN is a mixture of 3% amino acids and 20% dextrose (final concentration of 1.5% amino acids and 10% dextrose), which has an osmolarity of 500 mosm/L. The dextrose will provide 340 kcal/L, so 2.5 L of the mixture will provide 850 kcal. If 250 mL of 20% Intralipid is added to the regimen (adding 500 kcal), the total nonprotein calories will increase to 1,350 kcal/day. This should be close to the nonprotein caloric requirement of an average-size, unstressed adult (20 kcal/kg/day).

A FINAL WORD

The final word on parenteral nutrition is . . . *avoid* . . . whenever possible. For an explanation, see the first section of Chapter 48.

REFERENCES

Clinical Practice Guidelines

1. Singer P, Berger MM, Van den Berghe G, et al. ESPEN guidelines on parenteral nutrition: Intensive care. Clin Nutr 2009; 387–400.

2. Jacobi J, Bircher N, Krinsley J, et al. Guidelines for the use of insulin infusion for the management of hyperglycemia in critically ill patients. Crit Care Med 2012; 40:3251–3276.

Substrate Solutions

3. Andris DA, Krzywda EA. Nutrition support in specific diseases: back to basics. Nutr Clin Pract 1994; 9:28–32.

4. Souba WW, Klimberg VS, Plumley DA, et al. The role of glutamine in maintaining a healthy gut and supporting the metabolic response to injury and infection. J Surg Res 1990; 48:383–391.

5. De-Souza DA, Greene LJ. Intestinal permeability and systemic infections in critically ill patients: effect of glutamine. Crit Care Med 2005; 33:1125–1135.

6. Dechelotte P, Hasselmann M, Cynober L, et al. L-alanyl-L-glutamine dipeptide-supplemented total parenteral nutrition reduces infectious complications and glucose intolerance in critically ill patients: the French controlled, randomized, double-blind, multicenter study. Crit Care Med 2006; 34:598–604.

7. Fuentes-Orozco C, Anaya-Prado R, Gonzalez-Ojeda A, et al. L-alanyl-L-glutamine-supplemented parenteral nutrition improves infectious morbidity in secondary peritonitis. Clin Nutr 2004; 23:13–21.

8. Heyland D, Muscedere J, Wischmeyer PE, et al. A randomized trial of glutamine and antioxidants in critically ill patients. N Engl J Med 2013; 368:1489–1497.

9. Driscoll DF. Compounding TPN admixtures: then and now. J Parenter Enteral Nutr 2003; 27:433–438.

10. Warshawsky KY. Intravenous fat emulsions in clinical practice. Nutr Clin Pract 1992; 7:187–196.

11. Barr LH, Dunn GD, Brennan MF. Essential fatty acid deficiency during total parenteral nutrition. Ann Surg 1981; 193:304–311.

12. Alhazzani W, Jacobi J, Sindi A, et al. The effect of selenium therapy on mortality in patients with sepsis syndrome. Crit Care Med 2013; 41:1555–1564.

Complications

13. Padberg FT, Jr., Ruggiero J, Blackburn GL, et al. Central venous catheterization for parenteral nutrition. Ann Surg 1981; 193:264–270.

14. The Veterans Affairs Total Parenteral Nutrition Cooperative Study group. Perioperative total parenteral nutrition in postoperative patients. N Eng J Med 1991; 325:525–532.

15. Marik PE, Preiser J-C. Toward understanding tight glycemic control in the ICU. Chest 2010; 137:544–551.

16. Moghissi ES, Korytkowski MT, DiNardo M, et al. American Association of Clinical Endocrinologists, American Diabetes Association, American Association of Clinical Endocrinologists, and American Diabetes Association consensus statement on inpatient glycemic control. Diabetes Care 2009; 32:1119–1131.

17. McEvoy GK, ed. AHFS Drug Information, 2012. Bethesda, MD: American Society of Heath System Pharmacists, 2012:3201.

18. Knochel JP. The pathophysiology and clinical characteristics of severe hypophosphatemia. Arch Intern Med 1977; 137:203–220.

19. Talpers SS, Romberger DJ, Bunce SB, et al. Nutritionally associated increased carbon dioxide production. Excess total calories vs. high proportion of carbohydrate calories. Chest 1992; 102:551–555.

20. Carpentier YA, Dupont IE. Advances in intravenous lipid emulsions. World J Surg 2000; 24:1493–1497.

21. Schuster DP. ARDS: clinical lessons from the oleic acid model of acute lung injury. Am J Respir Crit Care Med 1994; 149:245–260.

22. Suchner U, Katz DP, Furst P, et al. Effects of intravenous fat emulsions on lung function in patients with acute respiratory distress syndrome or sepsis. Crit Care Med 2001; 29:1569–1574.

23. Battistella FD, Widergren JT, Anderson JT, et al. A prospective, randomized trial of intravenous fat emulsion administration in trauma victims requiring total parenteral nutrition. J Trauma 1997; 43:52–58.

24. Freund HR. Abnormalities of liver function and hepatic damage associated with total parenteral nutrition. Nutrition 1991; 7:1–5.

25. Phelps SJ, Brown RO, Helms RA, et al. Toxicities of parenteral nutrition in the critically ill patient. Crit Care Clin 1991; 7:725–753.

Peripheral Parenteral Nutrition

26. Culebras JM, Martin-Pena G, Garcia-de-Lorenzo A, et al. Practical aspects of peripheral parenteral nutrition. Curr Opin Clin Nutr Metab Care 2004; 7:303–307.

27. Anderson AD, Palmer D, MacFie J. Peripheral parenteral nutrition. Br J Surg 2003; 90:1048–1054.

Chapter 50

ADRENAL AND THYROID DYSFUNCTION

Judge a tree from its fruit, not from the leaves.

Euripedes
484–406 BC

Adrenal and thyroid disorders are rarely the primary reason for admission to an ICU. However, critical illness can influence adrenal and thyroid function, and there is concern that this influence can have a negative impact on outcomes. This chapter describes the spectrum of adrenal and thyroid disorders that occur in critically ill patients, and how to detect and manage each of these disorders.

ADRENAL SUPPRESSION IN THE ICU

The adrenal gland plays a major role in the adaptive response to stress. The adrenal cortex releases glucocorticoids and mineralocorticoids that promote glucose availability and maintain extracellular volume, while the adrenal medulla releases catecholamines that support the circulation. Attenuation or loss of this adrenal response leads to hemodynamic instability, volume depletion, and defective energy metabolism (1,2). Adrenal insufficiency can remain silent until the adrenal gland is called on to respond to a physiologic stress. When this occurs, adrenal insufficiency becomes an occult catalyst that speeds the progression of acute, life-threatening conditions.

The activity of the adrenal glands is governed by the release of adreno-corticotrophic hormone (ACTH) from the anterior pituitary gland, which, in turn, is governed by the production of corticotrophin-releasing hormone (CRH) in the hypothalamus (see Figure 50.1). Adrenal insufficiency can be the result of suppression at the hypothalamic-pituitary level, or primary suppression of adrenal gland activity.

Cortisol

Cortisol (hydrocortisone) is the major glucocorticoid released by the adrenal cortex. The daily production of cortisol in the normal (un-stressed) adult is 15–25 mg/day, and this can increase up to 350 mg/day during periods of maximum physiological stress (2).

PLASMA CORTISOL: About 90% of the cortisol in plasma is bound to *cortico-steroid-binding globulin* (CBG) and albumin, while the remaining 10% is the free or biologically active form (1,2). The commercial assay for plasma cortisol measures both bound and unbound fractions; i.e., *total* cortisol. This assay can be misleading in acutely ill patients because plasma levels of CBG fall by as much as 50% during an acute illness (2). In one study of ICU patients with sepsis, total cortisol levels were diminished in 40% of the patients, while free cortisol levels were consistently elevated (4).

Critically Ill Patients

Adrenal insufficiency is common in critically ill patients. The overall prevalence is 10–20% (1), but rates as high as 60% have been reported in patients with severe sepsis and septic shock (3). The adrenal suppression in critically ill patients *is often reversible*, and is called *critical illness-related corticosteroid insufficiency* (CIRCI) (1). The mechanisms involved in CIRCI are complex, and are shown in Figure 50.1 (1–3,5). The systemic inflammatory response plays a major role in CIRCI. *Suppression at the hypothalamic-pituitary level* is particularly prominent, and *is responsible for as many as 75% of the cases of adrenal suppression in patients with severe sepsis and septic shock* (3).

Predisposing Conditions

As mentioned, severe sepsis and septic shock are the leading causes of adrenal suppression in critically ill patients. Other infection-related causes of adrenal suppression include HIV infection, systemic fungal infections, and meningococcemia (which can precipitate adrenal hemorrhage) (2,5).

Noninfectious sources of adrenal suppression in ICU patients include: (a) abrupt discontinuation of chronic steroid therapy, (b) adrenal hemorrhage from disseminated intravascular coagulation (DIC) or anticoagulant therapy, and (c) drugs that inhibit the synthesis of cortisol (e.g., etomidate and ketoconazole) or accelerate the metabolism of cortisol (e.g., phenytoin or rifampin) (2,5).

Clinical Manifestations

The principal manifestation of adrenal suppression in critically ill patients is *hypotension that is refractory to volume resuscitation* (1–3). The typical electrolyte abnormalities that accompany adrenal insufficiency (i.e., hyponatremia and hyperkalemia) are uncommon in the adrenal suppression associated with critical illness.

Diagnosis

Adrenal suppression should be suspected in any ICU patient with

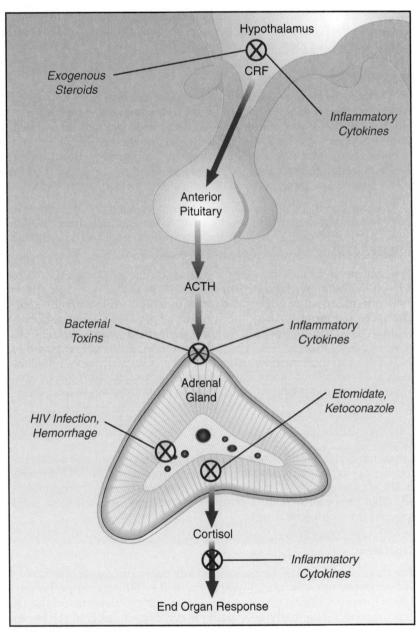

FIGURE 50.1 Mechanisms of adrenal suppression in ICU patients. CRF = cortico-trophin-releasing hormone; ACTH = adrenocorticotrophic hormone.

hypotension that does not respond to volume resuscitation. Unfortunately, the diagnosis of adrenal suppression in critically ill patients is steeped in uncertainty. (*Note:* The use of total cortisol levels to evaluate adrenal function is a major problem in critically ill patients because of the confounding influence of plasma proteins on total cortisol measurements, as mentioned previously.)

Rapid ACTH Stimulation Test

A popular (but often unnecessary) test of adrenal function in ICU patients is the rapid ACTH stimulation test, which can be performed at any time of the day or night. A blood sample is obtained for a baseline (random) plasma cortisol level, and the patient is given synthetic ACTH (Cosyntropin) intravenously in a dose of 250 μg. One hour after the ACTH injection, a second blood sample is obtained for a repeat plasma cortisol level. The interpretation of the test results is as follows (1,2):

> The best predictor of adrenal suppression in critically ill patients is a random plasma cortisol level < 10 μg/dL, *or* an increment in plasma cortisol of < 9 μg/dL after the intravenous injection of synthetic ACTH (250 μg).

The favorite approach to evaluating adrenal function in the ICU is to rely on the random plasma cortisol level. A level that is ≥35 μg/dL is evidence of normal or adequate adrenal function, while a baseline cortisol level that is below 10 μg/dL is evidence of adrenal suppression. A rapid ACTH stimulation test can be performed when the random serum cortisol level is 10–34 μg/dL. However, a normal response to ACTH (i.e., an increment in serum cortisol of ≥9 μg/dL) does not eliminate the possibility of secondary adrenal suppression due to hypothalamic-pituitary dysfunction (which may be more common than suspected in ICU patients).

Septic Shock

In patients with septic shock, plasma cortisol levels are not necessary for identifying patients who might benefit from corticosteroid therapy. In these patients, a trial of intravenous hydrocortisone is recommended when hypotension is refractory to volume resuscitation (and requires a vasopressor drug).

Treatment

The treatment of critical illness-related adrenal suppression is *intravenous hydrocortisone in a dose of 200–300 mg daily* (i.e., 50 mg every 6 hours, or 100 mg every 8 hours) (1). The addition of a mineralocorticoid (i.e., fludrocortisone, 50 μg orally once daily) is considered optional (1), because hydrocortisone has excellent mineralocorticoid activity (see Table 50.1).

Hydrocortisone can be discontinued after satisfactory resolution of the underlying condition. In septic shock, hydrocortisone can be discontinued when vasopressor therapy is no longer necessary, and serum lactate levels have normalized. A gradual taper of the hydrocortisone dose (over at least a few days) is recommended to prevent a rebound increase in proinflammatory mediators (1).

Table 50.1	Corticosteroid Comparisons		
Corticosteroid	Equivalent Doses	AIA Rank†	MCA Rank‡
Hydrocortisone	20 mg	4	1
Prednisone	5 mg	3	2
Methylprednisone	4 mg	2	2
Dexamethasone	0.75 mg	1	4

†Anti-inflammatory activity (1 = best, 4 = worst)
‡Mineralocorticoid activity (1 = best, 4 = worst)
From Reference 4.

EVALUATION OF THYROID FUNCTION

Laboratory tests of thyroid function can be abnormal in up to 90% of critically ill patients (6). In most cases, the abnormality is a consequence of non-thyroidal illness, and is not a sign of pathologic thyroid disease (6,7). This section describes the laboratory evaluation of thyroid function, and explains how to identify non-thyroidal illness as a cause of abnormal thyroid function tests.

Thyroxine (T_4) and Triiodothyronine (T_3)

Thyroxine (T_4) is the principal hormone secreted by the thyroid gland, but the active form is triiodothyronine (T_3), which is formed by deiodination of thyroxine in extrathyroidal tissues. Both T_3 and T_4 are extensively (> 99%) bound to plasma proteins (especially thyroxine-binding globulin), and less than 1% of either hormone is present in the free, or biologically active, form (8). Because of the potential for alterations in plasma proteins and protein binding in acute illness, free T_4 and T_3 levels are more reliable for assessing thyroid function in ICU patients. Free T_3 levels are not routinely available, *so free T_4 levels are used to evaluate thyroid function in acutely ill patients.*

Thyroid-Stimulating Hormone (TSH)

The plasma level of thyroid-stimulating hormone (TSH) is considered *the most reliable test of thyroid function*, and is useful for identifying non-thyroidal illness, and for distinguishing between primary and secondary thyroid disorders. Plasma TSH levels have a diurnal variation, with the lowest values in late afternoon, and the highest values around the hour of sleep. TSH levels can vary by as much as 40% over a 24-hour period (9), and this diurnal variation must be considered when interpreting changes in plasma TSH levels. The reference range for serum TSH is 0.3 – 4.5 mU/dL (10).

Primary vs. Secondary Thyroid Disorders

Because of the negative feedback exerted by the thyroid hormones on

TSH secretion, plasma TSH levels can distinguish primary from secondary thyroid disorders. For example, in patients with hypothyroidism, an elevated plasma TSH level is evidence of primary hypothyroidism, while a reduced TSH level is evidence of secondary hypothyroidism due to hypothalamic–pituitary dysfunction.

Non-Thyroidal Illness

Plasma TSH levels are normal in a majority of instances where abnormal thyroid function tests are the result non-thyroidal illness (6). However, plasma TSH levels can be depressed in 30%, and elevated in 10%, of these patients (6). TSH secretion can be depressed by sepsis, corticosteroids, and dopamine infusions (11), and these factors must be considered when interpreting plasma TSH levels.

Patterns of Abnormal Thyroid Function Tests

The interpretation of free T_4 and TSH levels is shown in Table 50.2.

Table 50.2	Patterns of Abnormal Thyroid Function Tests	
Condition	**Free T_4**	**TSH**
Normal Range	0.8–1.8 ng/dL	0.35–4.5 mU/mL
Non-Thyroidal Illness (severe)	↓	NL or ↓
Primary Hypothyroidism	↓	↑
Secondary Hypothyroidism	↓	↓
Primary Hyperthyroidism	↑	↓

Non-Thyroidal Illness

Acute, non-thyroidal illness is associated with low plasma levels of free T_3, as a result of impaired conversion of T_4 to T_3 in non-thyroidal tissue (6). With increasing severity of illness, both free T_3 and free T_4 levels are depressed, which is the pattern reported in 30–50% of ICU patients (6,7). As mentioned earlier, plasma TSH levels are normal in a majority of patients with non-thyroidal illness, but TSH levels can be depressed in selected conditions (e.g., sepsis, corticosteroid therapy, or dopamine infusions).

Thyroid Disorders

Primary thyroid disorders are characterized by reciprocal changes in free T_4 and TSH levels, while in secondary thyroid disorders (due to hypothalamic-pituitary dysfunction), free T_4 and TSH levels change in the same direction.

THYROTOXICOSIS

Thyrotoxicosis is almost always the result of primary hyperthyroidism.

Notable causes include autoimmune thyroiditis, and chronic therapy with amiodarone (12).

Clinical Manifestations

The principal manifestations of thyrotoxicosis are agitation, tachycardias (including atrial fibrillation), and fine tremors. *Elderly patients with hyperthyroidism can be lethargic* rather than agitated; this condition is called *apathetic thyrotoxicosis.* The combination of lethargy and atrial fibrillation is a frequently cited presentation for apathetic thyrotoxicosis in the elderly (13).

Thyroid Storm

An uncommon but severe form of hyperthyroidism known as *thyroid storm* can be precipitated by acute illness or surgery. This condition is characterized by hyperpyrexia (body temperatures can exceed 104°F), severe agitation or delirium, and severe tachycardia with high-output heart failure. Advanced cases are associated with obtundation or coma, generalized seizures, and hemodynamic instability. If overlooked and left untreated, the outcome is uniformly fatal (12).

Diagnosis

The plasma TSH assay is the most sensitive and specific diagnostic test for hyperthyroidism, and is recommended as the initial screening test for suspected hyperthyroidism (12). TSH levels are < 0.01 mU/dL in mild cases of hyperthyroidism, and TSH levels are undetectable in most cases of overt thyrotoxicosis (12). A normal TSH level (0.3–0.45 mmU/dL) excludes the diagnosis of hyperthyroidism (12).

Management

Table 50.3 includes the drugs and dosing regimens used for the treatment of thyrotoxicosis and thyroid storm.

β-Receptor Antagonists

Treatment with β-receptor antagonists relieves the tachycardia, agitation, and fine tremors in thyrotoxicosis. *Propranolol* has been the most widely used β-receptor antagonist in hyperthyroidism (see Table 50.3 for the dosing recommendations), but it is a non-selective β-receptor antagonist, which is not optimal for patients with asthma. More selective β-receptor antagonists like *metoprolol* (25–50 mg PO every 4 hours) or esmalol (see Table 15.1 for dosing recommendations) can be used for thyrotoxicosis. However, propranolol remains the drug of choice for treatment of thyroid storm (12).

Antithyroid Drugs

Two drugs are used to suppress thyroxine production: methimazole and propylthiouracil (PTU). Both are given orally. *Methimazole is preferred for the treatment of thyrotoxicosis, while PTU is favored for the treatment of thyroid storm* (12). Uncommon but serious side effects include cholestatic jaundice for methimazole, and fulminant hepatic necrosis, plus agranulocytosis, for PTU (12). (See Table 50.3 for the dosing regimens for each drug).

Table 50.3	Drug Therapy for Thyrotoxicosis and Thyroid Storm
Drug	**Dosing Regimens and Comments**
Propanolol	Dosing: 10–40 mg PO TID or QID for thyrotoxicosis, and 60–80 mg IV or PO every 4 hrs for thyroid storm.
	Comment: Blocks conversion of T_4 to T_3 in high doses. Use cautiously in patients with systolic heart failure. Use selective β-blocker in asthmatics.
Methimazole	Dosing: 10–20 mg PO once daily for thyrotoxicosis, and 60–80 mg PO once daily for thyroid storm.
	Comment: Blocks synthesis of T_4. Preferred to PTU for thyrotoxicosis, but not for thyroid storm.
Propylthiouracil	Dosing: 50–150 mg PO TID for thyrotoxicosis, and 500–1,000 mg PO loading dose, then 250 mg PO every 4 hrs for thyroid storm.
	Comment: Blocks both T_4 synthesis and the conversion of T_4 to T_3. Preferred to methimazole for thyroid storm.
Iodine	Dosing: 50 drops of saturated potassium iodide (250 mg iodine) PO every 6 hrs, for severe thyrotoxicosis or thyroid storm.
	Comment: Blocks synthesis and secretion of T_4. Used in combination with antithyroid drugs.
Hydrocortisone	Dosing: 300 mg IV as a loading dose, then 100 mg every 8 hrs, for thyroid storm only.
	Comment: Used for prophylaxis of the relative adrenal insufficiency in thyroid storm.

Dosing regimens from Reference 12.

Inorganic Iodine

In severe cases of hyperthyroidism, iodine (which blocks the synthesis and release of T_4) can be added to antithyroid drug therapy. The iodine is given orally as a saturated potassium iodide solution (Lugol's solution). In patients with an iodine allergy, lithium (300 mg orally every 8 hours) can be used as a substitute (14).

Special Concerns in Thyroid Storm

In addition to the above measures, the management of thyroid storm often requires aggressive volume resuscitation to replace fluid losses from vomiting, diarrhea, and heightened insensible fluid loss. Thyroid storm can accelerate glucocorticoid metabolism and create a relative adrenal insufficiency, and prophylactic therapy with intravenous hydrocortisone (300 mg IV as a loading dose, followed by 100 mg IV every 8 hours) is recommended for thyroid storm (12).

HYPOTHYROIDISM

Symptomatic hypothyroidism is uncommon, with a prevalence of only 0.3% in the general population (15). Most cases are the result of chronic autoimmune thyroiditis (Hashimoto's thyroiditis). Other causes include radioiodine, thyroidectomy, or hypothalamic-pituitary dysfunction from tumors and hemorrhagic necrosis (Sheehan's syndrome), and drugs (lithium, amiodarone).

Clinical Manifestations

The clinical manifestations of hypothyroidism are often subtle, and include dry skin, fatigue, muscle cramps, and constipation. Contrary to popular perception, obesity is not a consequence of hypothyroidism (15). More advanced cases of hypothyroidism can be accompanied by hyponatremia and a skeletal muscle myopathy, with elevations in muscle enzymes (creatine phosphokinase and aldolase), and an increase in the serum creatinine (from creatine released by skeletal muscle) that is not caused by renal dysfunction (16).

Effusions

The most common cardiovascular manifestation of hypothyroidism is pericardial effusion, which is the most common cause of an enlarged cardiac silhouette in patients with hypothyroidism (17). These effusions usually accumulate slowly and do not cause cardiac compromise. Pleural effusions are also common in hypothyroidism. The pleural and pericardial effusions in hypothyroidism are due to an increase in capillary permeability, and are exudative in quality.

Myxedema

Advanced cases of hypothyroidism are accompanied by an edematous appearance known as *myxedema*. This condition is mistaken for edema, but is caused by the intradermal accumulation of proteins (18). Myxedema is also associated with hypothermia and depressed consciousness. The latter condition is called *myxedema coma*, even though unresponsiveness is uncommon (18).

Diagnosis

Serum T_3 levels can be normal in hypothyroidism, but free T_4 levels are always reduced (15). Serum TSH levels are elevated (often above 10 mU/dL) in primary hypothyroidism, and are depressed in hypothyroidism due to hypothalamic-pituitary dysfunction.

Thyroid Replacement Therapy

The treatment for mild to moderate hypothyroidism is *levothyroxine* (T_4), which is given orally in a single daily dose of 50 to 200 µg (19). The initial dose is usually 50 µg/day, and this is increased in 50 µg/day increments every 3 to 4 weeks. The optimal replacement dose of levothyroxine is determined by monitoring the serum TSH level.

Intravenous thyroxine is recommended for severe hypothyroidism (at least initially), because of the risk of impaired gastrointestinal motility in severe hypothyroidism. One recommended regimen includes an initial intravenous dose of 250 µg, followed on the next day by a dose of 100 µg, and followed thereafter by a daily dose of 50 µg (19).

T_3 Replacement Therapy

Because the conversion of T_4 to T_3 (the active form of thyroid hormone) can be depressed in critically ill patients (18), oral therapy with T_3 can be used to supplement thyroxine (T_4) replacement therapy. In patients with depressed consciousness, T_3 can be given (via NG tube) in a dose of 25 µg every 12 hours until the patient awakens (20). Studies evaluating the benefits of T_3 supplementation have shown mixed results (15).

A FINAL WORD

Much Ado About Not Much

The major concern with adrenal and thyroid dysfunction in critically ill patients is the possibility of a negative impact on outcomes. However, the following observations suggest that this concern is unfounded.

1. Critical illness-related corticosteroid insufficiency (CIRCI) is common, but the benefits of corticosteroid replacement therapy in critically ill patients are inconsistent (1), and difficult to prove, and this creates doubt about the clinical significance of adrenal suppression in critically ill patients.

2. As for thyroid disorders, hypothyroidism and hyperthyroidism are uncommon in ICU patients, and non-thyroidal effects on thyroid function have no proven influence on clinical outcomes.

Based on these observations, it seems that the adrenal and thyroid dysfunction have very little impact on the overall fate of critically ill patients. (Lots of leaves, but little fruit.)

REFERENCES

Adrenal Insufficiency

1. Marik PE, Pastores SM, Annane D, et al. Recommendations for the diagnosis and management of corticosteroid insufficiency in critically ill adult patients:

consensus statement from an international task force by the American College of Critical Care Medicine. Crit Care Med 2008; 36L1937–1949.

2. Marik PE. Critical illness-related corticosteroid insufficiency. Chest 2009; 135:181–193.

3. Annane D, Maxime V, Ibrahim F, et al. Diagnosis of adrenal insufficiency in severe sepsis and septic shock. Am J Respir Crit Care Med 2006; 174:1319–1326.

4. Hamrahian AH, Oseni TS, Arafah BM. Measurements of serum free cortisol in critically ill patients. N Engl J Med 2004; 350:1629–1638.

5. Bornstein SR. Predisposing factors for adrenal insufficiency. N Engl J Med 2009; 360:2328–2339.

Evaluation of Thyroid Function

6. Umpierrez GE. Euthyroid sick syndrome. South Med J 2002; 95:506–513.

7. Peeters RP, Debaveye Y, Fliers E, et al. Changes within the thyroid axis during critical illness. Crit Care Clin 2006; 22:41–55.

8. Dayan CM. Interpretation of thyroid function tests. Lancet 2001; 357:619–624.

9. Karmisholt J, Andersen S, Laurberg P. Variation in thyroid function tests in patients with stable untreated subclinical hypothyroidism. Thyroid 2008; 18:303–308.

10. Hollowell JG, Stachling NW, Flanders WD, et al. Serum TSH, T(4), and thyroid antibodies in the United States population (1988-1994): National Health and Nutrition Examination Survey (NHANES III). J Clin Endocrinol Metab 2002; 87:489–499.

11. Burman KD, Wartofsky L. Thyroid function in the intensive care unit setting. Crit Care Clin 2001; 17:43–57.

Thyrotoxicosis

12. Bahn RS, Burch HB, Cooper DS, et al. Hyperthyroidism and other causes of thyrotoxicosis: Management guidelines of the American Thyroid Association and the American Association of Clinical Endocrinologists. Thyroid 2011; 21:593–646.

13. Klein I. Thyroid hormone and the cardiovascular system. Am J Med 1990; 88:631–637.

14. Migneco A, Ojetti V, Testa A, et al. Management of thyrotoxic crisis. Eur Rev Med Pharmacol Sci 2005; 9:69–74.

Hypothyroidism

15. Garber JR, Cobin RH, Gharib H, et al. Clinical practice guidelines for hypothyroidism in adults. Endocr Pract 2012; 18:988–1028.

16. Lafayette RA, Costa ME, King AJ. Increased serum creatinine in the absence of renal failure in profound hypothyroidism. Am J Med 1994; 96:298–299.

17. Ladenson PW. Recognition and management of cardiovascular disease related to thyroid dysfunction. Am J Med 1990; 88:638–641.

18. Myers L, Hays J. Myxedema coma. Crit Care Clin 1991; 7:43–56.

19. Toft AD. Thyroxine therapy. New Engl J Med 1994; 331:174–180.

20. McCulloch W, Price P, Hinds CJ, et al. Effects of low dose oral triiodothyronine in myxoedema coma. Intensive Care Med 1985; 11:259–262.

CRITICAL CARE DRUG THERAPY

*The desire to take medicine is, perhaps, the great feature
that distinguishes man from other animals.*

Sir William Ostler

Chapter 51

ANALGESIA AND SEDATION IN THE ICU

"Pain is perfect misery, the worst of evils . . .

John Milton
Paradise Lost

Contrary to popular perception, our principal function in patient care is not to save lives (since this is impossible on a consistent basis), but to *relieve pain and suffering*. And the patients that experience the greatest pain and suffering are the ones in the ICU. If you want an idea of how prepared we are to relieve pain and suffering in the ICU, take a look at Figure 51.1 (1). This might explain why most patients who are discharged from the ICU remember discomfort and unrelieved pain as a dominant experience during their ICU stay (2).

This chapter describes the use of intravenous analgesics and sedatives to achieve patient comfort in the ICU. Pertinent reviews, along with the most recent clinical practice guidelines on analgesia and sedation in the ICU, are included in the bibliography at the end of the chapter (3–5).

THE ICU EXPERIENCE

In patients who have been discharged from an ICU, surveys conducted at 6 months to 4 years after discharge show that 20–40% of the patients have no recollection of what happened during their ICU stay (2,6,7). This may be a reflection of the amnestic effects of benzodiazepines, because patients who have not been heavily sedated while in the ICU are more likely to recall experiences during the ICU stay (7). Regardless of the mechanism, amnesia for the ICU stay seems beneficial because it eliminates memories of a stressful experience.

Stressful Experiences in the ICU

It seems axiomatic that the ICU experience is stressful for a majority of patients. Several stressors have been identified by patients after discharge

Question: Does Diazepam Relieve Pain?

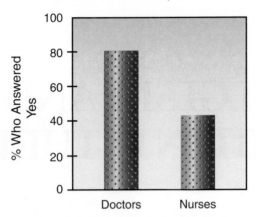

FIGURE 51.1 Percentage of housestaff physicians and ICU nurses who answered incorrectly when asked if diazepam (Valium) relieved pain.

from the ICU, and the major ones are (a) unrelieved pain, (b) inadequate sedation, (c) inability to communicate (in intubated patients), (d) difficulty sleeping, and (e) hallucinations and nightmares (2,6,7). The most frequently cited source of stress is painful procedures (8). Stressful experiences during the ICU stay can have prolonged neuropsychiatric effects. One study has reported that 25% of patients with stressful experiences in the ICU showed symptoms of post-traumatic stress disorder 4 years later (9).

Pain in Critically Ill Patients

Surveys indicate that 50–80% of ICU patients experience pain and discomfort while in the ICU (2,6,7). Surprisingly, the prevalence of pain is the same in surgical ICUs and medical ICUs (10).

Hypernociception

Critically ill patients experience pain more readily than healthy subjects (*hypernociception*). For example, *the most painful experiences for ICU patients are endotracheal suctioning, and being turned in bed* (8). In addition, 30–50% of critically ill patients *experience pain while at rest, without a noxious stimulus* (8,10). This type of pain typically involves the back and lower extremities.

The heightened pain experience in critically ill patients is attributed to immobility and systemic inflammation. (The rest pain experienced by ICU patients is similar to the myalgias experienced during a systemic infection.) Failure to recognize this heightened nociceptive state is a major source of inadequate pain relief in the ICU. Frequent pain assessments using pain intensity scales (described next) can help to correct problems with inadequate pain control in the ICU (3).

Monitoring Pain

Pain is defined as *"an unpleasant sensory or emotional experience"* (11), which highlights the subjective nature of pain. The pain sensation can be described in terms of intensity, duration, location, and quality, but pain intensity is the parameter most often monitored because it reflects the "unpleasantness" of pain.

Table 51.1	The Behavioral Pain Scale	
Item	**Description**	**Score**
Facial Expression	Relaxed	1
	Partially tightened	2
	Fully tightened	3
	Grimacing	4
Upper Limbs	No movement	1
	Partially bent	2
	Fully bent, fingers flexed	3
	Permanently retracted	4
Compliance with Ventilation	Tolerating ventilator	1
	Coughing, but tolerating ventilator	2
	Fighting ventilator	3
	Unable to control ventilation	4
		Total Score
	Score Interpretation	
	1 No pain	
	1–5 Acceptable pain control	
	12 Maximal pain	

From Reference 10.

Pain Intensity Scales

Pain intensity scales are used to determine the need for, and evaluate the effectiveness of, analgesic therapy. There are 6 different pain intensity scales, but only a few are needed to assess pain intensity in most ICU patients.

1. When patients can reliably self-report pain, the Numerical Ranking Scale can be used for pain assessment (12). This is a ruler with 10 equally spaced divider markings, numbered 1 (no pain) to 10 (maximum pain). The patient points to one of the numbered markings to indicate the severity of pain. A score of 3 or less is considered adequate pain control.

2. When patients are sedated and on a ventilator, the Behavioral Pain

Scale (BPS) shown in Table 51.1 is recommended for pain assessments (3). This scale evaluates pain intensity by elicited behaviors (i.e., facial expression, arm flexion, and tolerance of mechanical ventilation) (11). Scores can range from 3 (no pain) to 12 (maximum pain). A score of 5 or less represents adequate pain control (3).

Vital Signs

Vital signs (e.g., heart rate) show a poor correlation with patients' reports of pain intensity (the gold standard), and they can remain unchanged in the presence of pain (13). As a result, vital signs are not recommended for pain assessments (3).

OPIOID ANALGESIA

The natural chemical derivatives of opium are called *opiates*. Opiates and other substances that produce their effects by stimulating discrete opioid receptors in the central nervous system are called *opioids*. Stimulation of opioid receptors produces a variety of effects, including analgesia, sedation, euphoria, pupillary constriction, respiratory depression, bradycardia, constipation, nausea, vomiting, urinary retention, and pruritis (14). The term *narcotic* refers to a general class of drugs that blunt sensation and depress consciousness (i.e., *narcotize*).

Opioids are the most frequently used drugs for pain relief in the ICU (3,8), and are given intravenously as intermittent bolus doses or continuous infusions. Opioids also produce mild sedation but, unlike benzodiazepines, they have no amnestic effects (15).

Drugs and Dosing Regimens

The opioids used most often in the ICU are morphine, fentanyl, and hydromorphone. The recommended intravenous doses for each drug are shown in Table 51.2. It is important to emphasize that opioid dose requirements can vary widely in individual patients, and that *the effective dose of an opioid is determined by each patient's response, not by the recommended dose range of the drug.*

Fentanyl

Fentanyl has replaced morphine as the most popular opioid analgesic in ICUs (8). The advantages of fentanyl over morphine include a more rapid onset of action (because fentanyl is 600 times more lipid soluble than morphine), less risk of hypotension (because fentanyl does not promote histamine release) (16), and the absence of active metabolites. The relative lack of adverse hemodynamic effects is a major source of fentanyl's appeal in critically ill patients.

Morphine

Opioids are metabolized primarily in the liver, and the metabolites are excreted in the urine. Morphine has several active metabolites that can accumulate in renal failure. One metabolite (morphine 3-glucuronide) can produce central nervous system excitation with myoclonus and seizures (17), while another metabolite (morphine-6-glucuronide) has more potent analgesic effects than the parent drug (14). To avoid accumulation of these metabolites, *the maintenance dose of morphine should be reduced by 50% in patients with renal failure* (18). Fentanyl does not have active metabolites, and dose not require dose adjustments in renal failure.

Morphine also promotes the release of histamine, and this can produce systemic vasodilation and a decrease in blood pressure (14). Hypotension can occur, and is typically seen in patients with a hyperadrenergic state and increased peripheral vascular tone (4). Morphine-induced histamine release does not promote bronchoconstriction, and morphine doses of 1.5 mg/kg have been given to asthma patients without adverse consequences (19).

Hydromorphone

Hydromorphone is a morphine derivative that may produce more effective analgesia (according to a recent meta-analysis) (20). However, other than the lack of a need for dose alterations in renal failure, hydromorphone has no apparent clinical advantage over morphine in critically ill patients.

Table 51.2	Commonly Used Intravenous Opioids		
Feature	**Morphine**	**Hydromorphone**	**Fentanyl**
Onset	5–10 min	5–15 min	1–2 min
Bolus Dosing	2–4 mg q 1–2 hr	0.2–0.6 mg q 1–2 hr	0.35–0.5 µg/kg q 0.5–1 hr
Infusion rate	2–30 mg/hr	0.5–3 mg/hr	0.7–10 µg/kg/hr
PCA		1	4
Demand (bolus)	0.5–3 mg	0.1–0.5 mg	15–75 µg
Lockout Interval	10–20 min	5–15 min	3–10 min
Lipid Solubility	x	0.2x	600x
Active Metabolites	Yes	Yes	No
Histamine Release	Yes	No	No
Dose Adjustment for Renal Failure	↓50%	None	None

Dosing recommendations from Reference 3.

Remifentanil

Remifentanil is an ultra-short acting opioid that is given by continuous intravenous infusion, using the dosing regimen shown below.

Dosing Regimen: 1.5 µg/kg as a loading dose, followed by a continuous infusion at 0.5–15 µg/kg/hr (3).

Analgesic effects are lost within 10 minutes after stopping the drug infusion. The short duration of action is a reflection of drug metabolism; i.e., remifentanil is broken down by nonspecific esterases in plasma. Because drug metabolism does not take place in the liver or kidneys, dose adjustments are not necessary in renal or hepatic failure.

Remifentanil's short duration of action is most advantageous in conditions that require frequent evaluations of cerebral function (e.g., traumatic head injuries). The abrupt cessation of opioid activity can precipitate acute opioid withdrawal (5), which can be prevented by combining remifentanil with a longer-acting opioid.

Meperidine

Meperidine (Demerol, Pethidine) is an opioid analgesic that is no longer favored for pain control in the ICU because of the potential for *neurotoxicity*. Meperidine is metabolized in the liver to normeperidine, a metabolite that is slowly excreted by the kidneys (elimination half-life is 15–40 hours) (21). Accumulation of normeperidine can produce central nervous system excitation, with agitation, myoclonus, delirium, and generalized seizures (21). Since renal dysfunction is prevalent in ICU patients, there is a high risk for accumulation of the neurotoxic metabolite of meperidine in ICU patients.

Patient-Controlled Analgesia

For patients who are awake and capable of drug self-administration, *patient-controlled analgesia* (PCA) can be an effective method of pain control, and may be superior to intermittent opioid dosing. The PCA method uses an electronic infusion pump that can be activated by the patient. When pain is sensed, the patient presses a button connected to the pump to receive a small intravenous bolus of drug. After each bolus, the pump is disabled for a mandatory time period called the "lockout interval," to prevent overdosing. The opioid dosing regimens for PCA are shown in Table 51.2. The minimum lockout interval is determined by the time required to achieve peak drug effect (22). When writing orders for PCA, you must specify the initial loading dose (if any), the lockout interval, and the repeat bolus dose. PCA can be used alone or in conjunction with a low-dose opioid infusion.

Adverse Effects of Opioids

Respiratory Depression

Opioids produce a centrally mediated, dose-dependent decrease in respiratory rate and tidal volume (23,24), but *respiratory depression and hypoxemia are uncommon when opioids are given in the usual doses* (25). Opioid doses that impair arousal also impair ventilation and produce hypercapnia (23). Patients with sleep apnea syndrome or chronic hypercapnia are particularly prone to respiratory depression from opioids.

Cardiovascular Effects

Opioid analgesia is often accompanied by decreases in blood pressure and heart rate, which are the result of decreased sympathetic activity and increased parasympathetic activity. These effects are usually mild and well-tolerated, at least in the supine position (26). Decreases in blood pressure can be pronounced in patients with hypovolemia or heart failure (where there is an increased baseline sympathetic tone), or when opioids are given in combination with benzodiazepines (27). Opioid-induced hypotension is rarely a threat to tissue perfusion, and the blood pressure responds to intravenous fluids or small bolus doses of vasopressors.

Intestinal Motility

Opioids are well known for their ability to depress bowel motility via activation of opioid receptors in the GI tract. This is a source of troublesome constipation in cancer patients. In critically ill patients, impaired GI motility can promote reflux of enteral tube feedings into the oropharynx, creating a risk for aspiration pneumonia. Opioid-induced bowel hypomotility can be partially reversed with enteral naloxone (8 mg every 6 hours) without affecting opioid analgesia. In one small study (28), this approach resulted in fewer cases of aspiration pneumonia.

Nausea and Vomiting

Opioids can promote vomiting via stimulation of the chemoreceptor trigger zone in the lower brainstem (23). All opioids are equivalent in their ability to promote vomiting, but substituting one opioid for another sometimes resolves the problem.

NON-OPIOID ANALGESIA

The list of intravenous non-opioid analgesics is a very short one, and includes only three drugs: acetaminophen, ketorolac, and ibuprofen. These drugs are used primarily for pain control in the early postoperative period. They can be used alone for mild pain, but are used in combination with an opioid analgesic for moderate-to-severe pain. The goal of combination analgesic therapy is to reduce the opioid dose ("opioid sparing" effect) and hence reduce the risk of an opioid-related adverse effect. The intravenous dosing regimens for the non-opioid analgesics are presented in Table 51.3.

Ketorolac

Ketorolac is a nonsteroidal anti-inflammatory drug (NSAID) that was introduced in 1990 as the first parenteral analgesic agent for postoperative pain that does not produce respiratory depression (29). Ketorolac has a proven opioid sparing effect, and the dose of opioid analgesics can often be reduced by 25–50% (30).

Dosing Regimen

Ketorolac can be given by intravenous (IV) or intramuscular (IM) injection. The recommended dosing regimen for moderate-to-severe pain in adults is *30 mg IV or IM every 6 hrs,* for up to 5 days (31). A dose reduction of 50% is recommended for elderly patients (age ≥65 yrs), and for patients with a body weight < 50 kg. IM injection of ketorolac can produce hematomas (32), so IV bolus injection may be preferred.

Risk of Adversity

The beneficial actions of ketorolac and other NSAIDS are attributed to inhibition of prostaglandin production, but this also creates a risk for adverse effects, particularly gastric mucosal injury, upper GI hemorrhage, and impairment of renal function (31). These adverse effects are typically associated with excessive dosing or prolonged exposure to NSAIDS, and they are uncommon when ketorolac is given in the recommended doses, and the treatment period is limited to 5 days (32–34).

Table 51.3	Intravenous Non-Opioid Analgesia
Drug	**Dosing Regimens and Comments**
Keterolac	Dosing: 30 mg IV or IM every 6 hrs, for up to 5 days. Reduce dose by 50% for age ≥65 yrs or body weight <50 kg.
	Comment: Keterolac is an NSAID, and has anti-inflammatory and antipyretic effects. Serious complications are uncommon when treatment is limited to 5 days.
Ibuprofen	Dosing: 400–800 mg IV every 6 hrs.
	Comment: Ibuprofen is also an NSAID, with actions similar to kerotolac. Serious complications are uncommon when used for short-term pain relief.
Acetaminophen	Dosing: 1 gram IV every 6 hrs. Daily dose should not exceed 4 grams.
	Comment: No anti-inflammatory effects, which is a major disadvantage in critically ill patients.

Ibuprofen

Ibuprofen is very similar to ketorolac because (a) it is an NSAID that can be given intravenously, (b) it has an opioid sparing effect, and (c) it is safe when used for short-term pain control (35). The intravenous dose of ibuprofen is *400-800 mg IV every 6 hrs,* with a maximum daily dose of 3.2 grams (35). Unlike ketorolac, the treatment period for ibuprofen has no recommended time limit. Clinical trials of IV ibuprofen typically employ a treatment period of 24–48 hrs, and serious complications are uncommon over that time period.

Acetaminophen

Acetaminophen was approved for intravenous use in 2010, and is intended for the short-term treatment of pain and fever in postoperative patients who are unable to receive acetaminophen via the oral or rectal routes (36). The recommended dose for IV acetaminophen is *1 gram every 6 hrs*, with a maximum allowable dose of 4 grams daily (to prevent acetaminophen hepatotoxicity) (36). This dosing regimen has a documented opiate sparing effect in postoperative patients (37).

Disadvantages

Acetaminophen has no anti-inflammatory activity, which is a major disadvantage in critically ill patients. Furthermore, although the daily dose limitation of 4 grams is intended to avoid acetaminophen hepatotoxicity, the toxic dose of acetaminophen has not been evaluated in critically ill patients. For these reasons, IV acetaminophen is not the optimal choice for opiate-sparing analgesia in critically ill patients. (For a description of acetaminophen hepatotoxicity, see Chapter 54.)

Neuropathic Pain

Non-opioid analgesia is usually required for neuropathic pain (e.g., from diabetic neuropathy), and the recommended drugs for this type of pain are *gabapentin* and *carbamazepine* (3). Both drugs must be given enterally. Effective drug doses vary in individual patients, but typical doses are 600 mg every 8 hrs for gabapentin, and 100 mg every 6 hours for carbamazepine (oral suspension).

ANXIETY IN THE ICU

Anxiety and related disorders (agitation and delirium) are observed in as many as 85% of patients in the ICU (38). These disorders can be defined as follows.

1. Anxiety is characterized by exaggerated feelings of fear or apprehension that are sustained by internal mechanisms more than external events.

2. Agitation is a state of anxiety that is accompanied by increased motor activity.

3. Delirium is an acute confusional state that may, or may not, have agitation as a component. Although delirium is often equated with agitation, there is a hypoactive form of delirium that is characterized by lethargy. (Delirium is described in more detail in Chapter 44.)

The common denominator in these disorders is the *absence of a sense of well-being.*

Sedation

Sedation is the process of relieving anxiety and establishing a state of calm. This process includes general supportive measures (like frequent communication with patients and families), and drug therapy. The drugs used most often for sedation in ICUs are midazolam and propofol (3).

Table 51.4		Richmond Agitation Sedation Scale (RASS)
Score	Term	Description
+4	Combative	Overly combative or violent; immediate danger to staff
+3	Very agitated	Pulls on or removes tube(s)/catheter(s), or aggressive behavior
+2	Agitated	Frequent non-purposeful movement or patient-ventilator asynchrony
+1	Restless	Anxious or apprehensive but movements not aggressive or vigorous
0	Alert & calm	
−1	Drowsy	Not fully alert, but awakens for >10 sec, with eye contact, to voice
−2	Light sedation	Briefly awakens (<10 sec), with eye contact, to voice
−3	Moderate sedation	Any movement (but no eye contact) to voice
−4	Deep sedation	No respomse to voice, but movement to physical stimulation
−5	Unarousable	No response to voice or physical stimulation

To determine the RASS, proceed as follows:

Step 1 Observation: Observe the patient without interaction. If patient is alert, assign the appropriate score (0 to +4). If patient is not alert, go to Step 2.

Step 2 Verbal Stimulation: Address patient by name in a loud voice and ask the patient to look at you. Can repeat once if necessary. If patient responds to voice, assign the appropriate score (−1 to −3). If there is no response, go to Step 3.

Step 3 Physical Stimulation: Shake the patient's shoulder. If there is no response, rub the sternum vigorously. Assign the appropriate score (−4 to −5).

From Reference 39.

Monitoring Sedation

The routine use of sedation scales is instrumental in achieving effective sedation (3). The sedation scales that are most reliable in ICU patients are the Sedation-Agitation Scale (SAS) and the Richmond Agitation-Sedation Scale (RASS) (3), and the latter scale is shown in Table 51.4 (39). The RASS includes 4 possible scores for progressive agitation (+1 to +4) and 5 possible scores for progressive sedation (-1 to -5). The optimal RASS score is zero (alert and calm). The added advantage of RASS is the ability to monitor serial changes in a patient's mental state (40). This latter feature allows the RASS score to be used as the end-point of sedative drug therapy. (Sedative drug infusions can be titrated to achieve a RASS score of –1 to –2, which represents light sedation.)

BENZODIAZEPINES

Benzodiazepines are currently the most popular drugs for sedation in ICUs (3,8), but they are gradually losing ground to other sedatives because of problems with drug accumulation and excessive sedation.

Drug Profiles

Two benzodiazepines are used for sedation in ICUs: midazolam and lorazepam. (Diazepam is no longer used because of excessive sedation with prolonged use.) Both drugs are given intravenously, and a brief profile of each drug is presented in Table 51.5.

Midazolam

Midazolam (Versed) is a rapid-acting drug by virtue of its high lipid solubility. Sedative effects are apparent within 1–2 minutes after an intravenous (IV) injection of midazolam, and this makes midazolam the preferred benzodiazepine for rapid sedation (e.g., for a severely agitated or combative patient). The avid uptake of midazolam into tissues also results in rapid clearance from the bloodstream, resulting in a short duration of action (41). Because of the short-lived effect (1–2 hrs), midazolam is given as a continuous IV infusion, preceded by a bolus loading dose. However, because the brief drug effect is due to avid drug uptake into tissues, rather than drug elimination from the body, a continuous infusion of midazolam will result in progressive drug accumulation in tissues. To avoid excessive sedation from drug accumulation, midazolam infusions should be limited to ≤48 hrs (4).

Lorazepam

Lorazepam (Ativan) is a longer-acting drug than midazolam, with effects lasting up to 6 hours after a single intravenous dose (3). Lorazepam can given by intermittent IV injections, or by continuous IV infusion. The intravenous preparation of lorazepam contains propylene glycol, a solvent used to increase drug solubility in plasma. This solvent has adverse effects (see later), which is why the lorazepam dosing recommendations in Table 51.5 have a maximum allowable dose (2 mg for bolus doses of lorazepam, and 10 mg/hr for continuous infusions).

Metabolism

Benzodiazepines are metabolized in the liver. Midazolam is metabolized by the cytochrome P450 enzyme system, and drugs that interfere with this enzyme system (e.g., diltiazem, erythromycin) can inhibit midazolam metabolism and potentiate it effects. Midazolam has one active metabolite, 1-hydroxymidazolam, that is cleared by the kidneys, so alterations in renal function can also influence midazolam sedation. Lorazepam is metabolized by glucuronidation, and has no active metabolites.

Table 51.5	Sedation with Intravenous Benzodiazepines	
Feature	**Midazolam**	**Lorazepam**
Loading Dose	0.01–0.05 mg/kg	0.02–0.04 mg/kg (≤2 mg)
Onset of Action	2–5 min	15–20 min
Duration (after bolus)	1–2 hr	2–6 hr
Continuous Infusion	0.02–0.1 mg/kg/hr	0.01–0.1 mg/kg/hr (≤10 mg/hr)
Intermittent Bolus Dosing		0.02–0.06 mg/kg q 2–6 hr, prn
Lipophilicity	+++	++
Specific Concerns	Active Metabolites[†]	Propylene Glycol Toxicity[ξ]

[†]Active Metabolites prolong sedation, especially in renal failure.
[ξ]Lorazepam, 2 mg/mL, contains propylene glycol, 830 mg/mL. as a solvent.
Dosing recommendations from Reference 3.

Advantages

The advantages of sedation with benzodiazepines include the following.

1. Benzodiazepines have a dose-dependent amnestic effect that is distinct from the sedative effect. The amnesia extends beyond the sedation period (antegrade amnesia), and this may be responsible for the surprising percentage (up to 40%) of patients who, after discharge from the ICU, have no recollection of events during their ICU stay (2,6,7). As mentioned earlier, this amnesia should be beneficial because it eliminates memories of stressful experiences.

2. Benzodiazepines have anticonvulsant effects (see Chapter 45), which is always a benefit in critically ill patients.

3. Benzodiazepines are the sedatives of choice for drug withdrawal syndromes, including alcohol, opiate, and benzodiazepine withdrawal.

Disadvantages

The major disadvantages of sedation with benzodiazepines are (a) drug accumulation with prolonged sedation, and (b) the apparent tendency for benzodiazepines to promote delirium.

Prolonged Sedation

Maintaining sedation in ICU patients is often a long-term affair, especially in ventilator-dependent patients, and both midazolam and lorazepam accumulate in tissues with prolonged use. This produces deeper levels of sedation, and prolongs the time for awakening when the drugs are discontinued. This can result in delays in weaning patients from mechanical ventilation, and longer ICU stays (3,4). Prolonged sedation is more of a problem with midazolam, because of its greater lipid solubility, and the accumulation of its active metabolite. In one study of sedation in ICU patients, the time to emerge from sedation was 1,815 min (30.2 hours) for midazolam, versus 261 min (4.4 hr) for lorazepam (42).

SOLUTIONS: The following are some solutions to the problem of prolonged sedation with benzodiazepines:

1. Daily interruption of benzodiazepine infusions (until the patient awakens) curtails drug accumulation, and has been shown to shorten the duration of mechanical ventilation, and reduce the length of stay in the ICU (43). This is the accepted practice for limiting excessive sedation from benzodiazepines.

2. Titration of benzodiazepine infusions to maintain light levels of sedation, using routine monitoring with a sedation scale (SAS or RASS), has been proposed in the most recent guidelines on sedation in ICUs (3). This is a more logical solution to the problem than daily interruption of benzodiazepine infusions, and should be a standard practice.

3. The final solution to the problem is to avoid benzodiazepines for sedation, which is a current trend.

Delirium

The prevailing opinion is that the frequent appearance of delirium in ICU patients (described in Chapter 44) is at least partly due to the frequent use of benzodiazepines in ICU patients (3,4). Benzodiazepines produce their effects by binding to receptors for gamma-amino-butyric-acid (GABA), which are involved in the development of delirium (44), and sedation with drugs that do not involve GABA receptors is associated with fewer cases of delirium in ICU patients (see later). The role of benzodiazepines in promoting delirium will be a severe blow to their popularity if suitable alternatives are available.

Propylene Glycol Toxicity

Intravenous preparations of lorazepam contain propylene glycol (415 mg/mg lorazepam) to enhance drug solubility in plasma. Propylene glycol is converted to lactic acid in the liver, and excessive intake of propylene glycol can produce a toxidrome characterized by a metabolic (lactic) acidosis, delirium (with hallucination), hypotension, and (in severe cases) multiorgan failure. This toxidrome has been reported in 19–66% of patients receiving high-dose intravenous lorazepam for more than 2 days (45,46).

The maximum daily intake of propylene glycol that is considered safe is 25 mg/kg (47), or 17.5 g/day for a 70 kg adult. A lorazepam infusion at 2 mg/hr represents a daily intake of propylene glycol of 830 mg × 24 = 19.9 g/day, which exceeds the safe limit for a 70 kg adult. This highlights the risk of propylene glycol toxicity with lorazepam infusions that continue for 24 hrs or longer.

DIAGNOSIS: An unexplained metabolic acidosis during prolonged (> 24 hr) infusions of lorazepam should prompt a measurement of the serum lactate levels, and an elevated lactate should raise suspicion of propylene glycol toxicity. Plasma levels of propylene glycol can be measured, but the results may not be immediately available. An *elevated osmolal gap* can suggest the diagnosis because propylene glycol will elevate the osmolal gap. (See page 656 for a description of the osmolal gap).

Withdrawal Syndrome

Abrupt termination of prolonged benzodiazepine infusions can produce a withdrawal syndrome, characterized by agitation, disorientation, hallucinations, and seizures (48). However, this does not appear to be a common occurrence.

OTHER SEDATIVES

Concerns about the delayed emergence from sedation with benzodiazepines has led to the increasing popularity of two sedatives that allow rapid arousal: *propofol and dexmedetomidine.*

Propofol

Propofol (Deprivan) is a powerful sedative that exerts its effects by binding to GABA receptors (similar to benzodiazepines, but different receptors). It is used for induction of general anesthesia, and has become popular in ICUs because arousal is rapid when the drug infusion is stopped. A profile of this drug is presented in Table 51.6.

Actions and Uses

Propofol has sedative and amnestic effects, but no analgesic effects (49). A single intravenous bolus of propofol produces sedation within 1–2 minutes, and the drug effect lasts 5–8 minutes (49). Because of the short duration of action, propofol is given as a continuous infusion. When the infusion is stopped, awakening occurs within 10–15 minutes, even with prolonged infusions (49). Loading doses of propofol can be used in patients who are hemodynamically stable.

Propofol was originally intended for short-term sedation when rapid awakening is desired (e.g., during brief procedures), but it is being used for longer periods of time in ventilator-dependent patients, to avoid delays in weaning from ventilatory support. Propofol can be useful in neurosurgical patients and patients with head injuries because it reduces intracranial pressure (49), and the rapid arousal allows for frequent evaluations of mental status.

Preparation and Dosage

Propofol is highly lipophilic, and is suspended in a 10% lipid emulsion to enhance solubility in plasma. This lipid emulsion is almost identical to

10% Intralipid used in parenteral nutrition formulas, and it has a caloric density of 1 kcal/mL, which should be included as part of the daily caloric intake. *Propofol dosing is based on ideal rather than actual body weight,* and no dose adjustment is required for renal failure or moderate hepatic insufficiency (49). Loading doses are not advised in patients who are hemodynamically unstable (because of the risk of hypotension) (3).

Table 51.6	Sedation with Rapid-Arousal Drugs	
Feature	**Propofol**	**Dexmedetomidine**
Loading Dose	5 µg/kg/min over 5 min[†]	1 µg/kg over 10 min[†]
Onset of Action	1–2 min	5–10 min
Maintenance Infusion	5–50 µg/kg/min	0.2–0.7 µg/kg/hr
Time to Arousal	10–15 min	6–10 min
Respiratory Depression	Yes	No
Adverse Effects	Hypotension	Hypotension
	Hyperlipidemia	Bradycardia
	Propofol Infusion Syndrome	Sympathetic Rebound

[†]Use loading dose only in hemodynamically stable patients.
Dosing recommendations from Reference 3.

Adverse Effects

Propofol is well known for producing respiratory depression and hypotension (50). Because of the risk of respiratory depression, propofol infusions are recommended only for ventilator-dependent patients. Hypotension is attributed to systemic vasodilatation (4), and can be profound in conditions like hypovolemia and heart failure, where blood pressure is maintained by systemic vasoconstriction. Anaphylactoid reactions to propofol are uncommon but can be severe (49), and green urine is observed occasionally from harmless phenolic metabolites (49).

The lipid emulsion in propofol preparations can promote hypertriglyceridemia. The incidence is not known, but propofol infusions are the leading independent risk factor for hypertriglyceridemia in ICU patients (51). Monitoring triglyceride levels is often recommended during propofol infusions, but hypertriglyceridemia is common in ICU patients, and is not associated with adverse outcomes (51), so the merits of monitoring triglyceride levels are questionable.

Propofol Infusion Syndrome

Propofol infusion syndrome is a rare and poorly understood condition that is characterized by the abrupt onset of bradycardic heart failure, lactic acidosis, rhabdomyolysis, and acute renal failure (52). This syndrome almost always occurs during prolonged, high-dose propofol infusions (>4–6 mg/kg/hr for longer than 24–48 hrs) (53). The mortality rate is 30% (52). Avoiding propofol infusion rates above 5 mg/kg/hr for longer than 48 hrs is recommended to reduce the risk of this condition (53).

Dexmedetomidine

Dexmedetomidine is an alpha-2 receptor agonist that has sedative, amnestic, and mild analgesic effects, and does not depress ventilation. A brief profile of the drug is presented in Table 51.6. The most distinguishing feature of dexmedetomidine is the type of the sedation it produces, which is described next.

Cooperative Sedation

The sedation produced by dexmedetomidine is unique because *arousal is maintained, despite deep levels of sedation*. Patients can be aroused from sedation without discontinuing the drug infusion, and when awake, patients are able to communicate and follow commands. When arousal is no longer required, the patient is allowed to return to the prior state of sedation. This has been called *cooperative sedation* (5), and is similar to temporary awakening from sleep. In fact, the EEG changes in this type of sedation are similar to the EEG changes in natural sleep (5).

Cooperative sedation with dexmedetomidine is very different than the sedation produced by GABAergic drugs (benzodiazepines and propofol), where arousal occurs only after the drug is discontinued and the sedative effects abate. In fact, daily interruption of benzodiazepine sedation is aimed at achieving the type of sedation produced by dexmedetomidine; i.e., arousable and cooperative. Dexmedetomidine should be well suited for ventilator-dependent patients, because sedation can be continued during the transition period from mechanical ventilation to spontaneous breathing.

Delirium

Clinical studies have shown a lower prevalence of delirium in patients who are sedated with dexmedetomidine instead of midazolam (55), and based on these studies, *dexmedetomidine is recommended over benzodiazepines for the sedation of patients with ICU-acquired delirium* (3).

Adverse Effects

Dexmedetomidine produces dose-dependent decreases in heart rate, blood pressure, and circulating norepinephrine levels (sympatholytic effect) (5). Patients with heart failure and cardiac conduction defects are particularly susceptible to the sympatholytic actions of dexmedetomidine. Life-threatening bradycardia has been reported, primarily in patients treated with high infusion rates of dexmedetomidine (>0.7 µg/kg/min) together with a loading dose (56). Patients with cardiac conduction defects should not receive dexmedetomidine, and patients with heart failure or hemodynamic instability should not receive a loading dose of the drug.

Haloperidol

Haloperidol (Haldol) is a first-generation antipsychotic agent that has a long history of treating agitation and delirium (57–58).

Features

Haloperidol produces its sedative and antipsychotic effects by blocking dopamine receptors in the central nervous system. Following an intravenous bolus dose of haloperidol, sedation is evident in 10–20 minutes, and the effect lasts 3–4 hours. There is no respiratory depression, and hypotension is unusual in the absence of hypovolemia.

DOSING: The recommended dosing for intravenous haloperidol is shown in Table 51.7 (59,60). Because haloperidol has a delayed onset of action, midazolam can be given with the first dose of haloperidol to achieve more rapid sedation. Individual patients show a wide variation in serum drug levels after a given dose of haloperidol (61). If there is no evidence of a sedative response after 10 minutes, the dose should be doubled. If there is a partial response at 10–20 minutes, a second dose can be given along with 1 mg lorazepam (preferred to midazolam because of the longer duration of action) (61). Lack of response to a second dose of haloperidol should prompt a switch to another agent.

Table 51.7	Intravenous Haloperidol for the Agitated Patient
Severity of Anxiety	**Dose**
Mild	0.5–2 mg
Moderate	5–10 mg
Severe	10–20 mg

1. Administer dose by IV push.
2. Allow 10–20 min for response:
   a. If no response, double the drug dose, or
   b. Add lorazepam (1 mg)
3. If still no response, switch to another sedative.
4. Give ¼ of the loading dose every 6 hr for maintenance of sedation.

Adapted from References 59 and 60.

Adverse Effects

The adverse effects of haloperidol include: (a) extrapyramidal reactions, (b) neuroleptic malignant syndrome, and (c) ventricular tachycardia.

1. Extrapyramidal reactions (e.g., rigidity, spasmodic movements) are dose-related side effects of oral haloperidol therapy, but these reactions are uncommon when haloperidol is given intravenously (for unclear reasons) (61).
2. The neuroleptic malignant syndrome (described on pages 763–765) is

an idiosyncratic reaction to neuroleptic agents that consists of hyper-pyrexia, severe muscle rigidity, and rhabdomyolysis. This condition has been reported with intravenous haloperidol (62), but is rare.

3. The most publicized risk of therapy with haloperidol is prolongation of the QT interval on the electrocardiogram, which can trigger a polymorphic ventricular tachycardia (*torsade de pointes*, shown in Figure 15.8). This arrhythmia is reported in up to 3.5% of patients receiving intravenous haloperidol (63), which provides a reason to avoid haloperidol in patients with a prolonged QT interval.

A FINAL WORD

Improving the ICU Experience

It is not possible to completely eliminate the stress experienced by ICU patients because being critically ill is inherently stressful. However, the following considerations might help to reduce the "unpleasantness" of the ICU experience.

1. Critically ill patients experience pain in situations that are not normally painful. For example, being turned in bed is one of the most painful experiences reported by ICU patients, and up to 50% of patients experience pain at rest, without any noxious stimulus (8,10). This indicates that pain control is a full-time endeavor in ICU patients.

2. Unrelieved pain can be a source of agitation, so make sure that pain is relieved before considering a sedative drug for agitation.

3. When a benzodiazepine is used for prolonged (> 48 hrs) sedation, attention to preventing drug accumulation and prolonged sedation can result in a shorter time in the ICU. The preventive measures include daily interruption of drug infusions, or maintaining light sedation using a reliable sedation scale to guide adjustments in drug dosage.

4. Consider using dexmedetomidine for sedation, because this drug allows the patient to be aroused while still sedated (e.g., to help with repositioning or speak with family members). When arousal is no longer needed, the patient will resume the prior level of sedation. This is more like sleep than a drug-induced stupor.

5. Finally, communicate with patients (e.g., tell them what you are going to do before doing it), and allow some "down time" for patients to sleep.

REFERENCES

Introduction

1. Loper KA, Butler S, Nessly M, Wild L. Paralysed with pain: the need for education. Pain 1989; 37:315–316.

2. Rotondi AJ, Chelluri L, Sirio C, et al. Patients' recollections of stressful experiences while receiving prolonged mechanical ventilation in an intensive care unit. Crit Care Med 2002; 30:746–752.

Clinical Practice Guideline

3. Barr J, Fraser GL, Puntillo K, et al. Clinical practice guidelines for the management of pain. agitation, and delirium in adult patients in the intensive care unit. Crit Care Med 2013; 41:263–306.

Reviews

4. Devlin JW, Roberts RJ. Pharmacology of commonly used analgesics and sedatives in the ICU: benzodiazepines, propofol, and opioids. Crit Care Clin 2009; 25:431–449.

5. Panzer O, Moitra V, Sladen RN. Pharmacology of sedative-analgesic agents: dexmedetomidine, remifentanil, ketamine, volatile anesthetics, and the role of peripheral mu antagonists. Crit Care Clin 2009; 25:451–469.

The ICU Experience

6. Granja C, Lopes A, Moreira S, et al. Patients' recollections of experiences in the intensive care unit may affect their quality of life. Crit Care 2005; 9:R96–R109.

7. Samuelson KA, Lundberg D, Fridlund B. Stressful experiences in relation to depth of sedation in mechanically ventilated patients. Nurs Crit Care 2007; 12:93–104.

8. Payen J-F, Chanques G, Mantz J, et al, for the DOLOREA Investigators. Current practices in sedation and analgesia for mechanically ventilated critically ill patients. Anesthesiology 2007; 106:687–695.

9. Schelling G, Stoll C, Haller M, et al. Health-related quality of life and posttraumatic stress disorder in survivors of the acute respiratory distress syndrome. Crit Care Med 1998; 26:651–659.

10. Chanques G, Sebbane M, Barbotte E, et al. A prospective study of pain at rest: incidence and characteristics of an unrecognized symptom in surgical and trauma versus medical intensive care unit patients. Anesthesiology 2007; 107:858–860.

11. Pain terms: A list with definitions and notes on usage, recommended by the IASP subcommittee on taxonomy. Pain 1979; 6:249.

12. Ahlers S, van Gulik L, van der Veen A, et al. Comparison of different pain scoring systems in critically ill patients in a general ICU. Crit Care 2008; 12:R15. (An open source journal.)

13. Siffleet J, Young J, Nikoletti S, et al. Patients' self-report of procedural pain in the intensive care unit. J Clin Nurs 2007; 16:2142–2148.

Pain Control with Opioids

14. Pasternak GW. Pharmacological mechanisms of opioid analgesics. Clin Neuropharmacol 1993; 16:1–18.

15. Veselis RA, Reinsel RA, Feshchenko VA, et al. The comparative amnestic effects of midazolam, propofol, thiopental, and fentanyl at equisedative concentrations. Anesthesiology 1997; 87:749–764.

16. Rosow CE, Moss J, Philbin DM, et al. Histamine release during morphine and fentanyl anesthesia. Anesthesiology 1982; 56:93–96.

17. Smith MT. Neuroexcitatory effects of morphine and hydromorphone: evidence implicating the 3-glucuronide metabolites. Clin Exp Pharmacol Physiol 2000; 27:524–528.

18. Aronoff GR, Berns JS, Brier ME, et al. Drug Prescribing in Renal Failure: Dosing Guidelines for Adults. 4th ed. Philadelphia: American College of Physicians, 1999.

19. Eschenbacher WL, Bethel RA, Boushey HA, Sheppard D. Morphine sulfate inhibits bronchoconstriction in subjects with mild asthma whose responses are inhibited by atropine. Am Rev Resp Dis 1984; 130:363–367.

20. Felden L, Walter C, Harder S, et al. Comparative clinical effects of hydromorphone and morphine: a meta-analysis. Br J Anesth 2011; 107:319–328.

21. Latta KS, Ginsberg B, Barkin RL. Meperidine: a critical review. Am J Therap 2002; 9:53–68.

22. White PF. Use of patient-controlled analgesia for management of acute pain. JAMA 1988; 259:243–247.

23. Bowdle TA. Adverse effects of opioid agonists and agonist-antagonists in anaesthesia. Drug Safety 1998; 19:173–189.

24. Weil JV, McCullough RE, Kline JS, et al. Diminished ventilatory response to hypoxia and hypercapnia after morphine in normal man. N Engl J Med 1975; 292:1103–1106.

25. Bailey PL. The use of opioids in anesthesia is not especially associated with nor predictive of postoperative hypoxemia. Anesthesiology 1992; 77:1235.

26. Schug SA, Zech D, Grond S. Adverse effects of systemic opioid analgesics. Drug Safety 1992; 7:200–213.

27. Tomicheck RC, Rosow CE, Philbin DM, et al. Diazepam-fentanyl interaction—hemodynamic and hormonal effects in coronary artery surgery. Anesth Analg 1983; 62:881–884.

28. Meissner W, Dohrn B, Reinhart K. Enteral naloxone reduces gastric tube reflux and frequency of pneumonia in critical care patients during opioid alagesia. Crit Care Med 2003; 31:776–780.

Non-Opioid Analgesics

29. Buckley MM, Brogden RN. Ketorolac. A review of its pharmacodynamic and pharmacokinetic properties, and therapeutic potential. Drugs 1990; 39:86–109.

30. Gillis JC, Brogden RN. Ketorolac. A reappraisal of its pharmacodynamic and pharmacokinetic properties and therapeutic use in pain management. Drugs 1997; 53:139–188.

31. Ketorolac Tromethamine. In: McEvoy GK, ed. AHFS Drug Information, 2012. Bethesda: American Society of Health System Pharmacists, 2012:2139–2148.

32. Ready LB, Brown CR, Stahlgren LH, et al. Evaluation of intravenous ketorolac administered by bolus or infusion for treatment of postoperative pain. A double-blind, placebo-controlled, multicenter study. Anesthesiology 1994; 80:1277–1286.

33. Strom BL, Berlin JA, Kinman JL, et al. Parenteral ketorolac and risk of gastrointestinal and operative site bleeding. A postmarketing surveillance study. JAMA 1996; 275:376–382.

34. Reinhart DI. Minimising the adverse effects of ketorolac. Drug Safety 2000; 22:487–497.

35. Scott LJ. Intravenous ibuprofen. Drugs 2012; 72:1099–1109.

36. Yeh YC, Reddy P. Clinical and economic evidence for intravenous acetaminophen. Pharmacother 2012; 32:559–579.

37. Sinatra RS, Jahr JS, Reynolds LW, et al. Efficacy and safety of single and repeated administration of 1 gram intravenous acetaminophen injection (paracetamol) for pain management after major orthopedic surgery. Anesthesiology 2005; 102:822–831.

Anxiety in the ICU

38. Ely EW, Inouye SK, Bernard GR, et al. Delirium in mechanically ventilated patients: validity and reliability of the confusion assessment method for the intensive care unit (CAM-ICU). JAMA 2001;286:2703–2710.

39. Sessler CN Gosnell MS, Grap MJ, et al. The Richmond Agitation-Sedation Scale: validity and reliability in adult intensive care units. Am J Resp Crit Care Med 2002; 166:1338–1344.

40. Ely EW, Truman B, Shintani A, et al. Monitoring sedation status over time in ICU patients: reliability and validity of the Richmond Agitation-Sedation Scale (RASS). JAMA 2003; 289:2983–2991.

Benzodiazepines

41. Reves JG, Fragen RJ, Vinik HR, et al. Midazolam: pharmacology and uses. Anesthesiology 1985; 62:310–324.

42. Pohlman AS, Simpson KP, Hall JB. Continuous intravenous infusions of lorazepam versus midazolam for sedation during mechanical ventilatory support: a prospective, randomized study. Crit Care Med 1994; 22:1241–1247.

43. Kress JP, Pohlman AS, O'Connor MF, et al. Daily interruption of sedative infusions in critically ill patients undergoing mechanical ventilation. N Engl J Med 2000; 342:1471–1477.

44. Zaal IJ, Slooter AJC. Delirium in critically ill patients: epidemiology, pathophysiology, diagnosis and management. Drugs, 2012; 72:1457–1471.

45. Wilson KC, Reardon C, Theodore AC, Farber HW. Propylene glycol toxicity: a severe iatrogenic illness in ICU patients receiving IV benzodiazepines. Chest 2005; 128:1674–1681.

46. Arroglia A, Shehab N, McCarthy K, Gonzales JP. Relationship of continuous infusion lorazepam to serum propylene glycol concentration in critically ill adults. Crit Care Med 2004; 32:1709–1714.

47. Nordt SP, Vivero LE. Pharmaceutical additives. In: Nelson LS, Lewin NA, Howland MA, et al, eds. Goldfrank's Toxicological Emergencies. 9th ed, New York:McGraw Hill, 2011:803–816.

48. Shafer A. Complications of sedation with midazolam in the intensive care unit and a comparison with other sedative regimens. Crit Care Med 1998; 26:947–956.

Propofol

49. McKeage K, Perry CM. Propofol: a review of its use in intensive care sedation of adults. CNS drugs 2003; 17:235–272.

50. Riker RR, Fraser GL. Adverse events associated with sedatives, analgesics, and other drugs that provide patient comfort in the intensive care unit. Pharmacotherapy 2005; 25:8S–18S.

51. Devaud JC, Berger MM, Pannatier A. Hypertriglyceridemia: a potential side effect of propofol sedation in critical illness. Intensive Care Med 2012; 38:1990–1998.

52. Fong JT, Sylvia L, Ruthazer R, et al. Predictors of mortality in patients with suspected propofol infusion syndrome. Crit Care Med 2008; 36:2281–2287.

53. Fodale V, LaMonaca E. Propofol infusion syndrome: an overview of a perplexing disease. Drug Saf 2008; 31:293–303.

Dexmedetomidine

54. Bhana N, Goa KL, McClellan KJ. Dexmedetomidine. Drugs 2000; 59:263–268.

55. Riker RR, Shehabi Y, Bokesch PM, et al. SEDCOM (Safety and Efficacy of Dexmedetomidine Compared With Midazolam) Study Group: Dexmedetomidine vs. midazolam for sedation of critically ill patients. JAMA 2009; 301:489–499.

56. Tan JA, Ho KM. Use of dexmedetomidine as a sedative and analgesic agent in critically ill patients: a meta-analysis. Intensive Care Med 2010; 36:926–939.

Haloperidol

57. Haloperidol. In: McEvoy GK, ed. AHFS Drug Information, 2012. Bethesda: American Society of Health System Pharmacists, 2012:2542–2547.

58. Clinton JE, Sterner S,Steimachers Z, Ruiz E. Haloperidol for sedation of disruptive emergency patients. Ann Emerg Med 1987; 16:319–322.

59. Jacobi J, Fraser GL, Coursin DB, et al. Clinical practice guidelines for the sustained use of sedatives and analgesics in the critically ill adult. Crit Care Med 2002; 30:119–141.

60. Riker RR, Fraser GL, Cox PM. Continuous infusion of haloperidol controls agitation in critically ill patients. Crit Care Med 1994; 22:433–440.

61. Sanders KM, Minnema AM, Murray GB. Low incidence of extrapyramidal symptoms in the treatment of delirium with intravenous haloperidol and lorazepam in the intensive care unit. J Intensive Care Med 1989; 4:201–204.

62. Sing RF, Branas CC, Marino PL. Neuroleptic malignant syndrome in the intensive care unit. J Am Osteopath Assoc 1993; 93:615–618.

63. Sharma ND, Rosman HS, Padhi ID, et al. Torsade de Pointes associated with intravenous haloperidol in critically ill patients. Am J Cardiol 1998; 81:238–240.

Chapter 52

ANTIMICROBIAL THERAPY

*The danger with germ-killing drugs is that
they may kill the patient as well as the germ.*

J.B.S. Haldane

Antibiotic therapy is inescapable in the ICU, and the antibiotics used most often are included in the list shown below. Each of these will be presented in alphabetical order, as listed.

1. Aminoglycosides
2. Antifungal agents
3. Carbapenems
4. Cephalosporins
5. Fluoroquinolones
6. Penicillins
7. Vancomycin & Alternatives

AMINOGLYCOSIDES

The aminoglycosides are a group of antibiotics derived from cultures of *Streptomyces* (hence the name streptomycin for the first aminoglycoside). There are three aminoglycosides available for intravenous use in the United States: gentamicin, tobramycin, and amikacin (introduced in 1966, 1975, and 1981, respectively).

Activity & Clinical Uses

The aminoglycosides are bactericidal, and are among the most active antibiotics against Gram-negative aerobic bacilli (see Figure 52.1), including *Pseudomonas aeruginosa* (see Figure 52.2) (1,2). Amikacin is the most active of the aminoglycosides, probably because it has been in clinical use for a shorter period of time (giving microbes less time to develop resistance). Because of the risk of nephrotoxicity (see later), aminoglycosides are usually reserved for infections involving *Pseudomonas aeruginosa*. However, there is some evidence that, in cases of Gram-negative septicemia associated with neutropenia or septic shock, empiric antibiotic

923

coverage is more effective if an aminoglycoside is added to another drug with activity against Gram-negative aerobic bacilli (e.g., a carbapenem, cefepime, or piperacillin/tazobactam) (3).

Dosing Regimens

Aminoglycosides are given in one daily dose, which is based on body weight and renal function, as shown in Table 52.1.

Table 52.1	Aminoglycoside Dosing by Creatinine Clearance		
Cr CL (mL/min)	Gent/Tobra	Amikacin	Interval
≥80	7 mg/kg	20 mg/kg	24 hrs
60–79	5 mg/kg	15 mg/kg	24 hrs
40–59	4 mg/kg	12 mg/kg	24 hrs
20–39	4 mg/kg	12 mg/kg	48 hrs
10–19	3 mg/kg	10 mg/kg	48 hrs
<10	2.5 mg/kg	7.5 mg/kg	48 hrs

From Reference 1. Cr CL = creatinine clearance. Gent = gentamicin; Tobra = tobramycin.

Dosing by Body Weight

Aminoglycoside dosing is based on ideal body weight (see Appendix 2 for charts of ideal body weights). For obese patients, dosing should be based on an adjusted body weight (ABW), which is equivalent to the ideal body weight (IBW) plus 45% of the difference between the total body weight (TBW) and ideal body weight (1); i.e.,

$$ABW = IBW + 0.45 (TBW - IBW) \tag{52.1}$$

Dosing by Renal Function

The aminoglycosides are cleared by filtration in the kidneys, and dose adjustments are necessary when renal clearance is impaired. Note in Table 52.1 that the strength of the dose is progressively decreased with decreasing creatinine clearance, and at a creatinine clearance below 40 mL/min, the dosing interval increases to 48 hours. (Formulas for estimating the creatinine clearance are in the Appendix at the end of the book.) Hemodialysis for 6 hours will eliminate about 40–50% of the accumulated aminoglycoside, so 50% of a full dose should be given after each dialysis session (1).

Monitoring

Serum aminoglycoside levels should be monitored to determine if dosing is appropriate in individual patients. Target peak levels are 4–8 mg/L for gentamicin and tobramycin, and 15–20 mg/L for amikacin (4). Target

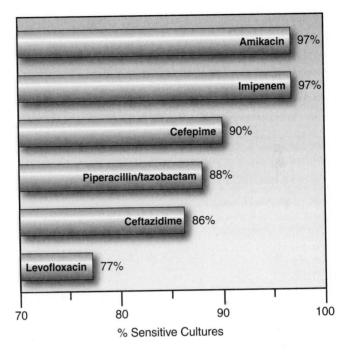

FIGURE 52.1 Antibiotic susceptibilities of Gram-negative aerobic bacilli isolated from abdominal infections in 37 hospitals in North America from 2005 to 2010. Data from Reference 2.

trough levels (obtained just before a dose) are 1–2 mg/L for gentamicin and tobramycin, and 5–10 mg/L for amikacin (4).

Adverse Effects

Nephrotoxicity is the principal adverse effect of aminoglycosides.

Nephrotoxicity

Aminoglycosides have been called *obligate nephrotoxins* because renal impairment will eventually develop in all patients if treatment is continued (5). The site of renal injury is the proximal tubules, and the risk of renal injury is the same with each of the aminoglycosides. The earliest signs of injury include cylindrical casts in the urine, proteinuria, and inability to concentrate urine (3). The urinary changes appear in the first week of drug treatment, and the serum creatinine begins to rise 5–7 days after the start of therapy. The renal impairment can progress to acute renal failure, which is usually reversible. Nephrotoxic effects are enhanced by hypovolemia and pre-existing renal disease (5,6).

Other Adverse Effects

Other adverse effects, which include ototoxicity and neuromuscular blockade, are rarely a problem. The ototoxicity can produce irreversible

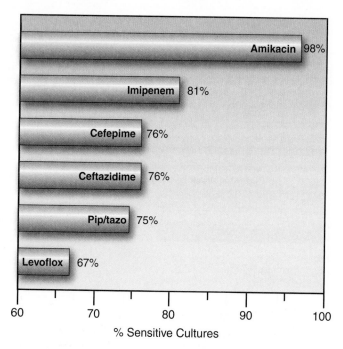

% Sensitive Cultures

FIGURE 52.2 Susceptibility of Pseudomonas aeruginosa to selected antibiotics. Data from a survey of abdominal infections in 37 hospitals in North America from 2005 to 2010. From Reference 2.

hearing loss and vestibular damage, but these changes are usually asymptomatic (5). Aminoglycosides can block acetylcholine release from presynaptic nerve terminals, but this is never clinically apparent with therapeutic dosing (4). There is a small risk that aminoglycosides will aggravate the neuromuscular blockade associated with myasthenia gravis and nondepolarizing muscle relaxants (7,8), and it is wise to avoid aminoglycosides in these conditions.

Comment

Aminoglycosides were once the darlings of the infectious disease community because they were the first antibiotics capable of treating serious Gram-negative infections. However, because of their nephrotoxicity, and the availability of less harmful drugs capable of treating serious Gram-negative infections, aminoglycosides should be reserved for *Pseudomonas* bacteremias in patients with neutropenia or septic shock.

ANTIFUNGAL AGENTS

Antifungal therapy in the critical care setting is primarily directed against *Candida* species, and this is the focus of the following presentation.

Amphotericin B

Amphotericin B (AmB) is a naturally occurring antibiotic that is fungicidal for most of the pathogenic fungi in humans (9). It is one of the most effective antifungal agents available, but is plagued by toxic reactions; i.e., infusion-related inflammatory responses, and nephrotoxicity. As a result, AmB is used mostly as a backup, for patients who are intolerant of, or refractory to, less toxic antifungal drugs (see Table 52.2) (10).

Dosing Regimen

AmB is available for intravenous use only, and contains a vehicle (sodium deoxycholate) to enhance solubility in plasma. It is given once daily in a dose of 0.5–1 mg/kg. The dose is initially delivered over a 4-hour time period, but can be delivered in one hour, if tolerated. Daily infusions are continued until a specified cumulative dose is achieved. The total AmB dose is determined by the type and severity of the fungal infection: it can be as little as 500 mg (for catheter-related candidemia) or as much as 4 grams (for life-threatening invasive aspergillosis).

Infusion-Related Inflammatory Response

Infusions of AmB are accompanied by fever, chills, nausea, vomiting, and rigors in about 70% of instances (11). This reaction is most pronounced with the initial infusion, and often diminishes in intensity with repeated infusions. The following measures are used to reduce the intensity of this reaction (11):

1. Thirty minutes before the infusion, give acetaminophen (10–15 mg/kg orally) and diphenhydramine (25 mg orally or IV). If rigors are a problem, premedicate with meperidine (25 mg IV).

2. If the premedication regimen does not give full relief, add hydrocortisone to the AmB infusate (0.1 mg/mL).

Central venous cannulation is preferred for AmB infusions to reduce the risk of infusion-related phlebitis, which is common when AmB is infused through peripheral veins (9).

Nephrotoxicity

AmB binds to cholesterol on the surface of renal epithelial cells and produces an injury that clinically resembles a renal tubular acidosis (distal type), with increased urinary excretion of potassium and magnesium (12). Azotemia is reported in 30–40% of patients during daily infusions of AmB (13), and can occasionally progress to acute renal failure that requires hemodialysis (14). The renal impairment from AmB usually stabilizes with continued infusions, and improvement is expected if AmB is discontinued. Hypovolemia aggravates the renal injury, and maintaining intravascular volume is important for mitigating the injury. An increase in the serum creatinine above 3.0 mg/dL should prompt cessation of AmB infusions for a few days (11).

ELECTROLYTE ABNORMALITIES: *Hypokalemia* and *hypomagnesemia* are common during AmB therapy, and the hypokalemia can be difficult to correct until the magnesium deficits are replaced (as described in Chapter 37). Oral magnesium (300–600 mg elemental magnesium daily) is recommended during AmB therapy, except for patients with progressive azotemia.

Lipid Preparations

Specialized lipid preparations of AmB have been developed to enhance AmB binding to fungal cell membranes and reduce binding to mammalian cells (thereby reducing the risk of renal injury). There are 2 lipid preparations, *liposomal amphotericin*, and *amphotericin B lipid complex*, and the recommended dose is 3–5 mg/kg daily (10). Both reduce the incidence of nephrotoxic reactions, and the decrease is greater with the liposomal preparation (15). Both preparations are costly.

Triazoles

The triazoles are synthetic antifungal agents that are less toxic alternatives to AmB for selected fungal infections. There are 3 drugs in this class, *fluconazole, itraconazole,* and *voriconazole,* but fluconazole is the one used for *Candida* infections.

Clinical Uses

Fluconazole is the drug of choice for infections involving *Candida albicans, C. tropicalis,* and *C. parapsilosis,* but not for infections involving *C. glabrata* or *C. krusei* (see Table 52.2) (10).

Table 52.2	Antifungal Therapy for Invasive Candidiasis	
Organism	**First-Line Drug**	**Alternate Drug**
Candida albicans	Fluconazole	Echinocandin
Candida tropicalis	Fluconazole	Echinocandin
Candida parapsilosis	Fluconazole	Amphotericin B
Candida glabrata	Echinocandin	Amphotericin B
Candida krusei	Echinocandin	Amphotericin B

Adapted from Reference 10.

Dosing Regimens

Fluconazole can be given orally or intravenously. The *usual dose is 400 mg daily*, given as a single dose. Doses of 800 mg daily are recommended for clinically unstable patients. The time to reach steady state levels after the start of therapy is 4–5 days, and this can be shortened by doubling the initial dose. Adjustments are necessary for renal impairment: if the creatinine clearance is < 50 mL/min, the dose should be reduced by 50% (9).

Drug Interactions

The triazoles inhibit the cytochrome P450 enzyme system in the liver, and they can potentiate the activity of several drugs. For fluconazole, the significant interactions include phenytoin, cisapride, and the statins (lovastatin, atorvastatin) (9).

Toxicity

Fluconazole is largely devoid of serious toxicity. Asymptomatic elevation of liver enzymes has been reported (9), and there are rare reports of severe and even fatal hepatic necrosis during fluconazole therapy in HIV patients (16).

Echinocandins

The echinocandins are antifungal agents that are active against a broader spectrum of *Candida* species than fluconazole (except *C. parapsilosis*) (10). The drugs in this class include *caspofungin, micafungin,* and *anidulafungin*. These agents can be used as alternatives to fluconazole for treating invasive candidiasis involving *C. albicans* and *C. tropicalis,* and are the preferred agents for infections involving *C. glabrata* and *C. krusei* (10). They are also preferred by some for prophylaxis of invasive candidiasis in unstable or immunocompromised patients (10).

Caspofungin

Caspofungin is the flagship drug in this class, and is equivalent to amphotericin for treating invasive candidiasis (17). The drug is given intravenously, and *the usual IV dose is 70 mg initially, then 50 mg daily thereafter.* Like all echinocandins, no dose adjustment is needed for renal insufficiency (18).

Others

Anidulafungin (200 mg IV on day 1, then 100 mg IV daily) and micafungin (100 mg IV daily) are equivalent to caspofungin (10), but there is much less clinical experience with these drugs.

Toxicity

The echinocandins are relatively non-toxic. Transient elevations in liver enzymes can occur, and there are occasional reports of hepatic dysfunction associated with these drugs (18).

CARBAPENEMS

The carbapenems have the broadest spectrum of antibacterial activity of any class of antibiotics currently available. There are 4 carbapenems available for clinical use: *imipenem, meropenem, doripenem,* and *ertapenem.* Some notable features of these drugs are included in Table 52.3. The following description is limited to imipenem and meropenem, which are currently the most popular carbapenems. Doripenem is largely indistinguishable from meropenem, and ertapenem is not active against *Pseudomonas aeruginosa*, which makes it the least desirable carbapenem for critically ill patients.

Table 52.3	The Carbapenems			
Feature	**Imipenem**	**Meropenem**	**Doripenem**	**Ertapenem**
Usual Dose	0.5 g q 6 hr	1 g q 8 hr	0.5 g q 8 hr	1 g q 24 hr
Seizure Risk	Yes	No[†]	No	Possibly
Pseudomonas Activity	Yes	Yes	Yes	No
Renal Dose Adjustment	Yes	Yes	Yes	Yes

[†]Meropenem does not cause seizures, but it can reduce serum levels of valproic acid, and will increase the risk of seizures in patients being treated with this anticonvulsant.

Spectrum of Activity

Imipenem and meropenem are active against all common bacterial pathogens except methicillin-resistant staphylococci (MRSA) and vancomycin-resistant enterococci (19). As demonstrated in Figures 52.1 and 52.2, imipenem is one of the most active agents for aerobic Gram-negative bacilli, and is also active against *Pseudomonas aeruginosa* (although less so). These agents also provide adequate coverage for pneumococci, methicillin-sensitive staphylococci, coagulase-negative staphylococci, and anaerobes, including *Bacteroides fragilis* and *Enterococcus faecalis*. Furthermore, acquired resistance to the carbapenems has increased much less than with other antimicrobials used in critical care (19).

Clinical Uses

Because of their broad spectrum of activity, imipenem and meropenem are well suited for empiric antibiotic coverage of suspected Gram-negative infections (e.g., abdominal infections), or mixed aerobic/anaerobic infections (e.g., pelvic infections). Imipenem has also been effective as single-agent empiric coverage for neutropenic patients with fever (20). Meropenem readily crosses the blood-brain barrier (21), and can be used for empiric antibiotic coverage of suspected Gram-negative meningitis.

Dosing Regimens

The carbapenems can only be given intravenously. Imipenem is inactivated by enzymes on the luminal surface the proximal renal tubules, so it is impossible to achieve high levels of the drug in urine. To overcome this problem, the commercial preparation of imipenem contains an enzyme inhibitor, cilastatin (22). The combination imipenem–cilastatin preparation is available as Primaxin. The *usual dose of imipenem–cilastatin is 500 mg IV every 6 hours.* In suspected *Pseudomonas* infections, the dose is doubled to 1 g every 6 hours. In renal failure, the dose should be reduced by 50–75% (23).

Meropenem does not require the cilastatin addition, and the usual dose is 1 gram IV every 8 hours, which can be increased to 2 grams every 8 hours for serious infections. A 50% dose reduction is recommended in patients with renal failure (23).

Adverse Effects

The major risk associated with imipenem is *generalized seizures,* which has been reported in 1–3% of patients receiving the drug (22). Most of the seizure cases are in patients with a history of a seizure disorder, or an intracranial mass, who did not receive an adjusted dose of imipenem for renal insufficiency (22).

There is little risk of seizures with meropenem (19,21). However, meropenem can reduce serum levels of valproic acid, and this can increase the risk of seizures in patients being treated with this anticonvulsant (19).

Cross-Reactivity

Patients with hypersensitivity reactions to penicillin can occasionally have a hypersensitivity reaction to carbapenems. The incidence of this cross-reactivity is not known, but the allergic reactions usually include a rash or urticaria, and are almost never life-threatening (24).

Comment

The ideal antibiotic would be effective against all pathogens and produce no adverse reactions. Meropenem comes closer to this ideal than any antibiotic currently available, with imipenem as a close second. These agents have been my personal favorites for several years because they cover almost everything, which simplifies the selection of empiric antibiotic coverage. Meropenem plus vancomycin (for MRSA) provides adequate empiric coverage for most patients in the ICU (unless there is a problem with vancomycin-resistant enterococci in your ICU). Add fluconazole for empiric coverage if invasive candidiasis is a possibility, and that should be it. The risk of seizures with imipenem is also overstated, and should not be a problem if you adjust the dose for renal insufficiency.

CEPHALOSPORINS

The first cephalosporin (cephalothin) was introduced in 1964, and this was followed by a small army of other cephalosporins. There are currently more than 20 cephalosporins available for clinical use (24,25). They are divided into *generations,* and some of the parenteral agents in the first four generations are shown in Table 52.4.

Table 52.4	The Generations of Parenteral Cephalosporins					
Agent	Generation	Gram⁺ Cocci˟	Gram⁻ Bacilli	*P. aeruginosa*	*B. fragilis*	*H. influenza*
Cefazolin (Ancef)	1	++++	++	—	—	++
Cefoxatin (Mefoxin)	2	++	++++	—	++	++
Ceftriaxone (Rocephin)	3	++	++++	—	—	++++
Ceftazidime (Fortaz)	3	—	++++	++++	—	++++
Cefepime (Maxipime)	4	++	++++	++++	—	++++

˟Does not include coagulase-negative or methicillin-resistant staphylococci, or enterococci.
Relative antibacterial activity is indicated by number of plus signs.
Adapted from Reference 24.

Generations of Cephalosporins

The *first-generation* cephalosporins are primarily active against aerobic Gram-positive cocci, but are not active against *Staphylococcus epidermidis* or methicillin-resistant strains of *S. aureus*. The popular intravenous agent in this group is cefazolin (Ancef).

The *second-generation* cephalosporins exhibit stronger antibacterial activity against Gram-negative aerobic and anaerobic bacilli of enteric origin. The popular parenteral agents in this group are cefoxatin (Mefoxin) and cefamandole (Mandol).

The *third-generation* cephalosporins have greater antibacterial activity against Gram-negative aerobic bacilli, including *P. aeruginosa* and *Hemophilus influenza*, but are less active against aerobic Gram-positive cocci than the first-generation agents. The popular parenteral agents in this group are ceftriaxone (Rocephin), and ceftazidime (Fortaz). Ceftriaxone is popular for the treatment of severe community-acquired pneumonia, primarily because it is active against penicillin-resistant pneumococci and *H. influenza*. Ceftazidime has been a popular anti-pseudomonal antibiotic, but is being eclipsed by a drug (cefepime) in the next generation of cephalosporins.

The *fourth-generation* cephalosporins retain activity against Gram-negative organisms, but add some Gram-positive coverage. The only drug in this generation is cefepime (Maxipime), which has the Gram-negative antibacterial spectrum of ceftazidime (i.e., it covers *P. aeruginosa*), but is also active against Gram-positive cocci (e.g. streptococci and methicillin-sensitive staphylococci).

There is a *fifth-generation* cephalosporin, ceftaroline, that is similar in activity to the fourth generation drugs, but is also active against methicillin-resistant *S. aureus* (MRSA) (25). This drug is not included in Table 52.4 because there is no clinical experience with the drug in ICUs, at least at the present time.

Dosing Regimens

The doses for the more popular parenteral cephalosporins are shown in Table 52.5, along with dose adjustments for renal failure. Note that the dose in renal failure is adjusted by extending the dosing interval rather than decreasing the amount of drug given with each dose (22). This is done to preserve concentration-dependent bacterial killing. Note also that ceftriaxone requires no dose adjustment in renal failure.

Table 52.5	Intravenous Dosing for Commonly Used Cephalosporins	
Drug	**Serious Infections**	**Renal Failure***
Cefazolin	1 g every 6 hr	1 g every 24 hr
Ceftriaxone	2 g every 12 hr	2 g every 12 hr
Ceftazidime	2 g every 8 hr	2 g every 48 hr
Cefepime	2 g every 8 hr	2 g every 24 hr

*From Reference 22.

Toxicity

Adverse reactions to cephalosporins are uncommon and nonspecific (e.g., nausea, rash, and diarrhea). There is a 5–15% incidence of cross-antigenicity with penicillin (24), and cephalosporins should be avoided in patients with a history of *serious* anaphylactic reactions to penicillin.

Comment

The only cephalosporins that continue to have some value in the ICU are ceftriaxone (for empiric therapy of serious community-acquired pneumonias) and cefepime (for empiric coverage of Gram-negative enteric pathogens).

THE FLUOROQUINOLONES

The fluoroquinolone era began in the mid-1980s with the introduction of norfloxacin. Since then, several fluoroquinolones have been introduced, but only three survive: ciprofloxacin, levofloxacin, and moxifloxacin.

Changing Spectrum of Activity

The fluoroquinolones are active against methicillin-sensitive staphylococci, and the newer agents (levofloxacin and moxifloxacin) are active against streptococci (including penicillin-resistant pneumococci), and "atypical" organisms like *Mycoplasma pneumoniae* and *Hemophilus influenza* (26). When first introduced, the fluoroquinolones were very active against Gram-negative aerobic bacilli, including *Pseudomonas aeruginosa*, but rapidly emerging resistance has reduced their activity against Gram-negative organisms, as shown in Figures 52.1 and 52.2.

The development of resistance in Gram-negative organisms has severely curtailed the use of fluoroquinolones in the ICU. Levofloxacin and moxifloxacin are used primarily for community-acquired pneumonia, exacerbations of chronic obstructive lung disease, and for uncomplicated urinary tract infections.

Dosing Regimens

Table 52.6 shows the intravenous dosing regimens for the quinolones. The newer quinolones have longer half-lives than ciprofloxacin, and require only one once-daily dosing. Dose adjustments are required for renal failure for all but moxifloxacin, which is metabolized in the liver (26).

Table 52.6	Intravenous Dosing Regimens for Fluoroquinolones	
Drug	Serious Infections	Renal Failure*
Ciprofloxacin	400 g every 8 hr	400 g every 18 hr
Levofloxacin	500 g every 24 hr	250 g every 48 hr
Moxifloxacin	400 g every 24 hr	400 g every 24 hr

*From Reference 22.

Drug Interactions

Ciprofloxacin interferes with the hepatic metabolism of theophylline and warfarin, and can potentiate the actions of both of these drugs (27,28). Ciprofloxacin causes a 25% increase in serum theophylline levels, and combined therapy has resulted in symptomatic theophylline toxicity (29). Although no dose adjustments are necessary, serum theophylline levels and prothrombin times should be monitored carefully when ciprofloxacin is given in combination with theophylline or warfarin.

Toxicity

The fluoroquinolones are relatively safe. Neurotoxic reactions (confusion, hallucinations, seizures) can develop days after starting quinolone therapy in 1–2% of patients (30). Prolongation of the QT interval and polymorphic ventricular tachycardia (*torsade de pointes*) have been reported with all quinolones except moxifloxacin, but is a rare occurrence (31).

Comment

The emerging resistance of Gram-negative pathogens to fluoroquinolones has just about eliminated fluoroquinolones from the ICU formulary. Levofloxacin is a popular antibiotic for community-acquired pneumonias, and is also used for exacerbations of COPD, but these conditions are often managed outside the ICU.

PENICILLINS

The penicillin discovered by Alexander Fleming in 1929 is benzylpenicillin, or penicillin G, which is (was) active against aerobic streptococci (*S. pneumoniae, S. pyogenes*) and anaerobic mouth flora. The emergence of penicillin-resistant pneumococci in recent years, along with broader spectrum drugs for treating anaerobic infections, has eliminated penicillin G from the ICU formulary.

Extended-Spectrum Penicillins

The penicillins in this category have an extended antibacterial spectrum that covers aerobic Gram-negative bacilli. This category includes the aminopenicillins (ampicillin and amoxicillin), the carboxypenicillins (carbenicillin and ticarcillin), and the ureidopenicillins (azlocillin, mezlocillin, and piperacillin). All groups are active against Gram-negative pathogens, but the latter two groups are active against *Pseudomonas aeruginosa* (32). These agents are also known as antipseudomonal penicillins. The most popular drug in this class is piperacillin, which is available in a special combination product (see next).

Piperacillin-Tazobactam

When used for serious Gram-negative infections, piperacillin is given in combination with tazobactam, a β-lactamase inhibitor that has synergistic activity when combined with piperacillin. The commercial product (Zosyn) contains piperacillin in an 8:1 ratio with tazobactam. The recommended dose of the combination product is 3.375 grams (3 grams piperacillin and 0.375 mg tazobactam) IV every 4–6 hours. In the presence of renal insufficiency, the dose should be changed to 2.25 grams every 8 hours (33).

Comment

Piperacillin-tazobactam is a favorite drug for empiric coverage of suspected Gram-negative infections in the ICU. However, Figures 52.1 and 52.2 show that there are more effective drugs than piperacillin/tazobactam for empiric coverage, and treatment, of Gram-negative infections in the ICU.

VANCOMYCIN & ALTERNATIVES

Vancomycin is the bedrock of antibiotic therapy in the ICU, and has been for several years.

Antibacterial Spectrum

Vancomycin is active against all Gram-positive cocci, including all strains of *Staphylococcus aureus* (coagulase-positive, coagulase-negative, methicillin-sensitive, methicillin-resistant) as well as aerobic and anaerobic streptococci (including pneumococcus and enterococcus) (34). It is the drug of choice for penicillin-resistant pneumococci, and is one of the most active agents against *Clostridium difficile*. Enterococci can be resistant to vancomycin. The prevalence of vancomycin-resistant enterococci (VRE) varies from 2% to 60%, depending on the species involved (34).

Clinical Use

Vancomycin is the drug of choice for infections caused by methicillin-resistant *Staphylococcus aureus* (MRSA) and *Staphylococcus epidermidis*. However, as much as $2/3$ of the vancomycin use in ICUs is not directed at a specific pathogen, but is used for empiric antibiotic coverage in patients with suspected infections (35). The popularity of vancomycin in empiric antibiotic regimens is a reflection of the prominent role played by MRSA and *S. epidermidis* in ICU-related infections.

Dosing Regimens

Vancomycin dosing is based on body weight and renal function.

Weight-Based Dosing

Standard dosing recommendations for vancomycin (1 gram IV every 12 hrs for normal renal function) frequently results in subtherapeutic vancomycin levels in blood. As a result, weight-based dosing is now recommended for vancomycin. The loading dose for most patients is 15–20 mg/kg, and a larger *loading dose of 25 – 30 mg/kg is recommended for critically ill patients* (36). Actual body weight can be used unless the weight is more than 20% above the upper limit of normal for ideal body weight. For overweight patients, an adjusted body weight should be calculated using Equation 52.1 (37).

After the loading dose, subsequent dosing is determined by renal function and the target vancomycin level in blood. An example of a vancomycin dosing nomogram based on body weight, renal function, and a target vancomycin blood level, is shown in Table 52.7. Most hospital pharmacies have nomograms, and will determine the appropriate vancomycin dose for you. After the dosing begins, serum vancomycin levels are used to adjust the dosing regimen.

DRUG LEVELS: Monitoring vancomycin blood levels is recommended when the drug is used to treat serious infections. Steady-state drug levels are usually reached after the fourth intravenous dose (36). Trough blood levels should be > 10 mg/L to prevent the development of resistance. For serious infections, *trough blood levels of 15–20 mg/L are recommended* (36).

Toxicity

Rapid administration of vancomycin can be accompanied by vasodilation, flushing, and hypotension (*red man syndrome*) as a result of histamine release from mast cells (34). The trigger for this release is unknown, but slowing the infusion rate (to less than 10 mg/min) usually corrects the problem.

Original reports of vancomycin-induced nephrotoxicity were likely due to impurities in the vancomycin preparation, or other nephrotoxic drugs, because recent reports are unable to confirm nephrotoxicity with vancomycin monotherapy (34). There is evidence of an immune-mediated thrombocytopenia in 20% of patients receiving vancomycin (38), and vancomycin-induced neutropenia has been reported in 2–12% of patients who receive the drug for more than 7 days (39).

Table 52.7	Vancomycin Dosing Nomogram			
Creatinine Clearance (mL/min)	Weight (kg)			
	60–69	70–79	80–89	90–99
>80	1,000 mg q 12 hr	1,250 mg q 12 hr	1,250 mg q 12 hr	1,500 mg q 12 hr
70–79	1,000 mg q 12 hr	1,250 mg q 12 hr	1,250 mg q 12 hr	1,250 mg q 12 hr
60–69	750 mg q 12 hr	1,000 mg q 12 hr	1,000 mg q 12 hr	1,250 mg q 12 hr
50–59	1,000 mg q 18 hr	1,000 mg q 18 hr	1,250 mg q 18 hr	1,250 mg q 18 hr
40–49	750 mg q 18 hr	1,000 mg q 18 hr	1,250 mg q 18 hr	1,250 mg q 18 hr
30–39	750 mg q 24 hr	1,000 mg q 24 hr	1,250 mg q 24 hr	1,250 mg q 24 hr
20–29	750 mg q 24 hr	1,000 mg q 36 hr	1,250 mg q 36 hr	1,250 mg q 36 hr
10–19	1,000 mg q 48 hr	1,000 mg q 48 hr	1,250 mg q 48 hr	1,250 mg q 48 hr
<10	Repeat dose when spot serum vancomycin <20 mg/L			

From UptoDate (www.uptodate.com). Accessed 6/2013.
Based on a target vancomycin level (trough) of 15–20 mg/L.

Comment

Vancomycin continues to be a solid performer in the ICU, but alternative drugs are needed for infections with vancomycin-resistant enterococci, and for patients who are unable to receive vancomycin (e.g., because of toxic reactions). There is also a need for a vancomycin replacement, to curb the current use of vancomycin, and slow the rate of microbial resistance.

Alternatives

The alternative antibiotics for vancomycin are included in Table 52.8.

Table 52.8	Alternatives to Vancomycin
Antibiotic	**Dosing Regimens and Comments**
Linezolid	Dosing: 400–600 mg IV every 12 hrs.
	Comment: Currently the closest to a replacement for vancomycin.
Daptomycin	Dosing: 4–6 mg/kg IV every 24 hrs.
	Comment: Ineffective for pneumonia (is inactivated by surfactants in the lung).
Quinupristin-Dalfopristin	Dosing: 7.5 mg/kg IV every 8–12 hrs.
	Comment: Use has been limited by side effects (e.g., painful arthralgias and myalgias).

Linezolid

Linezolid is a synthetic antibiotic that has the same spectrum of activity as vancomycin (including MRSA), but is also active against vancomycin-resistant enterococci (VRE) (34). The intravenous dose is *600 mg twice daily*. Linezolid has much better penetration into lung secretions than vancomycin, but original studies suggesting improved outcomes with linezolid in MRSA pneumonia have not been confirmed in a review of all available studies (40).

Linezolid could be used as a replacement for vancomycin, although resistance is already beginning to appear (34). Toxicity associated with linezolid includes thrombocytopenia (with prolonged use) (34), a partially-reversible optic neuropathy (41), and serotonin syndrome (see Table 42.3).

Daptomycin

Daptomycin is a naturally occurring antibiotic that is active against Gram-positive organisms, including MRSA and VRE (34). The recommended IV dose is 4–6 mg/kg given once daily. Dose reductions are recommended for creatinine clearance < 30 mL/min (34).

Daptomycin can be used to treat soft tissue infections or bacteremias involving MRSA and VRE (34). However, it cannot be used to treat pneumonias (42) because it is inactivated by surfactants in the lung. The major toxicity of daptomycin is a skeletal muscle myopathy, and monitoring of serum CPK levels is recommended during therapy with daptomycin (34).

Quinupristin-Dalfopristin

Quinupristin-dalfopristin is a combination of naturally occurring compounds that was the first antibiotic introduced for the treatment of VRE infections. The recommended dose is 7.5 mg/kg IV every 8 hours (34). The principal use of this drug is for infections involving VRE, and use has been curtailed because of troublesome side effects, including painful myalgias and arthralgias (34).

A FINAL WORD

A Simplified Approach

The first rule of antibiotics is try not to use them, and the second rule is try not to use too many of them for too long. If empiric antibiotic coverage is necessary, pending culture results, the combination of *vancomycin and meropenem* will provide adequate coverage for most infections. If invasive candidiasis is a concern, add *fluconazole or caspofungin*. You can then tailor antibiotic therapy according to the culture results, or discontinue antibiotics if the cultures are sterile (unless you suspect invasive candidiasis, when antifungal therapy should be continued until you have an answer). Remember that fever and leukocytosis are signs of systemic inflammation, not infection, and that only 25–50% of ICU patients with signs of systemic inflammation will have a documented infection (see page 266).

REFERENCES

Aminoglycosides

1. Craig WA. Optimizing aminoglycoside use. Crit Care Clin 2011; 27:107–111.

2. Babinchak T, Badal R, Hoban D, Hackel M, et al. Trends in susceptibility of selected gram-negative bacilli isolated from intra-abdominal infections in North America: SMART 2005-2010. Diag Micro Infect Dis 2013; 76:379–381.

3. Martinez JA, Cobos-Triqueros N, Soriano A, et al. Influence of empiric therapy with a beta-lactam alone or combined with an aminoglycoside on prognosis of bacteremia due to gram-negatice organisms. Antimicrob Agents Chemother 2010; 54:3590–3596.

4. Wallach J. Interpretation of diagnostic tests. 8th ed. Philadelphia: Lippincott, Williams & Wikins, 2007:1095.

5. Turnidge J. Pharmacodynamics and dosing of aminoglycosides. Infect Dis Clin N Am 2003; 17:503–528.

6. Wilson SE. Aminoglycosides: assessing the potential for nephrotoxicity. Surg Gynecol Obstet 1986; 171(Suppl):24–30.

7. Lippmann M, Yang E, Au E, Lee C. Neuromuscular blocking effects of tobramycin, gentamicin, and cefazolin. Anesth Analg 1982; 61:767–770.

8. Drachman DB. Myasthenia gravis. N Engl J Med 1994; 330:179–1810.

Antifungal Agents

9. Groll AH, Gea-Banacloche JC, Glasmacher A, et al. Clinical pharmacology of antifungal compounds. Infect Dis Clin N Am 2003; 17:159–191.

10. Limper AH, Knox KS, Sarosi GA, et al. An official American Thoracic Society statement: Treatment of fungal infections in adult pulmonary and critical care patients. Am J Respir Crit Care Med 2011; 183:96–128.

11. Bult J, Franklin CM. Using amphotericin B in the critically ill: a new look at an old drug. J Crit Illness 1996; 11:577–585.

12. Carlson MA, Condon RE. Nephrotoxicity of amphotericin B. J Am Coll Surg 1994; 179:361–381.

13. Walsh TJ, Finberg RW, Arndt C, et al. Liposomal amphotericin B for empirical therapy in patients with persistent fever and neutropenia. N Engl J Med 1999; 340:764–771.

14. Wingard JR, Kublis P, Lee L, et al. Clinical significance of nephrotoxicity in patients treated with amphotericin B for suspected or proven aspergillosis. Clin Infect Dis 1999; 29:1402–1407.

15. Wade WL, Chaudhari P, Naroli JL, et al. Nephrotoxicity and other adverse events among inpatients receiving liposomal amphotericin B and amphotericin B lipid complex. Diag Microbiol Infect Dis 2013; 76:361–367.

16. Gearhart MO. Worsening of liver function with fluconazole and a review of azole antifungal hepatotoxicity. Ann Pharmacother 1994; 28:1177–1181.

17. Mora-Duarte J, Betts R, Rotstein C, et al. Comparison of caspofungin and amphotericin B for invasive candidiasis. N Engl J Med 2002; 347:2020–2029.

18. Echinocandins. In: McEvoy GK, ed. AHFS Drug Information, 2012. Bethesda: American Society of Health-System Pharmacists, 2012:528–538.

Carbapenems

19. Baughman RP. The use of carbapenems in the treatment of serious infections. J Intensive Care Med 2009; 24:230–241.

20. Freifield A, Walsh T, Marshall D, et al. Monotherapy for fever and neutropenia in cancer patients: a randomized comparison of ceftazidime versus imipenem. J Clin Oncol 1995; 13:165–176.

21. Cunha B. Meropenem for clinicians. Antibiotics for Clinicans 2000; 4:59–66.

22. Hellinger WC, Brewer NS. Imipenem. Mayo Clin Proc 1991; 66:1074–1081.

22. Bennett WM, Aronoff GR, Golper TA, et al. eds. Drug prescribing in renal failure. 3rd ed. Philadelphia: American College of Physicians, 1994.

23. Carbapenems. In: McEvoy GK, ed. AHFS Drug Information, 2012. Bethesda: American Society of Health-System Pharmacists, 2012:166–182.

Cephalosporins

24. Asbel LE, Levison ME. Cephalosporins, carbapenems, and monobactams. Infect Dis Clin N Am 2000; 14:1–10.

25. Cephalosporins: General statement. In: McEvoy GK, ed. AHFS Drug Information, 2012. Bethesda: American Society of Health-System Pharmacists, 2012:68–83.

Fluoroquinolones

26. Rotschafer JC, Ullman MA, Sullivan CJ. Optimal use of fluoroquinolones in the intensive care setting. Crit Care Clin 2011; 27:95–106.

27. Walker RC, Wright AJ. The fluoroquinolones. Mayo Clin Proc 1991; 66:1249–1259.

28. Robson RA. The effects of quinolones on xanthine pharmacokinetics. Am J Med 1992; 92(Suppl 4A):22S–26S.

29. Maddix DS. Do we need an intravenous fluoroquinolone? West J Med 992; 157:55–59.

30. Finch C, Self T. Quinolones: recognizing the potential for neurotoxicity. J Crit Illness 2000; 15:656–657.

31. Frothingham R. Rates of torsade de pointes associated with ciprofloxacin, ofloxacin, levofloxacin, gatifloxacin, and moxifloxacin. Pharmacother 2001; 21:1468–1472.

Penicillins

32. Wright AJ. The penicillins. Mayo Clin Proc 1999; 74:290–307.

33. Piperacillin and Tazobactam. In: McEvoy GK, ed. AHFS drug information, 2012. Bethesda: American Society of Hospital Pharmacists, 2012:340–344.

Vancomycin

34. Nailor MD, Sobel JD. Antibiotics for gram-positive bacterial infections: vancomycin, teicoplanin, quinupristin/dalfopristin, oxazolidinones, daptomycin, dalbavancin, and telavancin. Infect Dis Clin N Am 2009; 23:965–982.

35. Ena J, Dick RW, Jones RN. The epidemiology of intravenous vancomycin usage in a university hospital. JAMA 1993; 269:598–605.

36. Rybak M, Lomaestro B, Rotschafer JC, et al. Therapeutic monitoring of vancomycin in adult patients: A consensus review of the American Society of Health System Pharmacists, the Infectious Disease Society of America, and the Society of Infectious Diseases Pharmacists. Am J Heath-Syst Pharm 2009; 66:82–98.

37. Leong JVB, Boro MS, Winter ME. Determining vancomycin clearance in an overweight and obese population. Am J Heath-Syst Pharm 2011; 68:599–603.

38. Von Drygalski A, Curtis B, Bougie DW, et al. Vancomycin-induced immune thrombocytopenia. N Engl J Med 2007; 356:904–910.

39. Black E, Lau TT, Ensom MHH. Vancomycin-induced neutropenia. Is it dose- or duration-related? Ann Pharmacother 2011; 45:629–638.

Alternatives to Vancomycin

40. Kali AC, Murthy MH, Hermsen ED, et al. Linezolid versus vancomycin or teicoplanin for nosocomial pneumonia: A systematic review and meta-analysis. Crit Care Med 2010; 38:1802–1808.

41. Rucker JC, Hamilton SR, Bardenstein D, et al. Linezolid-associated toxic optic neuropathy. Neurology 2006; 66:595–598.

42. Daptomycin. In: McEvoy GK, ed. AHFS drug information, 2012. Bethesda: American Society of Hospital Pharmacists, 2012:454–457.

Chapter 53

HEMODYNAMIC DRUGS

In the successful resuscitation of the shocked patient,
the physician achieves his or her greatest victory.

Evan Geller
1993

Pharmacological support of blood pressure and blood flow is one of the fundamental practices in the care of critically ill patients. This chapter describes the principal drugs that are used for circulatory support in the ICU, and includes only drugs that are administered by continuous intravenous infusion. The very last section of the chapter includes a brief comment on the shortcomings of circulatory support drugs in the critically ill.

CATECHOLAMINES

Catecholamines are drugs that promote blood flow and blood pressure by stimulating adrenergic receptors. The different types of adrenergic receptors are summarized in Table 53.1, and the effects of catecholamine drugs on adrenergic receptors is summarized in Table 53.2. Despite differences in adrenergic receptor activation and physiological responses, *no catecholamine drug has proven superior to the others for improving clinical outcomes* (1,2).

Table 53.1	Adrenergic Receptors and Associated Responses	
Alpha Receptors	**Beta-1 Receptors**	**Beta-2 Receptors**
Vasoconstriction	Cardioacceleration	Vasodilatation
Iris Dilatation	Increased Cardiac Contractility	Bronchodilatation
Piloerection		Increased Glycolysis
	Lipolysis	Uterine Relaxation

Table 53.2	Effects of Catecholamine Drugs on Adrenergic Receptors		
	Type of Receptor		
Catecholamine	**Alpha**	**Beta-1**	**Beta-2**
Dobutamine	—	++	+
Dopamine (Moderate Dose)	—	+++	+++
Dopamine (High Dose)	++	+++	+++
Epinephrine	+++	++++	+++
Norepinephrine	+++	+	—
Phenylephrine	+++	—	—

Dobutamine

Dobutamine is a synthetic catecholamine that is classified as an *inodilator* because it has positive inotropic and vasodilator effects.

Actions

Dobutamine is primarily a β_1-receptor agonist, but also has weak β_2-receptor agonist activity. The β_1-receptor stimulation produces an increase in heart rate and stroke volume, while the β_2-receptor stimulation produces peripheral vasodilatation (3,4). The stroke volume augmentation produced by dobutamine is shown in Figure 53.1 (4). Because the increase in stroke volume is accompanied by a decrease in systemic vascular resistance, the blood pressure is usually unchanged or slightly increased (3). The response to dobutamine, however, can vary widely in critically ill patients (5).

The cardiac stimulation produced by dobutamine is often accompanied by an increase in cardiac work and myocardial O_2 consumption (3). These effects can be deleterious in heart failure because cardiac work and myocardial energy needs are already heightened in the failing myocardium.

Clinical Uses

Dobutamine has been used to augment cardiac output in patients with decompensated heart failure due to systolic dysfunction. However, the unfavorable effects of dobutamine on myocardial energetics has created a preference for other inodilators in decompensated heart failure (see pages 250–251). Dobutamine remains the preferred inotropic agent for the treatment of myocardial depression associated with septic shock (1), but it usually must be combined with a vasoconstrictor agent (e.g., norepinephrine) to raise the blood pressure.

Dosing Regimen

Dobutamine is started at an infusion rate of 3–5 µg/kg/min (without a loading dose), and this can be increased in increments of 3–5 µg/kg/min, if necessary, to achieve the desired effect. (A pulmonary artery catheter is usually needed to guide dobutamine dosing.) The usual dose range is 5–20 µg/kg/min (3), but doses as high as 200 µg/kg/min have been used safely (5). Therapy should be driven by hemodynamic end-points, and not by pre-selected dose rates.

Adverse Effects

Dobutamine produces only mild increases in heart rate (5-15 beats/min) in most patients, but it occasionally causes significant tachycardia (rate increases > 30 beats/min) (3), which can be deleterious in patients with coronary artery disease. Like all positive inotropic agents, dobutamine is contraindicated in patients with hypertrophic cardiomyopathy.

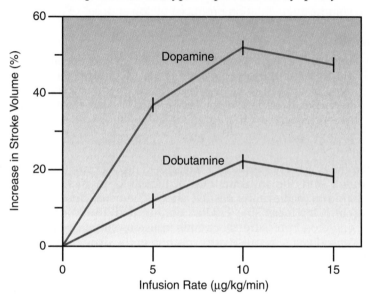

FIGURE 53.1 Stroke volume augmentation produced by equivalent doses of dobutamine and dopamine in post-cardiopulmonary bypass patients. Data from Reference 4.

Dopamine

Dopamine is an endogenous catecholamine that serves as a precursor for norepinephrine. When given as an exogenous drug, dopamine produces a variety of dose-dependent effects, as described next.

Actions

At *low infusion rates* (≤3 µg/kg/min), dopamine selectively activates dopamine-specific receptors in the renal and splanchnic circulations, which increases blood flow in these regions (6). Low-dose dopamine also directly affects renal tubular epithelial cells, causing an increase in both urinary sodium excretion (natriuresis) and urine output that are independent of the changes in renal blood flow (6). *The renal effects of low-dose dopamine are minimal or absent in patients with acute renal failure* (7).

At *moderate infusion rates* (3–10 µg/kg/min), dopamine stimulates β-receptors in the heart and peripheral circulation, producing an increase in myocardial contractility and heart rate, along with peripheral vasodilatation. The increase in stroke volume produced by dopamine is shown in Figure 53.1. Note the greater effect with dopamine compared to dobutamine at equivalent infusion rates.

At *high infusion rates* (> 10 µg/kg/min), dopamine produces a dose-dependent activation of α-receptors in the systemic and pulmonary circulations, resulting in progressive pulmonary and systemic vasoconstriction. This vasopressor effect increases ventricular afterload, and can reduce the stroke volume augmentation produced by lower doses of dopamine (4).

Clinical Uses

Dopamine can be used to manage patients with cardiogenic shock and septic shock, although other measures are favored in these conditions (i.e., mechanical assist devices are preferred for cardiogenic shock, and norepinephrine is preferred for septic shock). Low-dose dopamine is NOT recommended as a therapy for acute renal failure (see page 640).

Dosing Regimen

Dopamine is usually started at a rate of 3–5 µg/kg/min (without a loading dose), and the infusion rate is increased in increments of 3–5 µg/kg/min to achieve the desired effect. The usual dose range is 3–10 µg/kg/min for increasing cardiac output, and 10–20 µg/kg/min for increasing blood pressure. Dopamine infusions should be delivered into large, central veins, because extravasation of the drug through peripheral veins can produce extensive tissue necrosis.

Adverse Effects

Sinus tachycardia and atrial fibrillation are reported in 25% of patients receiving dopamine infusions (8). Other adverse effects of dopamine include increased intraocular pressure (9), splanchnic hypoperfusion, and delayed gastric emptying, which could predispose to aspiration pneumonia (10).

EXTRAVASATION OF VASOPRESSORS: The risk of tissue necrosis from extravasation of dopamine is a concern with all vasopressor (vasoconstrictor) drug infusions, and eliminating this risk is the reason that *large, central veins are recommended for all vasopressor drug infusions.* If dopamine or any other vasopressor drug escapes from a peripheral vein into the surrounding tissues, the tendency for ischemic tissue necrosis can be reduced by injecting *phentolamine* (an α-receptor antagonist) into the involved area.

The recommended injectate is a solution containing 5–10 mg phentolamine in 15 mL of isotonic saline (6).

Epinephrine

Epinephrine is an endogenous catecholamine that is released by the adrenal medulla in response to physiological stress. It is the most potent natural β-agonist.

Actions

Epinephrine stimulates both α-adrenergic and β-adrenergic receptors (β_1 and β_2 subtypes), and produces dose-dependent increases in heart rate, stroke volume, and blood pressure (11). Epinephrine is a more potent β_1-receptor agonist than dopamine, and produces a greater increase in stroke volume and heart rate than comparable doses of dopamine (12). This is demonstrated in Figure 53.2. The α-receptor stimulation produces a nonuniform peripheral vasoconstriction, with the most prominent effects in the subcutaneous, renal, and splanchnic circulations. Epinephrine also has several metabolic effects, including lipolysis, increased glycolysis, and increased lactate production (from β-receptor activation), and hyperglycemia from α-receptor-mediated inhibition of insulin secretion (11,13).

Clinical Uses

Epinephrine plays an important role in the resuscitation of cardiac arrest (see pages 330–332), and it is the drug of choice for hemodynamic support in anaphylactic shock (see pages 274–276). Epinephrine is also used for hemodynamic support in the early postoperative period following cardiopulmonary bypass surgery (4). Although epinephrine is as effec-

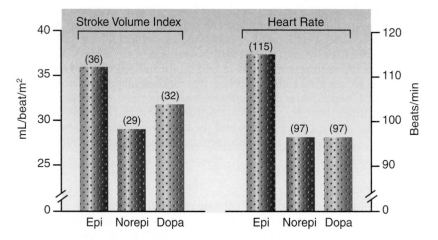

FIGURE 53.2 Cardiac effects of epinephrine (Epi), norepinephrine (Norepi), and dopamine (Dopa) at infusion rates needed to maintain a mean arterial pressure of 75 mm Hg in patients with septic shock. Data from Reference 12.

tive as other catecholamines in septic shock (12,13), concerns about side effects have limited its popularity in septic shock.

Dosing Regimen

The dosing regimens for epinephrine in cardiac arrest and anaphylactic shock are presented in Table 14.5 (see page 275). Epinephrine infusions are not preceded by a loading dose. The initial infusion rate is usually $1-2$ µg/min (or 0.02 µg/kg/min), and the rate is then increased in increments of $1-2$ µg/min to achieve the desired effect (11). The usual dose range for augmenting cardiac output or correcting hypotension is $5-15$ µg/min.

Adverse Effects

Epinephrine creates a greater risk of unwanted cardiac stimulation (which can be deleterious in patients with coronary artery disease) than the other catecholamine drugs (11,12). Other adverse effects include hyperglycemia, increased metabolic rate, and splanchnic hypoperfusion (which can damage the mucosal barrier in the bowel) (11–13). Epinephrine infusions are accompanied by an increase in serum lactate levels (11), but this is not an adverse effect because it reflects an increased rate of glycolysis (not tissue hypoxia), and the lactate can be used as an alternative fuel source (see page 187).

Norepinephrine

Norepinephrine is an endogenous catecholamine that normally functions as an excitatory neurotransmitter. When used as an exogenous drug, norepinephrine functions as a vasopressor.

Actions

The principal action of norepinephrine is α-receptor-mediated peripheral vasoconstriction. However, the adrenergic response to norepinephrine is altered in patients with septic shock (15). For example, norepinephrine infusions are usually accompanied by a decrease in renal blood flow (15), but in patients with septic shock, renal blood flow is increased by norepinephrine infusions (15,16). Similar alterations may also occur with splanchnic blood flow (i.e., normally reduced, but not in septic shock) (15). Norepinephrine is also a weak β_1-receptor agonist, but the effects of norepinephrine on stroke volume and heart rate can be comparable to dopamine (a more potent β_1-receptor agonist) in patients with septic shock (see Figure 53.2).

Clinical Uses

Norepinephrine is the preferred catecholamine for circulatory support in patients with septic shock. This preference is not based on improved outcomes, because the mortality rate in septic shock is the same regardless of the catecholamine used for circulatory support (1,2,12). Instead, norepinephrine is favored in septic shock because it has fewer adverse effects than dopamine or epinephrine (8,12).

Dosing Regimen

Norepinephrine infusions are usually started at a rate of 8–10 µg/min, and the dose rate is then titrated upward or downward to maintain a mean blood pressure of at least 65 mm Hg. The effective dose rate in septic shock varies widely in individual patients, but is usually below 40 µg/min. Hypotension that is refractory to norepinephrine usually prompts the addition of dopamine or vasopressin, but there is no evidence that this practice improves outcomes.

Adverse Effects

Adverse effects of norepinephrine include local tissue necrosis from drug extravasation, and intense systemic vasoconstriction with organ dysfunction when high dose rates are required. However, whenever high doses of a vasoconstrictor drug are required to correct hypotension, it is difficult to distinguish between adverse drug effects and adverse effects of the circulatory shock.

Phenylephrine

Phenylephrine is a potent vasoconstrictor that has very few applications in the ICU.

Actions

Phenylephrine in a pure α-receptor agonist that produces widespread vasoconstriction. The consequences of this vasoconstriction can include bradycardia, a decrease in cardiac stroke output (usually in patients with cardiac dysfunction), and hypoperfusion of the kidneys and bowel.

Clinical Uses

The principal use of phenylephrine is for the reversal of severe hypotension produced by spinal anesthesia. However, pure α-receptor agonists are not universally favored in this situation because they can aggravate the decrease in cardiac stroke output that occurs in spinal shock (17). Phenylephrine is not recommended for hemodynamic support in septic shock, although a clinical study comparing phenylephrine and norepinephrine for the early management of septic shock showed no differences in hemodynamic effects or clinical outcomes with the use of either drug (18).

Dosing Regimen

Phenylephrine can be given as intermittent IV doses. The initial IV dose is 0.2 mg, which can be repeated in increments of 0.1 mg to a maximum dose of 0.5 mg (17). Phenylephrine can be infused at an initial dose rate 0.1–0.2 mg/min, which is progressively decreased after the blood pressure is stabilized (17).

Adverse Effects

The principal adverse effects of phenylephrine are bradycardia, low cardiac output, and renal hypoperfusion. These effects are magnified in hypovolemic patients.

ADJUNCTIVE VASOPRESSORS

The following drugs can be added to vasopressor therapy with catecholamines in selected situations.

Vasopressin

Antidiuretic hormone (ADH) is an osmoregulatory hormone that is also called *vasopressin* because it produces vasoconstriction.

Actions

The vasoconstrictor effects of vasopressin are mediated by specialized vasopressin (V_1) receptors located on vascular smooth muscle. Vasoconstriction is most prominent in skin, skeletal muscle, and splanchnic circulations (19). Exogenous vasopressin does not increase blood pressure in healthy volunteers, but it can produce significant increases in blood pressure in patients with hypotension caused by peripheral vasodilatation (19). This type of hypotension occurs in septic shock, anaphylactic shock, autonomic insufficiency, and the hypotension associated with spinal and general anesthesia.

Other actions of vasopressin include enhanced water reabsorption in the distal renal tubules (mediated by V_2 receptors), and stimulation of ACTH release by the anterior pituitary gland (mediated by V_3 receptors). These actions are clinically silent when vasopressin is administered in the recommended doses (19).

Clinical Uses

Vasopressin can be used in the following clinical situations.

1. In the resuscitation of cardiac arrest, vasopressin can be given as a single IV dose (40 units) to replace the first or second dose of epinephrine (see page 332).

2. In cases of septic shock that are resistant, or refractory, to hemodynamic support with norepinephrine or dopamine, a vasopressin infusion can be used to raise the blood pressure and reduce the catecholamine requirement (catecholamine sparing effect) (19–20). Unfortunately, there is *no survival benefit* associated with the this practice (20).

3. In cases of hemorrhage from esophageal or gastric varices, vasopressin infusions can be used to promote splanchnic vasoconstriction and reduce the rate of bleeding.

Dosing Regimen

The plasma half-life of exogenous vasopressin is 5–20 min (17), so vasopressin must be given by continuous infusion to produce prolonged effects.

In septic shock, the recommended infusion rate is 0.01–0.04 units/hr, and a rate of 0.03 units/hr is most popular.

Adverse Effects

Adverse effects are uncommon with infusion rates < 0.04 units/hr (19). At higher infusion rates, unwanted effects can include consequences of excessive vasoconstriction (e.g., impaired renal and hepatic function), along with excessive water retention and hyponatremia.

Terlipressin

Terlipressin is a vasopressin analogue that has two advantages over vasopressin. First, it is a selective V_1 receptor agonist, and does not produce the side effects associated with stimulation of the other vasopressin receptors. Secondly, terlipressin has a much longer duration of action than vasopressin, and a single IV dose of 1–2 mg can raise the blood pressure for 5 hours (19). The long duration of action allows terlipressin to be given by intermittent IV dosing. Terlipressin is a potent splanchnic vasoconstrictor, and may prove valuable in the management of variceal bleeding. However, there is an increased risk of splanchnic ischemia with terlipressin, and ischemic effects cannot be reversed for 5 hours after the drug is administered. Like vasopressin, there is no survival advantage associated with the addition of terlipressin in patients with septic shock (20).

NITROVASODILATORS

Drugs that produce vasodilatation via nitric oxide–mediated relaxation of vascular smooth muscle are known as *nitrovasodilators* (21). There are two drugs that act in this manner: nitroglycerin and nitroprusside.

Nitroglycerin

Nitroglycerin is an organic nitrate that produces a dose-dependent dilation of arteries and veins (22,23).

Vasodilator Actions

The biochemical basis for the vasodilator actions of nitroglycerin is illustrated in Figure 53.3 Nitroglycerin (glyceryl trinitrate) binds to the surface of endothelial cells and releases inorganic nitrite (NO_2), which is converted to nitric oxide (NO) in the endothelial cells. The nitric oxide then moves out of the endothelial cells and into adjacent smooth muscle cells, where it produces muscle relaxation by promoting the formation of cyclic guanosine monophosphate (cGMP).

Venodilatation predominates at lower infusion rates of nitroglycerin (< 50 µg/min), while higher infusion rates produce arterial vasodilatation as well. Both of these effects are advantageous in patients with heart failure; i.e., the venodilatation reduces cardiac filling pressures (which

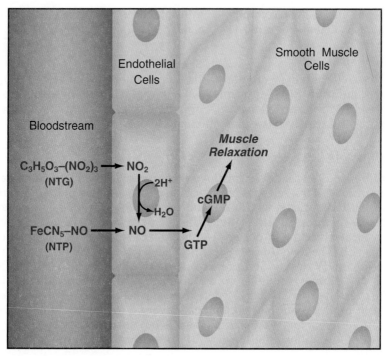

FIGURE 53.3 The biochemical basis for the vasodilator actions of nitroglycerin (NTG) and nitroprusside (NTP). Chemical symbols: nitroglycerin [$C_3H_5O_3$-$(NO_2)_3$], nitroprusside ($FeCN_5$-NO), inorganic nitrite (NO_2), nitric oxide (NO), guanosine triphosphate (GTP), cyclic guanosine monophosphate (cGMP).

reduces edema formation), and the arterial vasodilatation reduces ventricular afterload (which increases cardiac stroke output).

Antiplatelet Effects

Nitrates inhibit platelet aggregation, and nitric oxide is believed to mediate this effect as well (24). Because platelet thrombi play an important role in the pathogenesis of acute coronary syndromes, the antiplatelet actions of nitroglycerin have been proposed as the mechanism for the antianginal effects of the drug (24). This would explain why nitroglycerin's ability to relieve ischemic chest pain is not shared by other vasodilator drugs.

Clinical Uses

Nitroglycerin infusions are used to relieve chest pain in patients with unstable angina (see page 306), and to augment cardiac output in patients with decompensated heart failure (see pages 248–249).

Dosage and Administration

Nitroglycerin binds to soft plastics such as polyvinylchloride (PVC), which is a common constituent of the plastic bags and tubing used for intravenous infusions. *As much as 80% of the drug can be lost by adsorption to PVC* in standard intravenous infusion systems (22). Nitroglycerin does not bind to glass or hard plastics like polyethylene (PET), so drug loss via adsorption can be eliminated by using glass bottles and PET tubing. Drug manufacturers often provide specialized infusion sets to prevent nitroglycerin loss via adsorption.

DOSING REGIMEN When nitroglycerin adsorption is not a problem, the initial infusion rate is typically 5–10 µg/min, which can be increased in increments of 5–10 µg/min every 5 minutes until the desired effect is achieved. The effective dose is 5–100 µg/min in most cases, and infusion rates above 200 µg/min are rarely necessary unless nitrate tolerance has developed (see later).

Adverse Effects

The venodilating effects of nitroglycerin can promote hypotension in hypovolemic patients and in patients with acute right heart failure due to right ventricular infarction. In either of these conditions, aggressive volume loading is required prior to initiating a nitroglycerin infusion.

Nitroglycerin-induced increases in cerebral blood flow can lead to increased intracranial pressure (25), while increases in pulmonary blood flow can result in increased intrapulmonary shunting and worsening arterial oxygenation in patients with infiltrative lung disease (e.g., pneumonia or ARDS) (26).

METHEMOGLOBINEMIA: Nitroglycerin metabolism generates inorganic nitrites (see Fig. 53.3), which can oxidize the iron moieties in hemoglobin to produce methemoglobin. However, clinically apparent methemoglobinemia is not a common complication of nitroglycerin infusions, and occurs only at very high dose rates (25).

SOLVENT TOXICITY: Nitroglycerin does not readily dissolve in aqueous solutions, and nonpolar solvents such as ethanol and propylene glycol are required to keep the drug in solution. These solvents can accumulate during prolonged infusions. Both ethanol intoxication (27) and propylene glycol toxicity (28) have been reported as a result of nitroglycerin infusions. Propylene glycol toxicity may be more common than suspected because this solvent makes up 30–50% of some nitroglycerin preparations (25). (For a description of propylene glycol toxicity, see page 911–912).

NITRATE TOLERANCE: Tolerance to the vasodilator and antiplatelet actions of nitroglycerin is a well-described phenomenon, and can appear after only 24–48 hours of continuous drug administration (25). The underlying mechanism may be oxidative stress-induced endothelial dysfunction (29). The most effective measure for preventing or reversing nitrate tolerance is a daily drug-free interval of at least 6 hours (25).

Nitroprusside

Nitroprusside is a rapidly-acting vasodilator that is favored for the treatment of hypertensive emergencies. The popularity of this drug is limited by the risk of cyanide intoxication.

Actions

The vasodilator actions of nitroprusside, like those of nitroglycerin, are mediated by nitric oxide (21). The nitroprusside molecule contains one nitrosyl group (NO), which is released as nitric oxide when nitroprusside enters the bloodstream. The nitric oxide somehow ends up in endothelial cells, where it proceeds as shown in Figure 53.3.

Like nitroglycerin, nitroprusside dilates both arteries and veins, but it is less potent than nitroglycerin as a venodilator, and more potent as an arterial vasodilator. Nitroprusside has variable effects on cardiac output in subjects with normal cardiac function (30), but it consistently improves cardiac output in patients with decompensated heart failure (30,31).

Clinical Uses

The principal uses of nitroprusside are the treatment of hypertensive emergencies, where rapid blood pressure reduction is desirable, and management of acute, decompensated heart failure, as described on page 248.

Dosing Regimen

Nitroprusside infusions are started at 0.2 µg/kg/min, and then titrated upward every 5 minutes to the desired result. Control of hypertension usually requires infusion rates of 2–5 µg/kg/min, but *infusion rates should be kept below 3 µg/kg/min*, if possible, to limit the risk of cyanide intoxication (30). In renal failure, the infusion rate should be kept below 1 µg/kg/min to limit thiocyanate accumulation (described later) (30).

Cyanide Intoxication

Nitroprusside infusions carry a considerable risk of cyanide intoxication. In fact, *cyanide accumulation is common during therapeutic infusions of nitroprusside* (25,32,33). The origin of the cyanide is the nitroprusside molecule, which is a ferricyanide complex with 5 cyanide molecules bound to an oxidized iron core (see Figure 53.4). This cyanide is released in the bloodstream when nitroprusside breaks up to release nitric oxide and exert its vasodilator actions. The clearance mechanisms for the released cyanide are shown in Figure 53.4. Two chemical reactions help to remove cyanide from the bloodstream. One involves the binding of cyanide to the oxidized iron moiety in methemoglobin. The other reaction involves the transfer of sulfur from a donor molecule (thiosulfate) to cyanide to form a thiocyanate compound, which is then cleared by the kidneys. The latter (transulfuration) reaction is the principal mechanism for removing cyanide from the human body.

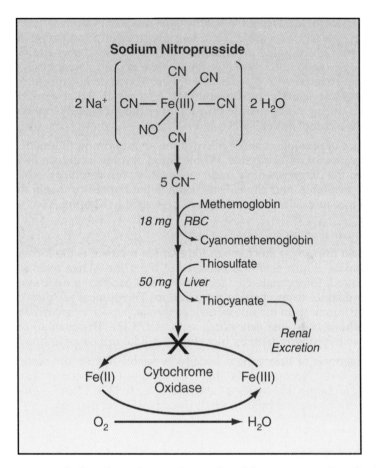

FIGURE 53.4 The fate of cyanide (CN) that is released from nitroprusside molecules. See text for explanation.

Healthy adults have enough methemoglobin to bind the cyanide in 18 mg of nitroprusside, and enough thiosulfate to bind the cyanide in 50 mg of nitroprusside (25). This means that healthy adults can detoxify 68 mg of nitroprusside. At a nitroprusside infusion rate of 2 µg/kg/minute (therapeutic dose) in an 80-kg adult, the 68 mg limit of detoxification is reached in 500 minutes (8.3 hours) after the start of the infusion. Thereafter, the cyanide released by nitroprusside will combine with the oxidized iron in cytochrome oxidase and block the utilization of oxygen in the mitochondria.

The capacity for cyanide removal is reduced by *thiosulfate depletion*, which is common in smokers and postoperative patients (25,32). To elim- inate the risk of thiosulfate depletion, thiosulfate can be routinely added to the nitroprusside infusate. About 500 mg of thiosulfate should be added for every 50 mg of nitroprusside (24).

CLINICAL MANIFESTATIONS: One of the early signs of cyanide accumulation is *nitroprusside tachyphylaxis* (25); i.e., progressively increasing requirements for nitroprusside to maintain the desired blood pressure. Signs of impaired oxygen utilization (i.e., an increase in central venous O_2 saturation, and an increase in plasma lactate levels) often do not appear until the late stages of cyanide intoxication (34). As a result, the absence of lactic acidosis during nitroprusside infusion does not exclude the possibility of cyanide accumulation (25,32).

Evidence of possible cyanide intoxication should prompt immediate discontinuation of nitroprusside. Whole blood cyanide levels can be used to confirm the diagnosis of cyanide intoxication, but results are not immediately available, and clinical suspicion is the impetus to begin detoxification measures. These measures are described in Chapter 55.

Thiocyanate Intoxication

The most important mechanism for cyanide removal is the formation of thiocyanate, which is slowly excreted in the urine. When renal function is impaired, thiocyanate can accumulate and produce a toxic syndrome that is distinct from cyanide intoxication. The clinical features of thiocyanate intoxication include *anxiety, confusion, pupillary constriction, tinnitus, hallucinations, and generalized seizures* (25,32). Thiocyanate can also promote hypothyroidism by blocking thyroidal uptake of iodine (32).

The diagnosis of thiocyanate toxicity is established by the serum thiocyanate level. Normal levels are below 10 mg/L, and clinical toxicity is usually accompanied by levels above 100 mg/L (32). Thiocyanate intoxication can be treated by hemodialysis or peritoneal dialysis.

A FINAL WORD

The Vasopressor Folly

One of the frustrating aspects of critical care practice is the continuing high mortality rates in circulatory shock, particularly septic shock, despite correction of the blood pressure with vasopressor drugs. The likely explanation for this is the probability that low blood pressure plays little or no role in the pathogenesis of circulatory shock, or in the clinical outcomes. This is consistent with observations in septic shock indicating that the pathological injury is a defect in oxygen utilization in mitochondria, and the culprit is uncontrolled inflammation, not a low blood pressure. In light of this explanation, the decrease in blood pressure that occurs in shock is more likely to be the *result* of the pathological cell injury (i.e., shock of the blood vessels) rather than a cause of the injury. Hypotension then becomes one of several consequences of cellular shock, and correcting the hypotension is not expected to correct the primary pathological process. After at least 50 years of focusing on vasopressor therapy in shock, it's time for a do-over.

REFERENCES

Reviews

1. Holmes CL, Walley KR. Vasoactive drugs for vasodilatory shock in ICU. Curr Opin Crit Care 2009; 15:398–402.

2. Beale RJ, Hollenberg SM, Vincent J-L, Parrillo JE. Vasopressor and inotropic support in septic shock: An evidence-based review. Crit Care Med 2004; 32(Suppl): S455–S465.

Dobutamine

3. Dobutamine hydrochloride. In McEvoy GK, ed. AHFS Drug Information, 2012. Bethesda: American Society of Health-System Pharmacists, 2012:1314–1316.

4. Steen PA, Tinker JH, Pluth JR, et al. Efficacy of dopamine, dobutamine, and epinephrine during emergence from cardiopulmonary bypass in man. Circulation 1978; 57:378–384.

5. Hayes MA, Yau EHS, Timmins AC, et al. Response of critically ill patients to treatment aimed at achieving supranormal oxygen delivery and consumption. Relationship to outcome. Chest 1993; 103:886–895.

Dopamine

6. Dopamine hydrochloride. In McEvoy GK, ed. AHFS Drug Information, 2012. Bethesda: American Society of Health-System Pharmacists, 2012:1314–1316.

7. Kellum JA, Decker JM. Use of dopamine in acute renal failure: A meta-analysis. Crit Care Med 2001; 29:1526–1531.

8. De Backer D, Biston P, Devriendt J, et al. Comparison of dopamine and norepinephrine in the treatment of shock. N Engl J Med 2010; 362:779–789.

9. Brath PC, MacGregor DA, Ford JG, Prielipp RC. Dopamine and intraocular pressure in critically ill patients. Anesthesiology 2000; 93:1398–1400.

10. Johnsom AG. Source of infection in nosocomial pneumonia. Lancet 1993; 341:1368 (Letter).

Epinephrine

11. Epinephrine. In McEvoy GK, ed. AHFS Drug Information, 2012. Bethesda: American Society of Health-System Pharmacists, 2012:1362–1368.

12. De Backer D, Creteur J, Silva E, Vincent J-L. Effects of dopamine, norepinephrine, and epinephrine on the splanchnic circulation in septic shock: Which is best? Crit Care Med 2003; 31:1659–1667.

13. Levy B. Bench-to-bedside review: Is there a place for epinephrine in septic shock? Crit Care 2005; 9:561–565.

Norepinephrine

14. Norepinephrine bitartrate. In: McEvoy GK, ed. AHFS Drug Information, 2012. Bethesda: American Society of Health System Pharmacists, 2012:1371–1374.

15. Bellomo R, Wan L, May C. Vasoactive drugs and acute kidney injury. Crit Care Med 2008; 36(Suppl):S179–S186.

16. Desairs P, Pinaud M, Bugnon D, Tasseau F. Norepinephrine therapy has no deleterious renal effects in human septic shock. Crit Care Med 1989; 17:426–429.

Phenylephrine

17. Phenylephrine hydrochloride. In: McEvoy GK, ed. AHFS Drug Information, 2012. Bethesda,: American Society of Health System Pharmacists, 2012:1306–1311.

18. Morelli A, Ertmer C, Rehberg S, et al. Phenylephrine versus norepinephrine for initial hemodynamic support of patients with septic shock: a randomized, controlled trial. Crit Care 2008; 12:R143.

Vasopressin

19. Treschan TA, Peters J. The vasopressin system: physiology and clinical strategies. Anesthesiology 2006; 105:599–612.

20. Polito A, Parisini E, Ricci Z, et al. Vasopressin for treatment of vasodilatory shock: an ESICM systematic review and meta-analysis. Intensive Care Med 2012; 38:9–19.

Nitroglycerin

21. Anderson TJ, Meredith IT, Ganz P, et al. Nitric oxide and nitrovasodilators: similarities, differences and potential interactions. J Am Coll Cardiol 1994; 24:555–566.

22. Nitroglycerin. In: McEvoy GK, ed. AHFS Drug Information, 2012. Bethesda: American Society of Health System Pharmacists, 2012:1824–1827.

23. Elkayam U. Nitrates in heart failure. Cardiol Clin 1994; 12:73–85.

24. Stamler JS, Loscalzo J. The antiplatelet effects of organic nitrates and related nitroso compounds in vitro and in vivo and their relevance to cardiovascular disorders. J Am Coll Cardiol 1991; 18:1529–1536.

25. Curry SC, Arnold-Cappell P. Nitroprusside, nitroglycerin, and angiotensin-converting enzyme inhibitors. In: Blumer JL, Bond GR, eds. Toxic effects of drugs used in the ICU. Crit Care Clin 1991; 7:555–582.

26. Radermacher P, Santak B, Becker H, Falke KJ. Prostaglandin F1 and nitroglycerin reduce pulmonary capillary pressure but worsen ventilation–perfusion distribution in patients with adult respiratory distress syndrome. Anesthesiology 1989; 70:601–606.

27. Korn SH, Comer JB. Intravenous nitroglycerin and ethanol intoxication. Ann Intern Med 1985; 102:274.

28. Demey HE, Daelemans RA, Verpooten GA, et al. Propylene glycol-induced side effects during intravenous nitroglycerin therapy. Intensive Care Med 1988; 14:221–226.

29. Münzel T, Gori T. Nitrate therapy and nitrate tolerance in patients with coronary artery disease. Curr Opin Pharmacol 2013; 13:251–259.

Nitroprusside

30. Sodium nitroprusside. In: McEvoy GK, ed. AHFS Drug Information, 2012. Bethesda: American Society of Health System Pharmacists, 2012:1811–1814.

31. Guiha NH, Cohn JN, Mikulic E, et al. Treatment of refractory heart failure with infusion of nitroprusside. New Engl J Med 1974; 291:587–592.

32. Hall VA, Guest JM. Sodium nitroprusside-induced cyanide intoxication and prevention with sodium thiosulfate prophylaxis. Am J Crit Care 1992; 2:19–27.

33. Robin ED, McCauley R. Nitroprusside-related cyanide poisoning. Time (long past due) for urgent, effective interventions. Chest 1992; 102:1842–1845.

34. Arieff AI. Is measurement of venous oxygen saturation useful in the diagnosis of cyanide poisoning? Am J Med 1992; 93:582–583.

TOXICOLOGIC EMERGENCIES

There are two things which Man cannot look at directly without flinching: the sun and death.

Francois De La Rochefoucauld
1630–1680

Chapter 54

PHARMACEUTICAL DRUG OVERDOSES

*Poisons and medicine are oftentimes the same substance
given with different intents.*

Peter Latham
1865

Prescription drug use in the United States is astronomical (see Figure 54.1), and among the massively consumed prescription drugs are "drugs of abuse" like opioid analgesics. The magnitude of the opioid prescribing frenzy is demonstrated by a recent estimate that the number of prescribed opioid analgesics in 2010 was enough to medicate every single adult in the United States for a period of one month (using typical doses) (1). As a result of the liberal prescribing practices for potentially dangerous drugs, prescription drugs have replaced "street drugs" as the principal offenders in toxic drug ingestions (2), and there has been an increase in the number of drug overdoses, as well as an increase in the number of fatal drug overdoses, in recent years (2a).

This chapter describes overdoses involving 5 pharmaceutical drugs: 3 prescription drugs (benzodiazepines, β-receptor antagonists, and opioids) and 2 over-the-counter drugs (acetaminophen and salicylates).

ACETAMINOPHEN

Acetaminophen is a ubiquitous analgesic-antipyretic agent that is included in over 600 commercial drug preparations. It is also a hepatotoxin, and is the *most common cause of acute liver failure in the United States* (3). Acetaminophen overdoses are responsible for half of the cases of acute liver failure in the United States, and *half of the overdoses are unintentional* (4). Because of the hepatotoxic risk, the Food and Drug Administration issued a mandate in 2009 for more prominent labeling of the risks associated with acetaminophen, and the recommended maximum dose of acetaminophen was reduced from 4 to 3.25 grams daily (5). The impact of these changes is unclear at the present time.

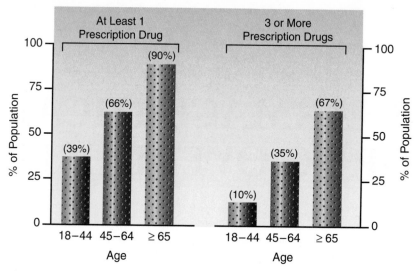

FIGURE 54.1 Prescription drug use in the United States in 2007–2010, by age group. Data from Health United States, 2012. DHHS Publication No. 2013-1232, May, 2013.

Toxic Mechanism

The toxicity of acetaminophen is related to its metabolism in the liver, and the metabolic pathways are shown Figure 54.2. The bulk of acetaminophen metabolism involves the formation of nontoxic sulfated conjugates, which are excreted in the urine. About 10% of the metabolism involves the oxidation of acetaminophen to form a toxic metabolite that is capable of producing oxidant cell injury. When the daily dose of acetaminophen is not excessive, the toxic metabolite is removed by conjugation with glutathione, an intracellular antioxidant. When the daily dose of acetaminophen exceeds 4 grams, the sulfated conjugation pathways become saturated, which diverts acetaminophen metabolism to the pathway with the toxic metabolite. The increased traffic in this pathway eventually depletes glutathione reserves, and when glutathione stores fall to 30% of normal, the toxic acetaminophen metabolite can accumulate and promote hepatocellular damage (3).

Toxic Dose

The toxic dose of acetaminophen can vary widely in individual patients, but is somewhere between 7.5 and 15 grams in most adults (6,7). However, several conditions can increase the susceptibility to acetaminophen hepatotoxicity, such as malnutrition, chronic illness, and chronic ethanol ingestion, and the toxic dose of acetaminophen may be lower in these patients. A general rule adopted by poison control centers is to recommend evaluation for acute ingestions of 10 grams of acetaminophen (20 extra-strength Tylenol tablets) (3). For patients who may have an increased susceptibility to acetaminophen hepatotoxicity, an acute ingestion of 4 grams of acetaminophen warrants an evaluation (3). The maximum recommended daily dose of acetaminophen is 3.25 grams (5).

Clinical Presentation

In the first 24 hours following a toxic ingestion, symptoms are either absent or nonspecific (e.g., nausea, vomiting, malaise), and liver enzymes do not begin to rise until 24–36 hours post-ingestion (6). Elevated aspartate aminotranferase (AST) is the most sensitive marker of acetaminophen toxicity; the rise in AST precedes the hepatic dysfunction, and peak levels are reached at 72–96 hours. Evidence of hepatic injury becomes apparent 24–48 hours after ingestion, with steadily rising liver enzymes, and the appearance of jaundice and a coagulopathy. Peak hepatic injury occurs at 3–5 days after the toxic ingestion, and hepatic encephalopathy may be evident at this time, along with acute, oliguric renal failure (mechanism unclear), and lactic acidosis (from reduced hepatic clearance) (3). Death from hepatic injury usually occurs 3–5 days post-ingestion. Patients who survive often recover completely, although recovery can be prolonged.

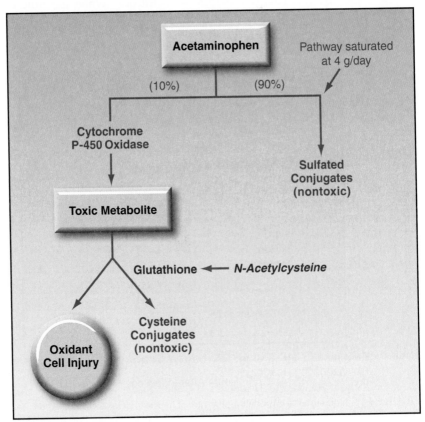

FIGURE 54.2 The hepatic metabolism of acetaminophen. See text for explanation.

Risk Assessment

In many cases of acetaminophen overdose, the initial encounter with the patient occurs within 24 hours after drug ingestion, when there are no manifestations of hepatic injury. The principal task at this time is to determine the risk of hepatocellular injury, and this involves two considerations: the time elapsed from the toxic ingestion, and the plasma level of acetaminophen. The ingested dose is not used to determine hepatotoxic risk because it is not possible to determine if the patient's recollection of the ingested dose is accurate. In addition, the toxic dose of acetaminophen can vary in individual patients.

Plasma Drug Levels

Plasma acetaminophen levels obtained from 4–24 hours after drug ingestion can be used to predict the risk of hepatotoxicity using the nomogram in Figure 54.3 (7). If the plasma level is in the high-risk region of the nomogram, the risk of developing hepatotoxicity is 60% or higher, and antidote therapy is warranted. The risk of hepatotoxicity is only 1–3% in the low-risk region of the nomogram, and this does not warrant antidote therapy (7). This nomogram is useful only when the time of drug ingestion can be identified, and when the plasma drug level can be measured between 4 and 24 hours post-ingestion.

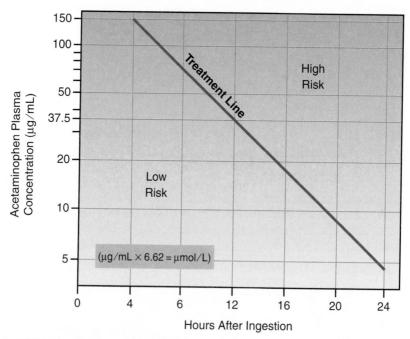

FIGURE 54.3 Nomogram for predicting the risk of hepatotoxicity according to the plasma acetaminophen level between 4 and 24 hours after ingestion. A plasma level that falls on, or above, the treatment line is an indication to begin antidotal therapy with N-acetylcysteine. Nomogram redrawn from Reference 7.

N-Acetylcysteine

Glutathione does not readily cross cell membranes, so exogenous glutathione is not a viable treatment option for acetaminophen hepatotoxicity. N-acetylcysteine (NAC) is a glutathione analogue that readily crosses cross cell membranes, and can serve as an intracellular glutathione surrogate (see Figure 54.2) (8). The cysteine residue in NAC contains a sulfhydryl group (SH), which is capable of reducing (and inactivating) the toxic acetaminophen metabolite.

Timing

NAC is most effective when therapy is started within 8 hours after ingestion; in this situation, NAC reduces the risk of hepatotoxicity to < 5% (3). NAC is less protective after 10 hours have elapsed, but some protection is provided for 24 hours after drug ingestion (6,9). NAC can also have beneficial effects after the onset of acetaminophen hepatotoxicity (3,10). Therefore, evidence of hepatotoxicity after 24 hours post-ingestion is an indication to begin NAC therapy (3).

Treatment Regimens

NAC can be given intravenously or orally using the dosing regimens shown in Table 54.1. Despite significant differences in total NAC dose and duration of therapy, the two dosing regimens are considered equally effective (13,14). The intravenous route is preferred because it is the most reliable mode of drug delivery, and is not as disagreeable as oral ingestion of NAC (see "Adverse Reactions").

EXTENDED TREATMENT: The standard duration of treatment is 21 hours for the IV regimen, and 72 hours for the oral regimen. However, because NAC can hasten the resolution of acetaminophen-induced liver injury (3), *treatment with NAC should be continued beyond the normal course of therapy if there is evidence of continued liver injury* (3). For the IV regimen, therapy is continued using the recommendations for the last 16 hours of the regimen. NAC can be discontinued when ALT levels have peaked and are improving, and when the INR is < 1.3 (3).

Adverse Reactions

Intravenous NAC can cause anaphylactoid reactions, and fatal reactions have been reported in asthmatics (15). Oral NAC has a very disagreeable taste (because of the sulfur content), and often causes nausea and vomiting. The oral NAC regimen produces diarrhea in about 50% of patients, but this usually resolves with continued therapy (16).

Activated Charcoal

Acetaminophen is rapidly absorbed from the GI tract, and activated charcoal (1 g/kg body weight) is recommended only if given within the first 4 hours after drug ingestion (17). However, following massive drug ingestions, charcoal can provide a benefit when given as late as 16 hours after drug ingestion (3). Activated charcoal does not curb the efficacy of oral NAC (3).

Table 54.1	Treatment of Acetaminophen Overdose with N-Acetylcysteine (NAC)

Intravenous Regimen:

Use 20% NAC (200 mg/mL) for each of the doses below and infuse in sequence.

1. 150 mg/kg in 200 mL D_5W over 60 min
2. 50 mg/kg in 500 mL D_5W over 4 hrs
3. 100 mg/kg in 1,000 mL D_5W over 16 hrs

Total dose: 300 mg/kg over 21 hrs

Oral Regimen:

Use 10% NAC (100 mg/mL) and dilute 2:1 in water or juice to make a 5% solution (50 mg/mL).

Initial dose: 140 mg/kg

Maintenance dosage: 70 mg/kg every 4 hrs for 17 doses

Total dose: 1,330 mg/kg over 72 hrs

From References 11 and 12.

BENZODIAZEPINES

Benzodiazepines are second only to opiates as the drugs most frequently involved in medication-related deaths (2). However, benzodiazepines are rarely fatal when ingested alone (18), and other respiratory depressant drugs (e.g., opiates) are almost always involved in benzodiazepine-related fatalities (2).

Clinical Features

Because overdoses involving benzodiazepines also involve other drugs, the clinical presentation can vary (according to the drugs ingested). Pure benzodiazepine overdoses produce deep sedation, but rarely result in coma (18). Respiratory depression (2–12% of cases), bradycardia (1–2% of cases) and hypotension (5–7% of cases) are also uncommon (18). Benzodiazepine intoxication can also produce an agitated confusional state (with hallucinations) that could be mistaken for alcohol withdrawal (18).

Involvement of benzodiazepines in an apparent overdose can be difficult to establish because there are no serum assays for benzodiazepines, and qualitative tests for benzodiazepines in urine are unreliable because of a limited spectrum of detection (19). Benzodiazepine involvement is usually based on the clinical history.

Management

The management of benzodiazepine overdose involves general supportive care, although an antidote is available.

Flumazenil

Flumazenil is a benzodiazepine antagonist that binds to benzodiazepine receptors, but does not exert any agonist actions (20). It is effective in reversing benzodiazepine-induced sedation, but is inconsistent in reversing benzodiazepine-induced respiratory depression (21).

DOSING REGIMEN: Flumazenil is given as an intravenous bolus. The initial dose is 0.2 mg, and this can be repeated at 1–6 minute intervals, if necessary, to a cumulative dose of 1 mg. The response is rapid, with onset in 1–2 minutes, and peak effect at 6–10 minutes (22). The effect lasts about one hour. Since flumazenil has a shorter duration of action than the benzodiazepines, sedation can return after 30–60 minutes. To reduce the risk of re-sedation, the initial bolus dose of flumazenil is often followed by a continuous infusion at 0.3–0.4 mg/hr (23).

ADVERSE REACTIONS: Flumazenil is safe to use in most patients. It can precipitate a benzodiazepine withdrawal syndrome in patients with a long-standing history of benzodiazepine use, but this is uncommon (24). Flumazenil can also precipitate seizures (a) in patients receiving benzodiazepines for seizure control, and (b) in mixed overdoses involving tricyclic antidepressants (25).

CLINICAL USE: Despite its effectiveness in reversing benzodiazepine-induced sedation, flumazenil is not a popular antidote. This is partly due to concerns about the risk of benzodiazepine withdrawal or seizures, and is partly due to the fact that benzodiazepine overdoses are rarely life-threatening.

β-RECEPTOR ANTAGONISTS

Intentional β-blocker overdoses are uncommon, but can be life-threatening. An effective antidote is available, if needed.

Toxic Manifestations

The typical manifestations of β-blocker overdose are *bradycardia* and *hypotension* (26). The bradycardia is usually sinus in origin, and is well tolerated. The hypotension can be due to peripheral vasodilatation (renin blockade), or a decrease in cardiac output, (β_1-receptor blockade). Hypotension that is sudden in onset is usually a reflection of a decrease in cardiac output and is an ominous sign.

Membrane-Stabilizing Effect

Excessive doses of β-blockers can exert a membrane-stabilizing effect that is independent of the β-receptor blockade. The principal consequence of this membrane-stabilizing effect is prolonged atrioventricular (AV) conduction, which can progress to complete heart block (27).

Neurotoxicity

Most β-blockers are lipophilic, and have a tendency to accumulate in lipid-rich tissues like the central nervous system. As a result, β-blocker overdose is often accompanied by lethargy, *depressed consciousness,* and *generalized seizures.* The latter manifestation is more prevalent than suspected, and has been reported in 60% of overdoses with propranolol (28). Like the prolonged AV conduction, the neurological manifestations are not the result of β-receptor blockade, and may be related to the membrane-stabilizing effect.

Glucagon

Glucagon is a regulatory hormone that acts in opposition to insulin by stimulating glycogen breakdown to raise blood glucose levels. In a seemingly unrelated role, glucagon antagonizes the cardiac depression produced by β-receptor antagonists.

Mechanism of Action

The illustration in Figure 54.4 shows how glucagon can correct the cardiac depression caused by β-blockers and calcium channel blockers. The glucagon receptor and β-receptor are linked to the adenyl cyclase enzyme on the inner surface of the cell membrane. Activation of each receptor-enzyme complex results in the hydrolysis of adenosine triphosphate (ATP) and the formation of cyclic adenosine monophosphate (cyclic AMP). The cyclic AMP then activates a protein kinase that promotes the inward movement of calcium through the cell membrane. The influx of calcium promotes interactions between contractile proteins to enhance the strength of cardiac contraction.

This sequence of reactions just described is responsible for the positive inotropic and chronotropic effects of β-receptor stimulation. Since the same reactions occur with activation of the glucagon receptor, glucagon has positive inotropic and chronotropic effects that are equivalent to β-receptor agonists. More importantly, the parallel orientation of the gluca-gon receptor and β-receptor allows glucagon to retain its cardiostimulatory effects when β-receptors are quiescent. This is the basis for gluca-gon's role as an antidote for β-blocker toxicity.

Clinical Use

Glucagon is indicated for the treatment of hypotension and *symptomatic* bradycardia associated with toxic exposure to β-blockers. When used in the appropriate doses, glucagon will elicit a favorable response in 90% of patients (29). Glucagon is *not* indicated for reversing the prolonged AV conduction or neurological abnormalities in β-blocker overdoses because these effects are not mediated by β-receptor blockade.

CALCIUM ANTAGONIST TOXICITY: Glucagon is also capable of antagonizing the effects of calcium channel blockers (30), as illustrated in Figure 54.4. However, glucagon is less effective in reversing the cardiac depression precipitated by calcium channel blocker overdoses. This is not unexpected, because glucagon and calcium blockers act at different sites in the pathways that modulate cardiac contractile strength.

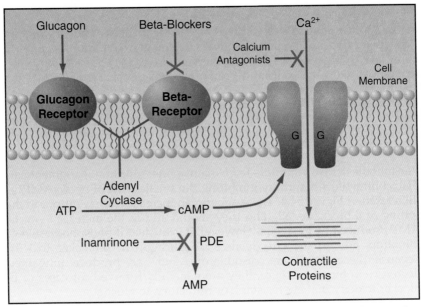

FIGURE 54.4 Mechanisms of drug-induced alterations in cardiac contractile strength. See text for explanation. Abbreviations: ATP=adenosine triphosphate; cAMP=cyclic adenosine monophosphate; PDE=phosphodiesterase; AMP=adenosine monophosphate.

Dosing Regimen

Dosing recommendations for glucagon are presented in Table 54.2. The effective dose of glucagon can vary in individual patients, but *a bolus dose of 3–5 mg IV should be effective in most adults* (28,29). The initial dose is 3 mg (or 0.05 mg/kg) as an IV bolus. The response to glucagon is usually evident within 3 minutes (30). If the response is not satisfactory, a second IV bolus dose of 5 mg (or 0.07 mg/kg) can be administered. The effects of glucagon can be short-lived (5 minutes), and so a favorable response should be followed by a continuous infusion (5 mg/hr). The chronotropic response to glucagon is optimal when the plasma ionized calcium is normal (31).

Table 54.2	Glucagon as an Antidote
Indications	**Dosing Regimen**
When the actions of β-receptor antagonists or calcium channel blockers result in: 1. Hypotension, or 2. Symptomatic Bradycardia	1. Start with 50 μg/kg (or 3 mg) as IV bolus. 2. If response is not satisfactory, give a second IV bolus of 70 μg/kg (or 5 mg). 3. Follow a satisfactory response with a continuous infusion at: 70 μg/kg/hr (or 5 mg/hr).

Adverse Effects

Nausea and vomiting are common at glucagon doses above 5 mg/hr. Mild hyperglycemia is common, and is the result of glucagon's actions to stimulate glycogenolysis. The insulin response to the hyperglycemia can drive potassium into cells and promote hypokalemia. Finally, glucagon stimulates catecholamine release from the adrenal medulla, and this can cause unwanted increases in blood pressure in patients with hypertension.

Phosphodiesterase Inhibitors

Phosphodiesterase inhibitors (e.g., inamrinone, milrinone) augment cardiac contractile strength by inhibiting the breakdown of cyclic AMP, as illustrated in Figure 54.4. These agents can increase cardiac output in the setting of β-blockade (32), and they should add to the increase in cyclic AMP produced by glucagon. However, it is unclear if phosphodiesterase inhibitors add to the effectiveness of glucagon in β-blocker toxicity. Because these drugs are vasodilators, and can produce unwanted decreases in blood pressure, they are generally reserved for cases of β-blocker toxicity that are resistant, or refractory, to glucagon.

OPIOIDS

Opiates are implicated in 75% of fatal drug overdoses in the United States (2a), and the problem is likely to grow rather than shrink. The adverse effects of opioids are described in Chapter 51; the following description focuses on the use of the narcotic antagonist, naloxone.

Clinical Features

The classic description of an opiate overdose is a patient who presents with stupor, pinpoint pupils, and slow breathing (bradypnea). However, these clinical findings are either absent or nonspecific, and it is not possible to identify an opiate overdose based on the clinical presentation or physical examination (33). The response to the narcotic antagonist, naloxone, is probably the most reliable method of identifying an opioid overdose.

Naloxone

Naloxone is a pure opioid antagonist; i.e., it binds to endogenous opioid receptors, but does not elicit any agonist responses. It is most effective in blocking mu receptors (primarily responsible for analgesia, euphoria, and respiratory depression) and less effective in blocking kappa receptors and delta receptors (32,33).

Dosing Regimen

Naloxone is usually given as an IV bolus, and the effect is apparent within 3 minutes. Alternate routes of delivery include intramuscular injection (onset in 15 minutes), intraosseous injection, intralingual injection, and endotracheal instillation (36). Reversing the sedative effects of opioids usually requires smaller doses of naloxone than reversing the respiratory depression.

DEPRESSED SENSORIUM: For patients with a depressed sensorium but no respiratory depression, the initial dose of naloxone should be *0.4 mg IV push*. This can be repeated in 2 minutes, if necessary. A total dose of 0.8 mg should be effective if the mental status changes are caused by an opioid derivative (24).

RESPIRATORY DEPRESSION: For patients who have evidence of respiratory depression (e.g., hypercapnia, respiratory rate < 12 breaths/min), the initial dose of naloxone should be *2 mg IV push*. If there is no response in 2–3 minutes, double the initial dose (i.e., give 4 mg IV bolus). If further doses are needed, each successive dose should be increased as shown in Table 54.3, until the dose reaches 15 mg (33). *Opioid overdose is unlikely if there is no response to a naloxone dose of 15 mg.*

The effects of naloxone last about 60–90 minutes, which is less than the duration of action of most opioids. Therefore, a favorable response to naloxone should be followed by repeat doses at one-hour intervals, or by a continuous infusion. For a continuous naloxone infusion, the hourly dose of naloxone should be two-thirds of the effective bolus dose (diluted in 250 or 500 mL of isotonic saline and infused over 6 hours) (37). To achieve steady-state drug levels in the early infusion period, a second bolus of naloxone (at one-half the original bolus dose) is given 30 minutes after the infusion is started. The duration of treatment varies (according to the drug and the dose ingested), but averages 10 hours (24).

Table 54.3	Naloxone Dosing Regimens
Depressed Sensorium	**Respiratory Depression**
1. Start with 0.4 mg IV bolus.	1. Start with 2 mg IV bolus.
2. If no response in 2–3 min, give another 0.4 mg IV bolus.	2. If no response in 2–3 min, give 4 mg IV bolus.
3. If no response in 2–3 min, give 2 mg IV bolus.	3. If no response in 2–3 min, give 10 mg IV bolus.
4. If no response in 2–3 min, STOP and reassess.	4. If no response in 2–3 min, give 15 mg IV bolus.
	5. If no response in 2–3 min, STOP and reassess.

Empiric Naloxone

Empiric therapy with naloxone (0.2–8 mg IV bolus) has been used in patients with altered mentation to identify occult cases of opioid overdose. However, this practice is effective in fewer than 5% of patients with altered mental status of unknown etiology (38). An alternative approach has been proposed where *empiric naloxone is indicated only for patients with pinpoint pupils and circumstantial evidence of opioid abuse* (e.g., needle tracks) (24,38). When naloxone is used in this manner, a favorable response (indicating an opioid overdose) is expected in about 90% of patients (38).

Adverse Reactions

Naloxone has few undesirable effects. The most common adverse reaction is the opioid withdrawal syndrome (anxiety, abdominal cramps, vomiting, and piloerection). There are case reports of acute pulmonary edema (most in the early postoperative period) and generalized seizures following naloxone administration (24), but these are rare occurrences.

SALICYLATES

Despite a steady decline in prevalence, salicylate intoxication is the 14th leading cause of drug-induced deaths in the United States (39).

Clinical Features

Ingestion of 10–30 grams of aspirin (150 mg/kg) can have fatal consequences. Once ingested, acetylsalicylic acid (aspirin) is promptly converted to *salicylic acid*, which is the active form of the drug. Salicylic acid is readily absorbed from the upper GI tract, and metabolism takes place in the liver. The hallmark of salicylate intoxication is the combination of a respiratory alkalosis and a metabolic acidosis.

Respiratory Alkalosis

Within hours after a toxic ingestion of aspirin, there is an increase in respiratory rate and tidal volume. This is the result of direct stimulation of brainstem respiratory neurons by salicylic acid, and the subsequent increase in minute ventilation results in a decrease in arterial PCO_2 (i.e., acute respiratory alkalosis).

Metabolic Acidosis

Salicylic acid is a weak acid that does not readily dissociate, and thus does not produce a metabolic acidosis. However, salicylic acid activates proteins in the mitochondria that uncouple oxidative phosphorylation, and this results in a marked increase in the anaerobic production of lactic acid, and this is the principal source of the metabolic acidosis in salicylate intoxication. The mixed metabolic acidosis-respiratory alkalosis produces an arterial blood gas with a low PCO_2, a low bicarbonate, and a normal pH (see Rule 3 on page 593). As the lactic acidosis progresses, the serum pH will eventually fall, which is a poor prognostic sign (40).

Other Features

Clinical features in the early stages of salicylate toxicity include nausea, vomiting, tinnitus, and agitation. Progression of the toxidrome is associated with neurologic changes (delirium, seizures, and progression to coma), fever (from the uncoupled oxidative phosphorylation), and acute respiratory distress syndrome (ARDS).

Diagnosis

The plasma salicylate level is used to confirm or exclude the diagnosis of salicylate toxicity. The therapeutic range of salicylates in plasma is 10–30 mg/L (0.7–2.2 mmol/L), and levels above 40 mg/L (2.9 mmol/L) are considered toxic (40). Plasma salicylate levels are usually elevated within 4–6 hours after a toxic ingestion.

Management

Management of salicylate toxicity includes general supportive care (i.e., fluids, vasopressors, and mechanical ventilation), if necessary. Multiple-dose activated charcoal is recommended, if it can be started within 2–3 hours of drug ingestion. The dosing regimen is 25 grams orally every 2 hours for 3 doses.

Alkalinization

Alkalinization of the urine to enhance salicylate excretion is the cornerstone of management for salicylate intoxication. Salicylic acid has a pK of 3 (the pK is the pH at which 50% of the acid is dissociated), which means that the acid will dissociate more readily as the pH rises. An alkaline pH in the urine will promote dissociation of salicylic acid in the renal tubules, and this essentially "traps" the salicylic acid in the renal tubular lumen, where it can be excreted in the urine. Bicarbonate infusions are used to raise the urine pH using the following regimen, which is summarized in Table 54.4.

Table 54.4	Protocol for Alkalinization of the Urine

1. Create a bicarbonate solution by adding 3 amps $NaHCO_3$ (44 mEq Na^+/amp).

2. Start with a bicarbonate loading dose of 1–2 mEq/kg.

3. Follow with infusion of the bicarbonate solution at 2–3 mL/kg/hr.

4. Maintain a urine output of 1–2 mL/kg/hr, and a urine pH of ≥7.5.

From References 40 and 41.

REGIMEN: Start IV bicarbonate therapy with 1–2 mEq/kg as an IV bolus, and follow with a continuous bicarbonate infusion. To create the bicarbonate infusate, add 3 ampules of 40% sodium bicarbonate (43 mEq/amp) to 1 liter of D_5W (129 mEq/L), and infuse this solution at 2–3 mL/kg/hr (40). The urine pH should be maintained at ≥7.5 (41). Treatment continues until the plasma salicylate levels fall below the toxic range.

HYPOKALEMIA: Bicarbonate infusions will lower the serum potassium (intracellular shift), and hypokalemia hampers the ability to alkalinize the urine. This is explained by the K^+-H^+ exchanger in the distal renal tubules, which releases H^+ into the tubular fluid as K^+ is reabsorbed. Since K^+ reabsorption is increased in the setting of hypokalemia, the extra H^+ released into the tubular fluid will hamper attempts to alkalinize the urine. Potassium should be added to the bicarbonate solution (40 mEq/L) to reduce the risk of hypokalemia.

Hemodialysis

Hemodialysis is the most effective method of clearing salicylates from the body (42). The indications for hemodialysis include a serum salicylate level > 100 mg/L, the presence of renal failure or ARDS, or progression of the toxidrome despite alkalinization therapy (39).

A FINAL WORD

Regulating Acetaminophen

If any over-the-counter drug deserves to be regulated, it's acetaminophen. Not because it is the leading cause of acute liver failure in the United States (which should be enough of a reason), but because *half* of the overdoses are unintentional, indicating a general lack of awareness of the toxic potential of acetaminophen (which can be fatal). The FDA has called for stronger warnings on drug packaging, but who reads that small print? Requiring a prescription that specifies how the drug should be used is the best way to ensure that acetaminophen is used safely in the general population.

Acetaminophen gained its popularity in the 1970s because of concerns about the toxicity of aspirin, and it looks like we moved from the frying pan into the fire.

REFERENCES

Introduction

1. Centers for Disease Control and Prevention. Vital signs: overdoses of pre-scribed opioid pain relievers—United States, 1999–2008. MMWR 2011; 60:1487–1492.

2. Centers for Disease Control and Prevention. National Vital Statistics System. 2010 Multiple Cause of Death File. Hyattsville, MD: US Department of Health and Human Services, Centers for Disease Control and Prevention; 2012.

2a. Jones CM, Mack KA, Paulozzi LJ. Pharmaceutical overdose deaths, United States, 2010. JAMA 2013; 309:657–659.

Acetaminophen

3. Hodgman M, Garrard AR. A review of acetaminophen poisoning. Crit Care Clin 2012; 28:499–516.

4. Larson AM, Polson J, Fontana RJ, et al. Acetaminophen-induced acute liver failure: results of a United States multicenter, prospective study. Hepatology 2005; 42:1364–1372.

5. Kuehn B. FDA focuses on drugs and liver damage. JAMA 2009; 302:369–370.

6. Hendrickson RG, Bizovi KE. Acetaminophen. In: Flomenbaum NE, et al., eds. Goldfrank's Toxicologic Emergencies. 8th ed. New York: McGraw-Hill, 2006; 523–543.

7. Rumack BH. Acetaminophen hepatotoxicity: the first 35 years. J Toxicol Clin Toxicol 2002; 40:3–20.

N-Acetylcysteine

8. Holdiness MR. Clinical pharmacokinetics of N-acetylcysteine. Clin Pharmacokinet 1991; 20:123–134.

9. Rumack BH, Peterson RC, Koch GG, et al. Acetaminophen overdose. 662 cases with evaluation of oral acetylcysteine treatment. Arch Int Med 1981; 141:380–385.

10. Harrison PM, Keays R, Bray GP, et al. Improved outcome of paracetamol-induced fulminant hepatic failure by late administration of acetylcysteine. Lancet 1990; 335:1572–1573.

11. Cumberland Pharmaceuticals. Acetadote Package Insert. 2006.

12. Smilkstein MJ, Knapp GL, Kulig KW, et al. Efficacy of oral N-acetylcysteine in the treatment of acetaminophen overdose. Analysis of the national multicenter study (1976 to 1985). N Engl J Med 1988; 319:1557–1562.

13. Howland MA. N-Acetylcysteine. In: Flomenbaum NE, et al., eds. Goldfrank's Toxicologic Emergencies. 8th ed. New York: McGraw-Hill, 2006; 544–549.

14. Buckley NA, Whyte IM, O'Connell DL, et al. Oral or intravenous N-acetylcysteine: which is the treatment of choice for acetaminophen (paracetamol) poisoning? J Toxicol Clin Toxicol 1999; 37:759–767.

15. Appelboam AV, Dargan PI, Knighton J. Fatal anaphylactoid reaction to N-acetylcysteine: caution in patients with asthma. Emerg Med J 2002; 19:594–595.

16. Miller LF, Rumack BH. Clinical safety of high oral doses of acetylcysteine. Semin Oncol 1983; 10:76–85.

17. Spiller HA, Krenzelok EP, Grande GA, et al. A prospective evaluation of the effect of activated charcoal before oral N-acetylcysteine in acetaminophen overdose. Ann Emerg Med 1994; 23:519–523.

Benzodiazepines

18. Gaudreault P, Guay J, Thivierge RL, Verdy I. Benzodiazepine poisoning. Drug Saf 1991; 6:247–265.

19. Wu AH, McCay C, Broussard LA, et al. National Academy of Clinical Biochemistry laboratory medicine practice guidelines: Recommendations for the use of laboratory tests to support poisoned patients who present to the emergency department. Clin Chem 2003; 49:357–379.

Flumazenil

20. Howland MA. Flumazenil. In: Flomenbaum NE, et al., eds. Goldfrank's Toxicologic Emergencies. 8th ed. New York: McGraw-Hill, 2006; 1112–1117.

21. Shalansky SJ, Naumann TL, Englander FA. Effect of flumazenil on benzodiazepine-induced respiratory depression. Clin Pharm 1993; 12:483–487.

22. Roche Laboratories. Romazicon (flumazenil) package insert. 2004.

23. Bodenham A, Park GR. Reversal of prolonged sedation using flumazenil in critically ill patients. Anaesthesia 1989; 44:603–605.

24. Doyon S, Roberts JR. Reappraisal of the "coma cocktail". Dextrose, flumazenil, naloxone, and thiamine. Emerg Med Clin North Am 1994; 12:301–316.

25. Haverkos GP, DiSalvo RP, Imhoff TE. Fatal seizures after flumazenil administration in a patient with mixed overdose. Ann Pharmacother 1994; 28:1347–1349.

ß-Receptor Antagonists

26. Newton CR, Delgado JH, Gomez HF. Calcium and beta receptor antagonist overdose: a review and update of pharmacological principles and management. Semin Respir Crit Care Med 2002; 23:19–25.

27. Henry JA, Cassidy SL. Membrane stabilising activity: a major cause of fatal poisoning. Lancet 1986; 1:1414–1417.

28. Weinstein RS. Recognition and management of poisoning with beta-adrenergic blocking agents. Ann Emerg Med 1984; 13:1123–1131.

29. Kerns W, 2nd, Kline J, Ford MD. Beta-blocker and calcium channel blocker toxicity. Emerg Med Clin North Am 1994; 12:365–390.

Glucagon

30. Howland MA. Glucagon. In: Flomenbaum NE, et al., eds. Goldfrank's Toxicologic Emergencies. 8th ed. New York: McGraw-Hill, 2006; 942–945.

31. Chernow B, Zaloga GP, Malcolm D, et al. Glucagon's chronotropic action is calcium dependent. J Pharmacol Exp Ther 1987; 241:833–837.

32. Travill CM, Pugh S, Noblr MI. The inotropic and hemodynamic effects of intravenous milrinone when reflex adrenergic stimulation is suppressed by beta adrenergic blockade. Clin Ther 1994; 16:783–792.

Opioids and Naloxone

33. Boyer EW. Management of opioid analgesic overdose. N Engl J Med 2012; 367:146–155.

34. Handal KA, Schauben JL, Salamone FR. Naloxone. Ann Emerg Med 1983; 12:438–445.

35. Howland MA. Opioid Antagonists. In: Flomenbaum NE, et al., eds. Goldfrank's Toxicologic Emergencies. 8th ed. New York: McGraw-Hill, 2006; 614–619.

36. Naloxone hydrochloride. In: McEvoy GK ed. AHFS Drug Information, 2012. Bethesda: American Society of Hospital Systems Pharmacists, 2012:2236–2239.

37. Goldfrank L, Weisman RS, Errick JK, et al. A dosing nomogram for continuous infusion intravenous naloxone. Ann Emerg Med 1986; 15:566–570.

38. Hoffman JR, Schriger DL, Luo JS. The empiric use of naloxone in patients with altered mental status: a reappraisal. Ann Emerg Med 1991; 20:246–252.

Salicylates

39. Bronstein AC, Spyker DA, Cantilena LR, et al. 2011 Annual Report of the American Association of Poison Control Centers' National Poison Data System (NPDS):29th Annual Report. Clin Toxicol 2012; 50:911–1164.

40. O'Malley GF. Emergency department management of the salicylate-poisoned patient. Emerg Med Clin N Am 2007; 25:333–346.

41. Proudfoot AT, Krenzelok EP, Vale JA. Position paper on urine alkalinization. J Toxicol Clin Toxicol 2004; 42:1–26.

42. Fertel BS, Nelson LS, Goldfarb DS. The underutilization of hemodialysis in patients with salicylate poisoning. Kidney Int 2009; 75:1349–1353.

Chapter 55

NONPHARMACEUTICAL TOXIDROMES

In clinical matters, ignorance can be dangerous,
but ignorance of ignorance can be fatal.

P.L.M.

This chapter describes toxic syndromes that are not the result of medications, and includes sections on carbon monoxide, cyanide, and the toxic alcohols (methanol and ethylene glycol). While these toxidromes will not be encountered often, they can be lethal if not recognized.

CARBON MONOXIDE

Carbon monoxide (CO) is a gaseous product of incomplete combustion involving organic (carbon-based) matter, and is one oxidation reaction shy of carbon dioxide: i.e., $2CO + O_2 \rightarrow 2 CO_2$. The principal source of CO poisoning is smoke inhalation during structural fires. The exhaust from automobile engines was once a major source of CO, but the catalytic converters that are mandated for all automobiles (and convert CO to CO_2) have reduced CO emissions by more than 95%.

Pathophysiology

Carbon monoxide binds to the heme moieties in hemoglobin (at the same site that binds oxygen) to produce *carboxyhemoglobin* (COHb). The affinity of CO for binding to hemoglobin is 200–300 times greater than the affinity of O_2, and CO pressures of only 0.4 mm Hg can fully saturate hemoglobin (2). The effects of COHb on systemic oxygenation are demonstrated in Figure 55.1. The curves in this graph show the relationship between oxygen tension (PO_2) and oxygen content when hemoglobin is normal (upper curve), and when COHb makes up 50% of the hemoglobin molecules (lower curve) (3). The arterial O_2 content (point A) decreases in proportion to the increase in COHb, reflecting the ability of CO to block O_2 binding to hemoglobin. The venous point (point V) on

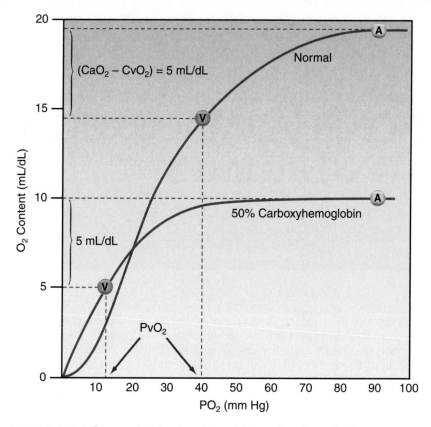

FIGURE 55.1 Influence of 50% carboxyhemoglobin on the relationship between oxygen tension (PO_2) and oxygen content.

both curves was identified by assuming a normal arteriovenous O_2 content difference ($CaO_2 - CvO_2 = 5$ mL/dL) for both curves. The venous PO_2 (PvO_2) is a close approximation of tissue PO_2, and it is much lower when COHb is present. This provides indirect evidence that CO poisoning can impair tissue oxygenation.

Other Effects

Carbon monoxide has toxic effects that are unrelated to COHb (4). These effects include: (a) inhibition of cytochrome oxidase, which impairs the ability to generate ATP from oxidative metabolism, (b) release of nitric oxide from platelets, which promotes the formation of *peroxynitrite*, a powerful oxidant capable of widespread cell injury, and (c) activation of neutrophils, which is an additional source of oxidant injury (see Figure 14.1). These effects may play an important role in CO poisoning, because there is a poor correlation between COHb levels and the severity of carbon monoxide poisoning (1,4).

Clinical Features

The following statements summarize the clinical manifestations of CO poisoning, which are variable and nonspecific.

1. There is no correlation between the clinical manifestations of CO poisoning and COHb levels in blood (1,4).

2. Headache (usually frontal) and dizziness are the earliest and most common complaints in CO poisoning (reported in 85% and 90% of patients, respectively) (4).

3. Progressive exposure to CO can produce ataxia, confusion, delirium, generalized seizures, and coma (4).

4. Cardiac effects of CO poisoning include elevated biomarkers with normal coronary angiography, and transient LV systolic dysfunction (5).

5. Advanced cases of CO poisoning can be accompanied by rhabdomyolysis, lactic acidosis, and acute respiratory distress syndrome (ARDS) (4).

6. The "cherry red" skin color in classic descriptions of CO poisoning (because COHb is a brighter shade of red than hemoglobin) is a rare finding (1).

Delayed Neurologic Sequelae

Acute CO intoxication can be followed by the emergence (within about one year) of a variety neurologic abnormalities, mostly involving cognitive deficits (from mild confusion to severe dementia) and parkinsonism (1,4,6). These occur most frequently following prolonged (≥ 24 hrs) exposure to CO, and in patients with loss of consciousness or COHb levels above 25% (1). The mechanism for these delayed reactions has not been identified.

Diagnosis

The diagnosis of CO poisoning is not possible based on signs and symptoms alone. The diagnosis is suspected when the presenting signs and symptoms are consistent with CO poisoning, and the clinical history identifies a likely source of CO exposure (e.g., a house fire). The diagnosis is confirmed by an elevated COHb level in blood.

Carboxyhemoglobin

The measurement of hemoglobin in its different forms (oxygenated and deoxygenated hemoglobin, methemoglobin, and carboxyhemoglobin) is based on light absorption; this method is known as *oximetry*, and is described in Chapter 21. The following statements summarize the use of oximetry to measure COHb levels in blood.

1. Pulse oximetry is NOT reliable for the detection of COHb. Pulse oximeters use 2 wavelengths of light to measure oxygenated and deoxygenated hemoglobin in blood. Light absorbance at one of the wavelengths (660 nm) is very similar for oxygenated hemoglobin

and COHb (see Figure 21.1 on page 410), so COHb is measured as oxygenated hemoglobin by pulse oximeters, and this results in spuriously high readings for O_2 saturation (1).

2. The measurement of COHb requires an 8-wavelength oximeter (known as a CO-oximeter) that is available in most clinical laboratories. This device measures the relative abundance of all 4 forms of hemoglobin in blood.

COHb levels are negligible (< 1%) in healthy nonsmokers, but smokers have COHb levels of 3–5% or even higher (1). The threshold for elevated COHb levels is 3–4% for nonsmokers, and 10% for smokers (1).

Treatment

The treatment for CO poisoning is inhalation of 100% oxygen. The elimination half-life of COHb is 320 minutes while breathing room air, and 74 minutes while breathing 100% oxygen (1), so only a few hours of breathing pure oxygen is needed to return COHb levels to normal.

Hyperbaric Oxygen

Hyperbaric oxygen has been advocated as a means of reducing the delayed neurologic sequelae in CO poisoning, but evidence of benefit has not been convincing (7).

Cyanide

House fires generate cyanide as well as carbon monoxide, and the possibility of cyanide poisoning must be considered in all patients with CO poisoning from a house fire. When smoke inhalation from a house fire is accompanied by a severe metabolic acidosis (pH < 7.2) or a markedly elevated serum lactate level (≥ 10 mmol/L), empiric treatment for cyanide poisoning is recommended (1). See the next section for the treatment of cyanide poisoning.

CYANIDE

Cyanide is a lethal toxin with a nefarious history. The Nazis used hydrogen cyanide gas (Zyklon-B) for mass murder in the 1940s, and in 1978, cyanide-laced fruit drinks were used for mass murder/suicide by Jim Jones and his followers. The principal source of cyanide poisoning is inhalation of hydrogen cyanide gas during domestic fires (8,9). Infusion of the vasodilator, *sodium nitroprusside*, is an additional source of cyanide toxicity in ICU patients (see Figure 53.4).

Pathophysiology

Cyanide ions have a high affinity for metalloproteins, including the oxidized iron (Fe^{3+}) in cytochrome oxidase and methemoglobin, and the cobalt in hydroxocobalamin (a precursor of vitamin B_{12}). Cytochrome oxidase is situated at the end of the electron-transport chain in mitochondria, and is the site where the electrons collected during ATP production are used to reduce oxygen to water (thereby clearing the way for continued ATP production). Cyanide-induced inhibition of cytochrome oxidase halts the process of oxidative metabolism in mitochondria. This halts the uptake of pyruvate into mitochondria, and results in excess production of lactic acid and a progressive metabolic (lactic) acidosis. The defect in cellular energy production is fatal if not corrected.

Cyanide Clearance

There are two endogenous mechanisms for clearing cyanide from the body, and these are shown in Figure 53.4 (see page 953). The principal mechanism is the transfer of sulfur from thiosulfate (S_2O_3) to cyanide, which forms thiocyanate (SCN). This is called a *transulfuration* reaction.

$$S_2O_3 + CN \rightarrow SCN + SO_3 \qquad (55.1)$$

Thiocyanate is then cleared by the kidneys. Thiocyanate can accumulate in patients with renal failure, and can cause an acute psychosis (10).

The second (minor) mechanism for cyanide clearance is the reaction of cyanide with methemoglobin to form cyanomethemoglobin; i.e.,

$$Hb\text{-}Fe^{3+} + CN \rightarrow Hb\text{-}Fe^{2+} - CN \qquad (55.2)$$

The hemoglobin-bound cyanide is eventually cleared via transulfuration. These two clearance mechanisms are easily overwhelmed, especially in the setting of thiosulfate deficiency (e.g., in smokers).

Clinical Features

Early signs of cyanide poisoning include agitation, tachycardia, and tachypnea, representing the compensatory stage of metabolic acidosis. Progressive cyanide accumulation eventually results in loss of consciousness, bradycardia, hypotension, and cardiac arrest. Plasma lactate levels are typically very high (> 10 mmol/L), and venous blood can look "arterialized" because of the marked decrease in tissue O_2 utilization. Progression is rapid after smoke inhalation, and the time from onset of symptoms to cardiac arrest can be less than 5 minutes (8).

Diagnosis

Cyanide poisoning is a clinical diagnosis. Whole blood cyanide levels can be used for documentation, but results are not immediately available, and cyanide antidotes must be given quickly for optimal results. The clinical diagnosis of cyanide poisoning is particularly challenging in victims of smoke inhalation, because many of the clinical features of cyanide poisoning are indistinguishable from carbon monoxide (CO) poisoning. As a general rule of thumb, *severe metabolic (lactic) acidosis and hemodynamic instability are the clinical features that distinguish cyanide poisoning from CO poisoning in victims of smoke inhalation* (8,9).

Treatment

Antidote therapy should begin immediately after cyanide poisoning is first suspected. The antidotes for cyanide poisoning are presented in Table 55.1.

Hydroxocobalamin

The antidote of choice for cyanide poisoning is *hydroxocobalamin*, a cobalt-containing precursor of vitamin B_{12} that combines with cyanide to form cyanocobalamin, which is then excreted in the urine. The recommended dose is *5 grams, as an IV bolus*. A second dose of 5 grams is recommended for patients with cardiac arrest (8). Hydroxocobalamin is relatively safe to use, but urine and other body fluids can have a reddish color for a few days.

Table 55.1	Antidotes for Cyanide Poisoning	
Agent	**Dosing Regimens and Comments**	
Hydroxocobalamin	Dosing:	5 grams as IV bolus. Give 10 g for cardiac arrest.
	Comment:	The antidote of choice for cyanide poisoning. May cause reddish color in urine for a few days.
Sodium Thiosulfate (25%)	Dosing:	50 mL (12.5 g) as IV bolus.
	Comment:	Used in combination with hydroxocobalamin. Avoid, if possible, in patients with renal failure.
Amyl Nitrate Inhalant	Dosing:	Inhale for 30 sec. each min, for up to 5 min.
	Comment:	Used only for temporary relief when IV access is not available. Contraindicated in smoke inhalation.

From References 8, 9.

Sodium Thiosulfate

Sodium thiosulfate converts cyanide to thiocyanate (see Equation 55.1), and is used in combination with hydroxocobalamin. The recommended dose is *12.5 grams as an IV bolus*. Since thiocyanate can accumulate in renal failure and cause an acute psychosis (10), *thiosulfate should not be used in patients with renal failure*. If thiosulfate is given before evidence of renal failure is available, watch for signs of thiocyanate toxicity (which is treated with hemodialysis).

Nitrates

Nitrates promote cyanide clearance by promoting the formation of methemoglobin. However, nitrates have undesirable side effects, and *are contraindicated in smoke inhalation* (because they cause a leftward shift in the oxyhemoglobin dissociation curve, and can aggravate the similar effect of carbon monoxide). The only role for nitrates in cyanide poisoning is the use of inhaled amyl nitrate as a temporary measure when IV access is not available.

Cyanide Antidote Kits

There are specialized antidote kits for cyanide poisoning (e.g., Akorn Cyanide Antidote Kit) that contain amyl nitrate for inhalation, sodium nitrite (300 mg in 10 mL) for IV injection, and sodium thiosulfate (12.5 g in 50 mL) for IV injection. These kits can be used as a source of thiosulfate, but they *do not contain hydroxocobalamin* (at least at the present time).

TOXIC ALCOHOLS

Ethylene glycol and methanol are common components of household, automotive, and industrial products, and they both produce toxidromes characterized by a metabolic acidosis. They are known as *toxic alcohols* (10), which is a misnomer, because it implies that ethanol is non-toxic. Toxic alcohols are the 12th leading source of toxic exposures in the United States (11).

Ethylene Glycol

Ethylene glycol is the main ingredient in many automotive antifreeze products. It has a sweet, agreeable taste, which makes it a popular method of attempted suicide.

Pathophysiology

Ethylene glycol is readily absorbed from the GI tract, and 80% of the ingested dose is metabolized in the liver. As shown in Figure 55.2, the metabolism of ethylene glycol involves the formation of a series of acids, with the participation of alcohol dehydrogenase and lactate dehydrogenase enzymes, and ends with the formation of oxalic acid (12). Each of the intermediate reactions involves the conversion of NAD to NADH, which promotes the conversion of pyruvate to lactate. As a result, serum lactate levels are also elevated in ethylene glycol poisoning (12). Each of the acid intermediates in ethylene glycol metabolism is a strong acid that readily dissociates, and can contribute to a metabolic acidosis. The oxalic acid also combines with calcium to form insoluble calcium oxalate crystals that precipitate in several tissues, and are particularly prominent in the renal tubules. These crystals can be a source of renal tubular injury.

Clinical Features

Early signs of ethylene glycol intoxication include nausea, vomiting, and apparent inebriation (altered mental status, slurred speech, and ataxia). Because ethylene glycol is odorless, there is no odor of alcohol on the breath. Severe cases are accompanied by depressed consciousness, coma, generalized seizures, renal failure, pulmonary edema, and cardiovascular collapse (12). Renal failure can be a late finding (24 hours after ingestion).

Laboratory studies show a metabolic acidosis with an elevated anion gap

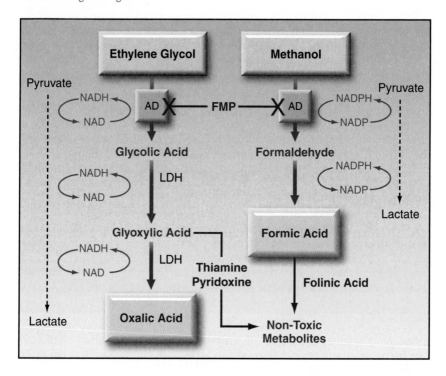

FIGURE 55.2 The metabolism of ethylene glycol and methanol in the liver. AD = alcohol dehydrogenase; LDH = lactate dehydrogenase; FMP = fomepizole.

and an elevated osmolal gap (see page 656 for a description of the osmolal gap). Serum lactate levels can be elevated (usually 5–6 mEq/L). A plasma assay for ethylene glycol is available, and a level > 20 mg/dL is considered toxic, but the results are not immediately available, and are not used in the decision to initiate therapy (12). (Plasma levels can be used to guide decisions about discontinuing therapy, as described later.)

CRYSTALLURIA: Calcium oxalate crystals can be visualized in the urine in about 50% of cases of ethylene glycol poisoning (14). The presence of calcium oxalate crystals is not specific for ethylene glycol poisoning, but *the shape of the crystals is more specific*; i.e., thin, monohydrate crystals, like the ones shown in Figure 55.3, are more characteristic of ethylene glycol poisoning than the box-shaped dihydrate crystals (12). Most hospital laboratories do not routinely inspect urine for crystals, so make sure to request a search for crystalluria when ethylene glycol toxicity is supected.

Treatment

The management of ethylene glycol poisoning involves measures to alter the metabolism of ethylene glycol, along with hemodialysis, if necessary.

FOMEPIZOLE: Fomepizole inhibits alcohol dehydrogenase, the enzyme involved in the initial step of ethylene glycol metabolism (see Figure

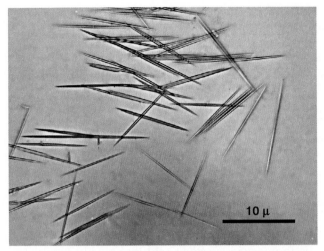

10 μ

FIGURE 55.3 Microscopic appearance of calcium oxalate monohydrate crystals. The presence of these thin, needle-shaped crystals in the urine is highly suggestive of ethylene glycol poisoning.

55.2). The recommended dosing regimen for both ethylene glycol and methanol poisoning is shown in Table 55.2. The best results are obtained if therapy begins within 4 hours of ingestion. Fomepizole should be continued until the metabolic acidosis has resolved, and the plasma level of ethylene glycol is in the non-toxic range (12).

Table 55.2	Dosing Regimen for Fomepizole

1. Start with an IV loading dose of 15 mg/kg.

2. Follow with a dose of 10 mg/kg IV every 12 hrs for 4 doses.

3. Then increase the dose to 15 mg/kg IV every 12 hrs[†], and continue until the following end-points are reached:

    (a) the plasma toxin level is <20 mg/dL,

    (b) the plasma pH is normal,

    (c) the patient is asymptomatic.

4. If more than one hemodialysis session is required, change the dose to 15 mg/kg IV every 4 hrs, until dialysis is no longer necessary.

[†]The increased dose represents compensation for a self-induced increase in metabolism.
From Reference 12.

HEMODIALYSIS: The clearance of ethylene glycol and all its metabolites is enhanced by hemodialysis. The indications for immediate hemodialysis include severe acidemia (pH < 7.1), and evidence of significant end-organ damage (e.g., coma, seizures, and renal insufficiency) (12). Multiple courses of hemodialysis may be necessary, and fomepizole dosing should be adjusted, if hemodialysis is continued, as indicated in Table 55.2.

ADJUNCTS: Thiamine (100 mg IV daily) and pyridoxine (100 mg IV daily) are recommended to divert glyoxylic acid to the formation of non-toxic metabolites (see Figure 55.2).

Methanol

Methanol (also known as *wood alcohol* because it was first distilled from wood) is a common ingredient in shellac, varnish, windshield washer fluid, and solid cooking fuel (Sterno) (12).

Pathophysiology

Like ethylene glycol, methanol is readily absorbed from the upper GI tract, and is metabolized by alcohol dehydrogenase in the liver. The principal metabolite is formic acid, a strong acid that readily dissociates and produces a metabolic acidosis with a high anion gap. Formic acid is also a mitochondrial toxin that inhibits cytochrome oxidase and blocks oxidative energy production. Tissues that are particularly susceptible to damage are the retina, optic nerve, and basal ganglia (12). Methanol metabolism promotes the conversion of pyruvate to lactate in the same manner described for ethylene glycol metabolism, and lactate production is increased further by the actions of formic acid on cytochrome oxidase activity.

Clinical Features

Early manifestations (within 6 hours of ingestion) include signs of apparent inebriation without the odor of alcohol on the breath (as in ethylene glycol intoxication). Later signs (6–24 hours after ingestion) include visual disturbances (e.g., scotoma, blurred vision, complete blindness), depressed consciousness, coma, and generalized seizures (12). Examination of the retina can reveal papilledema and generalized retinal edema. Visual disturbances are characteristic of methanol poisoning, and are not a feature of ethylene glycol poisoning.

Laboratory studies show a high-anion-gap metabolic acidosis and an elevated osmolal gap, similar to ethylene glycol poisoning. However, there is no crystalluria in methanol poisoning. A plasma assay for methanol is available, and a level above 20 mg/dL is considered toxic. However, the re-sults of the plasma assay are not immediately available, and are not used in the decision to initiate therapy.

Treatment

Treatment for methanol poisoning is the same as described for ethylene glycol poisoning, except for the following: (a) visual impairment is an indication for dialysis in methanol poisoning, and (b) folinic acid is used as adjunctive therapy in methanol poisoning, instead of thiamine and pyridoxine.

FOLINIC ACID: Folinic acid (leucovorin) can convert formic acid to non-toxic metabolites. The recommended dose is 1 mg/kg IV, up to 50 mg, at 4-hour intervals (12). Folic acid should be used if folinic acid is unavailable.

A FINAL WORD

The following points in this chapter deserve emphasis:

1. Carbon monoxide poisoning can be missed if you rely on pulse oximetry readings to detect O_2 desaturation. Detection of elevated carboxyhemoglobin levels requires an 8-wavelength CO-oximeter, which is available in most clinical laboratories.

2. A victim of smoke inhalation who has a severe metabolic acidosis should be treated empirically for cyanide poisoning.

3. Methanol and ethylene glycol poisoning should be considered in any patient who presents with a high-anion-gap metabolic acidosis of unclear etiology.

4. If ethylene glycol poisoning is a consideration, inspection of the urine for calcium oxalate monohydrate crystals can provide useful information.

REFERENCES

Carbon Monoxide

1. Hampson NB, Piantadosi CA, Thom SR, Weaver LK. Practice recommendations in the diagnosis, management, and prevention of carbon monoxide poisoning. Am J Resp Crit Care Med 2012; 186:1095–1101.

2. Guyton AC, Hall JE. Medical Physiology, 10th ed. Philadelphia: W.B. Saunders, Co, 2000:470.

3. Nunn JF. Nunn's Applied Respiratory Physiology. 4th ed. Oxford: Butterworth Heinemann, 1993:279–280.

4. Guzman JA. Carbon monoxide poisoning. Crit Care Clin 2012; 28:537–548.

5. Kalay N, Ozdogru I, Cetinkaya Y, et al. Cardiovascular effects of carbon monoxide poisoning. Am J Cardiol 2007; 99:322–324.

6. Choi IS. Delayed neurologic sequelae in carbon monoxide intoxication. Arch Neurol 1983; 40:433–435.

7. Buckley NA, Juurlick DN, Isbister G, et al. Hyperbaric oxygen for carbon monoxide poisoning. Cochrana Database Syst Rev 2011; 4:CD002041.

Cyanide

8. Anseeuw K, Delvau N, Burill-Putze G, et al. Cyanide poisoning by fire smoke inhalation: a European expert consensus. Eur J Emerg Med 2013; 20:2–9.

9. Baud FJ. Cyanide: critical issues in diagnosis and treatment. Hum Exp Toxicol 2007; 26:191–201.

Toxic Alcohols

10. Weiner SW. Toxic alcohols. In Nelson LS, Lewin NA, Howland MA, et al., eds. Goldfrank's Toxicologic Emergencies. 9th ed. New York: McGraw-Hill, 2006:1400–1410.

11. Bronstein AC, Spyker DA, Cantilena LR, Jr, et al. 2011 Annual Report of the American Association of Poison Control Centers' National Poison Data System (NPDS): 29th Annual Report. Clin Toxicol 2012; 50:911–1164.

12. Kruse PA. Methanol and ethylene glycol intoxication. Crit Care Clin 2012; 28:661–711.

APPENDICES

When you're through learning, you're through.

Vernon Law

APPENDICES

UNITS AND CONVERSIONS

The units of measurements in the medical sciences are taken from the metric system (centimeter, gram, second) and the Anglo-Saxon system (foot, pound, second). The metric units were introduced during the French Revolution and were revised in 1960. The revised units are called Système Internationale (SI) units and are currently the worldwide standard.

Part 1		Units of Measurement in the Système Internationale (SI)	
Parameter	**Dimensions**	**Basic SI Unit (Symbol)**	**Equivalencies**
Length	L	Meter (m)	1 inch = 2.54 cm
Area	L^2	Square meter (m²)	1 square centimeter (cm²) = 104 m²
Volume	L^3	Cubic meter (m³)	1 liter (L) = 0.001 m³ 1 milliliter (mL) = 1 cubic centimeter (cm³)
Mass	M	Kilogram (kg)	1 pound (lb) = 453.5 g 1 kg = 2.2 lbs
Density	M/L^3	Kilogram per cubic meter (kg/m³)	1 kg/m³ = 0.001 kg/dm³ Density of water = 1.0 kg/dm³ Density of mercury = 13.6 kg/dm³
Velocity	L/T	Meters per second (m/sec)	1 mile per hour (mph) = 0.4 m/sec
Acceleration	L/T^2	Meters per second squared (m/sec²)	1 ft/sec² = 0.03 m/sec²
Force	$M \times (L/T^2)$	Newton (N) = kg × (m/sec²)	1 dyne = 10^{-5} N

Part 2	Units of Measurement in the Système Internationale (SI)

Parameter	Dimensions	Basic SI Unit (Symbol)	Equivalencies
Pressure	$\dfrac{M \times (L/T^2)}{L^2}$	Pascal (Pa) = N/m^2	1 kPa = 7.5 mm Hg = 10.2 cm H_2O 1 mm Hg = 1×10^{-9} torr (See conversion table for kPa and cm H_2O)
Heat	$M \times (L/T^2) \times L$	Joule (J) = $N \times m$	1 kilocalorie (kcal) = 4184 J
Temperature	None	Kelvin (K)	$0°\,C = -273\,K$ (See conversion table for °C and °F)
Viscosity	M, 1/L, 1/T	Newton × second per square meter ($N \bullet sec/m^2$)	Centipoise (cP) = $10^{-3}\,N \bullet sec/m^2$
Amount of a substance	N	Mole (mol) = molecular weight in grams	Equivalent (Eq) = mol × valence

Part 1	Converting Units of Solute Concentration

1. For ions that exist freely in an aqueous solution, the concentration is expressed as milliequivalents per liter (mEq/L). To convert to millimoles per liter (mmol/L):

$$\frac{mEq/L}{valence} = mmol/L$$

   a. For a univalent ion like potassium (K^+), the concentration in mmol/L is the same as the concentration in mEq/L.

   b. For a divalent ion like magnesium (Mg^{++}), the concentration in mmol/L is one-half the concentration in mEq/L.

2. For ions that are partially bound or complexed to other molecules (e.g., plasma Ca^{++}), the concentration is usually expressed as milligrams per deciliter (mg/dL). To convert to mEq/L:

$$\frac{mg/dL \times 10}{mol\ wt} \times valence = mEq/L$$

where mol wt is molecular weight, and the factor 10 is used to convert deciliters (100 mL) to liters.

EXAMPLE: Ca^{++} has a molecular weight of 40 and a valence of 2, so a plasma Ca^{++} concentration of 8 mg/dL is equivalent to:
$$(8 \times 10/40) \times 2 = 4\ mEq/L.$$

Part 2	Converting Units of Solute Concentration

3. The concentration of uncharged molecules (e.g., glucose) is also expressed as milligrams per deciliter (mg/dL). To convert to (mmol/L):

$$\frac{mg/dL \times 10}{mol\ wt} = mmol/L$$

EXAMPLE: Glucose has a molecular weight of 180, so a plasma glucose concentration of 90 mg/dL is equivalent to: $(90 \times 10/180) = 5$ mmol/L.

4. The concentration of solutes can also be expressed in terms of osmotic pressure, which determines the distribution of water in different fluid compartments. Osmotic activity in aqueous solutions (called osmolality) is expressed as milliosmoles per kg water (mosm/kg H_2O or mosm/kg). The following formulas can be used to express the osmolality of solute concentrations (n is the number of nondissociable particles per molecule).

$$mmol/L \times n = mosm/kg$$

$$\frac{mEq/L}{valence} \times n = mosm/kg$$

$$\frac{mg/dL \times 10}{mol\ wt} \times n = mosm/kg$$

EXAMPLE:

a. A plasma Na^+ concentration of 140 mEq/L has the following osmolality:

$$\frac{140}{1} \times 1 = 140\ mosm/kg$$

b. A plasma glucose concentration of 90 mg/dL has the following osmolality:

$$\frac{90 \times 10}{180} \times 1 = 5\ mosm/kg$$

The sodium in plasma has a much greater osmotic activity than the glucose in plasma because osmotic activity is determined by the number of particles in solution, and is independent of the size of the particles (i.e., one sodium ion has the same osmotic activity as one glucose molecule).

Apothecary and Household Conversions	
Apothecary	**Household**
1 grain = 60 mg	1 teaspoonful = 5 mL
1 ounce = 30 mg	1 tablespoonful = 15 mL
1 fluid ounce = 30 mL	1 wineglassful = 60 mL
1 pint = 500 mL	1 teacupful = 120 mL
1 quart = 947 mL	

Temperature Conversions			
°C	°F	°C	°F
41	105.8	35	95
40	104	34	93.2
39	102.2	33	91.4
38	100.4	32	89.6
37	98.6	31	87.8
36	96.8	30	86
°F = (9/5 °C) + 32		°C = 5/9 (°F − 32)	

Pressure Conversions					
mm Hg	kPa	mm Hg	kPa	mm Hg	kPa
41	5.45	61	8.11	81	10.77
42	5.59	62	8.25	82	10.91
43	5.72	63	8.38	83	11.04
44	5.85	64	8.51	84	11.17
45	5.99	65	8.65	85	11.31
46	6.12	66	8.78	86	11.44
47	6.25	67	8.91	87	11.57
48	6.38	68	9.04	88	11.70
49	6.52	69	9.18	89	11.84
50	6.65	70	9.31	90	11.97
51	6.78	71	9.44	91	12.10
52	6.92	72	9.58	92	12.24
53	7.05	73	9.71	93	12.37
54	7.18	74	9.84	94	12.50
55	7.32	75	9.98	95	12.64
56	7.45	76	10.11	96	12.77
57	7.58	77	10.24	97	12.90
58	7.71	78	10.37	98	13.03
59	7.85	79	10.51	99	13.17
60	7.98	80	10.64	100	13.90

Kilopascal (kPa) = 0.133 × mm Hg; mm Hg = 7.5 × kPa

French Sizes

French Size	Outside Diameter*	
	Inches	mm
1	0.01	0.3
4	0.05	1.3
8	0.10	2.6
10	0.13	3.3
12	0.16	4.0
14	0.18	4.6
16	0.21	5.3
18	0.23	6.0
20	0.26	6.6
22	0.28	7.3
24	0.31	8.0
26	0.34	8.6
28	0.36	9.3
30	0.39	10.0
32	0.41	10.6
34	0.44	11.3
36	0.47	12.0
38	0.50	12.6

*Diameters can vary with manufacturers. However, a useful rule of thumb is OD (mm) $\times$ 3 = French size.

Gauge Sizes

Gauge Size	Outside Diameter*	
	Inches	mm
26	0.018	0.45
25	0.020	0.50
24	0.022	0.56
23	0.024	0.61
22	0.028	0.71
21	0.032	0.81
20	0.036	0.91
19	0.040	1.02
18	0.048	1.22
16	0.040	1.62
14	0.080	2.03
12	0.104	2.64

*Diameters can vary with manufacturers.

SELECTED REFERENCE RANGES

Part 1	Reference Ranges for Selected Clinical Laboratory Tests			
Substance	**Fluid***	**Traditional Units**	**× k =**	**SI Units**
Acetoacetate	P, S	0.3–3.0 mg/dL	97.95	3–30 µmol/L
Alanine amino-transferase (SGPT)	S	0–35 U/L	0.016	0–0.58 µkat/L
Albumin	S CSF	4–6 g/dL 11–48 mg/dL	10 0.01	40–60 g/L 0.11–0.48 g/L
Aldolase	S	0–6 U/L	16.6	0–100 nkat/L
Alkaline phosphatase	S	(F) 30–100 U/L (M) 45–115 U/L	0.016	0.5–1.67 µkat/L 0.75–1.92 µkat/L
Ammonia	P	10–80 µg/dL	0.587	5–50 µmol/L
Amylase	S	0–130 U/L	0.016	0–2.17 µkat/L
Aspartate amino-transferase (SGOT)	S	0–35 U/L	0.016	0–0.58 µkat/L
β-Hydroxybutyrate	S	<1.0 mg/dL	96.05	<100 µmol/L
Bicarbonate	S	22–26 mEq/L	1	22–26 mmol/L
Bilirubin: Total Conjugated	S S	0.1–1.0 mg/dL ≤0.2 mg/dL	17.1	2–18 µmol/L ≤4 µmol/L
Blood urea nitrogen (BUN)	P, S	8–18 mg/dL	0.367	3.0–6.5 mmol/L
Calcium: Total Ionized	S P	8.5–10.5 mg/dL 2.2–2.3 mEq/L	0.26 0.49	2.2–2.6 mmol/L 1.1–1.15 mmol/L

Part 2 | Reference Ranges for Selected Clinical Laboratory Tests

Substance	Fluid*	Traditional Units	x k =	SI Units
Chloride	P, S CSF U	95–105 mEq/L 120–130 mEq/L 10–200 mEq/L	1	95–105 mmol/L 120–130 mmol/L 10–200 mmol/L
Creatinine	S U	0.6–1.5 mg/dL 15–25 mg/kg/24h	0.09 0.009	0.05–0.13 mmol/L 0.13–0.22 mg/kg/24h
Cyanide: Nontoxic Lethal	WB	<5 µg/dL >30 µg/dL	3.8	<19 µmol/L >114 µmol/L
Fibrinogen	P	150–350 mg/dL	0.01	1.5–3.5 g/L
Fibrin split products	S	<10 µg/dL	1	<10 mg/L
Glucose (fasting)	P CSF	70–100 mg/dL 50–80 mg/dL	0.06	3.9–6.1 mmol/L 2.8–4.4 mmol/L
Lactate: Resting Exercise	P S	<2 mEq/L <4 mEq/L	1	<2 mmol/L <4 mmol/L
Lactate dehydrogenase (LDH)	S	50–150 U/L	0.017	0.82–2.66 µkat/L
Lipase	S	0–160 U/L	0.017	0–2.66 µkat/L
Magnesium	P	1.8–3.0 mg/dL 1.5–2.4 mEq/L	0.41 0.5	0.8–1.2 mmol/L 0.8–1.2 mmol/L
Osmolality	S	280–296 mosm/kg	1	280–296 mmol/kg
Phosphate	S	2.5–5.0 mg/dL	0.32	0.8–1.6 mmol/L
Potassium	P, S	3.5–5.0 mEq/L	1	3.5–5.0 mmol/L
Total protein	P, S CSF U	6–8 g/dL <40 mg/dL <150 mg/24h	10 0.01 0.01	60–80 g/L <0.4 mmol/L <1.5 g/24h
Sodium	P, S	135–147 mEq/L	1	135–147 mmol/L
Thyroxine: Total Free	S	4–11 µg/dL 0.8–2.8 mg/dL	12.9 0.49	51–142 nmol/L 10–36 pmol/L
Triiodothyronine (T3)	S	75–220 ng/dL	0.015	12–3.4 nmol/L

*P = Plasma; S = serum; U = urine; WB = whole blood; CSF = cerebrospinal fluid.

Adapted from the New England Journal of Medicine SI Unit Conversion Guide. Waltham, MA; Massachusetts Medical Society, 1992.

Desirable Weights (in lbs.) for Adults*

| Height | | Males | | |
Feet	Inches	Small Frame	Medium Frame	Large Frame
5	2	128–134	131–141	138–150
5	3	130–136	133–143	140–153
5	4	132–138	135–145	142–156
5	5	134–140	137–148	144–160
5	6	136–142	139–151	146–164
5	7	138–145	142–154	149–168
5	8	140–148	145–157	152–172
5	9	142–151	148–160	155–176
5	10	144–154	151–163	158–180
5	11	146–157	154–166	161–184
6	0	149–160	157–170	164–188
6	1	152–164	160–174	168–192
6	2	155–168	164–178	172–197
6	3	158–172	167–182	172–202
6	4	162–176	171–187	181–207

| Height | | Females | | |
Feet	Inches	Small Frame	Medium Frame	Large Frame
4	10	102–111	109–121	112–131
4	11	103–113	111–123	120–134
5	0	104–115	113–126	122–137
5	1	106–118	115–129	125–140
5	2	108–121	118–132	128–143
5	3	111–124	121–135	131–147
5	4	114–127	124–138	134–151
5	5	117–130	127–141	137–155
5	6	120–133	130–144	140–159
5	7	123–136	133–147	143–163
5	8	126–139	136–150	146–167
5	9	129–142	139–153	149–170
5	10	132–145	142–156	152–173
5	11	135–148	145–159	155–176
6	1	138–151	148–162	158–179

*Unclothed weights associated with the longest life expectancies. From the statistics bureau of the Metropolitan Life Insurance Company, 1983.

Body Mass Index

WEIGHT lbs	100	105	110	115	120	125	130	135	140	146	150	155	160	165	170	175	180	185	190	195	200	205	210	215
kg	45.5	47.7	50.0	52.3	54.5	56.8	59.1	61.4	63.6	65.9	68.2	70.5	72.7	75.0	77.3	79.5	81.8	84.1	86.4	88.6	90.9	93.2	95.5	97.7

Legend: ▇ Underweight ▇ Healthy Overweight Obese ▇ Extremely Obese

HEIGHT in / cm																								
5.'0" – 152.4	19	20	21	22	23	24	25	26	27	28	29	30	31	32	33	34	35	36	37	38	39	40	41	42
5.'1" – 154.9	18	19	20	21	22	23	24	25	26	27	28	29	30	31	32	33	34	35	36	36	37	38	39	40
5.'2" – 157.4	18	19	20	21	22	22	23	24	25	26	27	28	29	30	31	32	33	33	34	35	36	37	38	39
5.'3" – 160.0	17	18	19	20	21	22	23	24	24	25	26	27	28	29	30	31	32	32	33	34	35	36	37	38
5.'4" – 162.5	17	18	18	19	20	21	22	23	24	24	25	26	27	28	29	30	31	31	32	33	34	35	36	37
5.'5" – 165.1	16	17	18	19	20	20	21	22	23	24	25	25	26	27	28	29	30	30	31	32	33	34	35	35
5.'6" – 167.6	16	17	17	18	19	20	21	21	22	23	24	25	25	26	27	28	29	29	30	31	32	33	34	34
5.'7" – 170.1	15	16	17	18	18	19	20	21	22	22	23	24	25	25	26	27	28	29	29	30	31	32	33	33
5.'8 – 172.7	15	16	16	17	18	19	19	20	21	22	22	23	24	25	25	26	27	28	28	29	30	31	32	32
5.'9" – 175.2	14	15	16	17	17	18	19	20	20	21	22	22	23	24	25	25	26	27	28	28	29	30	31	31
5.'10" – 177.8	14	15	15	16	17	18	18	19	20	20	21	22	23	23	24	25	25	26	27	28	28	29	30	30
5.'11" – 180.3	14	14	15	16	16	17	18	18	19	20	21	21	22	23	23	24	25	25	26	27	28	28	29	30
6.'0" – 182.8	13	14	14	15	16	17	17	18	19	19	20	21	21	22	23	23	24	25	25	26	27	27	28	29
6.'1" – 185.4	13	13	14	15	15	16	17	17	18	19	19	20	21	21	22	23	23	24	25	25	26	27	27	28
6.'2" – 187.9	12	13	14	14	15	15	16	17	18	18	19	19	20	21	21	22	23	23	24	25	25	26	27	27
6.'3" – 190.5	12	13	13	14	15	15	16	16	17	18	18	19	20	20	21	21	22	23	23	24	25	25	26	26
6.'4" – 193.0	12	12	13	14	14	15	15	16	17	17	18	18	19	20	20	21	22	22	23	23	24	25	25	26

Peak Expiratory Flow Rates for Healthy Males

Age (yr)	Ht:	L/min			
		60"	65"	70"	75"
20		602	649	693	740
25		590	636	679	725
30		577	622	664	710
35		565	609	651	695
40		552	596	636	680
45		540	583	622	665
50		527	569	607	649
55		515	556	593	634
60		502	542	578	618
65		490	529	564	603
70		477	515	550	587

Peak Flow (L/min) = [3.95 − (0.0151 × Age)] × Ht (cm)

Regression equation from Leiner GC et al. Am Rev Respir Dis 1963; 88:646.

Peak Expiratory Flow Rates for Healthy Females

Age (yr)	Ht:	L/min 60"	65"	70"	75"
20		309	423	460	496
25		385	418	454	490
30		380	413	448	483
35		375	408	442	476
40		370	402	436	470
45		365	397	430	464
50		360	391	424	457
55		355	386	418	451
60		350	380	412	445
65		345	375	406	439
70		340	369	400	432

Peak Flow (L/min) = [2.93 − (0.0072 x Age)] × Ht (cm)

Regression equation from Leiner GC et al. Am Rev Respir Dis 1963; 88:646.

ADDITIONAL FORMULAS

This section includes formulas that deserve mention but are not included in any of the chapters.

Measures of Body Size

Ideal Body Weight*

Males: IBW (kg) = 50 + 2.3 (Ht in inches − 60)

Females: IBW (kg) = 45.5 + 2.3 (Ht in inches − 60)

Body Mass Index†

$$BMI = \frac{Wt\ (in\ lbs)}{Ht\ (in\ inches)^2\ \times 703}$$

Body Surface Area

Dubois Formula‡

BSA (m²) = Ht (in cm) + Wt (in kg)$^{0.425}$ × 0.007184

Jacobson Formula$^{\xi}$

$$BSA\ (m^2) = \frac{Ht\ (in\ cm) + Wt\ (in\ kg) - 60}{100}$$

*Devine BJ. Drug Intell Clin Pharm 1974; 8:650.

†Matz R. Ann Intern Med 1993; 118:232.

‡Dubois EF. Basal metabolism in health and disease. Philadelphia: Lea & Febiger, 1936.

$^{\xi}$Jacobson B. Medicine and clinical engineering. Englewood Cliffs, NJ: Prentice-Hall, 1977.

Creatinine Clearance

Cockroft Gault Equation (1):

$$Cr\ CL = \frac{(140 - Age) \times Weight\ (kg)}{SCr\ (mg/dL) \times 72} \quad (mL/min)$$

$$\times 0.85\ (for\ females)$$

MDMR Equation (2):

$$Cr\ CL = 170 \times SCr\ (mg/dL) \times Age^{-0.176}\ (mL/min/1.73\ m^2)$$

$$\times 0.762\ (for\ females)$$

$$\times 1.180\ (for\ African\ Americans)$$

SCr = serum creatinine; MDMR = Modification of Diet in Renal Disease; 1.73 m^2 is the body surface area of an average-sized adult.

(1) Cockcroft DW, Gault MH. Nephron. 1976; 16:31–41.

(2) Levey AS, Bosch JP, Lewis JB, et al. Ann Intern Med 1999; 130:461–470.

Index

Page numbers followed by f indicate figures and those followed by t indicate tables.